Contents

D1714281

Contributors and consultants

Gaylene Altman, RN, PhD
Faculty
University of Washington
Seattle

Helen C. Ballestas, RN, MS, CRRN
Nursing Faculty
New York Institute of Technology
Old Westbury

Kevin Carney, RN, CCTC
Lung Transplant Coordinator
Hospital of the University of Pennsylvania
Philadelphia

Ruth A. Chaplen, RN, MSN, CNS-BC, AOCN
Nurse Practitioner
Karmanos Cancer Institute
Clinical Instructor
Wayne State University
Detroit

Karen Demzien Connors, RN, MSN, CNE
Nursing Faculty
Central New Mexico Community College
Albuquerque

Marsha L. Conroy, RN, BA, MSN, APN
Nursing Instructor
Chamberlain College of Nursing
Columbus, Ohio

Kim Cooper, RN, MSN
Nursing Department Chair
Ivy Tech Community College
Terre Haute, Ind.

Anne W. Davis, RN, PhD
Professor of Nursing
East Central University
Ada, Okla.

Shirley Lyon Garcia, RN, BSN
Adjunct Nursing Faculty, PNE
McDowell Technical Community College
Marion, N.C.

Mary M. Kelly, MSN, CRNP-C
Nurse Practitioner
Abington (Pa.) Pulmonary & Critical Care
    Associates

Carla A.B. Lee, PhD, MN, ARNP, BC, FAAN
Adjunct Professor in Nursing and Nurse
    Anesthesia
Newman University
Wichita, Kan.

Jennifer M. Lee, RN, MSN, FNP-C
Nurse Practitioner
Greenville (S.C.) Hospital System

Susan Parsons, RN, PhD
Associate Professor of Nursing
Newman University
Wichita, Kan.

Roseanne Hanlon Rafter, MSN, APRN, BC
Director of Professional Nursing Practice
Chestnut Hill Hospital
Philadelphia

Allison J. Terry, RN, PhD, MSN
Director, Center for Nursing
Alabama Board of Nursing
Montgomery

Dawn Zwick, RN, MSN, CRNP
Adult Nurse Practitioner
Assistant Professor
Kent State University
North Canton, Ohio

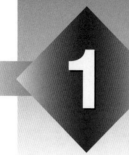

Part

1

Disorders

Acute respiratory distress syndrome

A form of noncardiogenic pulmonary edema that causes acute respiratory failure, acute respiratory distress syndrome (ARDS), also called *shock lung* or *adult respiratory distress syndrome*, results from increased permeability of the alveolocapillary membrane. Fluid accumulates in the lung interstitium, alveolar spaces, and small airways, causing the lung to stiffen. Effective ventilation is thus impaired, prohibiting adequate oxygenation of pulmonary capillary blood. Severe ARDS can cause intractable and fatal hypoxemia. Patients who recover, however, may have little or no permanent lung damage. (See *What happens in ARDS*, pages 4–5.)

CAUSES AND INCIDENCE

ARDS affects 10 to 14 people per 100,000, with a mortality rate of 36% to 52%. The mortality rate remains high in the geriatric population in those aged 60 to 69 as shown by studies of trauma patients. Trauma is the most common cause of ARDS, possibly because trauma-related factors, such as fat emboli, sepsis, shock, pulmonary contusions, and multiple transfusions, increase the likelihood of microemboli developing.

Other common causes of ARDS include anaphylaxis, aspiration of gastric contents, diffuse pneumonia (especially viral), drug overdose (for example, heroin, aspirin, and ethchlorvynol), idiosyncratic drug reaction (to ampicillin and hydrochlorothiazide), inhalation of smoke or noxious gases (such as nitrous oxide, ammonia, and chlorine), near-drowning, and oxygen toxicity. Less common causes of ARDS include coronary artery bypass grafting, hemodialysis, leukemia, acute miliary tuberculosis, pancreatitis, thrombotic thrombocytopenic purpura, uremia, and venous air embolism.

In ARDS, altered permeability of the alveolocapillary membrane causes fluid to accumulate in the interstitial space. If the pulmonary lymphatic glands can't remove this fluid, interstitial edema develops. The fluid collects in the peribronchial and peribronchiolar spaces, producing bronchiolar narrowing. Hypoxemia occurs as a result of fluid accumulation in alveoli and subsequent alveolar collapse, causing the shunting of blood through nonventilated lung regions. In addition, alveolar collapse causes a dramatic increase in lung compliance, which makes it more difficult to achieve adequate ventilation.

WHAT HAPPENS IN ARDS

These illustrations depict the process and progress of acute respiratory distress syndrome (ARDS).

1. The body responds to insult

Injury reduces normal blood flow to the lungs, allowing platelets to aggregate. These platelets release such substances as serotonin (S), bradykinin (B) and, especially, histamine (H), that inflame and damage the alveolar membrane and later increase capillary permeability. At this early stage, signs and symptoms of ARDS are undetectable.

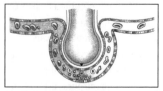

2. Fluid shift causes symptoms

Increased capillary permeability allows fluid to shift into the interstitial space. As a result, the patient may experience tachypnea, dyspnea, and tachycardia.

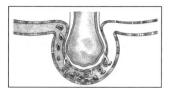

3. Pulmonary edema results

As capillary permeability continues to increase, shifting of proteins and fluid increases interstitial osmotic pressure and causes pulmonary edema. At this stage, the patient may experience increased tachypnea, dyspnea, and cyanosis. Hypoxia (usually unresponsive to increased FIO_2), decreased pulmonary compliance, and crackles and rhonchi may also develop.

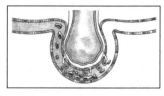

4. Alveoli collapse

Fluid in the alveoli and decreased blood flow damage surfactant in the alveoli, reducing the cells' ability to produce more surfactant. Without surfactant, alveoli collapse, impairing gas exchange. Look for thick, frothy sputum and marked hypoxemia with increased respiratory distress.

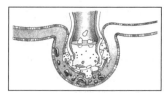

SIGNS AND SYMPTOMS

• Initially, rapid, shallow breathing and dyspnea within hours to days of the initial injury (sometimes after the patient's condition appears to have stabilized)

• Hypoxemia, which causes an increased drive for ventilation
• Intercostal and suprasternal retractions resulting from the effort required to expand the stiff lung

5. Gas exchange slows

The patient breathes faster, but sufficient oxygen (O_2) can't cross the alveolocapillary membrane. Carbon dioxide (CO_2), however, crosses more easily and is lost with every exhalation. Both O_2 and CO_2 levels in the blood decrease. Look for increased tachypnea, hypoxemia, and hypocapnia.

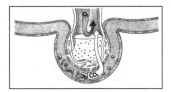

6. Metabolic acidosis occurs

Pulmonary edema worsens. Meanwhile, inflammation leads to fibrosis, which further impedes gas exchange. The resulting hypoxemia leads to metabolic acidosis. At this stage, look for increased partial pressure of arterial carbon dioxide, decreased pH and partial pressure of arterial oxygen, decreased bicarbonate (HCO_3^-) levels, and mental confusion.

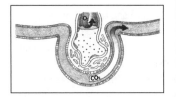

- Fluid accumulation, which produces crackles and rhonchi
- Restlessness, apprehension, mental sluggishness, and motor dysfunction
- Tachycardia, possibly with transient increased arterial blood pressure
- Hypotension
- Decreasing urine output
- Respiratory and metabolic acidosis
- Eventually, ventricular fibrillation or standstill

COMPLICATIONS

- Multisystem failure
- Pulmonary fibrosis
- Pneumothorax

DIAGNOSIS

- On room air, arterial blood gas (ABG) analysis initially shows decreased partial pressure of arterial oxygen (PaO_2) less than 60 mm Hg and partial pressure of arterial carbon dioxide ($PaCO_2$) less than 35 mm Hg. The resulting pH usually reflects respiratory alkalosis.
- ABG analysis shows respiratory acidosis (increasing $PaCO_2$ [more than 45 mm Hg]), metabolic acidosis (decreasing bicarbonate [less than 22 mEq/L]), and a decreasing PaO_2 despite oxygen therapy as ARDS becomes more severe.
- Pulmonary artery blood shows decreased oxygen saturation, reflecting tissue hypoxia.
- Serial chest X-rays initially show diffuse bilateral infiltrates that tend to be more peripheral and patchy, rather than the usual perihilar "bat wing" appearance of cardiogenic pulmonary edema.
- Later chest X-rays reveal ground-glass appearance and "whiteouts" of both lung fields as hypoxemia becomes irreversible.

Differential diagnosis must rule out cardiogenic pulmonary edema, pulmonary vasculitis, and diffuse pulmonary hemorrhage. To establish the etiology, laboratory work should include sputum Gram stain, culture and sensitivity tests, and blood cultures to detect infections; a toxicology screen for drug ingestion; and, when pancreatitis is a consideration, a serum amylase determination.

TREATMENT

When possible, treatment is designed to correct the underlying cause of ARDS as well as to prevent progression and the potentially fatal complications of hypoxemia and respiratory acidosis. Supportive medical care consists of administering humidified oxygen with continuous positive airway pressure. Hypoxemia that doesn't respond adequately to these measures requires ventilatory support with intubation, volume ventilation, and positive end-expiratory pressure (PEEP). Other supportive measures include fluid restriction, diuretics, and correction of electrolyte and acid-base abnormalities.

Drugs

• Sedatives, opioids, or neuromuscular blocking agents to optimize ventilation when ARDS requires mechanical ventilation
• Sodium bicarbonate to reverse severe metabolic acidosis, although in severe cases this may worsen the acidosis if carbon dioxide can't be cleared adequately

• Vasopressors and I.V. fluids to maintain blood pressure
• Antibiotics to treat infections
• Methylprednisolone infusions in early severe ARDS to significantly improve pulmonary and extrapulmonary organ dysfunction and reduce duration of mechanical ventilation and length of stay in the intensive care unit
• Anticoagulants and fibrinolytics (under study) to improve lung function and oxygenation in ARDS

SPECIAL CONSIDERATIONS

ARDS requires careful monitoring and supportive care.
• Frequently assess the patient's respiratory status. Be alert for retractions on inspiration. Note the rate, rhythm, and depth of respirations; watch for dyspnea and the use of accessory muscles of respiration. On auscultation, listen for adventitious or diminished breath sounds. Check for clear, frothy sputum, which may indicate pulmonary edema.
• Observe and document the hypoxemic patient's neurologic status (level of consciousness and mental status).
• Maintain a patent airway by suctioning, using sterile, nontraumatic technique. Ensure adequate humidification to help liquefy tenacious secretions.
• Closely monitor heart rate and blood pressure. Watch for arrhythmias that may result from hypoxemia, acid-base disturbances, or electrolyte imbalance. With pulmonary artery

catheterization, know the desired pressure levels. Check readings often and watch for decreasing mixed venous oxygen saturation.

• Monitor serum electrolytes and correct imbalances. Measure intake and output; weigh the patient daily.

• I.V. fluid management involves careful balancing. Fluids are necessary for oxygen and nutrient delivery; however, excessive fluid administration can worsen lung edema, further damaging gas exchange. Conservative fluid management has been shown to improve lung function as well as shorten duration of mechanical ventilation and I.V. care without increasing incidence of nonpulmonary organ failure.

• Check ventilator settings frequently, and empty condensate from tubing promptly to ensure maximum oxygen delivery. Monitor ABG studies and pulse oximetry. The patient with severe hypoxemia may need controlled mechanical ventilation with positive pressure. Give sedatives, as needed, to reduce restlessness.

• Because PEEP may decrease cardiac output, check for hypotension, tachycardia, and decreased urine output. Suction only as needed to maintain PEEP or use an in-line suctioning apparatus. Reposition the patient often and record an increase in secretions, temperature, or hypotension that may indicate a deteriorating condition. Monitor peak pressures during ventilation. Because of stiff, noncompliant lungs, the patient is at high risk for baro-

trauma (pneumothorax), which is evidenced by increased peak pressures, decreased breath sounds on one side, and restlessness.

• Prone positioning has been shown to reduce right ventricular overload. It permits an additional limitation in airway pressure (associated with a reduction in hypercapnia), reduces airway pressure, improves alveolar ventilation, and decreases right ventricular enlargement.

• Monitor nutrition, maintain joint mobility, and prevent skin breakdown.

• Accurately record calorie intake. Give tube feedings and parenteral nutrition, as ordered.

• Perform passive range-of-motion exercises or help the patient perform active exercises, if possible.

• Provide meticulous skin care.

• Plan patient care to allow periods of uninterrupted sleep.

• Provide emotional support. Warn the patient who's recovering from ARDS that recovery will take some time and that he will feel weak for a while.

• Watch for and immediately report all respiratory changes in the patient with injuries that may adversely affect the lungs (especially during the 2- to 3-day period after the injury when the patient may appear to be improving).

Acute respiratory failure in COPD

In patients with essentially normal lung tissue, acute respiratory failure

(ARF) usually means partial pressure of arterial carbon dioxide ($Paco_2$) above 50 mm Hg and partial pressure of arterial oxygen (Pao_2) below 50 mm Hg. These limits, however, don't apply to patients with chronic obstructive pulmonary disease (COPD), who usually have a consistently high $Paco_2$ and low Pao_2. In patients with COPD, only acute deterioration in arterial blood gas (ABG) values, with corresponding clinical deterioration, indicates ARF.

CAUSES AND INCIDENCE

The incidence of ARF increases markedly with age and is especially high among people age 65 and older.

ARF may develop in patients with COPD as a result of any condition that increases the work of breathing and decreases the respiratory drive. These conditions may result from respiratory tract infection (such as bronchitis or pneumonia), bronchospasm, or accumulated secretions secondary to cough suppression. Other common causes are related to ventilatory failure, in which the brain fails to direct respiration, and gas exchange failure, in which respiratory structures fail to function properly.

Central nervous system depression can occur due to head trauma or injudicious use of sedatives, opioids, tranquilizers, or oxygen. Cardiovascular disorders (myocardial infarction, heart failure, or pulmonary emboli) can result in untreated ventilation-perfusion ($\dot{V}\dot{Q}$) imbalances, which lead to right-to-left shunting, in which blood passes from the heart's right side to the left without being oxygenated. This unoxygenated blood reaches the arterial system and is distributed to the rest of the body. Likewise, hypoxemia deprives the myocardial tissue of oxygen and nutrients, possibly resulting in ischemia or a myocardial infarction. Thoracic abnormalities, such as chest trauma, pneumothorax, or thoracic or abdominal surgery can result in hypoventilation and resultant ARF in patients with COPD. Airway irritants, such as smoke and fumes, may produce hypoxia. Endocrine or metabolic disorders, such as myxedema or metabolic acidosis, place the patient with COPD at greater risk for ARF due to the patient's limited ability to compensate with the respiratory system. Also, noncompliance with prescribed bronchodilator or corticosteroid therapy can result in ARF in the COPD patient.

SIGNS AND SYMPTOMS

- Decreased Pao_2 (hypoxemia) and increased $Paco_2$ (hypercapnia) due to increased $\dot{V}\dot{Q}$ mismatch and reduced alveolar ventilation (as shown by ABGs); this rise in carbon dioxide lowers the pH.
- Increased, decreased, or normal respiratory rate, depending on the cause; shallow or deep respirations, or both; possible air hunger
- Possible cyanosis, depending on the hemoglobin (Hb) level and arterial oxygenation

- Crackles, rhonchi, wheezing, or diminished breath sounds as heard on auscultation
- Restlessness, confusion, loss of concentration, irritability, tremulousness, diminished tendon reflexes, papilledema, and eventual unresponsiveness (coma) as hypoxemia and hypercapnia occur
- Tachycardia, with increased cardiac output and mildly elevated blood pressure secondary to adrenal release of catecholamine, occurring early in response to low Pao_2
- Arrhythmias with myocardial hypoxia
- Elevated pressures on the right side of the heart, distended jugular veins, an enlarged liver, and peripheral edema due to pulmonary hypertension, which occurs secondarily to pulmonary capillary vasoconstriction
- Cardiac failure due to stress on the heart

COMPLICATIONS

- Tissue hypoxia
- Metabolic acidosis
- Multiple organ failure
- Cardiac arrest

DIAGNOSIS

- Progressive deterioration in ABG levels and pH, when compared with the patient's "normal" values, strongly suggests ARF in COPD. (In patients with essentially normal lung tissue, pH below 7.35 usually indicates ARF, but patients with COPD display an even greater deviation from this normal value, as they do with $Paco_2$ and Pao_2)

- Increased bicarbonate levels indicate metabolic alkalosis or reflect metabolic compensation for chronic respiratory acidosis.
- Abnormally low hematocrit (HCT) and Hb levels may be due to blood loss, indicating decreased oxygen-carrying capacity. Elevated levels may occur with chronic hypoxemia.
- Hypokalemia and hypochloremia may result from diuretic and corticosteroid therapies used to treat ARF.
- White blood cell count is elevated if ARF is due to bacterial infection; Gram stain and sputum culture can identify pathogens.
- Chest X-ray findings identify pulmonary pathologic conditions, such as emphysema, atelectasis, lesions, pneumothorax, infiltrates, or effusions.
- Arrhythmias on electrocardiogram commonly suggest cor pulmonale and myocardial hypoxia.

TREATMENT

ARF in patients with COPD is an emergency that requires cautious oxygen therapy (using nasal prongs or Venturi mask) to raise the Pao_2. In patients with chronic hypercapnia, oxygen therapy can cause hypoventilation by increasing $Paco_2$ and decreasing the respiratory drive, necessitating mechanical ventilation. The minimum fraction of inspired oxygen (Fio_2) required to maintain ventilation or oxygen saturation greater than 85% to 90% should be used. If significant uncompensated respiratory acidosis or unrefractory hypoxemia exists, mechanical ventilation (through an endotracheal [ET] or a tracheostomy tube) or noninvasive ventilation (with a face or nose mask) may be necessary. Postural drainage and chest physiotherapy is instituted to help clear secretions. For the non-ventilated patient retaining carbon dioxide, encourage him to cough and breathe deeply, teach him pursed-lip and diaphragmatic breathing to control dyspnea, and have him use an incentive spirometer.

Drugs

- Bronchodilators to relax bronchial smooth muscle and improve air flow
- Corticosteroids to decrease airway inflammation (often used for 10 to 14 days only)
- Anti-infectives specific to treat infection
- Antacids, histamine-2 receptor antagonists, or sucralfate in the intubated patient to prevent or treat stress

SPECIAL CONSIDERATIONS

- Because most patients with ARF are treated in an intensive care unit, orient them to the environment, procedures, and routines to minimize their anxiety.
- To reverse hypoxemia, administer oxygen at appropriate concentrations to maintain PaO_2 at a minimum of 50 to 60 mm Hg. Patients with COPD usually require only small amounts of supplemental oxygen. Watch for a positive re-

sponse—such as improvement in the patient's breathing, color, and ABG levels.
- Maintain a patent airway. If the patient is retaining carbon dioxide, encourage him to cough and to breathe deeply. Teach him to use pursed-lip and diaphragmatic breathing to control dyspnea. If the patient is alert, have him use an incentive spirometer; if he's intubated and lethargic, turn him every 1 to 2 hours. Use postural drainage and chest physiotherapy to help clear secretions.
- In an intubated patient, suction the trachea, as needed, after hyperoxygenation. Observe for a change in quantity, consistency, and color of sputum. Provide humidification to liquefy secretions.
- Observe the patient closely for respiratory arrest. Auscultate for breath sounds. Monitor ABG levels and report any changes immediately.
- Check the cardiac monitor for arrhythmias.
- If the patient requires mechanical ventilation:
– Check ventilator settings, cuff pressures, and ABG values often because the FIO_2 setting depends on ABG levels. Draw specimens for ABG analysis 20 to 30 minutes after every FIO_2 change or oximetry check.
– Prevent infection by using sterile technique while suctioning.
– Stress ulcers are common in the intubated patient. Check gastric secretions for evidence of bleeding if the patient has a nasogastric tube or

if he complains of epigastric tenderness, nausea, or vomiting. Monitor Hb level and HCT; check all stools for occult blood. Administer antacids, histamine-2-receptor antagonists, or sucralfate, as ordered.

⌦ PREVENTION

• *Prevent tracheal erosion, which can result from artificial airway cuff overinflation. Use the minimal leak technique and a cuffed tube with high residual volume (low-pressure cuff), a foam cuff, or a pressure-regulating valve on the cuff.*

• *To prevent oral or vocal cord trauma, make sure that the ET tube is positioned midline or moved carefully from side to side every 8 hours.*

• *To prevent nasal necrosis, keep the nasotracheal tube midline within the patient's nostrils and provide good hygiene. Loosen the tape periodically to prevent skin breakdown. Avoid excessive movement of any tubes; make sure the ventilator tubing is adequately supported.*

• *To reduce incidence of ventilator-associated pneumonia, provide frequent oral care.*

Adenovirus infection

Adenoviruses cause acute, self-limiting febrile infections, with inflammation of the respiratory or ocular mucous membranes, or both. (See *Major adenovirus infections*, page 12.)

CAUSES AND INCIDENCE

The adenovirus is an extremely hardy virus and can survive for long periods outside a host. It's endemic throughout the year. The adenovirus has 51 serotypes and is recognized as the causative agent of a variety of syndromes. It's transmitted through direct inoculation to the conjunctiva, fecal-oral route, aerosolized droplets, or exposure to infected tissue or blood. The virus is capable of infecting multiple organ systems, but most infections don't cause symptoms. The adenovirus is often cultured from the pharynx and stool of asymptomatic children, and most adults have measurable titers of antibodies from prior infection. These organisms are common and can remain latent for years; they infect almost everyone early in life, although maternal antibodies offer some protection during the first 6 months of life. The adenovirus has been associated with both sporadic and epidemic diseases.

The adenovirus produces cytolysis in tissues and induces a host inflammatory response, as well as cytokine production. When human cells are infected, one of three different interactions may occur. The first occurs when the virus enters the epithelial cells, replicates, and results in host cell death (lytic infection). The second is the asymptomatic chronic or latent infection as the virus enters the lymphoid tissue. Lastly, oncogenic transformation may occur in which adenoviral deoxyribonucleic acid (DNA) is then

MAJOR ADENOVIRUS INFECTIONS

Disease	Age-group	Clinical features
Acute febrile respiratory illness	Children	Nonspecific coldlike symptoms, similar to other viral respiratory illnesses: fever, pharyngitis, tracheitis, bronchitis, and pneumonitis
Acute respiratory disease	Adults (usually military recruits)	Malaise, fever, chills, headache, pharyngitis, hoarseness, and dry cough
Viral pneumonia	Children and adults	Sudden onset of high fever, rapid infection of upper and lower respiratory tracts, rash, diarrhea, and intestinal intussusception
Acute pharyngoconjunctival fever	Children (particularly after swimming in pools or lakes)	Spiking fever lasting several days, headache, pharyngitis, conjunctivitis, rhinitis, and cervical adenitis
Acute follicular conjunctivitis	Adults	Unilateral tearing and mucoid discharge; later, milder symptoms in other eye
Epidemic keratoconjunctivitis	Adults	Unilateral or bilateral ocular redness and edema, periorbital swelling, local discomfort, and superficial opacity of the cornea without ulceration
Hemorrhagic cystitis	Children (boys)	Adenovirus in urine, hematuria, dysuria, and urinary frequency
Diarrhea	Infants	Fever and watery diarrhea

integrated into the host cell's DNA, altering cellular transcription and leading to altered regulation of the cell and malignant transformation (this has mostly been seen in rodent tissue; a clear role in human oncogenesis hasn't been established).

SIGNS AND SYMPTOMS

The incubation period—usually lasting less than 1 week—is followed by acute illness lasting less than 5 days. Prolonged asymptomatic reinfection may occur. Clinical features vary, depending on the type of infection.

• Acute respiratory disease (predominantly serotypes 4 and 7), producing pharyngitis, pulmonary rhonchi and rales

• Super cold symptoms with adenovirus serotype 14 (may include lower respiratory tract infections, including tracheobronchitis, bronchiolitis, and pneumonia)

• Pharyngoconjunctival fever (predominantly serotypes 3, 4, and 7), producing pharyngitis, conjunctivitis, fever, and preauricular and cervical lymphadenopathy

• Epidemic keratoconjunctivitis (predominantly serotypes 8, 19, and 37), producing conjunctivitis, palpebral edema, vision haziness or impairment

• Acute hemorrhagic cystitis (serotypes 11 and 21) and nephritis, producing flank pain and hematuria

• Gastroenteritis (most commonly associated with serotypes 40 and 41, but others may be involved) with signs of dehydration

• Adenoviral infections occurring in immunocompromised hosts, causing dyspnea, dry cough, pulmonary rhonchi and crackles, grossly bloody urine, and diarrhea

COMPLICATIONS

• Acute conjunctivitis
• Sinusitis
• Pharyngitis
• Bronchiolitis
• Pneumonia
• Meningoencephalitis (rare)

DIAGNOSIS

• Definitive diagnosis requires isolation of the virus from respiratory or ocular secretions or fecal smears, or examination of tissue of other suspected sites.

• During epidemics, however, typical symptoms alone can confirm the diagnosis.

• Because adenoviral illnesses resolve rapidly, serum antibody titers aren't useful for diagnosis.

• Adenoviral infections cause lymphocytosis in children.

• Chest X-ray may show pneumonitis when adenoviruses cause respiratory disease.

TREATMENT

Supportive treatment includes bed rest, antipyretics, and analgesics. Ocular infections may require corticosteroids and direct supervision by an ophthalmologist. Hospitalization is required in cases of pneumonia (in infants) to prevent death and in epidemic keratoconjunctivitis (EKC) to prevent blindness.

Drugs

• Antiviral medications, such as ribavirin (Virazole), to inhibit viral DNA and protein synthesis

• Cidofovir (Vistide) for infection with cytomegalovirus retinitis

SPECIAL CONSIDERATIONS

• During acute illness, monitor respiratory status and intake and output. Give analgesics and antipyretics, as needed. Stress the need for bed rest.

• To help minimize the incidence of adenoviral infection, instruct all patients in proper handwashing to reduce fecal-oral transmission and eye inoculation.

• EKC can be prevented by sterilization of ophthalmic instruments, adequate chlorination in swimming pools, and avoidance of swimming pools during epidemics. Killed virus vaccine (not widely available) or a live oral virus vaccine can prevent adenoviral infection and are recommended for high-risk groups.

⊠ PREVENTION

• *Vaccination is available but is limited because of the increased risk of disease. It's used with the military population.*

• *Health care–associated infection can be prevented by effective isolation procedures, handwashing, and appropriate sterilization of instruments.*

• *Adequate chlorination of swimming pools may prevent breakouts that occur from such sources.*

• *In households with an infected patient, frequent handwashing and avoidance of towel and pillow sharing can help prevent infection with conjunctivitis.*

Asbestosis

Asbestosis is a form of pneumoconiosis characterized by diffuse interstitial fibrosis. It can develop as long as 15 to 20 years after regular exposure to asbestos has ended. Asbestos also causes pleural plaques and mesotheliomas of the pleura and the peritoneum. A potent cocarcinogen, asbestos increases the risk of lung cancer in cigarette smokers.

CAUSES AND INCIDENCE

Asbestosis occurs in 4 of every 10,000 people. It results from the inhalation of respirable asbestos fibers (50 microns or more in length and 0.5 micron or less in diameter), which assume a longitudinal orientation in the airway and move in the direction of airflow. The fibers penetrate respiratory bronchioles and alveolar walls. Sources include the mining and milling of asbestos, the construction industry, and the fireproofing and textile industries. Asbestos was also used in the production of paints, plastics, brake and clutch linings, and in shipbuilding.

Asbestos-related diseases develop in families of asbestos workers as a result of exposure to fibrous dust shaken off workers' clothing at home. Such diseases develop in the general public as a result of exposure to fibrous dust or waste piles from nearby asbestos plants, but exposures for occupants of typical buildings are quite low and not in a range associated with asbestosis.

Coughing attempts to expel the foreign matter. Mucus production and goblet cells are stimulated to protect the airway from the debris and aid in expectoration. Inhaled fibers become encased in a brown, proteinlike sheath that's rich in iron (ferruginous bodies or asbestos bodies) and is found in sputum and lung tissue. Chronic irritation by the fibers continues to affect the lower bronchioles and alveoli. The foreign material and inflammation swell airways, and fibrosis develops in response to the chronic irritation. Interstitial fibrosis may develop in lower lung zones, affecting lung parenchyma and pleurae. Raised hyaline plaques may form in parietal pleura, diaphragm, and pleura contiguous with the pericardium. Hypoxia develops as more alveoli and lower airways are affected.

SIGNS AND SYMPTOMS

• Dyspnea on exertion as a result of increased mucus production and airway narrowing
• Dyspnea at rest with extensive fibrosis
• Severe, nonproductive cough in nonsmokers or productive cough in smokers from chronic irritation of bronchial tree and mucus production
• Clubbed fingers due to chronic hypoxia
• Chest pain (commonly pleuritic) due to pleural irritation
• Recurrent respiratory infections as pulmonary defense mechanisms begin to fail
• Characteristic dry crackles at lung bases
• Pleural friction rub due to fibrosis
• Crackles on auscultation attributed to air moving through thickened sputum
• Decreased lung inflation due to lung stiffness
• Recurrent pleural effusions due to fibrosis
• Decreased forced expiratory volume due to diminished alveoli
• Decreased vital capacity due to fibrotic changes

COMPLICATIONS

• Pulmonary fibrosis
• Respiratory failure
• Pulmonary hypertension
• Right ventricular hypertrophy
• Cor pulmonale

DIAGNOSIS

• Chest X-rays show fine, irregular, and linear diffuse infiltrates; extensive fibrosis results in a "honeycomb" or "ground-glass" appearance, pleural thickening and calcification, with bilateral obliteration of costophrenic angles.
• In later stages, an enlarged heart with a classic "shaggy" heart border may be evident.
• Pulmonary function tests show:
– vital capacity, forced vital capacity, and total lung capacity—decreased
– forced expiratory volume in 1 second—decreased or normal
– carbon monoxide diffusing capacity—reduced when fibrosis destroys alveolar walls and thickens alveolocapillary membranes.
• Arterial blood gas analysis reveals:
– partial pressure of arterial oxygen—decreased
– partial pressure of arterial carbon dioxide—low due to hyperventilation.

TREATMENT

The goal of treatment is to relieve respiratory symptoms and, in advanced disease, manage hypoxemia and cor pulmonale. Respiratory symptoms may be relieved by chest physiotherapy techniques, such as controlled coughing and segmental bronchial drainage, chest percussion, and vibration. Aerosol therapy, inhaled mucolytics, and increased fluid intake (at least 3 qt [3 L] daily) may also relieve symptoms.

Diuretics, cardiac glycosides, and salt restriction may be indicated for patients with cor pulmonale. Hypoxemia requires oxygen administration by cannula or mask (1 to 2 L/minute) or by mechanical ventilation if arterial oxygen can't be maintained above 40 mm Hg. Respiratory infections require prompt administration of antibiotics.

Drugs

• Cough suppressants, such as guaifenesin with codeine (Robitussin AC) or dextromethorphan (Robitussin DM) are helpful if cough interrupts sleep; for severe cough, hydrocodone/homatropine (Hycodan)
• Bronchodilators, such as albuterol, if airflow is constricted

SPECIAL CONSIDERATIONS

• Teach the patient to prevent infections by avoiding crowds and people with infections and by receiving influenza and pneumococcal vaccines.
• Improve the patient's ventilatory efficiency by encouraging physical reconditioning, energy conservation in daily activities, and relaxation techniques.

Asthma

Asthma is a chronic inflammatory airway disorder characterized by airflow obstruction and airway hyperresponsiveness to a multiplicity of stimuli. This widespread but variable airflow obstruction is caused by bronchospasm, edema of the airway mucosa, and increased mucus production with plugging and airway remodeling.

CAUSES AND INCIDENCE

Although asthma strikes at any age, about 50% of patients are younger than age 10; twice as many boys as girls are affected in this age-group. One-third of patients develop asthma between ages 10 and 30, and the incidence is the same in both genders in this age group. Moreover, about one-third of all patients share the disease with at least one immediate family member.

Asthma may result from sensitivity to allergens; typically, patients are sensitive to specific external allergens. Allergens include animal dander (especially cat), food additives containing sulfites, ragweed, dust mites, house dust or mold, kapok or feather pillows, other sensitizing substances, and pollen.

Nonatopic, or nonallergic, asthma patients react to internal, nonallergenic factors; external substances can't be implicated in patients with nonatopic asthma. Nonatopic triggers include anxiety, coughing or laughing, emotional stress, endocrine changes, exposure to noxious fumes, fatigue, genetic factors, humidity variations, irritants, and temperature variations. Most episodes occur after a severe respiratory tract infection, especially in adults. Many patients with asthma, especially children, have both atopic and nonatopic asthma. A significant number of adults acquire an allergic form of asthma or exacerbate existing asthma from exposure to agents in the workplace. Irritants, such as chemicals in flour, acid anhydrides, toluene di-isocyanates, screw flies, river flies, and excreta of dust mites in carpet, have been identified as agents that trigger asthma.

There are two genetic influences identified with asthma, namely the ability of an individual to develop asthma and the tendency to develop hyperresponsiveness of the airways. Environmental factors interact with inherited factors to cause asthmatic reactions with associated bronchospasms.

In asthma, bronchial linings overreact to various stimuli, causing episodic smooth-muscle spasms that severely constrict the airways. IgE antibodies, attached to histamine-containing mast cells and receptors on cell membranes, initiate intrinsic asthma attacks. When exposed to an antigen, such as pollen, the IgE antibody combines with the antigen. (See *Pathophysiology of asthma*, page 18.)

On subsequent exposure to the antigen, mast cells degranulate and release mediators. Mast cells in the lung interstitium are stimulated to release histamine and leukotrienes. Histamine attaches to receptor sites in the larger bronchi, where it causes swelling in smooth muscles. Mucous membranes become inflamed, irritated, and swollen. The patient may experience dyspnea, prolonged expiration, and an increased respiratory rate.

Leukotrienes attach to receptor sites in the smaller bronchi and cause local swelling of the smooth muscle. Leukotrienes also cause prostaglandins to travel through the bloodstream to the lungs, where they enhance histamine's effect. A wheeze may be audible during coughing—the higher the pitch, the narrower the bronchial lumen. Histamine stimulates the mucous membranes to secrete excessive mucus, further narrowing the bronchial lumen. Goblet cells secrete viscous mucus that's difficult to cough up, resulting in coughing, rhonchi, and increased respiratory distress. Mucosal edema and thickened secretions further block the airways. (See *Looking at a bronchiole in asthma*, page 19.)

On inhalation, the narrowed bronchial lumen can still expand slightly, allowing air to reach the alveoli. On exhalation, increased intrathoracic pressure closes the bronchial lumen completely. Air enters but can't escape. The patient develops a barrel chest and hyperresonance to percussion.

Mucus fills the lung bases, inhibiting alveolar ventilation. Blood is shunted to alveoli in other lung

PATHOPHYSIOLOGY OF ASTHMA

In asthma, hyperresponsiveness of the airways and bronchospasms occur. These illustrations show the progression of an asthma attack.

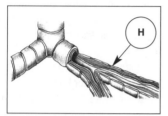

- Histamine (H) attaches to receptor sites in larger bronchi, causing swelling of the smooth muscles.

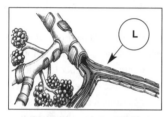

- Leukotrienes (L) attach to receptor sites in the smaller bronchi and cause swelling of smooth muscle there. Leukotrienes also cause prostaglandins to travel through the bloodstream to the lungs, where they enhance histamine's effects.

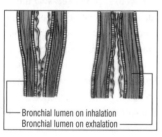

Bronchial lumen on inhalation
Bronchial lumen on exhalation

- Histamine stimulates the mucous membranes to secrete excessive mucus, further narrowing the bronchial lumen. On inhalation, the narrowed bronchial lumen can still expand slightly; however, on exhalation, the increased intrathoracic pressure closes the bronchial lumen completely.

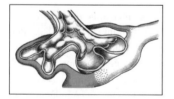

- Mucus fills lung bases, inhibiting alveolar ventilation. Blood is shunted to alveoli in other parts of the lungs, but it still can't compensate for diminished ventilation.

parts, but still can't compensate for diminished ventilation.

Hyperventilation is triggered by respiratory center stimulation, which in turn decreases partial pressure of arterial carbon dioxide ($Paco_2$) and increases pH, resulting in a respiratory alkalosis. As the

LOOKING AT A BRONCHIOLE IN ASTHMA

Asthma is characterized by bronchospasms, increased mucus secretion, and mucosal edema, which contribute to airway narrowing and obstruction. Shown here is a normal bronchiole in cross section and an obstructed bronchiole, as it occurs in asthma.

NORMAL BRONCHIOLE

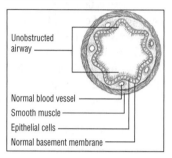

Unobstructed airway

Normal blood vessel
Smooth muscle
Epithelial cells
Normal basement membrane

OBSTRUCTED BRONCHIOLE

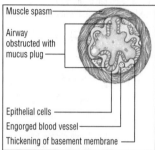

Muscle spasm

Airway obstructed with mucus plug

Epithelial cells
Engorged blood vessel
Thickening of basement membrane

---

airway obstruction increases in severity, more alveoli are affected. Ventilation and perfusion remain inadequate, and carbon dioxide retention develops. Respiratory acidosis results and respiratory failure occurs.

If status asthmaticus occurs, hypoxia worsens and expiratory flows and volumes decrease even further. If treatment isn't initiated, the patient begins to tire out. (See *Averting an asthma attack,* page 20.)

Acidosis develops as arterial carbon dioxide increases. The situation becomes life-threatening as no air becomes audible upon auscultation (a silent chest) and $Paco_2$ rises to over 70 mm Hg.

SIGNS AND SYMPTOMS

An acute asthma attack may begin dramatically, with simultaneous

onset of severe multiple symptoms, or insidiously, with gradually increasing respiratory distress. Asthma that occurs with cyanosis, confusion, and lethargy indicates the onset of life-threatening status asthmaticus and respiratory failure.

Signs and symptoms of asthma include:

- sudden dyspnea, wheezing, and tightness in the chest from bronchoconstriction
- coughing that produces thick, clear, or yellow sputum resulting from excess mucus production
- tachypnea, along with use of accessory respiratory muscles due to increasing air trapping and respiratory distress
- rapid pulse from increased workload of the heart due to the effects of hypoxemia and hyperinflation on the pulmonary vasculature

AVERTING AN ASTHMA ATTACK

The flowchart below shows pathophysiologic changes that occur with asthma. Treatments and interventions show where the physiologic cascade would be altered to stop an asthma attack.

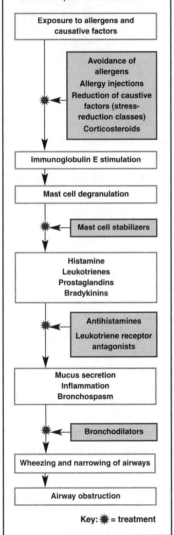

Key: ✳ = treatment

• hyperresonant lung fields from air trapping
• diminished breath sounds from obstruction and air trapping.

In 2007, the National Heart, Lung and Blood Institute of the National Institutes of Health modified the four classification levels of asthma severity based on the frequency of symptoms and exacerbation effects on activity level: intermittent asthma, mild persistent, moderate persistent, and severe persistent. (See *Asthma severity classifications*.)

COMPLICATIONS
• Status asthmaticus
• Respiratory failure

DIAGNOSIS
Patients with asthma commonly show these abnormalities in their test results:
• Pulmonary function tests reveal signs of airway obstruction (decreased peak expiratory flow rates and forced expiratory volume in 1 second [FEV_1]; the ratio of FEV_1 to forced vital capacity is a sensitive indicator, especially in childhood asthma), low-normal or decreased vital capacity, and increased total lung and residual capacity. However, pulmonary function studies may be normal between attacks.
• Pulse oximetry may reveal decreased arterial oxygen saturation (SaO_2).
• Arterial blood gas (ABG) analysis provides the best indication of the severity of an attack. In patients

with acutely severe asthma, the partial pressure of arterial oxygen (PaO_2) is less than 60 mm Hg, the $PaCO_2$ is 40 mm Hg or more, and pH is usually decreased.

• Complete blood count with differential reveals increased eosinophil count.

• Chest X-rays may show hyperinflation with areas of focal atelectasis.

Before initiating tests for asthma, rule out other causes of airway obstruction and wheezing. In children, such causes include cystic fibrosis, tumors of the bronchi or mediastinum, and acute viral bronchitis; in adults, other causes include obstructive pulmonary disease, heart failure, and epiglottiditis.

TREATMENT

Treatment of acute asthma aims to decrease bronchoconstriction, reduce bronchial airway edema, and increase pulmonary ventilation.

If a specific antigen is causing the asthma, the patient may be desensitized through a series of injections of limited amounts of that antigen. The aim is to curb his immune response to the antigen.

Low flow humidified oxygen may be used to treat dyspnea, cyanosis, and hypoxemia (however, the amount delivered should maintain PaO_2 between 65 and 85 mm Hg, as determined by ABG analysis. Mechanical ventilation may be used if the patient doesn't respond to initial ventilatory support and drugs, or if the patient develops respiratory

ASTHMA SEVERITY CLASSIFICATIONS

According to the National Heart, Lung and Blood Institute of the National Institutes of Health, the four classification levels of asthma severity include intermittent, mild persistent, moderate persistent, and severe persistent asthma.

Intermittent asthma
■ Daytime symptoms occur no more than twice per week.
■ Nighttime symptoms occur no more than twice per month.
■ Lung function testing by either peak expiratory flow (PEF) or forced expiratory volume in 1 second is 80% of predicted values or higher.
■ PEF varies no more than 20%.

Mild persistent asthma
■ Daytime symptoms occur 3 to 6 days per week.
■ Nighttime symptoms occur 3 to 4 times per month.
■ Lung function testing is 80% of predicted values or higher.
■ PEF varies 20% to 30%.

Moderate persistent asthma
■ Daytime symptoms occur daily.
■ Nighttime symptoms occur at least weekly.
■ Lung function testing is 60% to 80% of predicted values.
■ PEF varies more than 30%.

Severe persistent asthma
■ Daytime symptoms occur continually.
■ Nighttime symptoms occur frequently.
■ Lung function testing is 60% of predicted values.
■ PEF varies more than 30%.

failure. Relaxation exercises, such as yoga, can help increase circulation and help a patient recover from an asthma attack.

⚠ ALERT

Acute attacks that don't respond to treatment may require hospital care, an inhaled or subcutaneous beta$_2$-adrenergic agonist (in three doses over 60 to 90 minutes) and, possibly, oxygen for hypoxemia. If the patient responds poorly, a systemic corticosteroid and possibly subcutaneous epinephrine may help. Beta$_2$-adrenergic agonist inhalation continues hourly. I.V. aminophylline may be added to the regimen, and I.V. fluid therapy is started. A patient who doesn't respond to this treatment, whose airways remain obstructed, and who has increasing respiratory difficulty is at risk for status asthmaticus and may require mechanical ventilation.

⚠ ALERT

Treatment of status asthmaticus consists of aggressive drug therapy: a beta$_2$-adrenergic agonist by nebulizer every 30 to 60 minutes, possibly supplemented with subcutaneous epinephrine, an I.V. corticosteroid, I.V. aminophylline, oxygen administration, I.V. fluid therapy, and intubation and mechanical ventilation for hypercapnic respiratory failure (Paco$_2$ of 40 mm Hg or more).

Drugs

The goal of therapy is to control the asthma with minimal or no adverse reactions to the medication.

- Systemic corticosteroids (oral prednisone or methylprednisolone) for relief of symptoms
- Inhaled corticosteroids, such as beclomethasone, triamcinolone (Azmacort), or fluticasone (Flovent), which have anti-inflammatory action to decrease hyperresponsiveness and inhibit inflammatory cell migration
- Inhaled long-acting beta$_2$ agonists (also called *adrenergic stimulants*), such as salmeterol (Serevent Diskus) or formoterol (Foradil Aerolizer), which act as bronchodilators and prevent bronchospasm as well as exercised-induced asthma; they are frequently used in combination (salmeterol/fluticasone or Advair)
- Mast cell stabilizers, such as cromolyn sodium (Intal) and nedocromil (Tilade), which inhibit inflammatory cells and help prevent bronchoconstriction in asthma induced by cold air
- Leukotriene modifiers, such as montelukast (Singulair) and zileuton (Zyflo), which interfere with leukotriene mediator pathway; usually used in combination with inhaled corticosteroids
- Methylxanthines, such as sustained-released theophylline or I.V. aminophylline, which have mild to moderate bronchodilating activity
- Anticholinergics, such as ipratropium bromide (Atrovent), which are strong bronchodilators; this class may be combined with an adrenergic stimulant (albuterol/ipratropium or Combivent)

● Antibiotics to treat respiratory infections (stress the need to complete the prescribed course of antibiotic therapy)

SPECIAL CONSIDERATIONS

During an acute attack, follow these steps:

● First, assess the severity of asthma.
● Administer the prescribed treatments and assess the patient's response.
● Place the patient in high Fowler's position. Encourage pursed-lip and diaphragmatic breathing. Help him relax.

⚠ ALERT

Monitor the patient's vital signs. Keep in mind that developing or increasing tachypnea may indicate worsening asthma or drug toxicity. Blood pressure readings may reveal pulsus paradoxus, indicating severe asthma. Hypertension may indicate asthma-related hypoxemia.

● Administer prescribed humidified oxygen by nasal cannula at 2 L/minute to ease breathing and to increase SaO_2. Later, adjust oxygen according to the patient's vital signs and ABG levels.
● Anticipate intubation and mechanical ventilation if the patient fails to maintain adequate oxygenation.
● Monitor serum theophylline levels to ensure they're in the therapeutic range. Observe your patient for signs and symptoms of theophylline toxicity (vomiting, diarrhea, and headache), as well as for signs of subtherapeutic dosage (respiratory distress and increased wheezing).

● Observe the frequency and severity of your patient's cough, and note whether it's productive. Then auscultate the patient's lungs, noting adventitious or absent breath sounds. If his cough isn't productive and rhonchi are present, teach him effective coughing techniques. If the patient can tolerate postural drainage and chest percussion, perform these procedures to clear secretions. Suction an intubated patient, as needed.
● Treat dehydration with I.V. fluids until the patient can tolerate oral fluids, which will help loosen secretions.
● If conservative treatment fails to improve the airway obstruction, anticipate bronchoscopy or bronchial lavage when a lobe or larger area collapses.

During long-term care, follow these steps:

● Monitor the patient's respiratory status to detect baseline changes, to assess response to treatment, and to prevent or detect complications.
● Auscultate the lungs frequently, noting the degree of wheezing and quality of air movement.
● Review ABG levels, pulmonary function test results, and SaO_2 readings.
● If the patient is taking systemic corticosteroids, observe for complications, such as elevated blood glucose levels, friable skin, and bruising.

• Cushingoid effects resulting from long-term use of corticosteroids may be minimized by alternate-day dosage or use of prescribed inhaled corticosteroids.

• If the patient is taking corticosteroids by inhaler, watch for signs of candidal infection in the mouth and pharynx. Using an extender device and rinsing the mouth afterward may prevent this.

• Observe the patient's anxiety level. Keep in mind that measures that reduce hypoxemia and breathlessness should help relieve anxiety.

• Keep the room temperature comfortable and use an air conditioner or a fan in hot, humid weather.

• Control exercise-induced asthma by instructing the patient to use a bronchodilator or cromolyn 30 minutes before exercise. Also instruct him to use pursed-lip breathing while exercising.

All patients should know the following information:

• Teach the patient and his family to avoid known allergens and irritants.

• Describe to the patient prescribed drugs, including their names, dosages, actions, adverse effects, and special instructions.

• Teach the patient how to use a metered-dose inhaler. If he has difficulty using an inhaler, he may need an extender device to optimize drug delivery and lower the risk of candidal infection with orally inhaled corticosteroids.

• If the patient has moderate to severe asthma, explain how to use a peak flow meter to measure the degree of airway obstruction. Tell him to keep a record of peak flow readings and to bring it to medical appointments. Explain the importance of calling the physician immediately if the peak flow drops suddenly (may signal severe respiratory problems).

• Tell the patient to notify the physician if he develops a temperature above 100° F (37.8° C), chest pain, shortness of breath without coughing or exercising, or uncontrollable coughing. An uncontrollable asthma attack requires immediate attention.

• Teach the patient diaphragmatic and pursed-lip breathing as well as effective coughing techniques.

• Urge him to drink at least 3 qt (3 L) of fluids daily to help loosen secretions and maintain hydration.

Atelectasis

Atelectasis is incomplete expansion of lobules (clusters of alveoli) or lung segments, which may result in partial or complete lung collapse. Because parts of the lung are unavailable for gas exchange, unoxygenated blood passes through these areas unchanged, resulting in hypoxemia. Atelectasis may be chronic or acute. Many patients undergoing upper abdominal or thoracic surgery experience atelectasis to some degree. The prognosis depends on prompt removal of any airway obstruction, relief of hypoxemia, and reexpansion of the collapsed lung.

CAUSES AND INCIDENCE

The incidence and prevalence of atelectasis aren't well documented. Atelectasis commonly results from bronchial occlusion by mucus plugs. It's a problem in many patients with chronic obstructive pulmonary disease, bronchiectasis, or cystic fibrosis and in those who smoke heavily. (Smoking increases mucus production and damages cilia.) Atelectasis may also result from occlusion by foreign bodies, bronchogenic carcinoma, and inflammatory lung disease. The bronchial occlusion that occurs prevents air from entering the alveoli distal to the obstruction, causing an absorption atelectasis—the air present in the alveoli is absorbed gradually into the bloodstream and eventually the alveoli collapse.

Other causes include respiratory distress syndrome of the neonate (hyaline membrane disease), oxygen toxicity, and pulmonary edema, in which alveolar surfactant changes increase surface tension and permit complete alveolar deflation. Impaired production of surfactant can also cause absorption atelectasis, whereby increasing surface tension of the alveolus due to reduced surfactant leads to collapse.

External compression, which inhibits full lung expansion, or any condition that makes deep breathing painful, may also cause atelectasis. Such compression or pain may result from abdominal surgical incisions, rib fractures, pleuritic chest pain, tight dressings around the chest, stab wounds, impalement accidents, car accidents in which the driver slams into the steering column, thoracotomy, chest tubes, or obesity (which elevates the diaphragm and reduces tidal volume).

Prolonged immobility may also cause atelectasis by producing preferential ventilation of one area of the lung over another. Mechanical ventilation using constant small tidal volumes without intermittent deep breaths may also result in atelectasis. Central nervous system depression (as in drug overdose) eliminates periodic sighing and is a predisposing factor of progressive atelectasis.

SIGNS AND SYMPTOMS

Clinical effects vary with the cause of collapse, the degree of hypoxemia, and any underlying disease but generally include some degree of dyspnea. Atelectasis of a small area of the lung may produce only minimal symptoms that subside without specific treatment.

Massive collapse can produce:
- severe dyspnea
- anxiety, cyanosis
- diaphoresis
- peripheral circulatory collapse
- tachycardia
- arrhythmias
- substernal or intercostal retraction
- ompensatory hyperinflation of unaffected areas of the lung
- mediastinal shift to the affected side
- elevation of the ipsilateral hemidiaphragm.

COMPLICATIONS

- Acute pneumonia
- Bronchiectasis
- Hypoxemia and respiratory failure
- Pleural effusion and empyema
- Postobstructive drowning of the lung
- Sepsis

DIAGNOSIS

Diagnosis requires an accurate patient history, a physical examination, and chest X-rays.

- Auscultation reveals diminished or bronchial breath sounds.
- When much of the lung is collapsed, percussion reveals dullness.
- In widespread atelectasis, chest X-rays may show characteristic horizontal lines in the lower lung zones; however, extensive areas of "microatelectasis" may exist without abnormalities on the chest X-ray film.
- With segmental or lobar collapse, chest X-rays show characteristic dense shadows commonly associated with hyperinflation of neighboring lung zones.
- Bronchoscopy rules out an obstructing neoplasm or a foreign body.
- Arterial blood gas analysis may reveal respiratory acidosis and hypoxemia resulting from atelectasis.
- Pulse oximetry may show deteriorating levels of arterial oxygen saturation.

TREATMENT

Treatment includes incentive spirometry, frequent coughing, and deep-breathing exercises if the patient isn't ventilated; these exercises encourage deep inspiration and should be performed every 1 to 2 hours. If mechanical ventilation is used, tidal volume should be maintained at appropriate levels to ensure adequate expansion of the lungs. If atelectasis is secondary to mucus plugging, mucolytics, chest percussion, and postural drainage may be used, as can humidifying inspired air and maintaining adequate fluid intake. If these measures fail, bronchoscopy may be helpful in removing secretions. Humidity and bronchodilators can improve mucociliary clearance and dilate airways.

Atelectasis secondary to an obstructing neoplasm may require surgery or radiation therapy. Postoperative thoracic and abdominal surgery patients require analgesics to facilitate deep breathing, which minimizes the risk of atelectasis.

Drugs

- Mucolytics, such as N-acetylcysteine (Mucomyst), to decrease the viscosity of the sputum if the atelectasis is related to mucous plugging
- Bronchodilators, such as albuterol (Proventil, Ventolin) or metaproterenol (Alupent), to encourage sputum expectoration and improve ventilation in patients with underlying airflow problems
- Analgesics or consultation with pain management specialists to promote comfort if the atelectasis is due to inadequate pain control

- Anti-infectives to treat underlying infection

SPECIAL CONSIDERATIONS

- If mechanical ventilation is used, use the sigh mechanism on the ventilator, if appropriate, to intermittently increase tidal volume at the rate of 10 to 15 sighs/hour to encourage lung expansion.
- Use an incentive spirometer to encourage deep inspiration through positive reinforcement. Teach the patient how to use the spirometer, and encourage him to use it every 1 to 2 hours.
- Humidify inspired air and encourage adequate fluid intake to mobilize secretions. To promote loosening and clearance of secretions, encourage deep-breathing and coughing exercises and use postural drainage and chest percussion.
- If the patient is intubated or uncooperative, provide suctioning, as needed. Use sedatives with discretion because they depress respirations and the cough reflex as well as suppress sighing. However, the patient won't cooperate with treatment if he's in pain.
- Assess breath sounds and ventilatory status frequently; report changes immediately.
- Teach the patient about respiratory care, including postural drainage, coughing, and deep breathing.
- Encourage the patient to stop smoking and lose weight, as needed. Refer him to appropriate support groups for help.

- Provide reassurance and emotional support; the patient may be anxious due to hypoxia or respiratory distress.

⊠ PREVENTION

- *In a patient who's bedridden, encourage movement and deep breathing.*
- *Administer adequate analgesics.*
- *To prevent atelectasis, encourage the postoperative or other high-risk patient to cough and deep-breathe every 1 to 2 hours. To minimize pain during coughing exercises, splint the incision; teach the patient this technique as well. Gently reposition the patient often and encourage ambulation as soon as possible.*

Avian influenza

Avian influenza (flu) mainly infects birds, but it's of concern to humans, who have no immunity against it. The virus that causes this infection in birds can mutate and easily infect humans and potentially start a deadly worldwide epidemic. The first avian flu virus to infect humans directly occurred in Hong Kong in 1997 and has since spread across Asia. In October 2005 it was discovered in Turkey and Romania. About 161 people have been infected by H5N1 and the current death rate with confirmed infection is more than 50%. The H7N7 avian flu outbreak in the Netherlands resulted in 89 confirmed cases but only one death; an avian flu virus designated H9N2 infected three children in

Asia and all three recovered. Prognosis depends on the severity of infection as well as the type of avian flu virus that caused it.

CAUSES AND INCIDENCE

No cases of highly pathogenic H5N1 influenza have been reported in humans or birds in the United States. Frequently updated information on H5N1 avian influenza cases can be found on the Centers for Disease Control and Prevention website. Avian influenza A (H5N1) virus is commonly referred to as *bird flu virus*. Highly infective avian flu viruses, such as H5N1, have been shown to survive in the environment for long periods of time, and infection may be spread simply by touching contaminated surfaces. Birds who recover from flu can continue to shed the virus in their feces and saliva for as long as 10 days. Natural reservoirs for avian influenza A are considered to be the waterfowl (ducks and geese) in which most infections are believed to be asymptomatic. They also infect and cause disease in domestic poultry, but these often cause only minor disease. Avian influenza transmission to humans occurs through direct contact with infected poultry, with increased risk among those who are involved in slaughter, defeathering, and preparation of the birds for consumption. People at risk include those who are exposed to water and surfaces contaminated by bird droppings.

SIGNS AND SYMPTOMS

Symptoms of avian flu infection in humans depend on the particular strain of virus. In case of the H5N1 virus, infection causes more classic flulike symptoms, such as:
- headache
- malaise
- dry or productive cough
- sore throat
- temperature greater than 100.4° F (38° C)
- runny nose
- difficulty breathing
- diarrhea
- muscle aches.

COMPLICATIONS
- Conjunctivitis
- Pneumonia
- Acute respiratory distress
- Viral pneumonia
- Sepsis
- Organ failure

DIAGNOSIS
- The H5N1 virus is best identified by H5N1-specific reverse-transcriptase polymerase chain reaction (RT-PCR) performed at all state and many local public health laboratories.

⚠ ALERT
Viral culture of H5N1 should only be performed in a biosafety level 3 laboratory. If avian influenza is suspected, cultures shouldn't be ordered without guidance from a public health laboratory. Rapid influenza tests don't detect H5N1 avian influenza.

- Cultures obtained from oropharyngeal swabs, bronchoalveolar washes, or tracheal aspirates collected in the first 3 days of illness provide the best specimens for identification of the virus. Nasopharyngeal swabs may contain a low quantity of the virus.
- Serologic tests for avian H5N1 influenza can be performed but this is considered a second-line study.
- Chest X-rays, nasopharyngeal culture, and blood differential can also aid in diagnosis.

TREATMENT

It's currently recommended that people diagnosed with H5N1 infection be put in isolation and those in close contact should wear an N95 mask with ventilatory outflow.

Treatment is generally supportive, with oxygen administered for hypoxia and, possibly, ventilatory support. Supplemental I.V. fluids are administered for hydration and to support hemodynamic stability. Otherwise, the patient is treated symptomatically.

Drugs

- Antiviral therapy with neuraminidase inhibitors—the only specific therapy for human H5N1 disease. These agents work directly on the viral protein, decreasing the virulence of the infection. Early administration with oseltamivir phosphate (Tamiflu), and perhaps zanamivir (Relenza), may decrease the severity of the disease, if started within 48 hours after symptoms begin. Oseltamivir may also be prescribed for household contacts of people diagnosed with avian flu.
- Broad-spectrum antibiotics and aggressive fluid resuscitation to manage clinical signs of sepsis.

SPECIAL CONSIDERATIONS

- Tell patients to call their physician if they develop flulike symptoms within 10 days of handling infected birds or traveling to an area with a known avian flu outbreak.
- Those who work with birds who might be infected should use protective clothing and special breathing masks.
- Watch for signs and symptoms of complications.

⧉ PREVENTION

- *The first human vaccine against H5N1 avian influenza was approved by the FDA on April 17, 2007. Currently, the vaccine has been purchased by the federal government for the National Stockpile and isn't expected to become available to consumers. The Centers for Disease Control and Prevention have updated information about availability.*
- *Tell the patient that avoiding undercooked or uncooked meat reduces the risk of exposure to avian flu and other food-borne diseases.*
- *Teach the patient about proper disposal of tissues and proper handwashing technique.*

Bronchiectasis

A condition marked by chronic abnormal dilation of bronchi and destruction of bronchial walls, bronchiectasis can occur throughout the tracheobronchial tree or can be confined to one segment or lobe. However, it's usually bilateral and involves the basilar segments of the lower lobes. This disease has three forms: cylindrical (fusiform), varicose, and saccular (cystic). Bronchiectasis is irreversible once established.

CAUSES AND INCIDENCE

Bronchiectasis is relatively uncommon in the United States; however, bronchiectasis associated with cystic fibrosis occurs with a prevalence of 1 in 2,500 white births. Native Americans in Alaska have fourfold higher incidence of bronchiectasis than the general population.

The different forms of bronchiectasis may occur separately or simultaneously. In cylindrical bronchiectasis, the bronchi expand unevenly, with little change in diameter, and end suddenly in a squared-off fashion. In varicose bronchiectasis, abnormal, irregular dilation and narrowing of the bronchi give the appearance of varicose veins. In saccular bronchiectasis, many large dilations end in sacs. These sacs balloon into pus-filled cavities as they approach the periphery and are then called *saccules*. (See *Forms of bronchiectasis*.)

This disease results from conditions associated with repeated damage to bronchial walls and abnormal mucociliary clearance, which cause a breakdown of supporting tissue adjacent to airways. Such conditions include cystic fibrosis; immunologic disorders (agammaglobulinemia, for example); recurrent, inadequately treated bacterial respiratory tract infections, such as tuberculosis; and complications of measles, pneumonia, pertussis, or influenza. Bronchiectasis is also due to obstruction (by a foreign body—most common in children, tumor, or stenosis) in association with recurrent infection, as well as inhalation of corrosive gas or repeated aspiration of gastric juices into the lungs. Congenital anomalies are relatively uncommon causes, such as bronchomalacia, congenital bronchiectasis, immotile cilia syndrome, and Kartagener's syndrome, a variant of immotile cilia syndrome characterized by situs inversus, bronchiectasis, and either nasal polyps or sinusitis.

In bronchiectasis, hyperplastic squamous epithelium denuded of cilia replaces ulcerated columnar epithelium. Abscess formation involving all layers of the bronchial wall produces inflammatory cells and fibrous tissue, resulting in dilation and narrowing of the airways. Mucus plugs or fibrous tissue obliterates smaller bronchioles, whereas peribronchial lymphoid tissue becomes hyperplastic. Extensive vascular proliferation of bronchial circulation occurs and produces frequent hemoptysis.

SIGNS AND SYMPTOMS

Initially, bronchiectasis may be asymptomatic. When symptoms do arise, they're commonly attributed to other illnesses.
- Frequent bouts of infections, such as pneumonia and sinusitis, or history of hemoptysis
- Classic symptom: chronic cough that produces foul-smelling, mucopurulent secretions in amounts ranging from less than 10 ml/day in mild cases to more than 150 ml/day in more severe cases
- Coarse crackles during inspiration over involved lobes or segments
- Occasional wheezing
- Dyspnea
- Weight loss
- Anemia
- Malaise
- Clubbing of the fingers
- Recurrent fever, chills and other signs of infection

Advanced bronchiectasis may produce:
- chronic malnutrition

FORMS OF BRONCHIECTASIS

The three types of bronchiectasis are *cylindrical, fusiform (varicose),* and *saccular (cystic).* In cylindrical bronchiectasis, bronchioles are usually symmetrically dilated, whereas in fusiform bronchiectasis, bronchioles are deformed. In saccular bronchiectasis, large bronchi become enlarged and balloonlike.

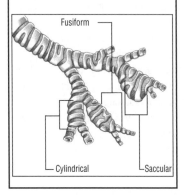

- right-sided heart failure
- cor pulmonale.

COMPLICATIONS
- Recurrent pneumonia requiring hospitalization
- Empyema
- Lung abscess
- Hemoptysis
- Progressive respiratory failure
- Cor pulmonale

DIAGNOSIS
- A history of recurrent bronchial infections, pneumonia, and hemoptysis in a patient whose chest X-ray

shows peribronchial thickening, areas of atelectasis, and scattered cystic changes suggests bronchiectasis.
- High-resolution computed tomography scanning may be used to confirm the diagnosis.

Other helpful laboratory tests include:
- sputum culture and Gram stain to identify predominant organisms
- complete blood count to detect anemia and leukocytosis
- pulmonary function tests to detect decreased vital capacity, expiratory flow rate, and hypoxemia. These tests also help determine the physiologic severity of the disease and the effects of therapy and help evaluate patients for surgery.

When cystic fibrosis is suspected as the underlying cause of bronchiectasis, sweat testing or genetic analysis is useful.

TREATMENT

The goals of treatment are to improve symptoms, reduce complications, control exacerbations, and reduce morbidity and mortality. Treatment typically includes antibiotics specific to culture results and may be administered until sputum production decreases. Bronchodilators, combined with postural drainage and chest percussion, help remove secretions if the patient has bronchospasm and thick, tenacious sputum. Bronchoscopy may be used to remove obstruction and secretions. Hypoxia requires oxygen therapy; severe hemoptysis commonly requires lobectomy, segmental resection, or bronchial artery embolization if pulmonary function is poor.

Drugs

- Antibiotics to treat infection, guided by sputum culture results; empiric therapy may be used as well with broad-spectrum anti-infectives
- Bronchodilators, such as albuterol (Proventil), to improve airflow by relieving bronchospasm
- Inhaled steroids, such as beclomethasone dipropionate (Beconase AQ Intranasal) or fluticasone propionate (Flovent), to reduce inflammation of airways
- Expectorants, such as guaifenesin (Guiatuss, Humibid LA), to help remove thickened secretions

SPECIAL CONSIDERATIONS

- Provide supportive care and help the patient adjust to the permanent changes in lifestyle that irreversible lung damage necessitates. Thorough teaching is vital.
- Administer antibiotics as ordered, and explain all diagnostic tests. Perform chest physiotherapy, including postural drainage and chest percussion designed for involved lobes, several times a day. The best times to do this are early morning and just before bedtime. Instruct the patient to maintain each position for 10 minutes, and then perform percussion and tell him to cough. Show family members how to perform postural drainage and percussion. Also teach the patient coughing and deep-breathing techniques to

promote good ventilation and the removal of secretions.

• Provide a warm, quiet, comfortable environment, and urge the patient to rest as much as possible. Encourage balanced, high-protein meals to promote good health and tissue healing and plenty of fluids (2 to 3 qt [2 to 3 L]) per day to hydrate and thin bronchial secretions). Give frequent mouth care to remove foul-smelling sputum. Teach the patient to dispose of all secretions properly. Instruct him to seek prompt attention for respiratory infections.

⧩ PREVENTION
• *Advise the patient to stop smoking, if appropriate, to avoid stimulating secretions and irritating the airways. Refer him to a local self-help group. Instruct him to seek prompt attention for respiratory infections.*

• *Tell the patient to avoid air pollutants and people with upper respiratory tract infections.*

• *Instruct the patient to take medications (especially antibiotics) exactly as prescribed.*

• *In children, stress the need for immunization to prevent childhood diseases.*

Chest trauma

Chest trauma accounts for almost one half of all trauma occurrences and almost one fourth of all trauma-related deaths. Chest trauma is commonly classified as penetrating or blunt, depending on the type of injury. *Penetrating* chest trauma involves an injury by a foreign object, such as a knife (most common stabbing injury), bullet (most common missile injury), pitch fork, or other pointed object that penetrates the thorax. These are considered open injuries because the thoracic cavity is exposed to pressure from the outside atmosphere. *Blunt* chest trauma, which is considered a closed chest injury, results from sudden compression or positive pressure inflicted by a direct blow to the organ and surrounding tissue. Blunt chest trauma commonly occurs in motor vehicle accidents (when the chest strikes the steering wheel), falls, or crushing injury.

Typically, penetrating chest trauma is fairly limited, usually involving isolated organs and lacerated tissues. In some cases, however, extensive tissue damage can occur if a bullet explodes in the chest cavity. Blunt chest trauma can cause extensive injury to the chest wall, lung, pleural space, and great vessels.

Injuries resulting from blunt chest trauma include pulmonary contusion, rib fractures, pneumothorax, hemothorax, and rupture of the diaphragm or great vessels. (See *Injuries Associated with Chest Trauma*, pages 36–41.) Blunt injuries are associated with multisystem organ injuries and carry a higher mortality rate than penetrating injuries.

CAUSES AND INCIDENCE

Motor vehicle accidents cause two-thirds of major chest trauma in the United States. Other common causes include sports and blast injuries and cardiopulmonary resuscitation. About 50% of these injuries affect the chest wall; 80% of those with significant blunt chest trauma also have extrathoracic injuries.

Chest trauma accounts for 70% of all trauma-related deaths in the United States. Injuries to the chest usually involve one or more of these conditions:

• hypoxemia resulting from airway alteration, damage to the chest muscles, lung parenchyma or ribs, severe hemorrhage, collapse of the lungs, or pneumothorax
• hypovolemia resulting from massive fluid loss
• cardiac failure resulting from an increase in intrathoracic pressure or

subsequent cardiac injury such as cardiac tamponade or contusion.

Tissue damage caused by penetrating trauma, such as an impaled object or foreign body, is related to the object size as well as the depth and velocity of penetration. For example, penetrating chest trauma by a bullet has many variables. The extent of injury depends on the distance at which the weapon was fired, the type of ammunition, the velocity of the ammunition, and the entrance and (if present) exit wounds. Additional factors to be considered when assessing the extent of a penetrating chest injury include the type of weapon; for example, the caliber, barrel, and length of a gun and the powder composition. An intact bullet causes less damage than a bullet that explodes on impact. A bullet that explodes within the chest may break up and scatter fragments, burn tissue, fracture bone, disrupt vascular structures, or cause a bullet embolism.

Injury resulting from blunt chest trauma is related to the amount of force, compression, and cavitation. Blunt force that strikes the chest wall at high velocity fractures the ribs and transfers that force to underlying organ and lung tissue. The direct impact of force is transmitted internally and the energy is dissipated to internal structures. The flexibility or elasticity of the chest wall directly affects the degree of injury. The first and second ribs take an enormous amount of blunt force to fracture and therefore are associated with significant intrathoracic injuries.

⚠ ALERT

Because the chest in the frail older person is inflexible and fragile, injury and mortality, even from minor chest trauma are more probable.

SIGNS AND SYMPTOMS

Signs and symptoms of blunt chest trauma depend on where the trauma initiates.

Rib fractures

- Tenderness
- Slight edema over the fracture site
- Pain that worsens with deep breathing and movement
- Shallow, splinted respirations

Sternal fractures

- Persistent chest pain, even at rest
- Severe dyspnea
- Cyanosis
- Agitation
- Extreme pain
- Subcutaneous emphysema

Flail chest

Multiple rib fractures within two or more places may cause flail chest, in which a portion of the chest wall "caves in," causing a loss of chest wall integrity and preventing adequate lung inflation. (See *Flail chest: Paradoxical breathing*, page 40.)

(Text continues on page 40)

INJURIES ASSOCIATED WITH CHEST TRAUMA

Injury	Pathophysiologic mechanism of injury
Pneumothorax	Blunt or penetrating injury allowing air to accumulate in the pleural space
Tension pneumothorax	Blunt or penetrating injury allowing air to accumulate in the pleural space without a way to escape, leading to complete lung collapse
Hemothorax	Blunt or penetrating trauma allowing blood to accumulate in the pleural space
Chylothorax	Blunt or penetrating trauma usually to the thoracic duct or lymphatics allowing lymphatic fluid to drain and accumulate in the pleural space
Pneumomediastinum	Blunt or penetrating trauma allowing air to accumulate in the mediastinum
Flail chest	Blunt trauma resulting in rib or sternal fractures leading to instability of the chest

Assessment findings	Treatment considerations
■ Dyspnea ■ Chest pain ■ Decreased or absent breath sounds ■ Chest X-ray positive for air between visceral and parietal pleura	■ Chest tube insertion
■ Severe dyspnea ■ Restlessness ■ Cyanosis ■ Tracheal shift to unaffected side ■ Distended jugular veins ■ Absence of breath sounds on affected side ■ Tachycardia ■ Hypotension ■ Distant heart sounds ■ Hypoxemia	■ Emergency lung reexpansion; possible thoracotomy for penetrating injury ■ Chest tube insertion
■ Dyspnea ■ Tachycardia ■ Tachypnea ■ Cool clammy skin ■ Hypotension ■ Diminished capillary refill ■ Absent breath sounds on affected side ■ Chest X-ray positive for blood accumulation	■ Chest tube insertion with possible autotransfusion
■ Chest X-ray positive for pleural effusion (although may not be evident for 2 to 4 weeks) after injury	■ Chest tube insertion ■ Possible thoracotomy to ligate thoracic duct
■ Dyspnea ■ Chest pain	■ Chest tube placement with repair of underlying injury
■ Dyspnea ■ Labored shallow respirations ■ Chest wall pain ■ Crepitus from body fragments (subcutaneous emphysema) ■ Asymmetrical (paradoxical) chest movements ■ Chest X-ray positive for fractures	■ Symptomatic and supportive care ■ Prevention of hemothorax and pneumothorax

(continued)

INJURIES ASSOCIATED WITH CHEST TRAUMA *(continued)*

Injury	Pathophysiologic mechanism of injury
Pulmonary contusion	Blunt trauma injuring lung tissue with the potential to cause respiratory failure
Tracheobronchial tear	Blunt trauma causing injury to the tracheobronchial tree, possibly leading to airway obstruction and tension pneumothorax
Diaphragmatic rupture	Blunt trauma causing a tear in the diaphragm, possibly allowing abdominal contents to herniate into the thorax
Cardiac contusion	Blunt trauma resulting in bruising of the cardiac muscle
Cardiac tamponade	Blunt or penetrating trauma allowing blood to accumulate in the pericardial sac, ultimately impairing venous return and cardiac output

Assessment findings	Treatment considerations
■ Dyspnea ■ Restlessness ■ Hemoptysis ■ Tachycardia ■ Crackles ■ Decreased lung compliance ■ Atelectasis ■ Arterial blood gas analysis revealing hypoxemia and hypercarbia ■ Chest X-ray revealing local or diffuse patchy, poorly outlined densities or irregular linear infiltrates	■ Intubation and mechanical ventilation ■ Hemodynamic monitoring ■ Possible thoracotomy if massive hemorrhage suspected
■ Dyspnea ■ Palpable fracture, hoarseness, and subcutaneous edema (laryngeal fracture) ■ Noisy breathing, labored respirations, and altered level of consciousness (tracheal injury) ■ Hemoptysis, subcutaneous emphysema, and possible tension pneumothorax (bronchial injury)	■ Emergency surgical repair of injury
■ Chest pain referred to the shoulder ■ Dyspnea ■ Diminished breath sounds ■ Bowels sounds audible in chest ■ Tachypnea ■ Chest X-ray positive for tear	■ Surgical repair
■ Chest discomfort ■ Electrocardiogram abnormalities (unexplained sinus tachycardia, atrial fibrillation, bundle branch block, ST segment changes) ■ Serial creatine kinase levels revealing possible cardiac muscle damage	■ Supportive and symptomatic care
■ Dyspnea ■ Midthoracic pain ■ Tachycardia ■ Tachypnea ■ Hypotension, distended jugular veins, and muffled heart sounds (Beck's triad) ■ Paradoxical pulse	■ Pericardiocentesis

(continued)

INJURIES ASSOCIATED WITH CHEST TRAUMA *(continued)*

Injury	Pathophysiologic mechanism of injury
Great vessel rupture	Blunt trauma resulting in injury to major blood vessels such as the aorta

Signs and symptoms include:
- bruised skin
- extreme pain caused by rib fracture and disfigurement
- paradoxical chest movements
- tachycardia
- hypotension
- respiratory acidosis

FLAIL CHEST: PARADOXICAL BREATHING

A patient with a blunt chest injury may develop flail chest, in which a portion of the chest "caves in." This results in paradoxical breathing, described below.

Inhalation
- Injured chest wall collapses in.
- Uninjured chest wall moves out.

Exhalation
- Injured chest wall moves out.
- Uninjured chest wall moves in.

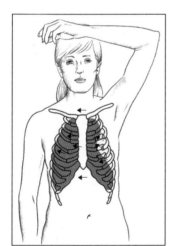
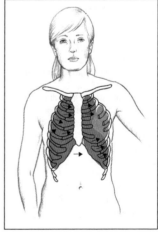

Assessment findings	Treatment considerations
▪ Dyspnea ▪ Hoarseness ▪ Stridor ▪ Absent femoral pulses ▪ Retrosternal or interscapular pain ▪ Widening mediastinum	▪ Transfusion ▪ Surgical repair

- cyanosis
- rapid, shallow respirations
- tension pneumothorax.

Tension pneumothorax
- Severe dyspnea
- Absent breath sounds (on the affected side)
- Agitation
- Jugular vein distention
- Tracheal deviation (away from the affected side)
- Cyanosis
- Shock

Hemothorax
- Respiratory distress
- Severe dyspnea with restlessness and pallor or cyanosis
- Asymmetrical chest movements
- Flat jugular veins
- Bloody sputum or hemoptysis
- Unilateral decreased fremitus and decreased chest expansion on inspiration
- Dullness over the area of fluid collection
- Unilateral diminished or absent breath sounds
- Hypotension and tachycardia

Myocardial contusions
- Tachycardia
- Ecchymosis
- Chest pain
- Electrocardiogram (ECG) abnormalities

Diaphragmatic rupture
- Severe respiratory distress
- Bowel sounds in the chest
- Decreased vital capacity

COMPLICATIONS
- Hemothorax
- Hemorrhagic shock
- Airway compromise
- Pneumothorax
- Tension pneumothorax
- Diaphragmatic rupture
- Arrhythmias
- Liver laceration
- Myocardial tears or rupture
- Cardiac tamponade
- Pulmonary artery tears
- Ventricular rupture
- Rupture of the aorta
- Bronchial, tracheal, or esophageal tears

DIAGNOSIS

A history of trauma with dyspnea, chest pain, and other typical clinical features suggest a blunt chest injury. To determine its extent, a physical examination and diagnostic tests are needed.

• In hemothorax, percussion reveals dullness. In tension pneumothorax, it reveals tympany. Auscultation may reveal a change in position of the loudest heart sound.

• Chest X-rays may confirm rib and sternal fractures, pneumothorax, flail chest, pulmonary contusions, lacerated or ruptured aorta, tension pneumothorax, diaphragmatic rupture, lung compression, or atelectasis with hemothorax.

• With cardiac damage, the ECG may show abnormalities, including unexplained tachycardias, atrial fibrillation, bundle-branch block (usually right), ST segment changes, and ventricular arrhythmias such as multiple premature ventricular contractions.

• Serial aspartate aminotransferase, alanine aminotransferase, lactate dehydrogenase, creatine kinase (CK), and CK-MB levels are elevated. However, cardiac enzymes fail to detect myocardial damage in up to 50% of patients.

• Retrograde aortography, computed tomography angiography, and transesophageal echocardiography reveal aortic laceration or rupture.

• Contrast studies and liver and spleen scans detect diaphragmatic rupture.

• Echocardiography, computed tomography scans, and cardiac and lung scans show the injury's extent.

TREATMENT

Blunt chest injuries call for controlling bleeding and maintaining a patent airway, adequate ventilation, and fluid and electrolyte balance. Further treatment depends on the specific injury and complications.

• Single fractured ribs are managed conservatively with mild analgesics and follow-up examinations to check for indications of a pneumothorax or hemothorax. To prevent atelectasis, the patient should perform incentive spirometry, deep breathing, and coughing for lung expansion. Intercostal nerve blocks may help with more severe fractures.

• Treatment for a pneumothorax involves inserting a spinal, 14G, or 16G needle into the second intercostal space at the midclavicular line to release pressure. Then the physician inserts a chest tube in the affected side to normalize pressure and reexpand the lung. The patient also receives oxygen and I.V. fluids. He may require intubation and mechanical ventilation.

• Shock related to hemothorax calls for I.V. infusion of lactated Ringer's or normal saline solution. If the patient loses more than 1,500 ml of blood or more than

30% of circulating blood volume, he'll also need a transfusion of packed red blood cells or an autotransfusion. He may also require intubation, mechanical ventilation, and possible thoracotomy. Chest tubes are inserted into the fifth or sixth intercostal space at the midaxillary line to remove blood.

• Treatment of flail chest may include endotracheal intubation and mechanical ventilation with positive pressure. The patient may also receive I.V. muscle relaxants. If the patient requires controlled ventilation, he'll receive a neuromuscular blocking agent. If an air leak occurs, the patient may need operative fixation of the flail chest.

• Pulmonary contusions are managed with colloids to replace volume and maintain oncotic pressure. (Steroid use is controversial.) The patient may also need endotracheal intubation and mechanical ventilation as well as antibiotics, diuretics, and analgesics.

• Myocardial contusions call for cardiac and hemodynamic monitoring to detect arrhythmias and prevent cardiogenic shock. Drug therapy depends on the type of arrhythmia. Treatment is similar to that for myocardial infarction.

• Immediate surgical repair is mandatory for myocardial rupture, septal perforation, and other cardiac lacerations. Less severe ventricular wounds require use of a digital or balloon catheter. Atrial wounds require a clamp or balloon catheter.

The patient with an aortic rupture or laceration who reaches the hospital alive needs immediate surgery, using synthetic grafts or anastomosis to repair the damage. Such a patient requires a large volume of I.V. fluids (usually lactated Ringer's solution) and whole blood along with oxygen at a very high rate. A pneumatic antishock garment is applied, and the patient is promptly transported to the operating room.

For a patient with a diaphragmatic rupture, a nasogastric tube is inserted to temporarily decompress the stomach, and the patient is prepared for surgical repair.

Drugs

• Mild analgesics for pain associated with fractures

• Analgesics and antibiotics to treat pneumothorax

• I.V. infusion of lactated Ringer's or normal saline solution for shock

• I.V. muscle relaxants to relieve muscle spasms in flail chat; neuromuscular blocking agents may be needed if the patient requires mechanical ventilation

• Antibiotics, diuretics, and analgesics for pulmonary contusions

• Antiarrhythmics, analgesics, and inotropic drugs such as dobutamine or dopamine for myocardial contusions

• Short-acting beta-blocking agents such as labetalol or esmolol (Brevibloc) to control the heart rate and decrease the mean arterial pressure for myocardial rupture, septal perforation, and other cardiac lacerations

SPECIAL CONSIDERATIONS

• Check all pulses and level of consciousness. Evaluate skin color and temperature, depth of respiration, use of accessory muscles, and length of inhalation compared to exhalation.

• Check pulse oximetry values for adequate oxygenation.

• Observe tracheal position. Look for distended jugular veins and paradoxical chest motion.

• Listen to heart and breath sounds carefully; palpate for subcutaneous emphysema (crepitation) or a lack of structural integrity of the ribs.

• Obtain a history of the injury. Unless severe dyspnea is present, have the patient locate the pain, and ask if he's having trouble breathing. Obtain laboratory studies (arterial blood gas analysis, cardiac enzyme studies, complete blood count, type, and crossmatch).

Simple rib fractures

• Have the patient cough and breathe deeply to mobilize secretions while splinting to decrease pain.

• Give adequate analgesics, encourage bed rest, and apply heat. Don't strap or tape the chest.

Severe fractures

• Administer intercostal nerve blocks.

• Obtain X-rays before and after the nerve blocks to rule out pneumothorax.

• Intubate the patient with excessive bleeding or hemopneumothorax.

• Chest tubes may be inserted to treat hemothorax and to assess the need for thoracotomy.

• To prevent atelectasis, turn the patient frequently and encourage coughing and deep-breathing exercises.

Pneumothorax

• Placement of a chest tube anterior to the midaxillary line at the fourth intercostal space may be required to aspirate as much air as possible from the pleural cavity and to reexpand the lungs.

• When time permits, insert chest tubes attached to water-seal drainage and suction.

Flail chest

• Place the patient in semi-Fowler's position.

• Reexpanding the lung is the first definitive care measure.

• Administer oxygen at a high flow rate under positive pressure.

• Suction the patient frequently and as completely as possible.

• Maintain acid-base balance.

• Observe carefully for signs of tension pneumothorax.

- Start I.V. therapy using lactated Ringer's or normal saline solution.

Hemothorax

- Treat shock with I.V. infusions of lactated Ringer's or normal saline solution.
- Administer packed red blood cells for blood losses greater than 1,500 ml or circulating blood volume losses exceeding 30%.
- Administer oxygen.
- The patient may need insertion of chest tubes in the fourth intercostal space anterior to the midaxillary line to remove blood.
- Monitor and document vital signs and blood loss.
- Watch for and respond immediately to falling blood pressure, rising pulse rate, and hemorrhage, all of which require a thoracotomy to stop bleeding.

Pulmonary contusion

- Give limited amounts of colloids (such as salt-poor albumin, whole blood, or plasma) as appropriate to replace volume and maintain oncotic pressure.
- Give analgesics, as necessary
- Monitor blood gas levels to ensure adequate ventilation; provide oxygen therapy, mechanical ventilation, and chest tube care.

Cardiac damage

- Close intensive care or telemetry may detect arrhythmias and prevent cardiogenic shock.

- Impose bed rest in semi-Fowler's position (unless the patient requires shock position); administer oxygen, analgesics, and supportive drugs to control heart failure or supraventricular arrhythmias, as needed.
- Watch for cardiac tamponade, which calls for pericardiocentesis.
- Provide essentially the same care as for a patient with a myocardial infarction.

⚠ ALERT
For myocardial rupture, septal perforation, and other cardiac lacerations, immediate surgical repair is mandatory. Less severe ventricular wounds require use of a digital or balloon catheter; atrial wounds require a clamp or balloon catheter.

⚠ ALERT
For patients with aortic rupture or laceration, immediate surgery is mandatory using synthetic grafts or anastomosis to repair the damage. Give large volumes of I.V. fluids (lactated Ringer's or normal saline solution) and whole blood, along with oxygen at very high flow rates, then transport the patient promptly to the operating room.

⚠ ALERT
For tension pneumothorax, the patient may need insertion of a 14G to 16G angiocatheter in the second intercostal space at the midclavicular line to release pressure in the chest. After this, insert a chest tube to normalize pressure and reexpand the lung. Administer oxygen

under positive pressure along with I.V. fluids.

Diaphragmatic rupture

• Insert a nasogastric tube to temporarily decompress the stomach, and prepare the patient for surgical repair.

Chronic bronchitis

Chronic bronchitis is inflammation of the bronchi caused by irritants or infection. The distinguishing characteristic of bronchitis is obstruction of airflow. In chronic bronchitis, a form of chronic obstructive pulmonary disease, hypersecretion of mucus and chronic productive cough are present during 3 months of the year for at least 2 consecutive years. Only a minority of patients with the clinical syndrome of chronic bronchitis develop significant airway obstruction.

CAUSES AND INCIDENCE

According to the National Center for Health Statistics, approximately 14 million people have chronic bronchitis, but this number may be underestimated. Chronic bronchitis develops when irritants are inhaled for a prolonged time. The irritants inflame the tracheobronchial tree, leading to increased mucus production and a narrowed or blocked airway. As the inflammation continues, changes in the cells lining the respiratory tract increase resistance in the small airways, and severe imbalance in the ventilation-perfusion ($\dot{V}/\dot{Q}$) ratio decreases arterial oxygenation.

Chronic bronchitis can result from a series of attacks of acute bronchitis or recurrent respiratory infections, or it may gradually evolve because of smoking or inhalation of air contaminated with other pollutants in the environment. Smoking is by far the most important of these factors; smoking impairs ciliary action and macrophage function, inflames airways, increases mucus production, destroys alveolar septa, and causes peribronchiolar fibrosis. The mucus-producing layer of the bronchial lining becomes thickened over time with such narrowing of the airway, whereby breathing becomes increasingly difficult. With immobilization of the cilia that sweep the air clean of foreign irritants, the bronchial passages become more vulnerable to further infection and the spread of tissue damage.

Chronic bronchitis causes hypertrophy and hyperplasia of airway smooth muscle and hyperplasia of the mucous glands, increased number of goblet cells, ciliary damage, squamous metaplasia of the columnar epithelium, and chronic leukocytic and lymphocytic infiltration of bronchial walls. (See *Changes in chronic bronchitis.*)

Hypersecretion of the goblet cells block the free movement of the cilia, which normally sweep dust, irritants, and mucus away from the airways. Accumulating mucus and debris impair the defenses and increase the likelihood of respiratory tract infections. (See *Mucus buildup in chronic bronchitis*, page 48.)

Additional effects include narrowing and widespread inflammation within the airways. Bronchial walls become inflamed and thickened from edema and accumulation of inflammatory cells, and smooth muscle bronchospasm further narrows the lumen. Initially, only large bronchi are involved, but eventually all airways are affected. Airways become obstructed and close, especially on expiration, trapping the gas in the distal portion of the lung. Consequent hypoventilation leads to a $\dot{V}/\dot{Q}$ mismatch and resultant hypoxemia and hypercapnia.

SIGNS AND SYMPTOMS

• Chronic bronchitis, insidious in onset, with productive cough and exertional dyspnea
• Upper respiratory infections associated with increased sputum production and worsening dyspnea, which take progressively longer to resolve
• Copious sputum (gray, white, or yellow)
• Weight gain due to edema
• Cyanosis
• Tachypnea
• Wheezing
• Prolonged expiratory time
• Use of the accessory muscles of respiration

CHANGES IN CHRONIC BRONCHITIS

In chronic bronchitis, irritants inflame the tracheobronchial tree over time, leading to increased mucus production and a narrowed or blocked airway. As the inflammation continues, goblet and epithelial cells hypertrophy. Because the natural defense mechanisms are blocked, the airways accumulate debris in the respiratory tract. The illllustrations here show these changes.

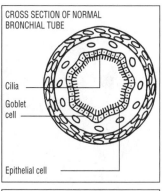

CROSS SECTION OF NORMAL BRONCHIAL TUBE

Cilia

Goblet cell

Epithelial cell

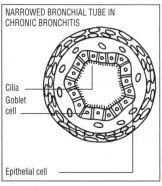

NARROWED BRONCHIAL TUBE IN CHRONIC BRONCHITIS

Cilia

Goblet cell

Epithelial cell

MUCUS BUILDUP IN CHRONIC BRONCHITIS

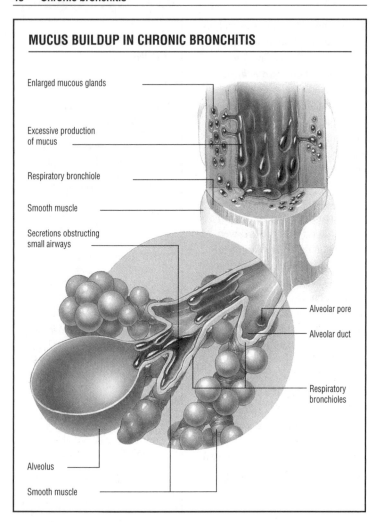

Enlarged mucous glands

Excessive production of mucus

Respiratory bronchiole

Smooth muscle

Secretions obstructing small airways

Alveolar pore

Alveolar duct

Respiratory bronchioles

Alveolus

Smooth muscle

COMPLICATIONS

- Recurrent respiratory tract infections
- Cor pulmonale
- Polycythemia
- Severe respiratory failure
- Death

DIAGNOSIS

- Physical examination reveals barrel chest, rhonchi and wheezes on auscultation, prolonged expiration, jugular vein distention, and pedal edema.

- Chest X-rays may show hyperinflation and increased bronchovascular markings.
- Pulmonary function tests show increased residual volume, decreased vital capacity and forced expiratory volumes, and normal static compliance and diffusing capacity.
- Arterial blood gas analysis shows decreased partial pressure of arterial oxygen (PaO_2) and normal or increased partial pressure of arterial carbon dioxide ($PaCO_2$).
- Electrocardiogram may show atrial arrhythmias; peaked P waves in leads II, III, and aV_F; and occasionally right ventricular hypertrophy.

TREATMENT

Treatment is designed to relieve symptoms and prevent complications. Because most patients receive outpatient treatment, they need comprehensive teaching to help them comply with therapy and understand the nature of this chronic, progressive disease. If programs in pulmonary rehabilitation are available, encourage patients to enroll.

- The patient will require adequate fluid intake and chest physiotherapy to mobilize secretions.
- Ultrasonic or mechanical nebulizer treatments may be necessary to loosen secretions and aid in mobilization.
- Urge the patient to stop smoking. Provide smoking cessation counseling or refer him to a program.
- Avoid other respiratory irritants, such as secondhand smoke, aerosol spray products, and outdoor air pol-

lution. In the home, an air conditioner with an air filter may be helpful.

Drugs

- Beta-agonist bronchodilators (albuterol or salmeterol), anticholinergic bronchodilators (ipratropium) , and corticosteroids (beclomethasone or triamcinolone) by metered-dose inhaler to relieve bronchoconstriction
- Antimicrobials to treat respiratory infections
- Antitussives and expectorants, such as guaifenesin with dextromethorphan (Humibid DM, Robitussin DM) and guaifenesin and codeine (Robitussin AC), to assist with mucus removal
- Bronchodilators, such as albuterol (Proventil, Ventolin), to assist in keeping airways open and improve oxygenation
- Influenza vaccination with rimantadine (Flumadine) or amantadine (Symmetrel) during flu epidemics to prevent infection with influenza A and B
- Antivirals to treat viral infections
- Analgesics and antipyretics, such as ibuprofen (Advil, Motrin), or acetaminophen (Tylenol, Aspirin-Free Anacin) to treat fever, malaise, and aches or pains

SPECIAL CONSIDERATIONS

- Teach the patient and his family how to recognize early signs of infection; warn the patient to avoid contact with people with respiratory infections. Pneumococcal vaccination and annual influenza vaccinations are important preventive measures.

• To promote ventilation and reduce air trapping, teach the patient to breathe slowly, prolong expirations to two to three times the duration of inspiration, and to exhale through pursed lips.

• To help mobilize secretions, teach the patient how to cough effectively. If the patient with copious secretions has difficulty mobilizing secretions, teach his family how to perform postural drainage and chest physiotherapy. If secretions are thick, urge the patient to drink 12 to 15 glasses of fluid per day. A home humidifier may be beneficial, particularly in the winter.

• Administer low concentrations of oxygen as ordered. Perform blood gas analysis to determine the patient's oxygen needs and to avoid carbon dioxide narcosis. If the patient is to continue oxygen therapy at home, teach him how to use the equipment correctly. The patient with a chronic lung condition rarely requires more than 2 to 3 L/minute to maintain adequate oxygenation. Higher flow rates will further increase the PaO_2, but the patient whose ventilatory drive is largely based on hypoxemia commonly develops markedly increased $PaCO_2$. In these cases, chemoreceptors in the brain are relatively insensitive to the increase in carbon dioxide. Teach the patient and his family that excessive oxygen therapy may eliminate the hypoxic respiratory drive, causing confusion and drowsiness, signs of carbon dioxide narcosis.

• Emphasize the importance of a balanced diet. Because the patient may tire easily when eating, suggest that he eat frequent, small meals and consider using oxygen, administered by nasal cannula, during meals.

• Help the patient and his family adjust their lifestyles to accommodate the limitations imposed by this debilitating chronic disease. Instruct the patient to allow for daily rest periods and to exercise daily as his physician directs.

• As the disease progresses, encourage the patient to discuss his fears.

⧁ PREVENTION

• *To help prevent chronic bronchitis, as well as the other chronic obstructive lung diseases, advise all patients, especially those with a family history or those in its early stages, not to smoke.*

• *Assist in early detection by urging periodic physical examinations, including spirometry and medical evaluation of a chronic cough, and urging patients to seek prompt treatment for recurring respiratory infections.*

Coal worker's pneumoconiosis

A progressive nodular pulmonary disease, coal worker's pneumoconiosis (CWP) occurs in two forms. Simple CWP is characterized by small lung opacities; in complicated

CWP, also known as *progressive massive fibrosis,* masses of fibrous tissue occasionally develop in the patient's lungs. The risk of developing CWP (also known as *black lung disease, coal miner's disease, miner's asthma, anthracosis,* and *anthracosilicosis*) depends upon the duration of underground exposure to coal dust (usually 20 years or longer), intensity of exposure (dust count and particle size), location of the mine, silica content of the coal (anthracite coal has the highest silica content), and the worker's susceptibility.

The prognosis varies. Simple asymptomatic disease is self-limiting, although progression to complicated CWP is more likely if CWP begins after a relatively short period of exposure. Complicated CWP may be disabling, resulting in severe ventilatory failure and cor pulmonale.

CAUSES AND INCIDENCE

The incidence of CWP is highest among anthracite coal miners in the eastern United States. CWP is caused by the chronic inhalation and prolonged retention of respirable coal dust particles (less than 5 microns in diameter). Inhaled coal dust enters the terminal bronchioles and is engulfed by alveolar and interstitial macrophages. These particles are expelled in the mucus or through the lymphatic system. When the system becomes overwhelmed, the dust-laden macrophages accumulate in the alveoli and may trigger an im

mune response, causing the fibroblasts to secrete reticulin, which entraps the macrophages. More reticulin is laid down as macrophages lyse; this is also further stimulated by coal that contains silica fibers. Arterioles can become strangulated from continued interstitial fibrosis. As more and more dying macrophages, fibroblasts, reticulin, and collagen are deposited, the vessels become compromised, and ischemic necrosis occurs.

Simple CWP results in the formation of coal macules (accumulations of macrophages laden with coal dust) around the terminal and respiratory bronchioles, surrounded by a halo of dilated alveoli. Macule formation leads to atrophy of supporting tissue, causing permanent dilation of small airways and forming focal areas of emphysema. The macules may continue to enlarge and form nodules when they coalesce.

Simple disease may progress to complicated CWP, involving one or both lungs. In this form of the disease, fibrous tissue masses enlarge and coalesce, causing gross distortion of pulmonary structures (destruction of vasculature alveoli and airways).

SIGNS AND SYMPTOMS

Simple CWP produces no symptoms, especially in nonsmokers. Symptoms of complicated CWP include:
- exertional dyspnea and hypoxia
- chronic cough that occasionally produces inky-black sputum (when

fibrotic changes undergo avascular necrosis and their centers cavitate)

- increasing dyspnea and a cough that produces milky, gray, clear, or coal-flecked sputum
- recurrent bronchial and pulmonary infections producing yellow, green, or thick sputum.

COMPLICATIONS

- Cor pulmonale
- Right ventricular hypertrophy
- Pulmonary hypertension
- Pulmonary tuberculosis

In cigarette smokers, chronic bronchitis, emphysema, and other respiratory disorders may also complicate the disease.

DIAGNOSIS

- Patient history reveals exposure to coal dust.
- Physical examination shows barrel chest, hyperresonant lungs with areas of dullness, diminished breath sounds, crackles, rhonchi, and wheezes.
- In simple CWP, chest X-ray shows small opacities (less than 10 mm in diameter). These may be present in all lung zones but are more prominent in the upper lung zones.
- In complicated CWP, one or more large opacities (1 to 5 cm in diameter), possibly exhibiting cavitation, are seen.
- Pulmonary function tests show:
- vital capacity that's normal in simple CWP but decreased in complicated CWP

- forced expiratory volume in 1 second that's decreased in complicated disease
- residual volume and total lung capacity that's normal in simple CWP but decreased in complicated CWP
- carbon monoxide diffusing capacity that's significantly decreased in complicated CWP as alveolar septa are destroyed and pulmonary capillaries are obliterated
- partial pressure of arterial carbon dioxide that may be increased with concomitant chronic obstructive pulmonary disease.

TREATMENT

There's no specific treatment. The goal of treatment is to relieve respiratory symptoms, manage hypoxia and cor pulmonale, and avoid respiratory tract irritants and infections. Treatment also includes careful observation for the development of tuberculosis. Chest physiotherapy techniques, such as controlled coughing and segmental bronchial drainage, combined with chest percussion and vibration help remove secretions.

Other measures include increased fluid intake (at least 3 qt [3 L] daily), respiratory therapy techniques, and intermittent positive pressure breathing. Diuretics, cardiac glycosides, and salt restriction may be indicated in cor pulmonale. In severe cases, it may be necessary to administer oxygen for hypoxemia by cannula or mask (1 to 2 L/minute) if the patient has chronic hypoxia; mechanical ventilation is used if arterial oxygen can't be maintained above 40 mm Hg.

Drugs

- Oxygen to treat hypoxia
- Antibiotics to treat respiratory infections
- Mucolytics, such as acetylcysteine (Mucomyst), to reduce the thickness of pulmonary secretions
- Bronchodilators, such as aminophylline, to reduce bronchospasm

SPECIAL CONSIDERATIONS

- Encourage the patient to stay active to avoid deterioration in his physical condition but to pace his activities and practice relaxation techniques.

⊵ PREVENTION

- *Teach the patient to prevent infections by avoiding crowds and people with respiratory infections and by receiving Pneumovax and annual influenza vaccines.*
- *Provide education to workers in the coal industry on methods to reduce exposure to coal dust in their particular work area. This may involve use of masks or respirators as indicated.*
- *Periodic evaluation of workers is needed to assess lung status and prevent further deterioration by continued exposure.*

Common cold

The common cold (also known as *acute coryza*) is an acute, usually afebrile viral infection that causes inflammation of the upper respiratory tract. It's the most common infectious disease, accounting for more time lost from school or work than any other cause. Although a cold is benign and self-limiting, it can lead to secondary bacterial infections.

CAUSES AND INCIDENCE

The common cold is more prevalent in children than in adults, in adolescent boys than in girls, and in women than in men. In temperate zones, it's more common in the colder months; in the tropics, it's more common during the rainy season. About 90% of colds stem from a viral infection of the upper respiratory passages and consequent mucous membrane inflammation; occasionally, colds result from a mycoplasmal infection. (See *What happens in the common cold*, page 54.)

More than 100 viruses can cause the common cold. Major offenders include rhinoviruses, coronaviruses, myxoviruses, adenoviruses, coxsackie viruses, and echoviruses. The mode of transmission is through direct invasion of the mucosa lining the upper airway. After invasion, the offending pathogen encounters various physical, mechanical, humoral, and cellular immune defenses. Incubation times vary with the specific pathogen before the appearance of symptoms. Transmission occurs through airborne respiratory droplets, contact with contaminated objects, and hand-to-hand transmission. Children acquire new strains from their

WHAT HAPPENS IN THE COMMON COLD

Virus-infected droplets enter the body and attack the cells lining the throat and nose. The virus particles then multiply rapidly.

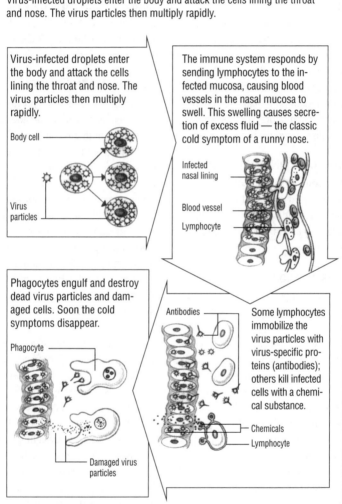

Virus-infected droplets enter the body and attack the cells lining the throat and nose. The virus particles then multiply rapidly.

Body cell

Virus particles

The immune system responds by sending lymphocytes to the infected mucosa, causing blood vessels in the nasal mucosa to swell. This swelling causes secretion of excess fluid — the classic cold symptom of a runny nose.

Infected nasal lining

Blood vessel

Lymphocyte

Phagocytes engulf and destroy dead virus particles and damaged cells. Soon the cold symptoms disappear.

Phagocyte

Damaged virus particles

Antibodies

Some lymphocytes immobilize the virus particles with virus-specific proteins (antibodies); others kill infected cells with a chemical substance.

Chemicals

Lymphocyte

schoolmates and pass them on to family members. Fatigue or drafts don't increase susceptibility. Reinfection (with productive cough) is common, but complications are rare. A cold is communicable for 2 to 3 days after the onset of symptoms.

Most symptoms (local swelling, erythema, edema, secretions, and fever) result from the inflammatory response and from toxin production from pathogens. An initial nasopharyngeal infection may spread to adjacent anatomical structures, producing symptoms of sinusitis, otitis media, epiglottiditis, laryngitis, tracheobronchitis, or pneumonia. Inflammatory narrowing of the epiglottis and larynx may result in a compromised airflow, especially in children. This inflammation may be threatening to those with congenital or acquired subglottic stenosis.

SIGNS AND SYMPTOMS

After a 1- to 4-day incubation period, the common cold produces:
- pharyngitis
- nasal congestion
- coryza
- headache
- burning, watery eyes
- feeling of fullness with a copious nasal discharge that commonly irritates the nose.

About 3 days after onset, major signs diminish, but the "stuffed up" feeling generally persists for about a week.

As the cold progresses, clinical features develop more fully. Additional effects may include:
- fever (in children)
- chills
- myalgia
- arthralgia
- malaise
- lethargy
- hacking, nonproductive, or nocturnal cough.

COMPLICATIONS
- Sinusitis
- Otitis media
- Pharyngitis
- Lower respiratory tract infection

DIAGNOSIS

No explicit diagnostic test exists to isolate the specific organism responsible for the common cold.
- Diagnosis rests on the typically mild, localized, and afebrile upper respiratory symptoms.
- Despite infection, white blood cell counts and differential are within normal limits.
- Diagnosis must rule out allergic rhinitis, measles, rubella, and other disorders that produce similar early symptoms.
- A temperature higher than 100° F (37.8° C), severe malaise, anorexia, tachycardia, exudate on the tonsils or throat, petechiae, and tender lymph glands may point to more serious disorders and require additional diagnostic tests.

TREATMENT

The primary treatments—fluids and rest—are purely symptomatic because the common cold has no cure.
- Fluids help loosen accumulated respiratory secretions and maintain hydration.
- Rest combats fatigue and weakness.
- Steam or vaporizers encourage expectoration and soothe irritated mucous membranes.
- In infants, saline nose drops and mucus aspiration with a bulb syringe may be beneficial.

- Warm facial packs can provide comfort, relieve congestion, and promote drainage in cases of rhinosinusitis.
- Encourage the patient to sleep with the head and shoulders slightly elevated, or the head of the crib or child's bed raised on blocks, to promote sinus and nasal drainage.

Drugs

- Aspirin, acetaminophen, or ibuprofen to help relieve fever, myalgia, and aches and pains

⚠ **ALERT**

In a child with a fever, acetaminophen (Tylenol, FeverAll) is the drug of choice. Also, the U.S. Food and Drug Administration strongly recommends that over-the-counter cough and cold medicines are contraindicated in children younger than 2 years old because they haven't been shown to be effective and can cause serious adverse effects or fatalities.

- Nasal decongestants, such as pseudoephedrine (Actifed, Afrin, Sudafed) or phenylephrine (Neo-Synephrine), to relieve congestion; these should be used in children older than 2 years of age
- Throat lozenges to relieve soreness
- Antitussives, such as guaifenesin and dextromethorphan (Benylin, Humibid DM, Mytussin, Robitussin DM), or codeine to relieve cough
- Antibiotics to treat specific infections and complications as indicated (such as sinusitis and ear infection)
- Anticholinergic agents, such as ipratropium (Atrovent), to reduce mucus in lungs and relax smooth muscles of large and medium bronchi; they may be used with short-acting beta$_2$-adrenergic bronchodilators
- Antihistamines, such as diphenhydramine (Benadryl, Benylin) or chlorpheniramine (Aller-Chlor, Chlo-Amine, Chlor-Trimeton), to reduce edema, bronchial constriction, mucous secretion, and smooth muscle contraction
- Adrenergic agonists, such as epinephrine (Adrenalin), to relieve severe bronchoconstriction
- Corticosteroids such as dexamethasone (Decadron) to decrease edema of the airway (such as in croup)

SPECIAL CONSIDERATIONS

- Emphasize that antibiotics don't cure the common cold.
- Tell the patient to maintain bed rest during the first few days, to use a lubricant on his nostrils to decrease irritation, to relieve throat irritation with hard candy or cough drops, to increase fluid intake, and to eat light meals.
- Warm baths or heating pads can reduce aches and pains but won't hasten a cure. Suggest hot or cold steam vaporizers. Commercial expectorants are available, but their effectiveness is questionable.
- Advise against overuse of nose drops or sprays because they may cause rebound congestion.

▣ PREVENTION
Warn the patient to minimize contact with people who have colds. To avoid spreading colds, teach the patient to wash his hands often and before touching his eyes, to cover coughs and sneezes, and to avoid sharing towels and drinking glasses.

Cor pulmonale

The World Health Organization defines chronic cor pulmonale as "hypertrophy of the right ventricle resulting from diseases affecting the function or the structure of the lungs, except when these pulmonary alterations are the result of diseases that primarily affect the left side of the heart or of congenital heart disease." Invariably, cor pulmonale follows some disorder of the lungs, pulmonary vessels, chest wall, or respiratory control center. For instance, chronic obstructive pulmonary disease (COPD) produces pulmonary hypertension, which leads to right ventricular hypertrophy and right-sided heart failure. Because cor pulmonale generally occurs late during the course of COPD and other irreversible diseases, the prognosis is generally poor. While cor pulmonale is usually a chronic progressive condition, it can have periods of acute exacerbation.

CAUSES AND INCIDENCE

Approximately 85% of patients with cor pulmonale have COPD, and 25% of patients with COPD eventu-

ally develop cor pulmonale. Other respiratory disorders that produce cor pulmonale include obstructive lung diseases (for example, bronchiectasis and cystic fibrosis), restrictive lung diseases (for example, pneumoconiosis, interstitial pneumonitis, scleroderma, and sarcoidosis), loss of lung tissue after extensive lung surgery, congenital cardiac shunts (such as a ventricular septal defect), pulmonary vascular diseases, (for example, recurrent thromboembolism, primary pulmonary hypertension, schistosomiasis, and pulmonary vasculitis), respiratory insufficiency without pulmonary disease (for example, in chest wall disorders such as kyphoscoliosis, neuromuscular incompetence due to muscular dystrophy, and amyotrophic lateral sclerosis, polymyositis, and spinal cord lesions above C6), obesity hypoventilation syndrome (pickwickian syndrome), upper airway obstruction, and living at high altitudes (chronic mountain sickness).

Pulmonary capillary destruction and pulmonary vasoconstriction (usually secondary to hypoxia) reduce the area of the pulmonary vascular bed. Thus, pulmonary vascular resistance is increased, causing pulmonary hypertension. To compensate for the extra work needed to force blood through the lungs, the right ventricle dilates and hypertrophies. In response to low oxygen content, the bone marrow produces more red blood cells (RBCs), causing erythrocytosis. When the hematocrit (HCT) exceeds

55%, blood viscosity increases, which further aggravates pulmonary hypertension and increases the hemodynamic load on the right ventricle. Right-sided heart failure is the result.

In COPD, increased airway obstruction makes airflow worse. The resulting hypoxia and hypercarbia can have vasodilatory effects on systemic arterioles. However, hypoxia increases pulmonary vasoconstriction. The liver becomes palpable and tender because it's engorged and displaced downward by the low diaphragm. Hepatojugular reflux may occur.

Compensatory mechanisms begin to fail, and larger amounts of blood remain in the right ventricle at the end of diastole, causing ventricular dilation. Increasing intrathoracic pressures impede venous return and raise pressure within the jugular vein. Peripheral edema can occur, and right ventricular hypertrophy increases progressively. The main pulmonary arteries enlarge, pulmonary hypertension increases, and heart failure occurs.

Cor pulmonale accounts for about 25% of all types of heart failure. It's most common in areas of the world where the incidence of cigarette smoking and COPD is high; cor pulmonale affects middle-age to elderly men more often than women, but incidence in women is increasing. In children, cor pulmonale may be a complication of cystic fibrosis, hemosiderosis, upper airway obstruction, scleroderma, extensive bronchiectasis, neurologic diseases affecting respiratory muscles, or abnormalities of the respiratory control center.

SIGNS AND SYMPTOMS

As long as the heart can compensate for the increased pulmonary vascular resistance, clinical features reflect the underlying disorder and occur mostly in the respiratory system.

Early
- Chronic, productive cough
- Exertional dyspnea
- Wheezing respirations
- Fatigue
- Weakness

Progressive
- Dyspnea at rest
- Tachypnea
- Orthopnea
- Dependent edema
- Distended jugular veins
- Hepatomegaly
- Right upper quadrant discomfort
- Tachycardia
- Decreased cardiac output
- Weight gain

COMPLICATIONS
- Right- and left-sided heart failure
- Hepatomegaly
- Edema
- Ascites
- Pleural effusions
- Thromboembolism

DIAGNOSIS
- Pulmonary artery pressure measurements show increased right ventricular and pulmonary artery

pressures stemming from increased pulmonary vascular resistance. Right ventricular systolic and pulmonary artery systolic pressures exceed 30 mm Hg; pulmonary artery diastolic pressure exceeds 15 mm Hg.

- Echocardiography or angiography indicates right ventricular enlargement; echocardiography can estimate pulmonary artery pressure while also ruling out structural and congenital lesions.
- Chest X-ray shows large central pulmonary arteries and suggests right ventricular enlargement by rightward enlargement of the heart's silhouette on an anterior chest film.
- Arterial blood gas (ABG) analysis shows decreased partial pressure of arterial oxygen (PaO_2) typically less than 70 mm Hg and usually no more than 90 mm Hg on room air.
- Electrocardiogram frequently shows arrhythmias, such as premature atrial and ventricular contractions and atrial fibrillation during severe hypoxia; it may also show right bundle-branch block, right axis deviation, prominent P waves and inverted T wave in right precordial leads, and right ventricular hypertrophy.
- Pulmonary function tests show results consistent with the underlying pulmonary disease.
- HCT is typically greater than 50%; other tests for hypercoagulability include homocysteine, protein C and S, and antithrombin III.
- Brain natriuretic peptide level is usually elevated.

TREATMENT

Treatment of cor pulmonale is designed to reduce hypoxemia, increase the patient's exercise tolerance and, when possible, correct the underlying condition. In addition to bed rest, treatment may include:

- administration of continuous oxygen by mask or cannula. This has been beneficial in concentrations ranging from 24% to 40%, depending on PaO_2, as necessary. In acute cases, therapy may also include mechanical ventilation; patients with underlying COPD generally shouldn't receive high concentrations of oxygen because of possible subsequent respiratory depression.
- a low-sodium diet and restricted fluid intake to help reduce edema
- phlebotomy to reduce the RBC count.

Depending on the underlying cause, some variations in treatment may be indicated. For example, a tracheotomy may be necessary if the patient has an upper airway obstruction.

Drugs

- Cardiac glycoside, such as digoxin (Lanoxin), to improve myocardial contraction, increase parasympathetic tone, and decrease heart rate
- Diuretics, such as furosemide (Lasix), to reduce edema
- Antimicrobials when respiratory infection is present; culture and sensitivity testing of a sputum specimen helps select an appropriate agent

- Calcium channel blockers (potent pulmonary artery vasodilators), such as nifedipine (Procardia, Adalat), diltiazem (Cardizem), or other agents, such as diazoxide, nitroprusside, hydralazine, angiotensin-converting enzyme inhibitors, or prostaglandins, used in primary pulmonary hypertension to reduce pulmonary vascular resistance and enhance cardiac output
- Anticoagulants, such as warfarin (Coumadin), to reduce the risk of thromboembolism
- Endothelin receptor antagonists, such as bosentan (Tracleer) or treprostinol (Remodulin), to provide direct vasodilation
- Steroids to reduce inflammation in the patient with a vasculitis autoimmune phenomenon or acute exacerbations of COPD

SPECIAL CONSIDERATIONS

- Plan diet carefully with the patient and staff dietitian. Because the patient may lack energy and tire easily when eating, provide small, frequent feedings rather than three heavy meals.
- Prevent fluid retention by limiting the patient's fluid intake to 1 to 2 qt (1 to 2 L) per day and providing a low-sodium diet.
- Monitor serum potassium levels closely if the patient is receiving diuretics. Low serum potassium levels can increase the risk of arrhythmias associated with cardiac glycosides.
- Watch the patient for signs of digoxin toxicity, such as complaints of anorexia, nausea, vomiting, and halos around visual images and color perception shifts. Monitor for cardiac arrhythmias. Teach the patient to check his radial pulse before taking digoxin or any cardiac glycoside. He should be instructed to notify the physician if he detects changes in pulse rate.
- Reposition bedridden patients often to prevent atelectasis.
- Provide meticulous respiratory care, including oxygen therapy, and pursed-lip breathing exercises for the patient with COPD. Periodically measure ABG levels and watch for signs of respiratory failure: changes in pulse rate, labored respirations, changes in mental status, and increased fatigue after exertion.

Before discharge, maintain these protocols:
- Make sure that the patient understands the importance of maintaining a low-sodium diet, weighing himself daily, and watching for increased edema. Teach him to detect edema by pressing the skin over a shin with one finger, holding it for a second or two, then checking for a finger impression. Increased weight, increased edema, or respiratory difficulty should be reported to the physician.
- Instruct the patient to plan for frequent rest periods and to do breathing exercises regularly.
- If the patient needs supplemental oxygen therapy at home, refer him to an agency that can help obtain the required equipment and, as necessary, arrange for follow-up examinations.

- If the patient has been placed on anticoagulant therapy, emphasize the need to watch for bleeding (epistaxis, hematuria, bruising) and to report signs to the physician. Also encourage him to return for periodic laboratory tests to monitor partial thromboplastin time, fibrinogen level, platelet count, HCT, hemoglobin level, and prothrombin time.

- Because pulmonary infection commonly exacerbates COPD and cor pulmonale, tell the patient to watch for and immediately report early signs of infection, such as increased sputum production, change in sputum color, increased coughing or wheezing, chest pain, fever, and tightness in the chest. Tell the patient to avoid crowds and people known to have pulmonary infections, especially during the flu season. The patient should receive Pneumovax and annual influenza vaccines.

- Warn the patient to avoid substances that may depress the ventilatory drive, such as sedatives and alcohol.

Croup

Croup is a severe inflammation and obstruction of the upper airway, occurring as acute laryngotracheobronchitis (most common), laryngitis, and acute spasmodic laryngitis; it must always be distinguished from epiglottiditis. It's derived from an old German word for "voice box" and refers to swelling around the larynx or vocal cords. Recovery is usually complete.

CAUSES AND INCIDENCE

Croup usually results from a viral infection but can also be caused by bacteria, allergies, and inhaled irritants. Parainfluenza viruses cause 75% of such infections; adenoviruses, respiratory syncytial virus (RSV), influenza, and measles viruses account for the rest. Croup is a childhood disease affecting more boys than girls (typically between ages 3 months and 5 years) and usually occurring during the winter. Up to 15% of patients have a strong family history of croup.

Croup is usually preceded by an upper airway infection that proceeds to laryngitis and then descends into the trachea (and sometimes the bronchi), causing inflammation of the mucosal lining and subsequent narrowing of the airway. Profound airway edema may lead to obstruction and seriously compromised ventilation. (See *How croup affects the upper airway*, page 62.)

The flexible larynx of a young child is particularly susceptible to spasm, which may cause complete airway obstruction. When the child's airway is significantly narrowed, he struggles to inhale air past the obstruction and into the lungs, producing the characteristic inspiratory stridor and suprasternal retractions, and the classic barking or seal-like cough. Cough is characterized by gradual onset of a low-grade fever. Worsening of symptoms at night and a cough are common. The airway obstruction increases, leading to retractions, restlessness, anxiety,

HOW CROUP AFFECTS THE UPPER AIRWAY

In croup, inflammatory swelling and spasms constrict the larynx, thereby reducing airflow. This cross-sectional drawing (from chin to chest) shows the upper airway changes caused by croup. Inflammatory changes almost completely obstruct the larynx (which includes the epiglottis) and significantly narrow the trachea.

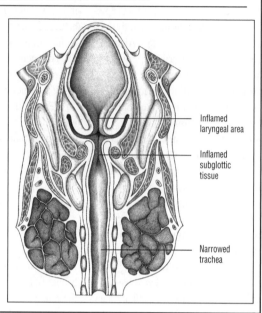

Inflamed laryngeal area

Inflamed subglottic tissue

Narrowed trachea

tachycardia, and tachypnea. Severe obstruction leads to respiratory exhaustion, hypoxemia, carbon dioxide accumulation, and respiratory acidosis.

SIGNS AND SYMPTOMS

The onset of croup usually follows an upper respiratory tract infection. Clinical features include:

- inspiratory stridor
- hoarse or muffled vocal sounds
- varying degrees of laryngeal obstruction and respiratory distress
- a characteristic sharp, barking, seal-like cough.

These symptoms may last only a few hours or persist for a day or two. As it progresses, croup causes inflammatory edema and, possibly, spasm, which can obstruct the upper airway and severely compromise ventilation.

Each form of croup has additional characteristics:

- In laryngotracheobronchitis, the symptoms seem to worsen at night. Inflammation causes edema of the bronchi and bronchioles as well as increasingly difficult expiration that frightens the child. Other characteristic features include fever, diffusely decreased breath sounds, expiratory rhonchi, and scattered crackles.
- Laryngitis, which results from vocal cord edema, is usually mild and produces no respiratory distress except in infants. Early signs include a

sore throat and cough, which rarely may progress to marked hoarseness, suprasternal and intercostal retractions, inspiratory stridor, dyspnea, diminished breath sounds, restlessness, and in later stages severe dyspnea and exhaustion.

• Acute spasmodic laryngitis affects a child between ages 1 and 3, particularly one with allergies and a family history of croup. It typically begins with mild to moderate hoarseness and nasal discharge, followed by the characteristic cough and noisy inspiration (that usually awaken the child at night), labored breathing with retractions, rapid pulse, and clammy skin. The child becomes anxious, which may lead to increasing dyspnea and transient cyanosis. These severe symptoms diminish after several hours but reappear in a milder form on the next 1 or 2 nights.

COMPLICATIONS

• Respiratory distress
• Respiratory arrest
• Epiglottiditis
• Bacterial tracheitis
• Atelectasis
• Dehydration

DIAGNOSIS

The clinical picture is characteristic, so the diagnosis should be suspected immediately.

• When bacterial infection is the cause, throat cultures may identify the organisms and their sensitivity to antibiotics and rule out diphtheria.

• On a posteroanterior X-ray examination of the chest, narrowing of the upper airway ("steeple sign") may be apparent.

• Laryngoscopy may reveal inflammation and obstruction in epiglottal and laryngeal areas. In evaluating the patient, assess for foreign body obstruction (a common cause of crouplike cough in a young child) as well as for masses and cysts.

⚠ ALERT

If you suspect epiglottiditis, don't compromise the child's airway by trying to assess the back of the throat with a tongue blade. Airway obstruction may occur; be prepared to assist with immediate tracheotomy in the event of obstruction.

TREATMENT

For most children with croup, home care with rest, cool mist humidification during sleep, and antipyretics, relieve symptoms. However, respiratory distress that's severe or interferes with oral hydration requires hospitalization and parenteral fluid replacement to prevent dehydration. Oxygen therapy may also be required. Increasing obstruction of the airway requires intubation and mechanical ventilation.

Inhaled racemic epinephrine and corticosteroids may be used to alleviate respiratory distress.

Drugs

• Antipyretics, such as acetaminophen (Tylenol), to reduce fevers

• Antibiotics for bacterial infections and after the specific pathogen is determined
• Corticosteroids, such as dexamethasone (Decadron) or prednisolone (Prelone), to reduce inflammation
• Bronchodilators, such as racemic epinephrine (AsthmaNefrin, microNefrin) to reduce congestion and edema of the airways

SPECIAL CONSIDERATIONS

• Monitor and support respiration, and control fever. Because croup is so frightening to the child and his family, also provide support and reassurance.
• Carefully monitor cough and breath sounds, hoarseness, severity of retractions, inspiratory stridor, cyanosis, respiratory rate and character (especially prolonged and labored respirations), restlessness, fever, and cardiac rate.
• Keep the child as quiet as possible. However, avoid sedation because it may depress respiration. If the patient is an infant, position him in an infant seat or prop him up with a pillow; place an older child in Fowler's position. If an older child requires a cool mist tent to help him breathe, explain why it's needed.
• Isolate patients suspected of having RSV and parainfluenza infections if possible. Wash your hands carefully before leaving the room to avoid transmission to other children, particularly infants. Instruct parents and others involved in the care of

these children to take similar precautions.
• Control fever with sponge baths and antipyretics. Keep a hypothermia blanket on hand for temperatures above 102° F (38.9° C). Watch for seizures in infants and young children with high temperatures. Give I.V. antibiotics, as ordered.
• Relieve sore throat with soothing, water-based ices, such as fruit sherbet and ice pops. Avoid thicker, milk-based fluids if the child is producing heavy mucus or has great difficulty in swallowing. Apply petroleum jelly or another ointment around the nose and lips to soothe irritation from nasal discharge and mouth breathing.
• Maintain a calm, quiet environment and offer reassurance. Explain all procedures and answer any questions.
• When croup doesn't require hospitalization:
– teach the parents effective home care. Suggest the use of a cool humidifier (vaporizer). To relieve croupy spells, tell parents to carry the child into the bathroom, shut the door, and turn on the hot water. Breathing in warm, moist air quickly eases an acute spell of croup.
– warn parents that ear infections and pneumonia are complications of croup, which may appear about 5 days after recovery. Stress the importance of immediately reporting earache, productive cough, high temperature, or increased shortness of breath.

✏ PREVENTION

- *Wash hands frequently to prevent a respiratory infection.*
- *Give diphtheria, tetanus, and pertussis;* Haemophilus influenzae *B; and measles, mumps, and rubella vaccines to children.*

Cryptogenic organizing pneumonia

Cryptogenic organizing pneumonia (COP), also known as *idiopathic bronchiolitis obliterans with organizing pneumonia* (BOOP), is one of several types of bronchiolitis obliterans. *Organizing pneumonia* refers to unresolved pneumonia, in which inflammatory alveolar exudate persists and eventually undergoes fibrosis. *Bronchiolitis obliterans* is a generic term used to describe an inflammatory disease of the small airways. In children, COP is considered one of the childhood interstitial lung diseases because of its pathophysiologic course.

CAUSES AND INCIDENCE

COP has no known cause. However, some forms may be associated with specific diseases or situations, such as bone marrow, heart, or heart-lung transplantation; collagen vascular diseases, such as rheumatoid arthritis and systemic lupus erythematosus; inflammatory diseases, such as Crohn's disease, ulcerative colitis, and polyarteritis nodosa; bacterial, viral, or mycoplasmal respiratory infections; inhalation of toxic gases; and drug therapy with amiodarone,

bleomycin, penicillamine, or lomustine.

Much debate exists about the various pathologies and classifications of bronchiolitis obliterans. Most patients are between ages 50 and 60. Incidence is equally divided between men and women. A smoking history doesn't seem to increase the risk of developing the disorder.

However, most patients share a common pathophysiologic feature of structural remodeling of the distal airspaces, leading to impaired gas exchange. This has been thought to be the sequela of persistent inflammation; however, tissue injury to the distal airspaces with aberrant wound healing has also been found to result in collagenous fibrosis. Adenoviral infection or exposure to organic dust can result in damage to the epithelial or endothelial layers and the associated basement membrane. The fibrinous exudate that usually forms from this is the base for subsequent repair and remodeling. Inflammation present in most types of COP are thought to be triggered by inflammatory events, such as infection or hypersensitivity. The end result is fibrotic remodeling of the airways that's eventually responsible for most of the morbidity and mortality.

SIGNS AND SYMPTOMS

The presenting symptoms of COP are usually subacute with flulike syndrome lasting for several weeks to several months.

- Flulike syndrome of fever
- Persistent and nonproductive cough
- Dyspnea (especially with exertion)
- Malaise
- Anorexia
- Weight loss
- Physical assessment findings of dry crackles
    Less common symptoms include:
- productive cough
- hemoptysis
- chest pain
- generalized aching
- night sweats.

COMPLICATIONS

- Respiratory failure
- Cor pulmonale
- Right-sided heart failure
- Death

DIAGNOSIS

Diagnosis begins with a thorough patient history meant to exclude any known cause of bronchiolitis obliterans or diseases with a pathology that includes an organizing pneumonia pattern.

- Chest X-ray usually shows bilateral patchy, diffuse airspace opacities with a ground-glass appearance that may migrate from one location to another. High-resolution computed tomography scans show areas of consolidation. Except for the migrating opacities, these findings are nonspecific and present in many other respiratory disorders.
- Pulmonary function tests may be normal or show reduced capacities.

The diffusing capacity for carbon monoxide is generally low.

- Arterial blood gas analysis usually shows mild to moderate hypoxemia at rest, which worsens with exercise.
- Blood tests reveal an increased erythrocyte sedimentation rate, an increased C-reactive protein level, an increased white blood cell count with a somewhat increased proportion of neutrophils, and a minor rise in eosinophils. Immunoglobulin (Ig) G and IgM levels are normal or slightly increased, and the IgE level is normal.
- Bronchoscopy reveals normal or slightly inflamed airways. Bronchoalveolar lavage fluid obtained during bronchoscopy shows a moderate elevation in lymphocytes and sometimes elevated neutrophil and eosinophil levels. Foamy-looking alveolar macrophages may also be found.
- Lung biopsy, thoracoscopy, or bronchoscopy is required to confirm the diagnosis of COP. Pathologic changes in lung tissue include plugs of connective tissue in the lumen of the bronchioles, alveolar ducts, and alveolar spaces.

These changes may occur in other types of bronchiolitis and in other diseases that cause organizing pneumonia. They also differentiate COP from constrictive bronchiolitis (characterized by inflammation and fibrosis that surrounds and may narrow or completely obliterate the bronchiolar airways). Although the pathologic findings in proliferative and constrictive bronchiolitis are different, the causes and presentations may overlap. Any known cause of bronchiolitis obliterans or organizing pneumonia must be ruled out before the diagnosis is made.

TREATMENT

Corticosteroids are the current treatment for COP, although the ideal dosage and duration of treatment remain topics of discussion. Relapse is common when steroids are tapered off or stopped. This usually can be reversed when steroids are increased or resumed. Occasionally, a patient may need to continue corticosteroids indefinitely, but should be placed on the lowest dose necessary to achieve benefit.

Oxygen is used to correct hypoxemia. The patient may need either no oxygen or a small amount of oxygen at rest and a greater amount when he exercises.

Other treatments vary, depending on the patient's symptoms, and may include inhaled bronchodilators, cough suppressants, and bronchial hygiene therapies.

COP is responsive to treatment and usually can be completely reversed with corticosteroid therapy. However, a few deaths have been reported, particularly in patients who had more widespread pathologic changes in the lung or patients who developed opportunistic infections or other complications related to steroid therapy.

Drugs

● Corticosteroids, such as methylprednisolone (Medrol) and prednisone, which are anti-inflammatory agents used in treating patients with COP
● Immunosuppressive-cytotoxic drugs, such as cyclophosphamide (Cytoxan) and hydroxychloroquine (Plaquenil), which have been used in the few cases of intolerance or unresponsiveness and have been shown to reduce inflammation; they may be used in patients who don't tolerate corticosteroids

SPECIAL CONSIDERATIONS

● Explain all diagnostic tests. The patient may experience anxiety and frustration because of the length of time and number of tests needed to establish the diagnosis.
● Explain the diagnosis to the patient and his family. This uncommon diagnosis may cause confusion and anxiety.
● Monitor the patient for adverse effects of corticosteroid therapy: weight gain, "moon face," glucose intolerance, fluid and electrolyte imbalance, mood swings, cataracts, peptic ulcer disease, opportunistic infections, and osteoporosis leading to bone fractures. In many cases, these effects leave the patient unable to tolerate the treatment. Teach the patient and his family about these adverse effects, emphasizing which reactions should be reported to the physician.
● Teach measures that may help prevent complications related to

treatment, such as infection control and improved nutrition.

• Teach breathing, relaxation, and energy conservation techniques to help the patient manage symptoms.

• Monitor oxygenation, both at rest and with exertion. The physician will probably prescribe an oxygen flow rate for use when the patient is at rest and a higher one for exertion. Teach the patient how to increase the oxygen flow rate to the appropriate level for exercise.

• If the patient needs oxygen at home, ensure continuity of care by making appropriate referrals to discharge planners, respiratory care practitioners, and home equipment vendors.

Cystic fibrosis

Cystic fibrosis is a chronic, progressive, inherited disease that affects the exocrine (mucus-secreting) glands. The disease is transmitted as an autosomal recessive trait; it's the most common fatal genetic disease in white children.

With improvements in treatment over the past decade, the average life expectancy has risen from age 16 to age 40 and older.

CAUSES AND INCIDENCE

Prevalence ranges from 1 case per 620 in a confined population with Dutch ancestry to 1 case per 90,000 in Asians. In the United States, the incidence of cystic fibrosis is highest in whites of northern European ancestry (1 in 3,200 live births) and lowest in blacks (1 in 15,000 live births). In Hispanics, prevalence is 1 case per 9,200. In Asian Americans, prevalence is 1 case per 31,000. The disease occurs equally in both genders.

The gene responsible for cystic fibrosis (located on chromosome 7) encodes a protein that involves chloride transport across epithelial membranes; more than 100 specific mutations of the gene are known. (See *Cystic fibrosis transmission link.*)

The gene responsible for cystic fibrosis encodes a membrane-associated protein called the *cystic fibrosis transmembrane regulator* (CFTR). The exact function of CFTR remains unknown, but it appears to help regulate chloride and sodium transport across epithelial membranes. CFTR resembles other transmembrane transport proteins, but in cystic fibrosis, it lacks the phenylalanine in the protein produced by normal genes. This regulator interferes with cyclic adenosine monophosphate-regulated chloride channels and transport of other ions by preventing adenosine triphosphate from binding to the protein or by interfering with activation by protein kinase. The mutation affects volume-absorbing epithelia (in the airways and intestines), salt-absorbing epithelia (in sweat ducts), and volume-excretory epithelia (in the pancreas). Lack of phenylalanine leads to dehydration, increasing the viscosity of mucous gland secretions and leading to obstruction of

CYSTIC FIBROSIS TRANSMISSION LINK

The chance that a relative of a person with cystic fibrosis or a person with no family history will carry the cystic fibrosis gene appears in the chart below.

Relative of affected person	Carrier chance
Brother or sister	2 in 3 (67%)
Niece or nephew	1 in 2 (50%)
Aunt or uncle	1 in 3 (33%)
First cousin	1 in 4 (25%)

No known family history	Carrier chance
Whites	1 in 25 (4%)
Blacks	1 in 65 (1.5%)
Asians	1 in 150 (0.67%)

glandular ducts. Cystic fibrosis has a varying effect on electrolyte and water transport. Causes of cystic fibrosis include abnormal coding found on as many as 350 CFTR alleles and autosomal recessive inheritance. The immediate causes of symptoms are increased viscosity of bronchial, pancreatic, and other mucous gland secretions and consequent destruction of glandular ducts. Cystic fibrosis accounts for almost all cases of pancreatic enzyme deficiency in children. (See *How cystic fibrosis affects the body*, pages 70–71.)

SIGNS AND SYMPTOMS

The clinical effects of cystic fibrosis may become apparent soon after birth or make take years to develop. They include major aberrations in sweat gland, respiratory, and GI functions.

- Hyponatremia and hypochloremia
- Wheezy respirations
- Dry, nonproductive, paroxysmal cough
- Dyspnea
- Tachypnea
- Barrel chest
- Cyanosis
- Clubbing of the fingers and toes
- Recurring bronchitis and pneumonia
- Nasal polyps and sinusitis
- Meconium ileus (abdominal distention, vomiting, constipation, dehydration, and electrolyte imbalance)
- Frequent, bulky, foul-smelling, and pale stool with a high fat content
- Poor weight gain
- Poor growth and development
- Ravenous appetite
- Distended abdomen
- Thin extremities
- Sallow skin with poor turgor
- Deficiency of fat-soluble vitamins (A, D, E, and K)

HOW CYSTIC FIBROSIS AFFECTS THE BODY

Because cystic fibrosis involves dysfunction of the exocrine glands, it affects multiple organ systems. The far-reaching effects prompt a multidisciplinary approach to the patient's care to allow for the best possible outcome.

Below is a summary of what cystic fibrosis does to the body, including collaborative management.

Effects on body systems
Respiratory system

- Thick secretions and dehydration occur as a result of ionic imbalance.
- Chronic airway infections by *Staphylococcus aureus, Pseudomonas aeruginosa,* and *Pseudomonas cepacia* may develop, possibly due to abnormal airway surface fluids and failure of lung defenses.
- Accumulation of thick secretions in the bronchioles and alveoli results in dyspnea.
- Stimulation of the secretion-removal reflex produces a paroxysmal cough.
- Barrel chest, cyanosis, and clubbing of fingers and toes result from chronic hypoxia.
- Obstructed glandular ducts occur leading to peribronchial thickening; this obstruction is due to increased viscosity of bronchial, pancreatic, and other mucous gland secretions.

Cardiovascular system

- Fatal shock and arrhythmias may result from hyponatremia and hypochloremia from sodium lost in sweat.
- Pulmonary hypertension can result in cardiac dysfunction in adult cystic fibrosis patients with severe lung disease.
- Pulmonary hypertension and cor pulmonale in cystic fibrosis are thought to be related to progressive destruction of the lung parenchyma and pulmonary vasculature and to pulmonary vasoconstriction secondary to hypoxemia.

Endocrine system

- Retention of bicarbonate and water due to the absence of cystic fibrosis transmembrane regulator chloride channel in the pancreatic ductile epithelia limits membrane function and leads to retention of pancreatic enzymes, chronic cholecystitis and cholelithiasis, and the ultimate destruction of the pancreas.
- Diabetes, pancreatitis, and hepatic failure can develop because of the disease's effects on the intestines, pancreas, and liver.

GI system

- Obstruction of the small and large intestines results from inhibited secretion of chloride and water and excessive absorption of liquid.

- Clotting problems
- Possible azoospermia and sterility in males
- Secondary amenorrhea in females
- In infants and children, rectal prolapse secondary to malnutrition and wasting of perirectal supporting tissues
- Signs of pancreatic insufficiency
- Cirrhosis
- Portal hypertension

■ Biliary cirrhosis occurs because of retention of biliary secretions.

■ Malnutrition and malabsorption of fat-soluble vitamins (A, D, E, and K) are caused by deficiencies of trypsin, amylase, and lipase from obstructed pancreatic ducts, preventing the conversion and absorption of fat and protein in the intestinal tract.

Genitourinary system

■ In males, a bilateral congenital absence of the vas deferens in accompanied by a lack of sperm in the semen.

■ In females, secondary amenorrhea and increased mucus in the reproductive tracts block the passage of ova.

Collaborative management

■ Pulmonary specialists and respiratory therapists assist with clearing airway secretions and maintaining a patent airway.

■ An endocrinologist may assist with managing diabetes as well as other pancreatic and reproductive disorders.

■ Nutritional specialists may be consulted to help with dietary measures (such as providing high-calorie meals that include the appropriate level of salt needed) and fluid therapy.

■ Physical and occupational therapists may be needed to help with activity management and energy conservation.

COMPLICATIONS

- Bronchiectasis
- Pneumonia
- Atelectasis
- Hemoptysis
- Dehydration
- Distal intestinal obstruction syndrome
- Malnutrition
- Nasal polyps
- Gastroesophageal reflux
- Rectal prolapse
- Cor pulmonale
- Diabetes
- Pancreatitis
- Cholecystitis

DIAGNOSIS

The Cystic Fibrosis Foundation has developed certain criteria for a definitive diagnosis: Two sweat tests using a pilocarpine solution (a sweat inducer) and either obstructive pulmonary disease, confirmed pancreatic insufficiency or failure to thrive, and a family history of cystic fibrosis.

The following test results may support the diagnosis:

- Chest X-rays indicate early signs of obstructive lung disease.

- Stool specimen analysis indicates the absence of trypsin, suggesting pancreatic insufficiency.

- Deoxyribonucleic acid testing can locate the presence of the delta F 508 deletion (found in about 70% of cystic fibrosis patients, although the disease can cause more than 100 other mutations). It allows prenatal diagnosis in families with a previously affected child.

- Pulmonary function tests reveal decreased vital capacity, elevated residual volume due to air entrapments, and decreased forced expiratory volume in 1 second. This test is used if pulmonary exacerbation already exists.

• Liver enzyme tests may reveal hepatic insufficiency.

• Sputum culture reveals organisms that cystic fibrosis patients typically and chronically colonize, such as *Staphylococcus* and *Pseudomonas*.

• Serum albumin measurement helps assess nutritional status.

• Electrolyte analysis assesses hydration status.

TREATMENT

The aim of treatment is to help the child lead as normal a life as possible. The type of treatment depends on the organ systems involved.

• To combat electrolyte losses in sweat, salt foods generously and, in hot weather, administer sodium supplements.

• Maintain a diet that's low in fat, but high in protein and calories, and provide supplements of water-miscible, fat-soluble vitamins (A, D, E, and K).

• Management of pulmonary dysfunction includes chest physiotherapy, postural drainage, and breathing exercises several times daily to aid removal of secretions from lungs.

• Antihistamines are contraindicated because they have a drying effect on mucous membranes, making expectoration of mucus difficult or impossible.

• Aerosol therapy includes intermittent nebulizer treatments before postural drainage to loosen secretions.

• Treatment of pulmonary infection requires broad-spectrum antimicrobials, oxygen therapy as needed, and loosening and removal of mucopurulent secretions.

• An intermittent nebulizer and postural drainage are used to relieve obstruction.

• Regular exercise increases physical fitness and upper body exercises, such as canoe paddling, may increase respiratory muscle endurance.

• Lung transplantation may be considered in some cases. Genetic research on curing cystic fibrosis by artificially inserting a "healthy" gene into a person through gene therapy is ongoing. The gene would be inserted by using an intranasal form. Research on correcting the disorder before birth is promising.

• Other areas of research include restoring salt transport in the cells and use of mucus-thinning drugs and nutritional supplementation.

Drugs

• Mucolytic agents, such as dornase alfa or DNase (Pulmozyme), which are a type of recombinant (genetically engineered) pulmonary enzymes given by aerosol nebulizer, to help thin airway mucus, thus improving lung function and reducing the risk of pulmonary infection

• Oral pancreatic enzymes, such as pancrelipase (Creon, Ultrase, and Viokase), which are given with meals and snacks to offset pancreatic enzyme deficiencies

• Bronchodilators, such as albuterol (Proventil, Ventolin), which are given to help open airways and improve air flow

• Antibiotics and other antimicrobials, which are used specific to the type of infection acquired by the patient

SPECIAL CONSIDERATIONS

• Throughout this illness, teach the patient and his family about the disease and its treatment. The Cystic Fibrosis Foundation can provide educational and support services.

• Although many males with cystic fibrosis are infertile, females may become pregnant (due to increased life expectancies). As a result, more cystic fibrosis patients are now facing difficult reproductive decisions.

Refer such patients (or the parents of an affected child) for genetic counseling so they can discuss family planning issues or prenatal diagnosis options if they're considering having more children.

• Be aware that some patients have recently undergone lung transplantation to reduce the effects of the disease. Also, aerosol gene therapy shows promise in reducing pulmonary symptoms.

• Research indicates that the genetic defect responsible for cystic fibrosis has also been identified in individuals experiencing some forms of unexplained pancreatitis.

Emphysema

Emphysema is one of several diseases usually labeled collectively as chronic obstructive pulmonary disease. It's the most common cause of death from respiratory disease in the United States. Emphysema appears to be more prevalent in men than in women; approximately 2 million Americans are affected with the disease. Postmortem findings reveal few adult lungs without some degree of emphysema.

CAUSES AND INCIDENCE

Emphysema may be caused by a genetic deficiency of alpha$_1$-antitrypsin (AAT) and by cigarette smoking. Genetically, 1 in 3,000 newborns are found with the disease, and 1% to 3% of all cases of emphysema are due to AAT deficiency. Cigarette smoking is thought to cause up to 20% of the cases. Other causative factors are unknown.

Primary emphysema has been linked to an inherited deficiency of the enzyme AAT, a major component of alpha$_1$-globulin. AAT inhibits the activation of several proteolytic enzymes; deficiency of this enzyme is an autosomal recessive trait that predisposes an individual to develop emphysema because proteolysis in lung tissues isn't inhibited.

Homozygous individuals have up to an 80% chance of developing lung disease; people who smoke have a greater chance of developing emphysema. Patients who develop emphysema before or during their early 40s and those who are nonsmokers are believed to have an AAT deficiency.

In emphysema, recurrent inflammation is associated with the release of proteolytic enzymes from lung cells. This causes irreversible enlargement of the air spaces distal to the terminal bronchioles. Enlargement of air spaces destroys the alveolar walls, which results in breakdown of elasticity and loss of fibrous and muscle tissue, thus making the lungs less compliant.

In normal breathing, the air moves into and out of the lungs to meet metabolic needs. A change in airway size compromises the lung's ability to circulate sufficient air. In patient's with emphysema, recurrent pulmonary inflammation damages and eventually destroys the alveolar walls, creating large air spaces. (See *Air trapping in emphysema*.)

The alveolar septa are initially destroyed, eliminating a portion of the capillary bed and increasing air volume in the acinus. This breakdown leaves the alveoli unable to recoil normally after expanding and

AIR TRAPPING IN EMPHYSEMA

After alveolar walls are damaged or destroyed, they can't support the airways and keep them open. The alveolar walls then lose their elastic recoil capability. Collapse then occurs on expiration.

Normal expiration
Normal expiration, as shown here, involves normal recoil and an open bronchiole.

Impaired expiration
Impaired expiration, as shown here, involves decreased elastic recoil and a narrowed bronchiole.

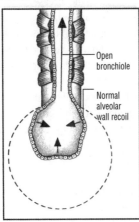

Open bronchiole

Normal alveolar wall recoil

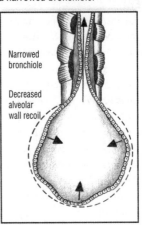

Narrowed bronchiole

Decreased alveolar wall recoil

results in bronchiolar collapse on expiration. The damaged or destroyed alveolar walls can't support the airways to keep them open.

The amount of air that can be expired passively diminishes, thus trapping air in the lungs and leading to overdistention. Hyperinflation of the alveoli produces bullae (air spaces) adjacent to pleura (blebs). Septal destruction also decreases airway calibration. Part of each inspiration is trapped because of increased residual volume and decreased calibration. Septal destruction may affect only the respiratory bronchioles and alveolar ducts, leaving alveolar sacs intact, or it can involve the entire acinus with more random damage and involve the lower lobes of the lungs.

SIGNS AND SYMPTOMS
- By history, long-time smoker
- Shortness of breath
- Chronic cough
- Anorexia with resultant weight loss and a general feeling of malaise
- Barrel chest
- Pursed-lip breathing

- Peripheral cyanosis, clubbed fingers and toes, and tachypnea
- Decreased tactile fremitus and decreased chest expansion
- Decreased breath sounds, crackles, and wheezing during inspiration
- Prolonged expiratory phase with grunting respirations
- Distant heart sounds

⚠ **ALERT**

Age-related changes in the respiratory system can worsen the symptoms of emphysema. Decreased peak airflow, gas exchange, and vital capacity can increase shortness of breath experienced by the patient as he ages. These changes can be complicated by smoking, which actually speeds up the process of aging in the lungs and further worsens symptoms. What's more, defense mechanisms in the lungs and immune system decrease, increasing the aging person's risk of pneumonia after bacterial or viral infection.

COMPLICATIONS

- Recurrent respiratory tract infections
- Cor pulmonale
- Respiratory failure
- Spontaneous pneumothorax
- Pneumomediastinum

DIAGNOSIS

- Chest X-rays in advanced disease may show a flattened diaphragm, reduced vascular markings at the lung periphery, overaeration of the lungs, a vertical heart, enlarged anteroposterior chest diameter, and large retrosternal air space.

- Pulmonary function tests typically indicate increased residual volume and total lung capacity, reduced diffusing capacity, and increased inspiratory flow.
- Arterial blood gas analysis usually shows reduced partial pressure of arterial oxygen and normal partial pressure of arterial carbon dioxide until late in the disease.
- Electrocardiography may reveal tall, symmetrical P waves in leads II, III, and aV_F; vertical QRS axis; and signs of right ventricular hypertrophy late in the disease.
- Red blood cell count usually demonstrates an increased hemoglobin level late in the disease when the patient has persistent severe hypoxia.

TREATMENT

Emphysema management usually includes bronchodilators such as aminophylline to promote mucociliary clearance; antibiotics to treat respiratory tract infection; and immunizations to prevent influenza and pneumococcal pneumonia.

Other treatment measures include adequate hydration and (in selected patients) and chest physiotherapy to mobilize secretions.

Some patients may require oxygen therapy (at low settings) to correct hypoxia. They may also require transtracheal catheterization to receive oxygen at home. Counseling about avoiding smoking and air pollutants is necessary.

Drugs

- Bronchodilators to prevent and control bronchospasm
- Corticosteroids to reduce bronchial inflammation
- Antibiotics to treat infections

SPECIAL CONSIDERATIONS

- Provide supportive care and help the patient adjust to lifestyle changes necessitated by a chronic illness.
- Answer the patient's questions about his illness as honestly as possible. Encourage him to express his fears and concerns about his illness. Remain with him during periods of extreme stress and anxiety.
- Include the patient and family members in care-related decisions. Refer the patient to appropriate support services, as needed.
- If ordered, perform chest physiotherapy, including postural drainage and chest percussion and vibration, several times daily.
- Provide the patient with a high-calorie, protein-rich diet to promote health and healing. Give small, frequent meals to conserve energy and prevent fatigue.
- Schedule respiratory treatments at least 1 hour before or after meals. Provide mouth care after bronchodilator therapy.
- Make sure the patient receives adequate fluids (at least 3 L [3.2 qt] a day) to loosen secretions.
- Encourage daily activity and provide diversionary activities, as appropriate. To conserve energy and prevent fatigue, assist the patient to alternate periods of rest and activity.
- Administer medications as ordered. Record the patient's response to these medications.
- Watch for complications, such as respiratory tract infections, cor pulmonale, spontaneous pneumothorax, respiratory failure, and peptic ulcer disease.

Epiglottiditis

Acute epiglottiditis, also known as *epiglottitis,* is an acute inflammation of the epiglottis that tends to cause airway obstruction. A critical emergency, epiglottiditis can be fatal unless it's recognized and treated promptly.

CAUSES AND INCIDENCE

Epiglottiditis usually results from infection with *Haemophilus influenzae* type B (Hib) and, occasionally, pneumococci and group A streptococci. It typically strikes children between ages 2 and 6 years. (However, immunosuppression can predispose adults to epiglottiditis.) Since the advent of the Hib vaccine, epiglottiditis is becoming more rare.

SIGNS AND SYMPTOMS

Sometimes preceded by an upper respiratory infection, epiglottiditis may rapidly progress to complete upper airway obstruction within 2 to 5 hours. Laryngeal obstruction results from inflammation and edema of the epiglottis. Accompanying symptoms include high temperature, stridor, sore throat, dysphagia, irritability, restlessness, and drooling. To relieve severe respiratory distress, the child with epiglottiditis may hyperextend his neck, sit up, and lean forward with his mouth open, tongue protruding, and nostrils flaring as he tries to breathe. He may develop inspiratory retractions and rhonchi.

DIAGNOSIS

• Lateral neck X-ray shows an enlarged ("thumbprint") epiglottis and distended hypopharynx.

• Direct laryngoscopy reveals the hallmark of acute epiglottiditis; a swollen, beefy-red epiglottis. The throat examination should follow X-rays and, in most cases, shouldn't be performed if significant obstruction is suspected or if immediate intubation isn't possible.

• Additional X-rays of the chest and cervical trachea help confirm the diagnosis.

• Blood or throat culture may show *H. influenzae* or other bacteria.

TREATMENT

A child with acute epiglottiditis and airway obstruction requires emergency hospitalization; he may need emergency endotracheal intubation or a tracheotomy with subsequent monitoring in an intensive care unit. Respiratory distress that interferes with swallowing necessitates parenteral fluid administration to prevent dehydration.

Drugs

• Parenteral antibiotics, usually a second- or third-generation cephalosporin, such as ceftriaxone sodium (Rocephin); if the child is allergic to penicillin, a quinolone or sulfa drug may be substituted

• Corticosteroids, such as dexamethasone (Decadron), to decrease inflammation of the throat

SPECIAL CONSIDERATIONS

• Keep equipment available in case of sudden complete airway obstruction to secure an airway. Be prepared to assist with intubation or tracheotomy, as necessary.

⚠ ALERT

• *Watch for increasing restlessness, rising cardiac rate, fever, dyspnea, and retractions, which may indicate the need for an emergency tracheotomy.*

• *Monitor blood gases for hypoxemia and hypercapnia.*

• After a tracheotomy, anticipate the patient's needs because he won't be able to cry or call out; provide emotional support. Reassure the patient and his family that the tracheotomy is a short-term intervention (usually from 4 to 7 days). Monitor the patient for rising temperature and pulse rate and for hypotension—signs of secondary infection.

• The bacterial infection causing epiglottiditis is contagious, and airborne or droplet precautions should be followed. Family members should be screened.

⊠ PREVENTION

• *Wash hands frequently to prevent infections.*

• *Administer the vaccine to children.*

F

Fat embolism syndrome

Fat embolism syndrome is a rare but potentially fatal problem. The syndrome involves pulmonary, cerebral, and cutaneous manifestations and occurs 24 to 48 hours after injury.

CAUSES AND INCIDENCE

Ninety percent of all cases of fat embolism syndrome occur after blunt trauma. Other causes include acute pancreatitis, diabetes mellitus, burns, joint reconstruction, liposuction, cardiopulmonary bypass, decompression sickness, sickle cell crisis, and pathologic fractures.

⚠ ALERT

Young men with fractures are at an increased risk for developing fat embolism syndrome.

The bone marrow from a fractured bone or other injured adipose tissue releases fatty globules that enter the systemic circulation through torn veins at the injury site. These fatty globules travel to the lungs, where they form an embolus that blocks pulmonary circulation. Lipase breaks down the trapped fat emboli into free fatty acids.

This process causes a local toxic effect that damages the epithelium, increases capillary permeability, and inactivates lung surfactant. The increased capillary permeability allows protein-rich fluid to leak into the interstitial space and alveoli, increasing workload of the right side of the heart and causing pulmonary edema. The decreased surfactant causes alveolar collapse, a decrease in functional reserve capacity, and ventilation-perfusion mismatch, leading to hypoxemia. Platelet aggregation on fat, normal injury-related platelet consumption, and platelet dilution through I.V. crystalloid administration all contribute to thrombocytopenia, petechiae and, possibly, disseminated intravascular coagulation. (See *How fat embolism threatens pulmonary circulation*, page 80.)

SIGNS AND SYMPTOMS

- Petechiae
- Increased respiratory rate
- Dyspnea
- Accessory muscle use
- Mental status changes
- Jaundice
- Fever
- Tachycardia

DIAGNOSIS

- Arterial blood gas analysis reveals partial pressure of arterial oxygen (PaO_2) less than 60 mm Hg; partial pressure of arterial carbon dioxide initially decreases and later increases.

HOW FAT EMBOLISM THREATENS PULMONARY CIRCULATION

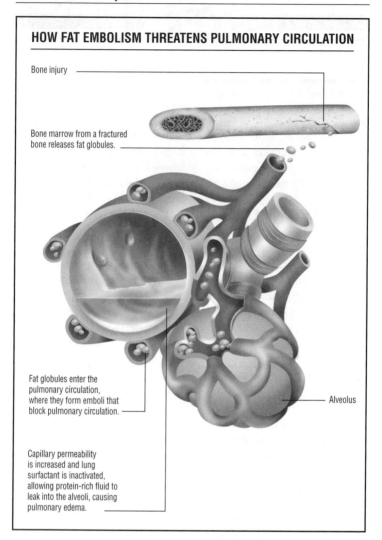

Bone injury

Bone marrow from a fractured bone releases fat globules.

Fat globules enter the pulmonary circulation, where they form emboli that block pulmonary circulation.

Capillary permeability is increased and lung surfactant is inactivated, allowing protein-rich fluid to leak into the alveoli, causing pulmonary edema.

Alveolus

• Chest X-ray is normal but later shows patchy areas of consolidation to complete "whiteout," if the condition progresses.

• Complete blood count shows decreased platelets and decreased hemoglobin.

• Ventilation-perfusion scans may be normal or may show subsegmental perfusion defects.

TREATMENT

• Supplemental oxygen and endotracheal intubation and mechanical ventilation may be necessary.

- I.V. fluids such as crystalloids (avoid colloids) may be used.

Drugs

- Corticosteroids to reduce inflammation and to prevent development of fat embolism syndrome

SPECIAL CONSIDERATIONS

- If mechanical ventilation is used, tidal volume should be maintained at appropriate levels to ensure adequate expansion of the lungs.
- Use an incentive spirometer to encourage deep inspiration through positive reinforcement. Teach the patient how to use the spirometer and encourage him to use it every 1 to 2 hours.
- Humidify inspired air and encourage adequate fluid intake to mobilize secretions. To promote loosening and clearance of secretions, encourage deep-breathing and coughing exercises, and use postural drainage and chest percussion.
- If the patient is intubated or unco-operative, provide suctioning, as needed. Use sedatives with discretion because they depress respirations and the cough reflex as well as suppress sighing. However, the patient won't cooperate with treatment if he's in pain.
- Assess breath sounds and ventilatory status frequently; report changes at once.
- Teach the patient about respiratory care, including postural drainage, coughing, and deep breathing.
- Provide reassurance and emotional support; the patient may be anxious due to hypoxia or respiratory distress.

Hantavirus pulmonary syndrome

Mainly occurring in the southwestern United States but not confined to that area, hantavirus pulmonary syndrome (HPS) is a viral disease first reported in May 1993. The syndrome, which rapidly progresses from flulike symptoms to respiratory failure and, possibly, death, is known for its high mortality. The hantavirus strain that causes disease in Asia and Europe—mainly hemorrhagic fever and renal disease—is distinctly different from the one currently described in North America.

CAUSES AND INCIDENCE

A member of the Bunyaviridae family, the genus *Hantavirus* (first isolated in 1977) is responsible for HPS. The Sin Nombre virus is the hantavirus primarily responsible for HPS. However, closely related strains (Bayou and Black Creek Canal viruses), found in the southeastern United States, produce a variant characterized by a greater degree of renal failure. The New York virus is the cause of cases in New York and Rhode Island.

Disease transmission is associated with exposure to aerosols (such as dust) contaminated by urine or feces from infected rodents, the primary reservoir for this virus. Data suggest that the deer mouse is the main source, but pinon mice, brush mice, and western chipmunks in close proximity to humans in rural areas are also sources. Hantavirus infections have been documented in people whose activities are associated with rodent contact, such as farming, hiking or camping in rodent-infested areas, and occupying rodent-infested dwellings.

Infected rodents manifest no apparent illness but shed the virus in feces, urine, and saliva. Human infection may occur from inhalation, ingestion (of contaminated food or water, for example), contact with rodent excrement, or rodent bites. Transmission from person to person or by mosquitoes, fleas, or other arthropods hasn't been reported.

The basic lesion of HPS infections is a generalized increase in capillary permeability resulting from endothelial damage. This stems from the immunologic response to viral antigens that penetrate the endothelium. This increased capillary permeability gives rise to widespread edema. The particular organs affected depend on the specific species of hantavirus; patients with HPS have edema concentrated in the pleura and lungs.

The endothelial cells appear swollen. An interstitial pneumonitis occurs, made up of edema fluid, mononuclear cells, and lymphocytes with polymorphonuclear leukocytes. Hyaline membranes appear, and as the disease progresses, the alveolar septa become increasingly fibrotic. The spleen also shows infiltration of immunocompetent cells. Severe cases present with noncardiogenic pulmonary edema accompanied by pulmonary capillary leak syndrome (the heart isn't directly affected). This pulmonary capillary leak syndrome is the primary defect responsible for both cardiopulmonary and renal dysfunction. Hypoxia also contributes to the state of shock.

SIGNS AND SYMPTOMS

Noncardiogenic pulmonary edema distinguishes the syndrome. Other signs and symptoms include:

- myalgia
- fever
- headache
- nausea
- vomiting
- cough
- respiratory distress that typically follows the onset of a cough
- a course typified by fever, hypoxia and, in some patients, serious hypotension
- rising respiratory rate (28 breaths/minute or more)
- increased heart rate (120 beats/minute or more).

COMPLICATIONS

- Respiratory failure
- Death

DIAGNOSIS

Despite ongoing efforts to identify clinical and laboratory features that distinguish HPS from other infections with similar features, diagnosis currently is based on clinical suspicion along with a process of elimination developed by the Centers for Disease Control and Prevention and the Council of State and Territorial Epidemiologists. Serologic testing for hantavirus can also be performed. (See *Screening for hantavirus pulmonary syndrome,* page 84.)

Laboratory tests usually reveal an elevated white blood cell count with a predominance of neutrophils, myeloid precursors, and atypical lymphocytes; an elevated hematocrit; a decreased platelet count; an elevated partial thromboplastin time; and a normal fibrinogen level. Usually, laboratory findings demonstrate only minimal abnormalities in renal function, with serum creatinine levels no higher than 2.5 mg/dl. Chest X-rays eventually show bilateral diffuse infiltrates in almost all patients (findings consistent with acute respiratory distress syndrome).

TREATMENT

Primarily supportive, treatment consists of maintaining adequate oxygenation, monitoring vital signs, and intervening to stabilize the patient's heart rate and blood pressure.

SCREENING FOR HANTAVIRUS PULMONARY SYNDROME

The Centers for Disease Control and Prevention (CDC) has developed a screening procedure to track cases of *Hantavirus* pulmonary syndrome. The screening criteria identify potential and actual cases.

Potential cases
For a diagnosis of possible *Hantavirus* pulmonary syndrome, a patient must have one of the following:
■ febrile illness (temperature equal to or above 101° F (38.3° C) occurring in a previously health person and characterized by unexplained acute respiratory distress syndrome
■ bilateral interstitial pulmonary infiltrates that develop within 1 week of hospitalization with respiratory compromise that requires supplemental oxygen
■ an unexplained respiratory illness resulting in a death and autopsy findings demonstrating noncardiogenic pulmonary edema without an identifiable specific cause of death.

Exclusions
Of the patients who meet the criteria for having potential *Hantavirus* pulmonary syndrome, the CDC excludes those who have any of the following:
■ a predisposing underlying medical condition (for example, severe underlying pulmonary disease), solid tumors or hematologic cancers, congenital or acquired immunodeficiency disorders, or medical conditions or treatment—such as rheumatoid arthritis or organ transplantation—requiring immunosuppressive drug therapy (for example, steroids or cytotoxic chemotherapy)
■ an acute illness that provides a likely explanation for the respiratory illness (for example, a recent major trauma, burn, or surgery; recent seizures or his history of aspiration; bacterial sepsis; another respiratory disorder such as a respiratory syncytial virus in young children; influenza; or legionella pneumonia).

Confirmed cases
Cases of confirmed *Hantavirus* pulmonary syndrome must include the following:
■ at least one serum or tissue specimen available for laboratory testing for evidence of hantavirus infection
■ in a patient with compatible clinical illness, serologic evidence (presence of hantavirus-specific immunoglobulin [Ig] M or rising titers of IgG), polymerase chain reaction for hantavirus ribonucleic acid, or positive immunohistochemistry for hantavirus antigen.

Drugs
• Vasopressors, such as dopamine or epinephrine, to treat hypotension
• Fluid volume replacement to combat fluid loss (with precautions not to overhydrate the patient)
• Ribavirin (an antiviral drug) in aerosol form for children (efficacy in adults has not been proven) to combat the virus

SPECIAL CONSIDERATIONS
• Frequently assess the patient's respiratory status and arterial blood gas values.
• Monitor the patient's serum electrolyte levels, and correct imbalances as appropriate.
• Maintain a patent airway by suctioning; ensure adequate humidification, and check ventilator settings frequently.

- If the patient has hypoxemia, assess his neurologic status, heart rate, and blood pressure frequently.
- Administer drug therapy and monitor the patient's response.
- Provide I.V. fluid therapy based on results of hemodynamic monitoring.
- Provide emotional support for the patient and his family.
- Report cases of HPS to the appropriate state health department.

⧉ PREVENTION

- *Caution patients against having contact with rodents or aerosolized rodent urine or excreta. Explain that dead rodents shouldn't be handled without wearing protection and taking proper precautions.*
- *Provide patients with prevention guidelines, such as making dwellings as rodent-proof as possible and following cleanliness and maintenance procedures to help prevent dwellings from attracting small rodents.*

Hemothorax

In hemothorax, blood from damaged intercostal, pleural, mediastinal, and (infrequently) lung parenchymal vessels enters the pleural cavity. Depending on the amount of bleeding and the underlying cause, hemothorax may be associated with varying degrees of lung collapse and mediastinal shift. Pneumothorax—air in the pleural cavity—commonly accompanies hemothorax.

CAUSES AND INCIDENCE

Hemothorax usually results from blunt or penetrating chest trauma; in fact, about 25% of patients with such trauma have hemothorax. In some cases, it results from thoracic surgery, pulmonary infarction, neoplasm, dissecting thoracic aneurysm, or a complication of tuberculosis or anticoagulant therapy. (See *Looking at a hemothorax,* page 86.)

SIGNS AND SYMPTOMS

Signs and symptoms include:
- chest pain
- tachypnea
- asymmetrical chest movements
- flat jugular veins
- bloody sputum (in massive hemothorax)
- unilateral decreased fremitus
- decreased chest expansion on inspiration
- unilateral diminished or absent breath sounds
- mild to severe dyspnea, depending on the amount of blood in the pleural cavity and associated pathologic conditions
- anxiety, restlessness, cyanosis, and possibly stupor (if respiratory failure occurs)
- marked blood loss produces hypotension and shock
- expansion and stiffening of the affected side of the chest, contrasted with normal rising and falling of the unaffected side.

LOOKING AT A HEMOTHORAX

The illustration below shows a hemothorax with blood in the right pleural cavity.

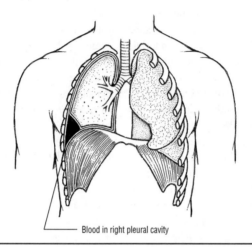

Blood in right pleural cavity

COMPLICATIONS

- Mediastinal shift
- Ventilatory compromise
- Lung collapse
- Cardiopulmonary arrest

DIAGNOSIS

- Characteristic clinical signs and a history of trauma strongly suggest hemothorax.
- Percussion and auscultation reveal dullness and decreased to absent breath sounds over the affected side.
- Thoracentesis yields blood or serosanguineous fluid; chest X-rays show pleural fluid with or without mediastinal shift.
- Arterial blood gas (ABG) analysis may reveal respiratory failure.
- Hemoglobin levels may be decreased, depending on the amount of blood lost.

TREATMENT

Treatment is designed to stabilize the patient's condition, stop the bleeding, evacuate blood from the pleural space, and reexpand the lung. Mild hemothorax usually clears in 10 to 14 days, requiring only observation for further bleeding. In severe hemothorax, thoracentesis not only serves as a diagnostic tool but also removes fluid from the pleural cavity.

After confirmation of the diagnosis, a chest tube is inserted into the sixth intercostal space at the posterior axillary line. Suction may be used; a large-bore chest tube is used to prevent clot blockage. If the chest tube doesn't improve the patient's condition, he may need a thoracotomy to evacuate blood and clots and to control bleeding.

Drugs

• Analgesics to control pain
• If necessary, intracostal nerve block to control pain, depending on the severity of the pain

SPECIAL CONSIDERATIONS

• Give oxygen by face mask or nasal cannula.
• Give I.V. fluids and blood transfusions as ordered to treat shock; monitor pulse oximetry and ABG levels often.
• Explain all procedures to the patient to help allay his fears.
• Assist with thoracentesis; warn the patient not to cough during this procedure.

• Carefully observe chest tube drainage, and record the volume drained at least every hour.
• Milk the chest tube (only if necessary and according to facility and physician protocols) to keep it open and free from clots. If the tube is warm and full of blood and the bloody fluid level in the water-seal bottle is rising rapidly, report this at once; the patient may need immediate surgery.
• Watch the patient closely for pallor and gasping respirations, and monitor his vital signs diligently. Falling blood pressure and rising pulse and rising respiratory rates may indicate shock or massive bleeding.

Idiopathic pulmonary fibrosis

Idiopathic pulmonary fibrosis (IPF) is a chronic and usually fatal interstitial pulmonary disease. About 50% of patients with IPF die within 5 years of diagnosis. Once thought to be a rare condition, it's now diagnosed with much greater frequency. IPF has been known by several other names over the years, including cryptogenic fibrosing alveolitis, diffuse interstitial fibrosis, idiopathic interstitial pneumonitis, and Hamman-Rich syndrome.

CAUSES AND INCIDENCE

IPF results from a cascade of events that involve inflammatory, immune, and fibrotic processes in the lung. However, despite many studies and hypotheses, the stimulus that begins the progression remains unknown. Speculation has revolved around viral and genetic causes, but no strong evidence has been found to support either theory. However, it's clear that chronic inflammation plays an important role.

Inflammation develops the injury, and fibrosis ultimately distorts and impairs the structure and function of the alveolocapillary gas exchange surface. Interstitial inflammation consists of an alveolar septal infiltrate of lymphocytes, plasma cells, and histiocytes. Fibrotic areas are composed of dense acellular collagen. Areas of honeycombing form, made up of cystic fibrotic air spaces, frequently lined with bronchiolar epithelium and filled with mucus. Smooth-muscle hyperplasia may occur in areas of fibrosis and honeycombing. (See *End-stage idiopathic pulmonary fibrosis*.)

IPF occurs in men slightly more often than in women and in smokers more often than in nonsmokers.

⚠ ALERT

IPF occurs most commonly in people between the ages of 50 to 70.

SIGNS AND SYMPTOMS

The usual presenting signs and symptoms of IPF are dyspnea and a dry, hacking, often paroxysmal cough. Most patients have had these for anywhere from several months to 2 years before seeking medical help. Other signs and symptoms include:

• cyanosis
• end-expiratory crackles, especially in the bases of the lungs (usually heard early in the disease)
• bronchial breath sounds (typically appear later in the disease, when airway consolidation develops)
• rapid, shallow breathing, especially with exertion
• clubbing of fingers and toes

END-STAGE IDIOPATHIC PULMONARY FIBROSIS

The illustrations below show the condition of the lungs in a patient with end-stage idiopathic pulmonary fibrosis. Note the honeycombed pattern formed by cystic fibrotic air space in the close-up inset.

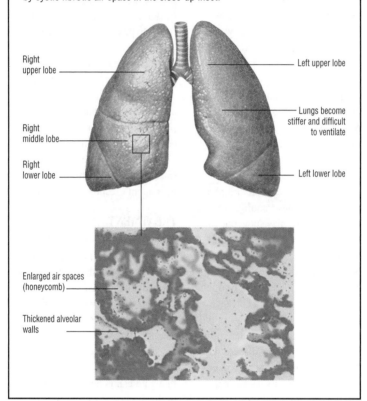

Right upper lobe

Left upper lobe

Lungs become stiffer and difficult to ventilate

Right middle lobe

Right lower lobe

Left lower lobe

Enlarged air spaces (honeycomb)

Thickened alveolar walls

- pulmonary hypertension (augmented S_2 and S_3 gallop)
- profound hypoxemia and severe, debilitating dyspnea (in advanced disease).

COMPLICATIONS

- Respiratory failure
- Chronic hypoxemia
- Pulmonary hypertension
- Cor pulmonale
- Polycythemia

DIAGNOSIS

Diagnosis begins with a thorough patient history to exclude more common causes of interstitial lung disease. A lung biopsy using a thoracoscope or bronchoscope—an improvement over the open lung biopsies that were previously performed to diagnose IPF—helps in the diagnosis. Histologic features of the biopsy tissue depend on the stage of the disease as well as on other factors that aren't yet completely understood. Typically, the alveolar walls appear swollen with chronic inflammatory cellular infiltrate composed of mononuclear cells and polymorphonuclear leukocytes. In the early stages, intra-alveolar inflammatory cells may be found. As the disease progresses, excessive collagen and fibroblasts fill the interstitium. In advanced stages, alveolar walls are destroyed, replaced by honeycombing cysts.

Chest X-rays may show one of four distinct patterns: interstitial, reticulonodular, ground glass, or honeycomb. Although chest X-rays help identifying the presence of an abnormality, they don't correlate well with histologic findings or pulmonary function tests in determining the severity of the disease. They also don't help distinguish inflammation from fibrosis. However, serial X-rays may help track the progression of the disease.

High-resolution computed tomography scans provide superior views of the four patterns seen on X-ray film and are used routinely to help establish the diagnosis of IPF. Research is currently underway to determine whether the four patterns of abnormality seen on these scans correlate with responsiveness to treatment.

Pulmonary function tests show reductions in vital capacity and total lung capacity as well as impaired diffusing capacity for carbon monoxide. Arterial blood gas (ABG) analysis and pulse oximetry reveal hypoxemia, which may be mild when the patient is at rest early in the disease but may become severe later in the disease. Oxygenation always deteriorates—usually to a severe level—with exertion. Serial pulmonary function tests (especially carbon monoxide diffusing capacity) and ABG values may help track the course of the disease and the patient's response to treatment.

TREATMENT

No known cure exists for IPF, although interferon-gamma-1B has shown some promise in treating the disease. Lung transplantation may be successful for younger, otherwise healthy individuals. In the early stages of the disease, oxygen therapy can prevent the problems related to dyspnea and tissue hypoxia, although it can't change the pathology of the disease process. The patient may require little or no supplemental oxygen while at rest initially, but he'll need more as the disease progresses and during exertion.

Drugs

• Glucocorticoids such as prednisone (Deltasone, Orasone, Sterapred) to reverse increased capillary permeability and suppress polymorphonuclear activity, decreasing inflammation

- Immunosuppressants, such as azathioprine (Imuran) and cyclophosphamide (Cytoxan), to lower autoimmune activity and reduce inflammation when corticosteroids aren't effective
- Antiviral cytokines such as interferon gamma-1b (Actimmune) to stimulate the immune system and inhibit proliferation of fibroblasts and to suppress production of the connective-tissue matrix protein
- Antioxidants such as N-acetylcysteine (Acetadote) to restore glutathione levels in lung tissue and bronchoalveolar lavage fluid

SPECIAL CONSIDERATIONS

- Explain all diagnostic tests to the patient, who may feel anxious and frustrated over the many tests required to establish the diagnosis.
- Monitor the patient's oxygenation level, both at rest and with exertion. The physician may prescribe one oxygen flow rate for use when the patient is at rest and a higher one for use during exertion to maintain adequate oxygenation. Tell the patient to increase his oxygen flow rate to the appropriate level for exercise.
- As IPF progresses, keep in mind that the patient will require more oxygen. He may need a nonrebreathing mask to supply high oxygen percentages. Eventually, maintaining adequate oxygenation may become impossible, despite maximum oxygen flow.
- Because most patients will need oxygen at home, make appropriate referrals to discharge planners, respiratory care practitioners, and home equipment vendors to ensure continuity of care.
- Teach breathing, relaxation, and energy conservation techniques to help the patient manage severe dyspnea.
- Encourage the patient to be as active as possible, and refer him to a pulmonary rehabilitation program.
- Monitor the patient for adverse reactions to drug therapy.
- Teach the patient about prescribed medications, especially adverse effects. Teach the patient and family members infection prevention techniques.
- Encourage good nutritional habits. The patient may require small, frequent meals with high nutritional value if dyspnea interferes with eating.
- Provide emotional support for the patient and family members as they deal with the patient's increasing disability, dyspnea, and probable death.

Influenza

Influenza—also called the grippe or the flu—is an acute, highly contagious infection of the respiratory tract that results from three different types of myxovirus influenzae. It occurs sporadically or in epidemics (usually during the colder months). Epidemics tend to peak within 3 weeks of initial cases and subside within a month.

Although influenza affects all age groups, its incidence is highest in schoolchildren. However, its effects are most severe in the very young, the elderly, and those suffering from chronic disease. In these groups, influenza may even lead to death. The catastrophic pandemic of 1918 was responsible for an estimated 20 million deaths. The most recent pandemics (in 1957, 1968, and 1977) began in mainland China.

CAUSES AND INCIDENCE

Transmission of influenza occurs through inhalation of respiratory droplets from an infected person or by indirect contact with a contaminated object, such as a drinking glass or other item contaminated with respiratory secretions. The influenza virus then invades the epithelium of the respiratory tract, causing inflammation and desquamation. (See *How influenza viruses multiply*.)

One of the remarkable features of the influenza virus is its capacity to undergo antigenic variation into several distinct strains, allowing it to infect new populations that have little or no immunologic resistance. Antigenic variation occurs as antigenic drift (minor changes that happen yearly or every few years) or antigenic shift (major changes that lead to pandemics). Influenza viruses are classified into three groups. Type A, the most prevalent, strikes every year, with new serotypes causing epidemics every 3 years. Type B also strikes annually but causes epidemics only every 4 to 6 years. Type C is endemic and causes only sporadic cases. Each year, tens of millions of people in the United States get the flu; about 114,000 people require hospitalization, and about 36,000 people die from the disease.

SIGNS AND SYMPTOMS

After an incubation period of 24 to 48 hours, flu symptoms begin to appear, including:
- sudden onset of chills
- fever ranging from 101° to 104° F (38° to 40° C)
- headache
- malaise
- myalgia (particularly in the back and limbs)
- nonproductive cough.

Occasionally, a patient may develop laryngitis, hoarseness, conjunctivitis, rhinitis, or rhinorrhea. Signs and symptoms usually subside in 3 to 5 days, although coughing and weakness may persist longer. Children typically run higher fevers than adults and are also more likely to experience cervical adenopathy and croup. In some patients—especially elderly patients—lack of energy and easy fatigability may persist for several weeks. Fever that lasts longer than 5 days signals the onset of complications. The most common complication is pneumonia, which occurs as primary influenza virus pneumonia or secondary to bacterial infection.

COMPLICATIONS
- Pneumonia
- Myositis

HOW INFLUENZA VIRUSES MULTIPLY

An influenza virus, classified as type A, B, or C, contains the genetic material ribonucleic acid (RNA), which is covered and protected by protein. RNA is arranged in genes that carry the instruction for viral replication. This genetic material has an extraordinary ability to mutate, causing the generation of new serologically distinct strains of influenza virus. Being a virus, the pathogen can't reproduce or carry out chemical reactions on its own. It needs a host cell.

After attaching to the host cell, the viral RNA enters the host cell and uses host components to replicate its genetic material and protein, which are then assembled into the new virus particles. These newly produced viruses can burst forth to invade other healthy cells.

The viral invasion destroys the host cells, impairing respiratory defenses, especially the mucociliary transport system, and predisposing the patient to secondary bacterial infection.

1. VIRUS ATTACHES TO HOST

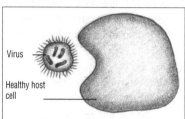

Virus

Healthy host cell

2. VIRAL RNA ENTERS HOST CELL

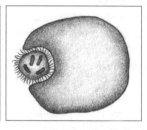

3. VIRAL RNA REPLICATES WITHIN HOST CELL

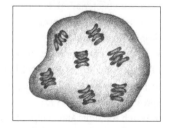

4. NEW VIRUS PARTICLES ARE ASSEMBLED AND RELEASED

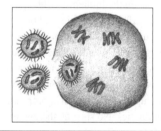

- Exacerbation of chronic obstructive pulmonary disease
- Reye's syndrome
- Myocarditis (rare)
- Pericarditis (rare)
- Transverse myelitis (rare)
- Encephalitis (rare)

DIAGNOSIS

At the beginning of an influenza epidemic, early cases are usually mistaken for other respiratory disorders. Because signs and symptoms of influenza aren't pathognomonic, isolation of the influenza virus through nose and throat cultures and increased serum antibody titers help confirm the diagnosis. Rapid diagnostic methods for detecting influenza are now available and help confirm this diagnosis.

After these measures confirm an influenza epidemic, diagnosis requires only observation of clinical signs and symptoms. Uncomplicated cases show a decreased white blood cell count with an increase in lymphocytes.

TREATMENT

Treatment of uncomplicated influenza includes bed rest, adequate fluid intake, aspirin or acetaminophen (in children) to relieve fever and muscle pain, and dextromethorphan or another antitussive to relieve nonproductive coughing. Prophylactic antibiotics aren't recommended because they have no effect on the influenza virus.

In influenza complicated by pneumonia, patients require supportive care (fluid and electrolyte supplements, oxygen, and assisted ventilation) and treatment of bacterial superinfection with appropriate antibiotics. No specific therapy exists for cardiac, central nervous system, or other complications.

Drugs

• Antiviral drugs, such as oseltamivir (Tamiflu), zanamivir (Relenza), amantadine (Symmetrel), and rimantadine (Flumadine), to inhibit neuraminidase, decreasing the release of viruses from infected cells and viral spread; these drugs must administered within 48 hours of the onset of signs and symptoms and reduce the severity of symptoms and the length of illness by an average of 1.5 days

• Influenza virus vaccine (Fluarix, Fluvirin, Fluzone), intranasal vaccine (FluMist), or influenza virus vaccine H5N1 to provide immunization and prevent the spread of influenza A and B viruses

SPECIAL CONSIDERATIONS

• Provide care to relieve signs and symptoms; the patient may require hospitaliztion if complications occur.

• Advise the patient to increase his fluid intake. Warm baths or heating pads may relieve myalgia. Give him nonopioid analgesics-antipyretics as ordered.

• Screen visitors to protect the patient from bacterial infection and the visitors from influenza. Use droplet precautions.

• Teach the patient proper disposal of tissues and proper hand-washing technique to prevent the virus from spreading.

• Watch for signs and symptoms of developing pneumonia, such as crackles, another temperature rise, or coughing accompanied by purulent or bloody sputum.

• Help the patient to gradually resume his normal activities.

• Inform people receiving the vaccine of possible adverse effects (discomfort at the vaccination site, fever, malaise and, rarely,

Guillain-Barré syndrome). Influenza vaccine (inactivated) is recommended for women who are pregnant and who will be in the second or third trimester during influenza season.

• Live attenuated influenza vaccine, available as a nasal spray, has different criteria and contraindications for use vary than the inactivated, injectable vaccine. Recipients of live attenuated influenza vaccine may shed influenza virus for up to 21 days post-immunization.

▷ PREVENTION

• *Educate patients about influenza immunizations. For high-risk patients and health care personnel, suggest annual inoculations at the start of the flu season (late autumn). The vaccine administered each year is based on the previous year's virus and is usually about 75% effective.*

• *Keep in mind that the vaccines are made from chicken embryos; because of this, they must not be given to people who are hypersensitive to eggs. For these people, amantadine is an effective alternative, but it must be started before the flu season begins and continue throughout the season.*

Inhalation injury

Inhalation injuries result from trauma to the pulmonary system after inhalation of either toxic substances or nontoxic gases that interfere with cellular respiration. Substances that may cause such injuries include fog, mist, fumes, dust, gas, vapor, and smoke. Inhalation injuries commonly accompany burns.

CAUSES AND INCIDENCE

Inhalation injuries can result from several causes, including thermal inhalation, chemical inhalation, and carbon monoxide poisoning. In children, about 50% of all burn deaths are related to inhalation injuries.

Thermal inhalation

Pulmonary complications remain the leading cause of death following thermal trauma. This type of trauma often results from inhalation of hot air or steam. The mortality rate exceeds 50% when inhalation injury accompanies burns of the skin. However, if a patient may have been trapped with flames in a confined area, suspect inflammation injury even if the patient doesn't have visible surface burns.

The entire respiratory tract is at risk for damage from thermal inhalation injury; however, injury rarely progresses to the lungs. The upper airway, where inhaled hot air or steam rapidly cools, typically suffers the greatest damage because reflective closure of the vocal cords and laryngeal spasm usually prevent full inhalation of the hot air or steam. This reaction also helps prevent injury to the lower respiratory tract. Steam inhalation causes more harm than hot air inhalation because water holds heat longer than dry air.

Chemical inhalation

Burning different materials can release a variety of gases, and the acids and alkalis released can produce chemical burns when inhaled. These inhaled substances can reach the respiratory tract as insoluble gases and lead to permanent damage.

Synthetic materials can also produce toxic gases. Some plastics, for instance, can produce toxic vapors when burned or even just heated. Some substances, such as ammonia, can cause pulmonary damage even when not burned if they are inhaled in a powder or liquid form. The inhalation of small amounts of noxious chemicals can also damage the alveoli and bronchi.

Irritating gases—including chlorine, hydrogen chloride, nitrogen dioxide, phosgene, and sulfur dioxide—combine with air in the lungs to form corrosive acids. These acids can then denature proteins and cause cellular damage and edema in pulmonary tissues. Smoke inhalation injuries generally fall into this category. Although chemical burns to the airway are similar in many ways to skin burns, they don't cause pain because the tracheobronchial tree isn't sensitive to pain.

Carbon monoxide poisoning

Carbon monoxide is a colorless, odorless, tasteless gas produced by combustion and oxidation. Poisoning can occur from inhaling small amounts of this chemical asphyxiant over a long period of time or large amounts over a short time. Accidental poisoning can result from exposure to a gas heater, smoke from a wood fire, or a gas lamp, gas stove, or charcoal grill used in a small, poorly ventilated area.

Although not directly toxic to the respiratory system, carbon monoxide (as well as similar gases such as hydrogen cyanide) interferes with cellular respiration. Because carbon monoxide has a greater attraction to hemoglobin than oxygen does, carbon monoxide binds with hemoglobin when it enters the bloodstream, forming carboxyhemoglobin. The carboxyhemoglobin reduces the oxygen-carrying capacity of hemoglobin, which results in decreased oxygenation to cells and tissues.

SIGNS AND SYMPTOMS

Physical findings with an inhalation injury vary depending upon the gas or substance inhaled and the duration of the exposure

Thermal inhalation

The entire respiratory tract has the potential to be damaged by this type of inhalation injury, but injury rarely progresses to the lungs. Signs and symptoms may include:
• ulcerations
• erythema and edema of the mouth and epiglottis
• stridor
• wheezing
• crackles
• increased secretions
• hoarseness
• shortness of breath

- facial and lip burns
- burned nasal hairs
- laryngeal edema.

Chemical inhalation

The most common effects of smoke or chemical inhalation include:
- atelectasis
- pulmonary edema
- tissue anoxia
- respiratory distress secondary to hypoxia.

Carbon monoxide poisoning

Because the carboxyhemoglobin that forms in the blood from carbon monoxide poisoning reduces the oxygen carrying capacity of hemoglobin, the patient's face may have a bright red flush and his lips may be cherry red. Other specific signs and symptoms vary with the concentration of carboxyhemoglobin.

Signs and symptoms of mild carbon monoxide poisoning that result in increased carboxyhemoglobin levels (from 11% to 20% carbon monoxide) include:
- headache
- decreased cerebral function
- decreased visual acuity
- slight shortness of breath.
Moderate poisoning (from 21% and 41%) can cause:
- headache
- tinnitus
- nausea
- drowsiness
- dizziness
- altered mental status
- confusion
- stupor

- irritability
- hypotension
- tachycardia
- ECG changes
- changes in skin color.
Severe poisoning (from 41% to 60%) causes:
- coma
- convulsions
- generalized instability.
Levels over 60% are fatal.

COMPLICATIONS

- Tracheitis
- Tracheal stenosis
- Tracheomalacia
- Chronic airway disease

DIAGNOSIS

- Initial laboratory studies, including electrolytes, liver function studies, blood urea nitrogen and creatinine levels, and a complete blood count, provide a baseline for analysis.
- Carboxyhemoglobin levels help confirm the diagnosis.
- Arterial blood gas levels provide information on the patient's acid-base, ventilation, and oxygenation status.
- Cardiac monitoring allows detection of ischemic changes; a depressed ST segment may indicate carbon monoxide poisoning.
- Chest X-rays reveal evidence of pulmonary injury 24 to 36 hours after the inhalation and establish a baseline for treatment.
- Fiberoptic bronchoscopy and direct laryngoscopy reveal erythema, edema, ulceration, and soot deposi-

tion and evaluate the extent of injury to the tracheobronchial tree.

TREATMENT

Treatment for inhalation injury includes obtaining a history of the exposure to identify the toxic agent and immediately providing the patient with oxygen. If the patient demonstrates severe respiratory distress or an altered mental state, he may require intubation and mechanical ventilation. Upper airway edema requires emergency endotracheal intubation.

The preferred treatment for carbon monoxide poisoning is administration of 100% humidified oxygen until carboxyhemoglobin levels fall to the nontoxic range of 10%. Although its use for carbon monoxide poisoning is controversial, hyperbaric oxygen therapy lowers carboxyhemoglobin levels more rapidly than humidified oxygen.

Fluid resuscitation helps manage inhalation injury, but the patient will require careful monitoring of his fluid status because of the risk of developing pulmonary edema. Chest physical therapy may help remove necrotic tissue.

Drugs

• Bronchodilators, such as nebulized albuterol (Proventil, Ventolin), racemic epinephrine 2.25% (microNefrin, AsthmaNefrin, Racepinephrine), terbutaline (Brethine), and epinephrine (Adrenaline, EpiPen), to relax smooth muscles and relieve bronchoconstriction

• Antibiotics to treat specific infections

SPECIAL CONSIDERATIONS

• Remove the patient's clothing, taking care to prevent self-contamination if there may be any toxic substance on the patient's clothing.
• Establish I.V. access for medication, blood product, and fluid administration.
• Obtain laboratory specimens to evaluate ventilation and oxygenation status and establish baseline values as ordered.
• Obtain chest X-rays, ECG, and pulmonary function studies as ordered.
• Implement cardiac monitoring to assess for ischemic changes or arrhythmias.
• Monitor for signs of pulmonary edema, which may accompany fluid resuscitation.
• If bronchospasms occur, provide oxygen, bronchodilators (using a nebulizer) and, possibly, aminophylline as ordered.
• Closely monitor fluid balance and intake and output.
• Administer antibiotics as prescribed.
• Assess lung sounds frequently; immediately notify the physician of any changes in lung sounds or oxygenation status.
• Offer support and teaching as appropriate to the patient and his family.
• Monitor laboratory studies for changes that may indicate multisystem complications.

⫸ PREVENTION

● *Teach the patient and his family how to decrease the risk of inhalation injuries, including the importance of functioning fire and smoke alarms, recognizing and reducing fire hazards, how to "stop, drop, and roll" in the event of fire, and how to formulate a proper fire exit plan in both the home and workplace.*

● *To help prevent chemical inhalation injury, teach the patient and his family the importance of properly storing chemicals, keeping such items out of reach of children, and using protective equipment and ventilation when working with chemicals.*

Laryngeal cancer

The most common form of laryngeal cancer is squamous cell cancer (95%); rare forms include adenocarcinoma, sarcoma, and others. Such cancer may be intrinsic or extrinsic. An intrinsic tumor is on the true vocal cord and doesn't tend to spread because underlying connective tissues lack lymph nodes. An extrinsic tumor is on some other part of the larynx and tends to spread early.

CAUSES AND INCIDENCE

In laryngeal cancer, major predisposing factors include smoking and alcoholism; minor factors include chronic inhalation of noxious fumes and familial tendency. Cancer of the larynx rarely occurs in nonsmokers.

Laryngeal cancer is classified according to its location. It can occur in the supraglottis (false vocal cords), glottis (true vocal cords), or subglottis (downward extension from vocal cords [rare]). The ratio of male to female incidence is 10:1, and most victims are between ages 50 and 65. The five-year survival rate is 65%. (See *Looking at laryngeal cancer*.)

SIGNS AND SYMPTOMS

Signs and symptoms of laryngeal cancer include:

- hoarseness that persists longer than 3 weeks
- lump in the throat or pain or burning in the throat when drinking citrus juice or hot liquid
- dysphagia
- dyspnea
- cough
- enlarged cervical lymph nodes
- pain radiating to the ear.

COMPLICATIONS

- Airway obstruction
- Metastasis
- Pain
- Difficulty swallowing

DIAGNOSIS

- Laryngoscopy shows the presence of the tumor.
- Xeroradiography, biopsy, laryngeal tomography, computed tomography scans, or laryngography define the borders of the lesion.
- Chest X-rays detect metastases. (See *Staging laryngeal cancer,* pages 102–103.)

TREATMENT

Early lesions are treated with surgery or radiation; advanced lesions, with surgery, radiation, and chemotherapy. In early stages, laser surgery can excise precancerous lesions; in advanced stages it can help relieve obstruction caused by tumor

LOOKING AT LARYNGEAL CANCER

This illustration shows a carcinoma of the right false vocal cord.

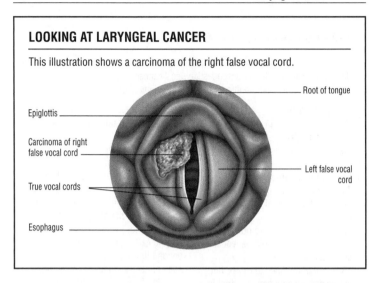

Root of tongue

Epiglottis

Carcinoma of right false vocal cord

True vocal cords

Esophagus

Left false vocal cord

growth. Surgical procedures vary with tumor size and can include cordectomy, partial or total laryngectomy, supraglottic laryngectomy, or total laryngectomy with laryngoplasty. The goal is to eliminate the cancer and preserve speech. If speech preservation isn't possible, speech rehabilitation may include esophageal speech or prosthetic devices; surgical techniques to construct a new voice box are still experimental.

Drugs

● Chemotherapeutic drugs, such as cisplatin; the combination of irinotecan, 5-Fluorouracil, and leucovorin (IFL); methotrexate; mitomycin; or the combination of paclitaxel, ifosfamide, and cisplatin (TIP), to slow tumor growth
● Analgesics to reduce pain

SPECIAL CONSIDERATIONS

Provide psychological support and good preoperative and postoperative care to minimize complications and speed recovery.

Before a partial or total laryngectomy, take these steps:
● Instruct the patient to maintain good oral hygiene. If appropriate, instruct a male patient to shave off his beard.
● Encourage the patient to express his concerns before surgery. Help him choose a temporary nonspeaking communication method, such as writing.
● If appropriate, arrange for a laryngectomee to visit the patient. Explain postoperative procedures (suctioning, nasogastric [NG] feeding, laryngectomy tube care) and their results (breathing through the neck, speech alteration). Also, prepare the

STAGING LARYNGEAL CANCER

The TNM (tumor, node, metastasis) classification system developed by the American Joint Committee on Cancer describes laryngeal cancer stages and guides treatment. The T stages cover supraglottic, glottic, and subglottic tumors.

Primary tumor

TX — primary tumor unassessible

T0 — no evidence of primary tumor

Tis — carcinoma in situ

Supraglottic tumor stages

T1 — tumor confined to one subsite in supraglottis; vocal cords retain motion

T2 — tumor extends to other sites in supraglottis or to glottis; vocal cords retain motion

T3 — tumor confined to larynx, but vocal cords lose motion; or tumor extends to the postcricoid area, the pyriform sinus, or the pre-epiglottic space, and vocal cords lose motion; or both

T4 — tumor extends through thyroid cartilage or extends to tissues beyond the larynx (such as the oropharynx or soft tissues of the neck) or both

T4a — tumor invades through the thyroid cartilage or invades tissues beyond the larynx (trachea, soft tissues of neck including deep extrinsic muscle of the tongue, strap muscles, thyroid, or esophagus)

T4b — tumor invades prevertebral space, encases carotid artery, or invades mediastinal structures

Glottic tumor stages

T1 — tumor confined to vocal cords, which retain normal motion; may involve anterior or posterior commissures

T2 — tumor extends to supraglottis or subglottis or both; vocal cords may lose motion

T3 — tumor confined to larynx, but vocal cords lose motion

T4 — tumor extends through thyroid cartilage or extends to tissues beyond the larynx (such as the oropharynx or soft tissues of the neck) or both

T4a — tumor invades through the thyroid cartilage or invades tissues beyond the larynx (trachea, soft tissues of neck including deep extrinsic muscle of the tongue, strap muscles, thyroid, or esophagus) or both

T4b — tumor invades prevertebral space, encases carotid artery, or invades mediastinal structures.

Subglottic tumor stages

T1 — tumor confined to subglottis

T2 — tumor extends to vocal cords; vocal cords may lose motion

T3 — tumor confined to larynx with vocal cord fixation

T4 — tumor extends through cricoid or thyroid cartilage or extends to tissues beyond the larynx, or both

T4a — tumor invades through the thyroid cartilage or invades tissues beyond the larynx (trachea, soft tissues of neck including deep extrinsic muscle of the tongue, strap muscles, thyroid, or esophagus) or both

T4b — tumor invades prevertebral space, encases carotid artery, or invades mediastinal structures

patient for other functional losses: He won't be able to smell, blow his nose, whistle, gargle, sip, or suck on a straw.

After a partial laryngectomy, take these steps:

● Give I.V. fluids and, usually, tube feedings in the initial postoperative

Regional lymph nodes

NX — regional lymph nodes can't be assessed
N0 — no evidence of regional lymph node metastasis
N1 — metastasis in a single ipsilateral lymph node, 3 cm or less in greatest dimension
N2 — metastasis in one or more ipsilateral lymph nodes, or in bilateral or contralateral nodes, larger than 3 cm but less than 6 cm in greatest dimension
N3 — metastasis in a node larger than 6 cm in greatest dimension

Distant metastasis

MX — distant metastasis unassessible
M0 — no evidence of distant metastasis
M1 — distant metastasis

Staging categories

Laryngeal cancer progresses from mild to severe as follows:
Stage 0 — Tis, N0, M0
Stage I — T1, N0, M0
Stage II — T2, N0, M0
Stage III — T3, N0, M0; T1, N1, M0; T2, N1, M0; T3, N1, M0
Stage IVA — T4, N0, M0; T4, N1, M0; Any T, N2, M0
Stage IVB — any T, N3, M0
Stage IVC — any T, any M, MI

period; then resume oral fluids. Keep the tracheostomy tube (inserted during surgery) in place until edema subsides

• Keep the patient from using his voice until he has medical permission (usually 2 to 3 days postoperatively). Then caution him to whisper until healing is complete.

After a total laryngectomy, follow these steps:
• As soon as the patient returns to his bed, place him on his side and elevate his head 30 to 45 degrees. When you move him, remember to support his neck.
• The patient will probably have a laryngectomy tube in place until his stoma heals (about 7 to 10 days). This tube is shorter and thicker than a tracheostomy tube but requires the same care. Watch for crusting and secretions around the stoma, which can cause skin breakdown. To prevent crust formation, provide adequate room humidification. Remove crusting with petroleum jelly, antimicrobial ointment, and moist gauze.
• Teach stoma care.
• Watch for and report complications, including fistula formation (redness, swelling, secretions on the suture line), carotid artery rupture (bleeding), and tracheostomy stenosis (constant shortness of breath). A fistula may form between the reconstructed hypopharynx and the skin. This eventually heals spontaneously, but healing may take weeks or months. Carotid artery rupture usually occurs in patients who have had preoperative radiation, particularly those with a fistula that constantly bathes the carotid artery with oral secretions.

⚠ ALERT

If carotid rupture occurs, apply pressure to the site; call for help immediately and take the patient to the operating room for carotid ligation.

- Tracheostomy stenosis occurs weeks to months after laryngectomy; treatment includes fitting the patient with successively larger tracheostomy tubes until he can tolerate insertion of a large one. If the patient has a fistula, feed him through an NG tube; otherwise, food will leak through the fistula and delay healing. Monitor vital signs (be especially alert for fever, which indicates infection). Record fluid intake and output, and watch for dehydration.
- Give frequent mouth care.
- Suction gently; unless ordered otherwise. Don't attempt deep suctioning, which could penetrate the suture line. Suction through both the tube and the patient's nose because the patient can no longer blow air through his nose; suction his mouth gently.
- After insertion of a drainage catheter (usually connected to a wound-drainage system or a GI drainage system), don't stop suction without the practitioner's consent. After catheter removal, check dressings for drainage.
- Give analgesics as ordered.
- If the patient has an NG feeding tube, check tube placement and elevate the patient's head to prevent aspiration.
- Reassure the patient that speech rehabilitation may help him speak again. Encourage contact with the International Association of Laryngectomees and other sources of support.
- Support the patient through the grieving process. If the depression seems severe, consider a psychiatric referral.

Legionnaires' disease

Legionnaires' disease is an acute bronchopneumonia produced by a gram-negative bacillus, *Legionella pneumophila*. It derives its name and notoriety from the peculiar, highly publicized disease that struck 182 people (29 of whom died) at an American Legion convention in Philadelphia in July 1976. This disease may occur epidemically or sporadically, usually in late summer or early fall. Its severity ranges from a mild illness, with or without pneumonitis, to multilobar pneumonia, with a mortality rate as high as 15%. A milder, self-limiting form (Pontiac syndrome) subsides within a few days but leaves the patient fatigued for several weeks. This form mimics Legionnaires' disease but produces few or no respiratory symptoms, no pneumonia, and no fatalities.

CAUSES AND INCIDENCE

L. pneumophila is an aerobic, gram-negative bacillus that's probably transmitted by an airborne route. In past epidemics, it has spread through cooling towers or evaporation condensers in air-conditioning systems. However, *Legionella* bacilli also flourish in soil and excavation sites. The disease doesn't spread from person to person.

Legionnaires' disease is most likely to affect:
• middle-age and elderly people
• immunocompromised patients (particularly those receiving corticosteroids, for example, after a transplant) or those with lymphoma or other disorders associated with delayed hypersensitivity
• patients with a chronic underlying disease, such as diabetes, chronic renal failure, or chronic obstructive pulmonary disease
• those with alcoholism
• cigarette smokers
• those on a ventilator for extended periods.

SIGNS AND SYMPTOMS

The multisystem clinical features of Legionnaires' disease follow a predictable sequence, although the onset of the disease may be gradual or sudden. After a 2- to 10-day incubation period, nonspecific, prodromal signs and symptoms appear, including:
• diarrhea
• anorexia
• malaise
• diffuse myalgias and generalized weakness
• headache
• recurrent chills
• unremitting fever that develops in 12 to 48 hours, with a temperature that may reach 105° F (40.6° C)

• nonproductive cough (initially); may eventually produce grayish, nonpurulent, and occasionally blood-streaked sputum
• nausea and vomiting
• disorientation
• mental sluggishness
• confusion
• mild temporary amnesia
• pleuritic chest pain
• tachypnea
• dyspnea
• fine crackles.

COMPLICATIONS
• Hypotension
• Delirium
• Heart failure
• Arrhythmias
• Acute respiratory failure
• Renal failure
• Shock (usually fatal)

DIAGNOSIS

The patient history focuses on possible sources of infection and predisposing conditions. Additional tests reveal the following:
• Chest X-rays show patchy, localized infiltration, which progresses to multilobar consolidation (usually involving the lower lobes), pleural effusion and, in fulminant disease, opacification of the entire lung.
• Auscultation reveals fine crackles, progressing to coarse crackles as the disease advances.
• Abnormal findings include leukocytosis, increased erythrocyte sedimentation rate, an increase in liver enzyme levels (alanine aminotransferase, aspartate aminotransferase,

and alkaline phosphatase), hyponatremia, decreased partial pressure of arterial oxygen and, initially, decreased partial pressure of arterial carbon dioxide. Bronchial washings and blood, pleural fluid, and sputum tests rule out other infections.

• Definitive tests include direct immunofluorescence of respiratory tract secretions and tissue, culture of *L. pneumophila*, and indirect fluorescent antibody testing of serum comparing acute samples with convalescent samples drawn at least 3 weeks later. A convalescent serum showing a fourfold or greater rise in antibody titer for *Legionella* confirms the diagnosis.

TREATMENT

Antibiotic treatment begins as soon as Legionnaires' disease is suspected and diagnostic material is collected; it shouldn't await laboratory confirmation. Supportive therapy includes administration of antipyretics, fluid replacement, circulatory support with pressor drugs, if necessary, and oxygen administration by mask, cannula, or mechanical ventilation.

Drugs

• Antibiotics, such as erythromycin (Ery-Tab, Erythrocin, EES) or doxycycline (Doryx, Bio-Tab) plus rifampin (Rifadin, Rimactane), tetracycline, or ciprofloxacin (Cipro), to inhibit bacterial growth

SPECIAL CONSIDERATIONS

• Closely monitor the patient's respiratory status. Evaluate chest wall expansion, depth and pattern of respirations, cough, and chest pain. Watch for restlessness as a sign of hypoxemia, which requires suctioning, repositioning, or more aggressive oxygen therapy.

• Continually monitor the patient's vital signs, oximetry or arterial blood gas values, level of consciousness, and dryness and color of lips and mucous membranes. Watch for signs of shock (decreased blood pressure, thready pulse, diaphoresis, and clammy skin).

• Keep the patient comfortable. Provide mouth care frequently. If necessary, apply soothing cream to the nostrils.

• Replace fluids and electrolytes as needed. The patient with renal failure may require dialysis.

• Provide mechanical ventilation and other respiratory therapy as needed. Teach the patient how to cough effectively, and encourage deep-breathing exercises. Stress the need to continue these until recovery is complete.

• Give antibiotic therapy as indicated, and observe carefully for adverse effects.

⧉ PREVENTION

Heating water above 140° F (60° C) or treating water with ultraviolet light or copper-silver ionization may help prevent contamination of water with L. pneumophila.

Lung cancer

Even though it's largely preventable, lung cancer is the most common cause of cancer death in both men and women. Lung cancer usually develops within the wall or epithelium of the bronchial tree. Its most common types are epidermoid (squamous cell) carcinoma, small-cell (oat cell) carcinoma, adenocarcinoma, and large-cell (anaplastic) carcinoma. Although the prognosis is usually poor, it varies with the extent of metastasis at the time of diagnosis and the cell type growth rate. Only about 13% of patients with lung cancer survive 5 years after diagnosis.

CAUSES AND INCIDENCE

Most experts agree that lung cancer is attributable to inhalation of carcinogenic pollutants by a susceptible host. Any smoker older than age 40, especially if he began to smoke before age 15, has smoked a whole pack or more per day for 20 years, or works with or near asbestos, is susceptible.

Pollutants in tobacco smoke cause progressive lung cell degeneration. Lung cancer is 10 times more common in smokers than in nonsmokers; 90% of patients with lung cancer are smokers. Cancer risk is determined by the number of cigarettes smoked daily, the depth of inhalation, how early in life smoking began, and the nicotine content of cigarettes. Two other factors also increase susceptibility: exposure to carcinogenic industrial and air pollutants (asbestos, uranium, arsenic, nickel, iron oxides, chromium, radioactive dust, and coal dust) and familial susceptibility.

Lung cancer begins with the transformation of one epithelial cell of the airway. The bronchi, as well as certain portions of the bronchi, such as the segmental bifurcations and sites of mucus production, are thought to be more vulnerable to injury from carcinogens. (See *Looking at a lung abscess,* page 108.)

As a lung tumor grows, it can partially or completely obstruct the airway, resulting in lobar collapse distal to the tumor. A lung tumor can also hemorrhage, causing hemoptysis. Early metastasis may occur to other thoracic structures, such as hilar lymph nodes or the mediastinum. Distant metastasis can occur to the brain, liver, bone, and adrenal glands. (See *Tumor infiltration in lung cancer,* page 109.)

SIGNS AND SYMPTOMS

Because early-stage lung cancer usually produces no symptoms, this disease is usually in an advanced state at diagnosis. Late-stage signs and symptoms for epidermoid and small-cell carcinoma include:

- smoker's cough
- hoarseness
- wheezing
- dyspnea
- hemoptysis
- chest pain.

For adenocarcinoma and large-cell carcinoma, late-stage indications include:

- fever
- weakness

LOOKING AT A LUNG ABSCESS

The photograph below shows a lung abscess with a purulent exudate that is contained by a fibrous wall.

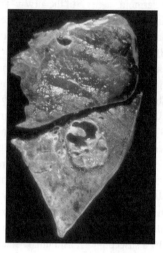

Image from Rubin, E., and Farber, J.L. *Pathology,* 3rd ed. Philadelphia: Lippincott Williams & Wilkins, 1999.

- weight loss
- anorexia
- shoulder pain.

Hormonal paraneoplastic syndromes

In addition to their obvious interference with respiratory function, lung tumors may also alter the production of hormones that regulate body function or homeostasis, resulting in the specific signs and symptoms of hormonal paraneoplastic syndromes.

- Large-cell carcinoma can cause gynecomastia.
- Large-cell carcinoma and adenocarcinoma can result in hypertrophic pulmonary osteoarthropathy (bone and joint pain from cartilage erosion due to abnormal production of growth hormone).
- Small-cell carcinoma can lead to Cushing's and carcinoid syndromes.
- Epidermoid tumors can cause hypercalcemia.

Metastatic signs and symptoms

Metastatic signs and symptoms vary greatly, depending on the effect of tumors on intrathoracic and distant structures.

- Bronchial obstruction can cause hemoptysis, atelectasis, pneumonitis, and dyspnea.
- Cervical thoracic sympathetic nerve involvement can lead to

TUMOR INFILTRATION IN LUNG CANCER

The illustrations below show a lung tumor projecting into the bronchi and metastasis to the hilar and carinal lymph nodes.

Right lung—Anterior view

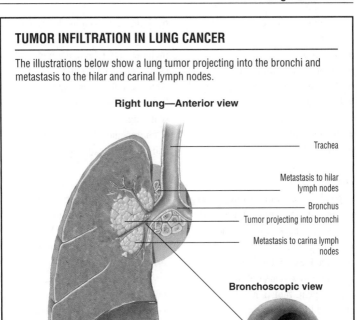

Trachea

Metastasis to hilar lymph nodes

Bronchus

Tumor projecting into bronchi

Metastasis to carina lymph nodes

Bronchoscopic view

Tumor projecting into bronchi

miosis, ptosis, exophthalmos, and reduced sweating.

• Chest wall invasion include piercing chest pain, increasing dyspnea, and severe shoulder pain that radiated down the arm.

• Esophageal compression can cause dysphagia.

• Local lymphatic spread can result in cough, hemoptysis, stridor, and pleural effusion.

• Pericardial involvement can cause pericardial effusion, tamponade, and arrhythmias.

• Phrenic nerve involvement can lead to dyspnea, shoulder pain, and a unilateral paralyzed diaphragm with paradoxical motion.

• Recurrent nerve invasion can result in hoarseness and vocal cord paralysis.

• Vena caval obstruction can cause venous distention and edema of face, neck, chest, and back.

Distant metastasis may involve any part of the body, most commonly the central nervous system, liver, and bone, leading to a variety of signs and symptoms.

COMPLICATIONS

• Anorexia
• Cachexia

- Clubbing of fingers and toes
- Dysphagia
- Dyspnea
- Esophageal compression
- Hypertrophic osteoarthropathy
- Hypoxemia
- Phrenic nerve paralysis
- Pleural effusion
- Tracheal obstruction

DIAGNOSIS

Typical clinical findings may strongly suggest lung cancer, but firm diagnosis requires further evidence.

- A chest X-ray usually shows an advanced lesion, but it can detect a lesion up to 2 years before symptoms appear. It also indicates tumor size and location.
- Sputum cytology, which is 75% reliable, requires a specimen coughed up from the lungs and tracheobronchial tree, not postnasal secretions or saliva.
- Spiral or helical computed tomography (CT) of the chest may help to delineate the tumor's size and its relationship to surrounding structures.
- Magnetic resonance imaging differentiates vascular abnormalities from tumor.
- Bronchoscopy can locate the tumor site. Bronchoscopic washings provide material for cytologic and histologic examination. The flexible fiberoptic bronchoscope increases the test's effectiveness.
- Percutaneous needle biopsy of the lungs uses biplane fluoroscopic visual control to detect peripherally located tumors. This allows firm diagnosis in 80% of patients.
- Mediastinoscopy with tissue biopsy of accessible metastatic sites includes supraclavicular and mediastinal node and pleural biopsy. Directed-needle biopsy may be performed in conjunction with CT scanning.
- Thoracentesis allows chemical and cytologic examination of pleural fluid.

Additional studies include preoperative mediastinoscopy or mediastinotomy to rule out involvement of mediastinal lymph nodes (which would preclude curative pulmonary resection).

Other tests to detect metastasis include bone scan, bone marrow biopsy (recommended in small-cell carcinoma), CT scan of the brain or abdomen, and positron emission tomography.

After histologic confirmation, staging determines the extent of the disease and helps in planning the treatment and predicting the prognosis. (See *Staging lung cancer*.)

TREATMENT

Recent treatment, which consists of combinations of surgery, radiation, and chemotherapy, may improve the prognosis and prolong survival. Nevertheless, because treatment usually begins at an advanced stage, it's largely palliative.

Surgery is the preferred treatment for stage I, stage II, or selected stage III squamous cell cancer; adenocarcinoma; and large-cell carcinoma, unless the tumor is

STAGING LUNG CANCER

Using the TNM (tumor, node, metastasis) classification system, the American Joint Committee on Cancer stages lung cancer as follows.

Primary tumor

TX — primary tumor can't be assessed or malignant tumor cells detected in sputum or bronchial washings but undetected by X-ray or bronchoscopy

T0 — no evidence of primary tumor

Tis — carcinoma in situ

T1 — tumor 3 cm or less in greatest dimension, surrounded by normal lung or visceral pleura; no bronchoscopic evidence of cancer closer to the center of the body than the lobar bronchus

T2 — tumor larger than 3 cm; one that involves the main bronchus and is 2 cm or more from the carina; one that invades the visceral pleura; or one that's accompanied by atelectasis or obstructive pneumonitis that extends to the hilar region but doesn't involve the entire lung

T3 — tumor of any size that extends into neighboring structures, such as the chest wall, diaphragm, or mediastinal pleura; tumor in the main bronchus that doesn't involve but is less than 2 cm from the carina; or tumor that's accompanied by atelectasis or obstructive pneumonitis of the entire lung

T4 — tumor of any size that invades the mediastinum, heart, great vessels, trachea, esophagus, vertebral body, or carina; or tumor with malignant pleural effusion

Regional lymph nodes

NX — regional lymph nodes can't be assessed

N0 — no detectable metastasis to lymph nodes

N1 — metastasis to the ipsilateral peribronchial or hilar lymph nodes or both

N2 — metastasis to the ipsilateral mediastinal or subcarinal lymph nodes or both

N3 — metastasis to the contralateral mediastinal or hilar lymph nodes, the ipsilateral or contralateral scalene lymph nodes, or the supraclavicular lymph nodes

Distant metastasis

MX — distant metastasis can't be assessed

M0 — no evidence of distant metastasis

M1 — distant metastasis

Staging categories

Lung cancer progresses from mild to severe as follows:

Occult carcinoma — TX, N0, M0

Stage 0 — Tis, N0, M0

Stage I — T1, N0, M0; T2, N0, M0

Stage II — T1, N1, M0; T2, N1, M0

Stage IIIa — T1, N2, M0; T2, N2, M0; T3, N0, M0; T3, N1, M0; T3, N2, M0

Stage IIIb — any T, N3, M0; T4, any N, M0

Stage IV — any T, any N, M1

---

nonresectable or other conditions rule out surgery.

Surgery may include partial removal of a lung (wedge resection, segmental resection, lobectomy, or radical lobectomy) or total removal (pneumonectomy or radical pneumonectomy). A less invasive form of surgery that's used for small (1½" [3.8 cm] or less) tumors is video-assisted thoracic surgery (VATS). VATS requires small incisions and causes less pain than other types of surgery.

Preoperative radiation therapy may reduce tumor bulk to allow for surgical resection. Preradiation chemotherapy helps improve response rates. Radiation therapy is ordinarily recommended for stage I and stage II lesions, if surgery is contraindicated, and for stage III lesions when the disease is confined to the involved hemithorax and the ipsilateral supraclavicular lymph nodes. Generally, radiation therapy is delayed until 1 month after surgery to allow the wound to heal; it's then directed to the part of the chest most likely to develop metastases. High-dose radiation therapy or radiation implants may also be used.

In laser therapy, laser energy is directed through a bronchoscope to destroy local tumors.

Drugs

- Combinations of the chemotherapeutic agents paclitaxel, gemcitabine, docetaxel, irinotecan, and vinorelbine with cisplatin or carboplatin (to improve tolerability and improve action) to attack the tumor
- Any of several chemotherapeutic agents used individually to treat small-cell and non–small-cell lung cancers
- Bevacizumab (Avastin) to stop a tumor from creating a new blood supply, preventing the tumor from receiving the oxygen and nutrients it needs to grow

- Erlotinib (Tarceva) to block chemicals that signal the cancer cells to grow and divide

SPECIAL CONSIDERATIONS

Comprehensive supportive care and patient teaching can minimize complications and speed recovery from surgery, radiation, and chemotherapy. Before surgery:

- Supplement and reinforce the information given to the patient by the health care team about the disease and the surgical procedure.
- Explain expected postoperative procedures, such as insertion of an indwelling catheter, use of an endotracheal tube or chest tube (or both), dressing changes, and I.V. therapy.
- Teach the patient how to perform coughing, deep diaphragmatic breathing, and range-of-motion (ROM) exercises.
- Reassure the patient that he will receive analgesics and proper positioning to control postoperative pain.
- Inform the patient that he may take nothing by mouth beginning after midnight the night before surgery, that he'll shower with a soap-like antibacterial agent the night or morning before surgery, and that he'll be given preoperative medications, such as a sedative and an anticholinergic to dry secretions.

After thoracic surgery:

- Maintain a patent airway, and monitor the patient's chest tubes to reestablish normal intrathoracic pressure and prevent postoperative and pulmonary complications.

• Check vital signs every 15 minutes during the 1st hour after surgery, every 30 minutes during the next 4 hours, and then every 2 hours. Watch for and report abnormal respiration and other changes.

• Suction the patient as needed, and encourage him to begin deep breathing and coughing as soon as possible. Check secretions often. Initially, sputum will be thick and dark with blood, but it should become thinner and grayish yellow within a day.

• Monitor and record closed chest drainage. Keep chest tubes patent and draining effectively; fluctuation in the water-seal chamber on inspiration and expiration indicates that the chest tube is patent. Watch for air leaks, and report them immediately. Position the patient on the surgical side to promote drainage and lung reexpansion.

• Watch for and report foul-smelling discharge and excessive drainage on dressings. The dressing is typically removed after 24 hours, unless the wound appears infected.

• Monitor the patient's intake and output, and maintain adequate hydration.

• Watch for and report signs and symptoms of infection, shock, hemorrhage, atelectasis, dyspnea, mediastinal shift, and pulmonary emboli.

• To prevent pulmonary emboli, apply antiembolism stockings and encourage ROM exercises.

If the patient is receiving chemotherapy and radiation:
• Explain possible adverse effects of radiation and chemotherapy
• Ask the dietary department to provide soft, nonirritating foods high in protein, and encourage the patient to eat high-calorie between-meal snacks.
• Give antiemetics and antidiarrheals as needed.
• Schedule patient care activities in a way that helps the patient conserve his energy.
• During radiation therapy, administer skin care to minimize skin breakdown. If the patient receives radiation therapy in an outpatient setting, warn him to avoid tight clothing, exposure to the sun, and harsh ointments on his chest. Teach him exercises to help prevent shoulder stiffness.

⚝ PREVENTION

• *If the patient smokes, explain the benefits of quitting and encourage him to quit. If he wants to quit, refer him to the American Cancer Society or other smoking-cessation program, or suggest group therapy, individual counseling, or smoking-cessation products.*

• *If the patient has a recurring or chronic respiratory infection or chronic lung disease and detects any change in the character of a cough, encourage him to see his practitioner promptly for evaluation.*

Mesotheliomas

Mesotheliomas, which originate in the serosal lining of the pleural cavity, account for less than 10% of all cancer-related deaths. Incidence is high, however, in asbestos workers and their immediate families and among people who live along major routes used for transporting large quantities of asbestos.

CAUSES AND INCIDENCE

Sarcomatous, epithelial, and mixed are the three major types of mesothelioma. Pleural mesothelioma usually begins at the lower part of the chest as discrete plaques and nodules that come together and produce a sheetlike neoplasm. The tumor may invade the diaphragm and encase the surface of the lung and interlobar fissures. From there, the pleural lymphatics carry it to the pleural surface. Signs and symptoms result from pleural effusion, restricted lung function, tumor mass, infection, and advanced disease. The tumor may also grow along drainage and thoracotomy tracts. As the disease progresses, it often extends into the chest wall and mediastinum and may extend into the esophagus, ribs, vertebra, brachial plexus, and superior vena cava. Most malignant mesotheliomas have complex karyotypes, with rearrangement of many chromosomes. A loss of a single copy on chromosome 22 is the most common abnormality.

The link between mesotheliomas and asbestos exposure is well established. The shipbuilding, construction, ceramics, paper milling, auto parts, railroad, and insulation industries are all associated with asbestos exposure. Smoking alone doesn't increase the risk for developing a mesothelioma; however, coupled with asbestos exposure, smoking increases the risk by about 50%. Mesotheliomas rarely result from chronic inflammation, radiation, or recurrent lung infection.

Mesotheliomas have a latency period of 20 to 45 years from exposure to tumor discovery. They typically occur in people older than 50 years and are invariably fatal. With trimodality treatment, median survival is 11 months, with some patients surviving 16 to 19 months and a few as long as 5 years. Without treatment, mesothelioma is fatal in 4 to 8 months.

SIGNS AND SYMPTOMS

The patient's history typically reveals asbestos exposure at some time in his life. Signs and symptoms of mesothelioma may not appear until 20 to 45 years after exposure to asbestos and include:

- chest pain
- dyspnea
- cough
- hoarseness
- anorexia
- weight loss
- weakness
- fatigue
- elevated temperature
- shortness of breath
- finger clubbing
- dullness over lung fields
- diminished breath sounds.

COMPLICATIONS

- Severe dyspnea
- Infection
- Complications of immobility (skin breakdown)

DIAGNOSIS

- Chest X-rays show nodular, irregular, unilateral pleural thickening and varying degrees of unilateral pleural effusion.
- A computed tomography scan of the chest defines the tumor's extent.
- Open pleural biopsy to obtain a specimen and histologic study confirm the diagnosis.

TREATMENT

No standard treatment exists for a mesothelioma. Surgery, radiation therapy, chemotherapy, and a combination of treatments can prolong survival but are mainly palliative.

Pleurectomy is the procedure of choice if surgery is performed, often followed by postoperative radiation

therapy. Chemotherapy can help control tumor cell reproduction, although the most successful combination—cisplatin and mitomycin—is quite toxic; the recently approved pemetrexed and cisplatin combination is usually tolerated well.

Drugs

- Antineoplastic agent combinations—including cisplatin (Platinol-AQ) or carboplatin combined with pemetrexed (Altima); cisplatin or carboplatin combined with gemcitabine (Gemzar); methotrexate and vincristine; cisplatin, vinblastine, and mitomycin (Mutamycin); cisplatin and doxorubicin (Doxil); cisplatin and raltitrexed; and cisplatin and doxorubicin combined with cyclophosphamide or ifosfamide—to interfere with cell reproduction
- Vitamin B_{12} and folic acid to avoid adverse effects of pemetrexed's interference with normal vitamin B_{12} and folic acid metabolism

SPECIAL CONSIDERATIONS

- Listen to the patient's fears and concerns. Give clear, concise explanations of all procedures and actions, and remain with the patient during periods of severe anxiety. Encourage him to identify actions that promote comfort; then perform these actions as possible, and encourage the patient and his family to help. Include the patient in decisions about his care whenever possible.
- Administer ordered pain medication as required; monitor and document the medication's effectiveness.

• Perform comfort measures, such as repositioning and relaxation techniques.

• Monitor respiratory status. Provide oxygen as ordered, and help the patient into a comfortable position (such as Fowler's position) that allows maximal chest expansion to relieve respiratory distress.

• If the patient develops limited mobility, turn him frequently and provide skin care, particularly over bony prominences. Encourage him to be as active as possible.

• Take steps to prevent infection. Follow strict sterile technique when suctioning, changing dressings or I.V. tubing, and performing any type of invasive procedure. Monitor the patient's body temperature and white blood cell count closely.

• Monitor I.V. fluid intake to avoid circulatory overload and pulmonary congestion.

• Detect treatment complications by observing and listening to the patient and monitoring laboratory studies and vital signs. Report any complications that occur, and take appropriate nursing measures to prevent or alleviate complications.

Parainfluenza

Parainfluenza refers to any of a group of respiratory illnesses caused by paramyxoviruses, a subgroup of the myxoviruses. Affecting both the upper and lower respiratory tracts, these self-limiting diseases resemble influenza but are milder and seldom fatal. They primarily affect young children.

CAUSES AND INCIDENCE

Parainfluenza is transmitted by direct contact or by inhalation of contaminated airborne droplets. Paramyxoviruses occur in four forms—Para 1 to 4—that are linked to several diseases: croup (Para 1, 2, 3); acute febrile respiratory illnesses (1, 2, 3); the common cold (1, 3, 4); pharyngitis (1, 3, 4); bronchitis (1, 3); and bronchopneumonia (1, 3). Para 3 ranks second to respiratory syncytial viruses as the most common cause of lower respiratory tract infections in children. Para 4 rarely causes symptomatic infections in humans.

Parainfluenza is rare among adults but widespread among children, especially males. By age 8, most children demonstrate antibodies to Para 1 and Para 3. Most adults have antibodies to all four types as a result of childhood infections and subsequent multiple exposures. Re-infection is usually less severe and affects only the upper respiratory tract. Incidence rises in the winter and spring.

Upon exposure, the major site of virus binding and subsequent infection is the respiratory epithelium. The virus causes airway inflammation, necrosis and sloughing of respiratory epithelium, edema, excessive mucus production, and interstitial infiltration of the lung. Edema of the mucus layer causes swelling (occurring in the vocal cords, larynx, trachea, and bronchi), leading to obstruction of airway inflow and stridor.

SIGNS AND SYMPTOMS

After a short incubation period (usually 3 to 6 days), signs and symptoms emerge that are similar to those of other respiratory diseases, including:

- chills
- muscle pain
- nasal discharge
- reddened throat (with little or no exudate)
- sudden fever.

COMPLICATIONS

- Croup
- Laryngotracheobronchitis
- Bronchiolitis
- Pneumonia

DIAGNOSIS

Parainfluenza infections are usually clinically indistinguishable from similar viral infections. A swab of nasal secretions allows for rapid viral testing. Although isolation of the virus and serum antibody titers can differentiate parainfluenza from other respiratory illnesses, it's rarely performed.

TREATMENT

Depending on the severity of signs and symptoms, treatment can range from no treatment to bed rest and use of antipyretics, analgesics, and antitussives. Complications, such as croup and pneumonia, require appropriate treatment. Corticosteroids and nebulization help control respiratory symptoms and reduce airway edema.

Drugs

• Corticosteroids, such as dexamethasone (Decadron, Solurex, Dexasone), prednisone (Deltasone, Orasone, Meticorten, Sterapred), and prednisolone (Delta-Cortef, Articulose-50, Econopred), to reduce airway inflammation; budesonide (Pulmicort Respules, Turbuhaler) given via inhaler for the same purpose
• Sympathomimetics such as epinephrine (AsthmaNefrin, microNefrin, S-2) to reverse upper airway edema

SPECIAL CONSIDERATIONS

• Throughout the illness, monitor respiratory status and temperature, and ensure adequate fluid intake and rest.

⊠ PREVENTION

• *The easiest and most effective way to prevent the spread of infection is to practice good hand washing.*

Pharyngitis

The most common throat disorder, pharyngitis is an acute or chronic inflammation of the pharynx. It frequently accompanies the common cold.

CAUSES AND INCIDENCE

Viruses account for 40% to 60% of pharyngitis cases and bacteria cause 5% to 40% of cases, with allergies, trauma, toxins, and neoplasias accounting for the rest. The most common bacterial cause is group A beta-hemolytic streptococci; others include *Mycoplasma* and *Chlamydia*.

The peak incidence of bacterial and viral pharyngitis occurs in children ages 4 to 7 years; it's rare in children younger than 3 years. Noninfectious pharyngitis is widespread among adults who live or work in dusty or very dry environments, use their voices excessively, habitually use tobacco or alcohol, or suffer from chronic sinusitis, persistent coughs, or allergies.

With infectious pharyngitis, bacteria or viruses may directly invade the pharyngeal mucosa, causing inflammation. Other viruses, such as rhinovirus, cause nasal secretions, which in turn irritate the mucosa. Streptococcal infections release extracellular toxins and proteases,

ACUTE PHARYNGITIS

The illustration below shows acute pharyngitis along with tonsillitis.

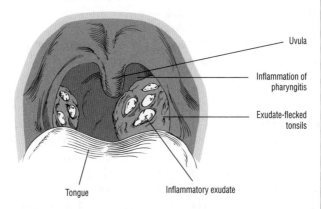

Uvula

Inflammation of pharyngitis

Exudate-flecked tonsils

Tongue   Inflammatory exudate

From Weber, J., and Kelly, J. *Health Assessment in Nursing,* 2nd ed. Philadelphia: Lippincott Williams & Wilkins, 2003.

which can cause such complications as rheumatic fever, heart valve damage, and acute glomerulonephritis. (See *Acute pharyngitis*.)

SIGNS AND SYMPTOMS

Typically, the patient complains of:
- a sore throat
- slight difficulty swallowing (swallowing saliva hurts more than swallowing food)
- sensation of a lump in the throat
- a constant and aggravating urge to swallow
- headache
- muscle and joint pain (especially in bacterial pharyngitis)
- mild fever
- pharyngeal wall appears fiery red, with swollen,
- exudate-flecked tonsils and lymphoid follicles

- acutely inflamed throat with patches of white and yellow follicles (bacterial pharyngitis)
- strawberry red tongue
- enlarged, tender cervical lymph nodes.

COMPLICATIONS

- Otitis media
- Sinusitis
- Mastoiditis
- Rheumatic fever
- Nephritis
- Glomerulonephritis
- Toxic shock syndrome
- Pneumonia

DIAGNOSIS

- A throat culture can identify any bacterial organisms causing inflammation, but it may not detect other causative organisms.

• Rapid strep tests generally detect group A streptococcal infections, but they miss the fairly common streptococcal groups C and G.

• Computed tomography scanning can identify the location of abscesses.

• A white blood cell (WBC) count is used to determine atypical lymphocytes; an elevated total WBC count is present.

TREATMENT

Treatment for acute viral pharyngitis is usually symptomatic and consists mainly of resting, gargling with warm saline solution, sucking throat lozenges that contain a mild anesthetic, drinking plenty of fluids, and taking analgesics as needed. If the patient can't swallow fluids, he may need I.V. hydration.

Suspected bacterial pharyngitis requires rigorous treatment with penicillin or another broad-spectrum antibiotic because *Streptococcus* (the most likely infecting organism) could lead to the development of acute rheumatic fever. Antibiotic therapy should continue for 48 hours until culture results are back. If the culture or a rapid strep test is positive for group A beta-hemolytic streptococci, or if bacterial infection is suspected despite negative culture results, penicillin therapy should continue for 10 days.

Chronic pharyngitis requires the same supportive measures as acute pharyngitis but with greater emphasis on eliminating the underlying cause, such as an allergen. Preventive measures include adequate humidification and avoiding excessive exposure to air conditioning. In addition, the patient should be urged to stop smoking.

Drugs

• Antimicrobials appropriate to the specific causative agent to combat infection

• Corticosteroids, such as dexamethasone (Decadron) or prednisone (Deltasone, Orasone, Sterapred), to reduce airway edema in cases of airway obstruction

• Antifungals, such as nystatin (Mycostatin) or fluconazole (Diflucan), to combat oral thrush

• Antivirals, such as acyclovir (Zovirax), famciclovir (Famvir), ganciclovir (Cytovene, Vitrasert), and foscarnet (Foscavir), for a severe mucocutaneous HSV infection or an immunocompromised patient

SPECIAL CONSIDERATIONS

• Administer analgesics and warm saline gargles, as ordered and as appropriate.

• Encourage the patient to drink plenty of fluids. Scrupulously monitor intake and output, and watch for signs of dehydration.

• Provide meticulous mouth care to prevent dry lips and oral pyoderma, and maintain a restful environment.

• Obtain throat cultures, and administer antibiotics as needed. If the patient has acute bacterial pharyngitis, emphasize the importance of completing the full course of antibiotic therapy. Tell him to call his practitioner if he experiences any adverse reactions.

• Inform the patient and his family that in the case of positive streptococcal infection, the family should undergo throat cultures regardless of the presence or absence of symptoms. Those with positive cultures require penicillin therapy.

• Teach the patient with chronic pharyngitis steps he can take to minimize environmental sources of throat irritation such as using a humidifier in the bedroom.

• Refer the patient to a self-help group to stop smoking if appropriate.

• Tell the parents of a school-age child with infectious pharyngitis that the child should receive at least 24 hours of therapy before returning to school.

• A patient who has exhibited three or more documented bacterial infections within 6 months may need daily penicillin prophylaxis during the winter months; carriers who live in closed or semiclosed communities may also need treatment.

Pleural effusion and empyema

Pleural effusion is an excess of fluid in the pleural space. Normally, this space contains a small amount of extracellular fluid that lubricates the pleural surfaces. Increased production or inadequate removal of this fluid results in pleural effusion. Empyema is the accumulation of pus and necrotic tissue in the pleural

space. Blood (hemothorax) and chyle (chylothorax) may also collect in this space.

CAUSES AND INCIDENCE

The balance of osmotic and hydrostatic pressures in parietal pleural capillaries normally results in fluid movement into the pleural space. Balanced pressures in visceral pleural capillaries promote reabsorption of this fluid. Excessive hydrostatic pressure or decreased osmotic pressure can cause excessive amounts of fluid to pass across intact capillaries. The result is a transudative pleural effusion, an ultrafiltrate of plasma containing low concentrations of protein. Such effusions can result from heart failure, hepatic disease with ascites, peritoneal dialysis, hypoalbuminemia, and disorders resulting in overexpanded intravascular volume. (See *Lung compression in pleural effusion,* page 122.)

Exudative pleural effusions result when capillaries exhibit increased permeability with or without changes in hydrostatic and colloid osmotic pressures, allowing protein-rich fluid to leak into the pleural space. Exudative pleural effusions occur with tuberculosis, subphrenic abscess, pancreatitis, bacterial or fungal pneumonitis or empyema, malignancy, pulmonary embolism with or without infarction, collagen disease (lupus erythematosus and rheumatoid arthritis), myxedema, and chest trauma.

Empyema is usually associated with infection in the pleural space.

LUNG COMPRESSION IN PLEURAL EFFUSION

The illustration below shows displacement of the heart and lung compression in pleural effusion.

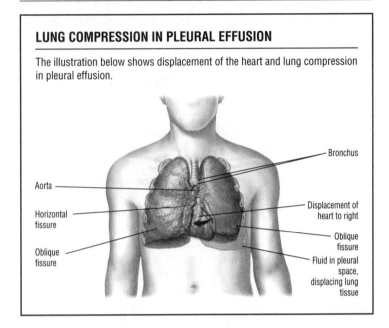

Such infection may be idiopathic or may be related to pneumonitis, carcinoma, perforation, or esophageal rupture.

Pleural effusion affects 1.3 million people each year. Morbidity and mortality are directly related to the cause, the stage of disease at the time of onset, and findings in the pleural fluid analysis. Patients with malignant pleural effusion have a poor prognosis, with a life expectancy of 3 to 6 months.

SIGNS AND SYMPTOMS

The patient's history characteristically shows underlying pulmonary disease. Signs and symptoms include:

- dyspnea (with effusion)
- pleuritic chest pain (with pleurisy)
- general feeling of malaise (with empyema)
- tracheal has deviation
- fever (with empyema)
- decreased tactile fremitus (with a large amount of effusion)
- dullness over the effused area that doesn't change with respiration.
- diminished or absent breath sounds over the effusion
- a pleural friction rub during both inspiration and expiration
- bronchial breath sounds, sometimes with the patient's pronunciation of the letter "e" sounding like the letter "a."

COMPLICATIONS

- Atelectasis
- Infection
- Hypoxemia

DIAGNOSIS

Chest X-rays show radiopaque fluid in dependent regions (usually with fluid accumulation of more than 250 ml). A negative tuberculin skin test helps rule out tuberculosis as a cause. A pleural biopsy can help confirm tuberculosis or cancer if thoracentesis doesn't provide a definitive diagnosis in exudative pleural effusion.

Analysis of fluid aspirated during thoracocentesis can provide the following information:

• In transudative effusion, fluid usually has a specific gravity less than 1.015 and contains less than 3 g/dl of protein.

• Exudative effusion has a ratio of protein in the fluid to serum of greater than or equal to 0.5, pleural fluid lactate dehydrogenase (LD) of greater than or equal to 200 IU, and a ratio of LD in pleural fluid to LD in serum of greater than or equal to 0.6.

• In empyema, aspirated fluid contains acute inflammatory white blood cells and microorganisms and shows leukocytosis.

• In empyema and rheumatoid arthritis, which can be the cause of an exudative pleural effusion, fluid shows an extremely decreased pleural fluid glucose level.

• Pleural effusion that results from esophageal rupture or pancreatitis usually has fluid amylase levels higher than serum levels.

• Aspirated fluid may also be tested for lupus erythematosus cells, antinuclear antibodies, and neoplastic cells and analyzed for color and consistency; acid-fast bacillus, fungal and bacterial cultures, and triglycerides (in chylothorax).

TREATMENT

Depending on the amount of fluid present, symptomatic pleural effusion may require either thoracentesis to remove fluid or careful monitoring of the patient's own reabsorption of the fluid. Hemothorax requires drainage to prevent fibrothorax formation.

Pleural effusions associated with lung cancer commonly reaccumulate quickly. If a chest tube is inserted to drain the fluid, a sclerosing agent, such as talc, may be injected through the tube to cause adhesions between the parietal and visceral pleura, thereby obliterating the potential space for fluid to recollect.

Treatment of empyema requires insertion of one or more chest tubes after thoracentesis to allow purulent material to drain, and possibly decortication (surgical removal of the thick coating over the lung) or rib resection to allow open drainage and lung expansion. Empyema also requires parenteral antibiotics. Associated hypoxia requires oxygen administration.

Drugs

• Antimicrobials specific to the type of organism involved to combat the infecting organism

• Diuretics, such as furosemide (Lasix) or spironolactone (Aldactone), as needed to promote diuresis

SPECIAL CONSIDERATIONS

• Explain thoracentesis to the patient. Before the procedure, tell him to expect a stinging sensation from the local anesthetic and a feeling of pressure when the needle is inserted. Instruct him to tell you immediately if he feels uncomfortable or has difficulty breathing during the procedure.

• Reassure the patient during thoracentesis. Remind him to breathe normally and to avoid sudden movements, such as coughing or sighing. Monitor his vital signs, and watch for syncope. If fluid is removed too quickly, the patient may suffer bradycardia, hypotension, pain, pulmonary edema, or even cardiac arrest.

⚠ ALERT

After thoracentesis, watch for respiratory distress and signs of pneumothorax (sudden onset of dyspnea and cyanosis).

• Administer oxygen and, in empyema, antibiotics, as ordered.

• Encourage the patient to perform deep-breathing exercises to promote lung expansion. Use an incentive spirometer to promote deep breathing.

• Provide meticulous chest tube care, and use sterile technique for changing dressings around the tube insertion site in empyema. Ensure tube patency by watching for fluctuations of fluid or air bubbling in the water-seal chamber. Continuous bubbling may indicate an air leak. Record the amount, color, and consistency of any tube drainage.

• If the patient has open drainage through a rib resection or intercostal tube, use hand and dressing precautions. Because weeks of such drainage are usually necessary to obliterate the space, make visiting nurse referrals for the patient who will be discharged with the tube in place.

• If pleural effusion was a complication of pneumonia or influenza, advise prompt medical attention for upper respiratory infections.

Pleurisy

Pleurisy, also known as pleuritis, is an inflammation of the visceral and parietal pleurae that line the inside of the thoracic cage and envelop the lungs.

CAUSES AND INCIDENCE

Pleurisy develops as a complication of pneumonia, tuberculosis, viruses, systemic lupus erythematosus, rheumatoid arthritis, uremia, Dressler's syndrome, certain cancers, pulmonary infarction, and chest trauma. Pleuritic pain is caused by the inflammation or irritation of sensory nerve endings in the parietal pleura. As the lungs inflate and deflate, the visceral pleura covering the lungs moves against the fixed parietal pleura lining the pleural space, causing pain. This disorder usually begins suddenly. The normal pleural space contains approximately 1 ml of fluid, balancing hydrostatic and oncotic forces (in the visceral and parietal pleural vessels) and lymphatic drainage. Pleural effusions result when a disruption occurs in this balance.

In the United States, the estimated incidence is 1 million cases per year. Most are caused by heart failure, malignancy, infections, and pulmonary emboli.

SIGNS AND SYMPTOMS

Signs and symptoms of pleurisy include:

- sudden, sharp, stabbing pain that worsens on inspiration
- shallow, rapid breathing
- dyspnea
- pleural friction rub—a coarse, creaky sound heard during late inspiration and early expiration—directly over the area of pleural inflammation.
- coarse vibrations over the affected area.

COMPLICATIONS

- Permanent adhesions that can restrict lung expansion

DIAGNOSIS

- Electrocardiography rules out coronary artery disease as the source of the patient's pain.
- Chest X-rays can identify pneumonia.
- Ultrasonography of the chest and thoracentesis may aid in diagnosis.

TREATMENT

Treatment is directed at the underlying cause; bacterial infections are treated with appropriate antibiotics, tuberculosis requires special treat

ment, and viral infections may be permitted to run their course. Treatment also includes measures to relieve signs and symptoms, such as anti-inflammatory agents, analgesics, and bed rest. Severe pain may require an intercostal nerve block of two or three intercostal nerves. Pleurisy with pleural effusion calls for thoracentesis as a therapeutic and diagnostic measure.

Drugs

- Antimicrobials specific to the type of organism involved to combat the infecting organism
- Analgesics to relieve pain
- Antitussives to relieve cough

SPECIAL CONSIDERATIONS

- Stress the importance of bed rest, and plan your care to allow the patient as much uninterrupted rest as possible.
- Asses the patient for pain every 3 hours, and administer antitussives and pain medication as ordered, but be careful not to overmedicate. Pain relief allows for maximum chest expansion. If the pain requires an opioid analgesic, warn the patient who's about to be discharged to avoid overuse because such medication depresses coughing and respiration.
- Encourage the patient to take deep breaths and to cough. To minimize pain, apply firm pressure at the site of the pain while the patient coughs.
- Encourage the use of incentive spirometry every hour and instruct the patient on proper use.

• Place the patient in high Fowler's position to help lung expansion. Positioning him on the affected side may aid in splinting.

• Assess the patient's respiratory status at least every 4 hours to detect early signs of compromise. Monitor for such complications as fever, increased dyspnea, and changes in breath sounds.

• Plan your care to allow the patient as much uninterrupted rest as possible.

• Pain can impair the patient's mobility, so help him perform active and passive range-of-motion exercises to prevent contractures and promote muscle strength.

• If the patient needs thoracentesis, remind him to breathe normally and avoid sudden movements, such as coughing or sighing, during the procedure. Monitor his vital signs, and watch for syncope. Also watch for indications that fluid is being removed too quickly: bradycardia, hypotension, pain, pulmonary edema, and cardiac arrest. Reassure the patient throughout the procedure.

⚠ ALERT

After thoracentesis, watch for respiratory distress and signs of pneumothorax (sudden onset of dyspnea and cyanosis).

• Throughout therapy, listen to the patient's fears and concerns, and answer any questions he may have. Remain with him during periods of extreme stress and anxiety. Encourage him to identify actions and care measures that help make him comfortable and relaxed. Perform these

measures, and encourage the patient to do so as well.

• Whenever possible, include the patient in care decisions, and include family members in all phases of the patient's care.

Pneumonia

Pneumonia is an acute infection of the lung parenchyma that commonly impairs gas exchange. The prognosis is generally good for people who have normal lungs and adequate host defenses before the onset of pneumonia; however, pneumonia is the sixth leading cause of death in the United States.

CAUSES AND INCIDENCE

Pneumonia can be classified in several ways. Classification by microbiologic etiology includes viral, bacterial, fungal, protozoan, mycobacterial, mycoplasmal, and rickettsial pneumonia. Classification by location looks at the part of the anatomy affected: Bronchopneumonia involves distal airways and alveoli; lobular pneumonia, part of a lobe; and lobar pneumonia, an entire lobe. (See *Pneumonia in two locations*.) Classification by type focuses on whether the pneumonia is primary or secondary: Primary pneumonia results from inhalation or aspiration of a pathogen and includes pneumococcal and viral pneumonia; secondary pneumonia may follow initial lung damage from a noxious chemical or other insult (superinfection) or may result

PNEUMONIA IN TWO LOCATIONS

These two illustrations show consolidation associated with lobar pneumonia (shown on the left) and bronchopneumonia (shown on the right).

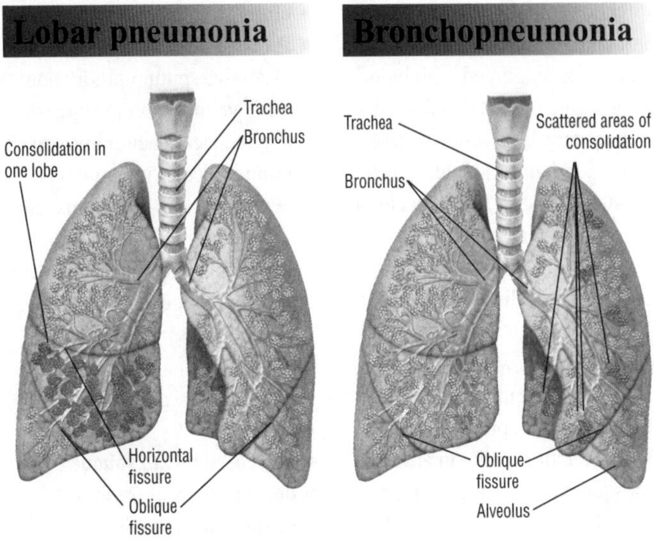

Lobar pneumonia

- Trachea
- Bronchus
- Consolidation in one lobe
- Horizontal fissure
- Oblique fissure

Bronchopneumonia

- Trachea
- Scattered areas of consolidation
- Bronchus
- Oblique fissure
- Alveolus

from hematogenous spread of bacteria from a distant focus. Aspiration pneumonia results from inhaling a foreign substance, such as food particles or vomit, into the lungs. Several other classification systems also exist.

Predisposing factors for bacterial and viral pneumonia include chronic illness and debilitation, cancer (particularly lung cancer), abdominal and thoracic surgery, atelectasis, common colds or other viral respiratory infections such as acquired immunodeficiency syndrome, chronic respiratory diseases (chronic obstructive pulmonary disease, asthma, bronchiectasis, and cystic

fibrosis), influenza, smoking, malnutrition, alcoholism, sickle cell disease, tracheostomy, exposure to noxious gases, aspiration, and immunosuppressive therapy.

Predisposing factors for aspiration pneumonia include old age, debilitation, artificial airway use, nasogastric (NG) tube feedings, impaired gag reflex, poor oral hygiene, and a decreased level of consciousness.

⚠ ALERT

In elderly or debilitated patients, bacterial pneumonia may follow influenza or a common cold. In children ages 2 to 3, respiratory viruses are the most common cause of pneumonia. In school-age children, mycoplasmal pneumonia is more common.

In bacterial pneumonia, which can occur in any part of the lungs, an infection initially triggers alveolar inflammation and edema. Capillaries become engorged with blood, causing stasis. As the alveolocapillary membrane breaks down, alveoli fill with blood and exudate, resulting in atelectasis. In severe bacterial infections, the lungs assume a heavy, liverlike appearance, as in acute respiratory distress syndrome (ARDS).

Viral infection, which typically causes diffuse pneumonia, first attacks bronchiolar epithelial cells, causing interstitial inflammation and desquamation. It then spreads to the alveoli, which fill with blood and fluid. In advanced infection, a hyaline membrane may form. As with bacterial infection, severe viral infection may clinically resemble ARDS.

In aspiration pneumonia, aspiration of gastric juices or hydrocarbons triggers similar inflammatory changes and also inactivates surfactant over a large area. Decreased surfactant leads to alveolar collapse. Acidic gastric juices may directly damage the airways and alveoli. Particles with the aspirated gastric juices may obstruct the airways and reduce airflow, which, in turn, leads to secondary bacterial pneumonia. (See *Causes of pneumonia,* pages 130–133.)

SIGNS AND SYMPTOMS

Signs and symptoms of pneumonia include:
- pleuritic chest pain
- cough
- chills
- fever
- excessive sputum production: creamy yellow sputum suggests staphylococcal pneumonia; green sputum indicates pneumonia caused by *Pseudomonas* organisms; currant jelly sputum indicates *Klebsiella* organisms; clear sputum indicates that that the patient doesn't have an infective process
- crackles
- wheezing
- rhonchi
- decreased breath sounds
- decreased vocal fremitus
- diffuse, fine crackles
- localized or extensive consolidation and pleural effusion
- headache
- sweating
- loss of appetite
- excess fatigue
- confusion (in older people).

COMPLICATIONS
- Septic shock
- Hypoxemia
- Respiratory failure
- Empyema
- Lung abscess
- Bacteremia
- Endocarditis
- Pericarditis
- Meningitis

DIAGNOSIS

- Chest X-rays disclose infiltrates, confirming the diagnosis.
- Sputum specimens for Gram stain and culture and sensitivity tests show acute inflammatory cells.
- White blood cell count is elevated in bacterial pneumonia and normal or low in viral or mycoplasmal pneumonia.
- Blood cultures reflect bacteremia and help to determine the causative organism.
- Arterial blood gas (ABG) levels vary depending on the severity of the pneumonia and the underlying lung state.
- Bronchoscopy or transtracheal aspiration allows the collection of material for culture.
- Pleural fluid may be collected for culturing.
- Pulse oximetry may show reduced arterial oxygen saturation.

TREATMENT

Antimicrobial therapy varies with the causative agent. Therapy should be reevaluated early in the course of treatment. Supportive measures include humidified oxygen therapy for hypoxemia, mechanical ventilation for respiratory failure, a high-calorie diet and adequate fluid intake, bed rest, and an analgesic to relieve pleuritic chest pain. Patients with severe pneumonia on mechanical ventilation may require positive end-expiratory pressure to promote adequate oxygenation.

Drugs

- Antimicrobials or antifungals depending on the specific causative organism to combat the infecting organism
- Analgesics to relieve pain

SPECIAL CONSIDERATIONS

- Provide supportive care to increase the patient's comfort, avoid complications, and speed recovery.
- Maintain a patent airway and adequate oxygenation. Monitor pulse oximetry and ABG levels, especially if the patient is hypoxemic. Administer supplemental oxygen if the partial pressure of arterial oxygen drops below 55 mm Hg; give oxygen cautiously if the patient has an underlying chronic lung disease.
- Teach the patient how to cough and perform deep-breathing exercises to clear secretions; encourage him to do so often. In severe pneumonia that requires endotracheal intubation or tracheostomy (with or without mechanical ventilation), provide thorough respiratory care. Suction often, using sterile technique, to remove secretions.
- Obtain sputum specimens as needed, using suctioning if the patient can't produce specimens independently. Collect specimens in a sterile container and deliver them promptly to the microbiology laboratory.
- Administer antibiotics as ordered and pain medication as needed; record the patient's response to medications. Fever and dehydration

(Text continues on page 134)

CAUSES OF PNEUMONIA

Characteristics

Viral pneumonias

Influenza

- Prognosis poor even with treatment
- 50% mortality from cardiopulmonary collapse
- Signs and symptoms: cough (initially nonproductive; later, purulent sputum), marked cyanosis, dyspnea, high fever, chills, substernal pain and discomfort, moist crackles, frontal headache, myalgia

Adenovirus

- Insidious onset
- Generally affects young adults
- Good prognosis: usually clears without residual effects
- Signs and symptoms: sore throat, fever, cough, chills, malaise, small amounts of mucoid sputum, retrosternal chest pain, anorexia, rhinitis, adenopathy, scattered crackles, rhonchi

Respiratory syncytial virus

- Most prevalent in infants and children
- Complete recovery in 1 to 3 weeks
- Signs and symptoms: listlessness, irritability, tachypnea with retraction of intercostal muscles, slight sputum production, fine moist crackles, fever, severe malaise, possibly cough or croup

Measles (rubeola)

- Signs and symptoms: fever, dyspnea, cough, small amounts of sputum, coryza, rash, cervical adenopathy

Chickenpox (varicella)

- Uncommon in children but present in 30% of adults with varicella
- Signs and symptoms: characteristic rash, cough, dyspnea, cyanosis, tachypnea, pleuritic chest pain, hemoptysis and rhonchi 1 to 6 days after onset of rash

Cytomegalovirus

- Difficult to distinguish from other nonbacterial pneumonias. In adults with healthy lung tissue, resembles mononucleosis and is generally benign; in neonates, occurs as devastating multisystemic infection; in immunocompromised hosts, varies from clinically inapparent to fatal infection
- Signs and symptoms: fever, cough, shaking chills, dyspnea, cyanosis, weakness, diffuse crackles

Diagnostic tests	Treatment
■ Chest X-ray: diffuse bilateral broncho-pneumonia radiating from hilus ■ White blood cell (WBC) count: normal to slightly elevated ■ Sputum smears: no specific organisms	■ Supportive treatment for respiratory failure includes endotracheal intubation and ventilator assistance; for fever, hypothermia blanket or antipyretics; for influenza A, amantadine (Symmetrel) or rimantadine (Flumadine).
■ Chest X-ray: patchy distribution of pneumonia, more severe than indicated by physical examination ■ WBC count: normal to slightly elevated	■ Treatment goal is to relieve symptoms.
■ Chest X-ray: patchy bilateral consolidation ■ WBC count: normal to slightly elevated	■ Supportive treatment includes humidified air, oxygen, antimicrobials (typically given until viral cause is confirmed), and aerosolized ribavirin (Virazole).
■ Chest X-ray: reticular infiltrates, sometimes with hilar lymph node enlargement ■ Lung tissue specimen: characteristic giant cells	■ Supportive treatment includes bed rest, adequate hydration, antimicrobials and, if necessary, assisted ventilation.
■ Chest X-ray: more extensive pneumonia than indicated by examination; bilateral, patchy, diffuse, nodular infiltrates ■ Sputum analysis: predominant mononuclear cells and characteristic intranuclear inclusion bodies	■ Supportive treatment includes adequate hydration and, in critically ill patients, oxygen therapy. ■ Patients who are immunocompromised also receive I.V. acyclovir (Zovirax).
■ Chest X-ray: in early stages, variable patchy infiltrates; later, bilateral, nodular, and more predominant in lower lobes ■ Percutaneous aspiration of lung tissue, transbronchial biopsy or open lung biopsy: typical intranuclear and cytoplasmic inclusions on microscopic examination (the virus can be cultured from lung tissue)	■ Supportive treatment includes adequate hydration and nutrition, oxygen therapy, and bed rest. ■ Disease is more severe in patients who are immunocompromised, warranting ganciclovir (Cytovene) or foscarnet. (Foscavir)

(continued)

CAUSES OF PNEUMONIA *(continued)*

Characteristics

Protozoan pneumonia

Pneumocystis carinii
- Occurs in immunocompromised patients
- Symptoms: dyspnea, nonproductive cough, anorexia, weight loss, fatigue, low-grade fever

Bacterial pneumonias

Streptococcus
- Caused by *Streptococcus pneumoniae*
- Signs and symptoms: sudden onset of a single, shaking chill and sustained temperature of 102° to 104° F (38.9° to 40° C); commonly preceded by upper respiratory tract infection

Klebsiella
- More likely in patients with chronic alcoholism, pulmonary disease, and diabetes
- Signs and symptoms: fever and recurrent chills; cough producing rusty, bloody, viscous sputum (currant jelly); cyanosis of lips and nail beds from hypoxemia; shallow, grunting respirations

Staphylococcus
- Commonly occurs in patients with viral illness, such as influenza or measles, and in those with cystic fibrosis
- Signs and symptoms: temperature of 102° to 104° F, recurrent shaking chills, bloody sputum, dyspnea, tachypnea, hypoxemia

Aspiration pneumonia

- Results from vomiting and aspiration of gastric or oropharyngeal contents into trachea and lungs or from ineffective swallowing muscles
- Noncardiogenic pulmonary edema possible with damage to respiratory epithelium from contact with gastric acid
- Subacute pneumonia possible with cavity formation
- Lung abscess possible if foreign body present
- Signs and symptoms: crackles, dyspnea, cyanosis, hypotension, tachycardia

Diagnostic tests	Treatment
■ Fiber-optic bronchoscopy: obtains specimen for histology studies ■ Chest X-ray: for specific infiltrations, nodular lesions, or spontaneous pneumothorax	■ Antimicrobial therapy consists of cotrimoxazole (Bactrim, Septra) or pentamidine therapy. ■ Supportive treatment includes oxygen, improved nutrition, and mechanical ventilation.
■ Chest X-ray: areas of consolidation, commonly lobar ■ WBC count: elevated ■ Sputum culture: possibly gram-positive *S. pneumoniae*	■ Antimicrobial therapy consists of penicillin G or, if the patient is allergic to penicillin, erythromycin (E-mycin); therapy is begun after obtaining culture specimen, but without waiting for results, and continues for 7 to 10 days.
■ Chest X-ray: typically, but not always, consolidation in the upper lobe that causes bulging of fissures ■ WBC count: elevated ■ Sputum culture and Gram stain: possibly gram-negative cocci *Klebsiella*	■ Antimicrobial therapy consists of an aminoglycoside and, in serious infections, a cephalosporin.
■ Chest X-ray: multiple abscesses and infiltrates; frequently empyema ■ WBC count: elevated ■ Sputum culture and Gram stain: possibly gram-positive staphylococci	■ Antimicrobial therapy consists of nafcillin or oxacillin (Bactocill) for 14 days if staphylococci are producing penicillinase. ■ A chest tube drains empyema.
■ Chest X-ray: location of areas of infiltrates (suggests diagnosis)	■ Antimicrobial therapy consists of penicillin G or clindamycin (Cleocin). ■ Supportive therapy includes oxygen therapy, suctioning, coughing, deep breathing, adequate hydration, and I.V. corticosteroids.

⧉ PREVENTION
PREVENTING PNEUMONIA

Taking the following steps can help prevent pneumonia:

- Advise patients to avoid using antibiotics indiscriminately during minor viral infections because doing so may result in upper airway colonization with antibiotic-resistant bacteria. If a patient does use antibiotics indiscriminately and then develops pneumonia, the organisms producing the pneumonia may require treatment with more toxic antibiotics.
- Encourage high-risk patients— such as those with COPD, chronic heart disease, or sickle cell disease—to receive pneumococcal vaccination (Pneumovax) and annual influenza vaccinations.

- Urge all bedridden and postoperative patients to perform deep-breathing and coughing exercises frequently. Reposition such patients often to promote full aeration and drainage of secretions. Encourage early ambulation in postoperative patients.
- To prevent aspiration during nasogastric tube feedings, elevate the patient's head, check the tube's position, and administer the formula slowly. Don't give large volumes at one time; this could cause vomiting. Keep the patient's head elevated for at least 30 minutes after the feeding. Check for residual formula at 4- to 6-hour intervals.

may require I.V. fluids and electrolyte replacement.

• Maintain adequate nutrition to offset a hypermetabolic state secondary to infection. Ask the dietary department to provide a high-calorie, high-protein diet consisting of soft, easy-to-eat foods. Encourage the patient to eat. As necessary, supplement oral feedings with nasogastric tube feedings or parenteral nutrition. Monitor fluid intake and output. Consider limiting the use of milk products because they may increase sputum production.

• Provide a quiet, calm environment for the patient, with frequent rest periods.

• Give emotional support by explaining all procedures (especially intubation and suctioning) to the patient and his family. Encourage family visits. Provide diversionary activities appropriate to the patient's age.

• To control the spread of infection, dispose of secretions properly. Tell the patient to sneeze and cough into a disposable tissue; tape a lined bag to the side of the bed for used tissues. (See *Preventing pneumonia*.)

Pneumothorax

A pneumothorax is an accumulation of air or gas between the parietal and visceral pleurae. The amount of air or gas trapped in the intrapleural space determines the degree of lung collapse. In tension pneumothorax, the air in the pleural space is under higher pressure than air in adjacent lung and vascular structures. Without prompt treatment, tension or large pneumothorax results in fatal pulmonary and circulatory impairment.

CAUSES AND INCIDENCE

A pneumothorax can be classified as spontaneous, traumatic, or tension. A spontaneous pneumothorax usually occurs in an otherwise healthy adult between the ages of 20 and 40. It may result from air leaking from ruptured congenital blebs adjacent to the visceral pleural surface, near the apex of the lung. Secondary spontaneous pneumothorax is a complication of underlying lung disease, such as chronic obstructive pulmonary disease, asthma, cystic fibrosis, tuberculosis, and whooping cough. Spontaneous pneumothorax may also occur in interstitial lung disease, such as eosinophilic granuloma or lymphangiomyomatosis.

A traumatic pneumothorax may result from insertion of a central venous line, thoracic surgery, or a penetrating chest injury, such as a gunshot or knife wound. It may also follow a transbronchial biopsy or it may occur during thoracentesis or a closed pleural biopsy. When traumatic pneumothorax follows a penetrating chest injury, it frequently coexists with hemothorax (blood in the pleural space).

In tension pneumothorax, positive pleural pressure develops as a result of traumatic pneumothorax. When air enters the pleural space through a tear in lung tissue and can't leave by the same vent, each inspiration traps air in the pleural space, resulting in positive pleural pressure. This, in turn, causes collapse of the ipsilateral lung and marked impairment of venous return, which can severely compromise cardiac output and may cause a mediastinal shift. Decreased filling of the great veins of the chest results in diminished cardiac output and lowered blood pressure. (See *Tension pneumothorax,* page 136.)

A pneumothorax can also be classified as open or closed. In open pneumothorax (usually the result of trauma), air flows between the pleural space and the outside of the body. In closed pneumothorax, air reaches the pleural space directly from the lung. (See *Open Pneumothorax,* page 136, and *Closed pneumothorax,* page 137.)

SIGNS AND SYMPTOMS

Signs and symptoms of an open pneumothorax include:

- sudden, sharp chest pain exacerbated by chest movement, breathing or coughing
- asymmetrical chest wall movement
- cyanosis
- shortness of breath
- hyperresonance or tympany
- respiratory distress
- absent breath sounds on the affected side
- chest rigidity on the affected side

TENSION PNEUMOTHORAX

In tension pneumothorax, air in the pleural space is under higher pressure than air in the adjacent lung. As the first illustration shows, air can enter the pleural space from the pleural rupture site on inspiration. However, once the air enters the pleural space, the rupture site acts as a one-way valve to present air from escaping on expiration, as shown in the second illustration.

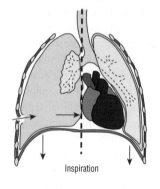

Inspiration

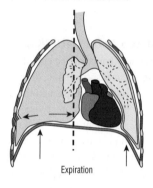

Expiration

- tachycardia
- crackling beneath the skin.

  Signs and symptoms of a closed pneumothorax include:

- sudden, sharp chest pain exacerbated by chest movement, breathing or coughing
- asymmetrical chest wall movement

OPEN PNEUMOTHORAX

Open pneumothorax results when atmospheric air (positive pressure) flows directly into the pleural cavity (negative pressure). As the air pressure in the pleural cavity becomes positive, the lung collapses on the affected side, resulting in decreased total lung capacity, vital capacity, and lung compliance.

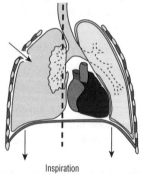

Inspiration

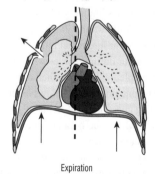

Expiration

CLOSED PNEUMOTHORAX

A closed pneumothorax occurs when air enters the pleural space from within the lung, causing increased pleural pressure that prevents lung expansion during normal inspiration. Spontaneous pneumothorax is another type of closed pneumothorax.

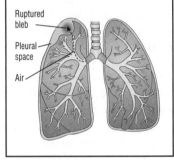

Ruptured bleb

Pleural space

Air

- cyanosis
- shortness of breath
- hyperresonance or tympany
- respiratory distress.

Signs and symptoms of a tension pneumothorax include:

- decreased cardiac output
- hypotension
- compensatory tachycardia
- tachypnea
- lung collapse
- mediastinal shift and tracheal deviation to the opposite side
- cardiac arrest.

COMPLICATIONS

- Fatal pulmonary and circulatory impairment

DIAGNOSIS

- A chest X-ray showing air in the pleural space and, possibly, mediastinal shift confirm the diagnosis.
- Arterial blood gas analysis shows a pH below 7.35, partial pressure of arterial oxygen below 80 mm Hg, and partial pressure of arterial carbon dioxide above 45 mm Hg.

TREATMENT

Treatment is conservative for spontaneous pneumothorax in which no signs of increased pleural pressure (indicating tension pneumothorax) appear, lung collapse is less than 30%, and the patient shows no signs of dyspnea or other indications of physiologic compromise. Such treatment consists of bed rest, careful monitoring of blood pressure and pulse and respiratory rates, oxygen administration and, possibly, needle aspiration of air with a large-bore needle attached to a syringe. If more than 30% of the lung is collapsed, treatment to reexpand the lung includes placing a thoracostomy tube in the second or third intercostal space in the midclavicular line (or in the fifth or sixth intercostal space in the midaxillary line), connected to a water-seal or low suction pressures.

Recurring spontaneous pneumothorax requires thoracotomy and pleurectomy; these procedures prevent recurrence by causing the lung to adhere to the parietal pleura. Traumatic and tension pneumothoraces require chest tube drainage; traumatic pneumothorax may also require surgery.

Drugs

- Antimicrobials specific to the causative agent if suspected empyema is present to combat the infecting organism

SPECIAL CONSIDERATIONS

- Urge the patient to control coughing and gasping during thoracotomy. However, after the chest tube is in place, encourage him to cough and breathe deeply (at least once an hour) to promote lung expansion.
- If the patient is undergoing chest tube drainage, watch for continuing air leakage (bubbling), indicating the lung defect has failed to close; this may require surgery. Also watch for increasing subcutaneous emphysema by checking around the neck or at the tube insertion site for crackling beneath the skin. If the patient is on a ventilator, watch for difficulty in breathing in time with the ventilator as well as pressure changes on ventilator gauges.
- Change dressings around the chest tube insertion site according to your facility's policy. Don't reposition or dislodge the tube. If it dislodges, immediately place a petroleum gauze dressing over the opening to prevent rapid lung collapse and notify the practitioner.
- Secure the chest tube drainage apparatus appropriately. Tape connections securely.
- Monitor the patient's vital signs frequently after thoracotomy. Also, for the first 24 hours, assess respiratory status by checking breath sounds hourly. Observe the chest tube site for leakage, noting the amount and color of drainage. Help the patient walk as ordered (usually on the first postoperative day) to promote deep inspiration and lung expansion.
- To reassure the patient, explain what pneumothorax is, what causes it, and all diagnostic tests and procedures. Make him as comfortable as possible. (The patient with pneumothorax is usually most comfortable sitting upright.)

⚠ ALERT

Watch for pallor, gasping respirations, and sudden chest pain. Monitor the patient's vital signs at least every hour for signs of shock, increasing respiratory distress, or mediastinal shift. Listen for breath sounds over both lungs. Falling blood pressure and rising pulse and respiratory rates may indicate tension pneumothorax, which can be fatal without prompt treatment.

Pulmonary edema

Pulmonary edema is the accumulation of fluid in the extravascular spaces of the lung. In cardiogenic pulmonary edema, fluid accumulation results from elevations in pulmonary venous and capillary hydrostatic pressures. A common complication of cardiac disorders, pulmonary edema can occur as a chronic condition or it can develop quickly, leading to cause death.

CAUSES AND INCIDENCE

Pulmonary edema generally results from left-sided heart failure due to arteriosclerotic, hypertensive, cardiomyopathic, or valvular cardiac disease. In such disorders, the compromised left ventricle can't maintain adequate cardiac output; increased pressures are transmitted to the left atrium, pulmonary veins, and pulmonary capillary bed. This increased pulmonary capillary hydrostatic force promotes transudation of intravascular fluids into the pulmonary interstitium, decreasing lung compliance and interfering with gas exchange. If colloid osmotic pressure decreases, the hydrostatic force that regulates intravascular fluids (the natural pulling force) is lost because there's no opposition. Fluid flows freely into the interstitium and alveoli, impairing gas exchange and leading to pulmonary edema. Decreased serum colloid osmotic pressure may occur as a result of nephrosis, protein-losing enteropathy, extensive burns, hepatic disease, or nutritional deficiency. (See *How pulmonary edema develops,* page 140.)

A blockage of the lymph vessels can result from compression by edema or tumor fibrotic tissue and by increased systemic venous pressure. Hydrostatic pressure in the large pulmonary veins increases, the pulmonary lymphatic system can't drain correctly into the pulmonary veins, and excess fluid moves into the interstitial space. Pulmonary edema then results from fluid accumulation. Impaired lung lymphatic drainage may occur from Hodgkin's lymphoma or obliterative lymphangitis after radiation.

Capillary injury, such as occurs in acute respiratory distress syndrome or with inhalation of toxic gases, increases capillary permeability and can also lead to pulmonary edema. The injury causes plasma proteins and water to leak out of the capillary and move into the interstitium, increasing interstitial oncotic pressure, which is normally low. As interstitial oncotic pressure begins to equal capillary oncotic pressure, the water begins to move out of the capillary and into the lungs, resulting in pulmonary edema.

Other factors that may predispose the patient to pulmonary edema include excessive infusion of I.V. fluids; mitral stenosis, which impairs left atrial emptying; pulmonary veno-occlusive disease; and kidney failure

SIGNS AND SYMPTOMS
The early signs and symptoms of pulmonary edema, which reflect interstitial fluid accumulation and diminished lung compliance, include:
- dyspnea on exertion
- paroxysmal nocturnal dyspnea
- orthopnea
- coughing
- tachycardia
- tachypnea
- dependent crackles
- jugular vein distention
- diastolic (S3) gallop.

HOW PULMONARY EDEMA DEVELOPS

The first illustration shows normal alveoli; the second shows how pulmonary edema develops.

Normal Alveoli

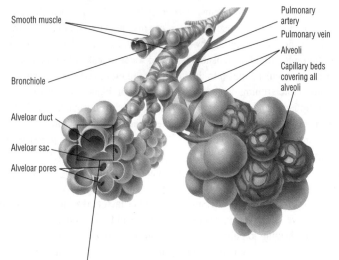

Smooth muscle

Bronchiole

Alveloar duct

Alveloar sac

Alveloar pores

Pulmonary artery

Pulmonary vein

Alveoli

Capillary beds covering all alveoli

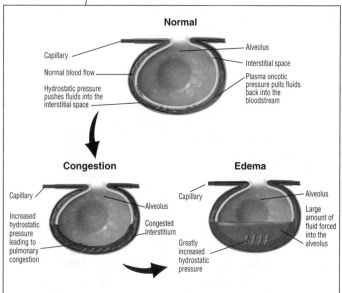

Normal

Capillary

Normal blood flow

Hydrostatic pressure pushes fluids into the interstitial space

Alveolus

Interstitial space

Plasma oncotic pressure pulls fluids back into the bloodstream

Congestion

Capillary

Increased hydrostatic pressure leading to pulmonary congestion

Alveolus

Congested interstitium

Greatly increased hydrostatic pressure

Edema

Capillary

Alveolus

Large amount of fluid forced into the alveolus

Indications of severe pulmonary edema include:

- intensification of early signs and symptoms if alveoli and bronchioles fill with fluid
- rapid, labored respirations, with more diffuse crackles and coughing that produces frothy, bloody sputum
- increased tachycardia and possible arrhythmias
- cold, clammy, diaphoretic, cyanotic skin
- falling cardiac output, marked by falling blood pressure and thready pulse.

Indications of severe heart failure with pulmonary edema may also include signs and symptoms of hypoxemia, including:

- anxiety
- restlessness
- changes in level of consciousness.

COMPLICATIONS

- Respiratory failure
- Respiratory acidosis
- Cardiac arrest

DIAGNOSIS

- Clinical features point to a working diagnosis of pulmonary edema.
- Arterial blood gas (ABG) analysis usually shows hypoxia; the partial pressure of arterial carbon dioxide is variable, and profound respiratory alkalosis and acidosis may occur.
- Chest X-rays show diffuse haziness of the lung fields and, commonly, cardiomegaly and pleural effusions.
- Ultrasonography (echocardiogram) may show weak heart muscle,

leaking or narrow heart valves, and fluid surrounding the heart.

- Pulmonary artery catheterization helps identify left-sided heart failure by showing elevated pulmonary wedge pressures; this helps rule out acute respiratory distress syndrome, in which pulmonary wedge pressure is usually normal.

TREATMENT

Treatment measures for pulmonary edema aim to reduce extravascular fluid, improve gas exchange and myocardial function and, if possible, correct any underlying pathologic conditions.

Administration of high concentrations of oxygen by a cannula, a face mask and, if the patient fails to maintain an acceptable partial pressure of arterial oxygen level, assisted ventilation improves oxygen delivery to the tissues and usually improves acid-base disturbances.

Drugs

- Diuretics, such as furosemide (Lasix) and bumetanide, to promote diuresis, reducing extravascular fluid
- Preload reducers such as nitroglycerin (Nitro-Bid, Deponit, Nitrol) to decrease pulmonary venous return, pulmonary capillary hydrostatic pressure, and fluid transudation into the pulmonary alveoli
- Afterload reducers such as captopril (Capoten) and angiotensin-converting enzyme inhibitors such as enalapril (Vasotec) to reduce systemic vascular resistance, increase cardiac output, and improve renal perfusion, promoting diuresis

- Catecholamines, such dobutamine (Dobutrex) and dopamine (Intropin), to produce vasodilation and increase inotropic state
- Phosphodiesterase enzyme inhibitors such as milrinone (Primacor), which are positive inotropic agents and vasodilators, to reduce afterload and preload and increase cardiac output
- Vasodilator drugs such as nitroprusside (Nitropress), which are potent direct smooth-muscle–relaxing agents, to reduce preload and afterload in acute episodes of pulmonary edema
- Morphine to reduce anxiety and dyspnea as well as to dilate the systemic venous bed, promoting blood flow from pulmonary circulation to the periphery

SPECIAL CONSIDERATIONS

- Carefully monitor the vulnerable patient for early signs of pulmonary edema, especially tachypnea, tachycardia, and abnormal breath sounds. Report any abnormalities. Assess for peripheral edema and weight gain, which may also indicate that fluid is accumulating in tissue.
- Administer oxygen as ordered.
- Monitor the patient's vital signs every 15 to 30 minutes while administering nitroprusside in dextrose 5% in water by I.V. drip. Protect the nitroprusside solution from light by wrapping the bottle or bag with aluminum foil, and discard unused solution after 4 hours. Watch for arrhythmias in the patient receiving cardiac glycosides and for

marked respiratory depression in the patient receiving morphine.

- Assess the patient's condition frequently, and record his response to treatment. Monitor ABG levels, oral and I.V. fluid intake, urine output and, in the patient with a pulmonary artery catheter, pulmonary end-diastolic and wedge pressures. Check the cardiac monitor often. Report changes immediately.
- Carefully record the time and amount of morphine given.
- Reassure the patient, who will be anxious as a result of hypoxia and respiratory distress. Explain all procedures. Provide emotional support to his family as well.

Pulmonary embolism

The most common pulmonary complication in hospitalized patients, pulmonary embolism is an obstruction of the pulmonary arterial bed by a dislodged thrombus, heart valve vegetation, or foreign substance. Although pulmonary infarction that results from embolism may be so mild as to be asymptomatic, massive embolism (more than 50% obstruction of pulmonary arterial circulation) and the accompanying infarction can be rapidly fatal. (See *Pulmonary emboli*.)

CAUSES AND INCIDENCE

Pulmonary embolism generally results from dislodged thrombi originating in the leg veins. More than half of such thrombi arise in the deep veins of the legs. Other less

PULMONARY EMBOLI

The illustration below shows multiple emboli in small branches of the left pulmonary artery and a single embolus in a branch of the right pulmonary artery. An area of infarction is also visible.

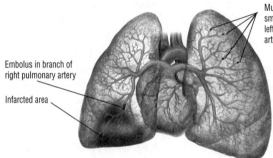

Multiple emboli in small branches of left pulmonary artery

Embolus in branch of right pulmonary artery

Infarcted area

common sources of thrombi are the pelvic veins, renal veins, hepatic vein, right side of the heart, and upper extremities. Such thrombus formation results directly from vascular wall damage, venostasis, or hypercoagulability of the blood. Trauma, clot dissolution, sudden muscle spasm, intravascular pressure changes, or a change in peripheral blood flow can cause the thrombus to loosen or fragment. Then the thrombus—now called an embolus—floats to the heart's right side and enters the lung through the pulmonary artery. There, the embolus may dissolve, continue to fragment, or grow.

By occluding the pulmonary artery, the embolus prevents alveoli from producing enough surfactant to maintain alveolar integrity. As a result, alveoli collapse and atelectasis develops. If the embolus enlarges, it may clog most or all of the pulmonary vessels and cause death.

Rarely, the emboli contain air, fat, bacteria, amniotic fluid, talc (from drugs intended for oral administration that are injected I.V. by addicts), or tumor cells.

Predisposing factors for pulmonary embolism include long-term immobility, chronic pulmonary disease, heart failure or atrial fibrillation, thrombophlebitis, polycythemia vera, thrombocytosis, autoimmune hemolytic anemia, sickle cell disease, varicose veins, recent surgery, advanced age, pregnancy, lower-extremity fractures or surgery, burns, obesity, vascular injury, cancer, I.V. drug abuse, or hormonal contraceptives.

SIGNS AND SYMPTOMS
Total occlusion of the main pulmonary artery is rapidly fatal;

smaller or fragmented emboli produce signs and symptoms that vary with the size, number, and location of the emboli. Typically, the first indication of pulmonary embolism is dyspnea, which may be accompanied by anginal or pleuritic chest pain. Other signs and symptoms include:

- tachycardia
- productive cough (sputum may be blood-tinged)
- low-grade fever
- pleural effusion
- pleural friction rub
- signs of circulatory collapse (weak, rapid pulse and hypotension)
- hypoxia (restlessness and anxiety)
  Less common signs include:
- massive hemoptysis
- chest splinting
- leg edema
- cyanosis, syncope, and distended jugular veins (with a large embolus).

COMPLICATIONS

- Pulmonary infarction
- Death

DIAGNOSIS

- A patient history should reveal predisposing conditions for pulmonary embolism, in particular Virchow's triad of factors that lead to deep vein thrombosis (DVT) formation: stasis, endothelial injury, and hypercoagulability. The history may reveal such risk factors as persistent immobility (such as long car or plane trips), cancer, pregnancy, hy-

percoagulability, previous DVT, or pulmonary emboli.

- Chest X-rays help rule out other pulmonary diseases and can show areas of atelectasis, an elevated diaphragm and pleural effusion, a prominent pulmonary artery and, occasionally, the characteristic wedge-shaped infiltrate suggestive of pulmonary infarction, or focal oligemia of blood vessels.
- A lung scan shows perfusion defects in areas beyond occluded vessels; however, it doesn't rule out microemboli.
- Pulmonary angiography is the most definitive test but requires a skilled angiographer and radiologic equipment; it also poses some risk to the patient. Its use depends on the uncertainty of the diagnosis and the need to avoid unnecessary anticoagulant therapy in a high-risk patient.
- Electrocardiography may show right axis deviation; right bundle-branch block; tall, peaked P waves; depression of ST segments and T-wave inversions (indicative of right-sided heart strain); and supraventricular tachyarrhythmias in extensive pulmonary embolism. A pattern sometimes observed is S1, Q3, and T3 (S wave in lead I, Q wave in lead III, and inverted T wave in lead III).
- Auscultation occasionally reveals a right ventricular S_3 gallop and an increased intensity of a pulmonic component of S_2. Also, crackles and a pleural rub may be heard at the embolism site.

- Arterial blood gas (ABG) analysis showing a decreased partial pressure of arterial oxygen and partial pressure of arterial carbon dioxide are characteristic of pulmonary embolism but don't always occur.
- If pleural effusion is present, thoracentesis may rule out empyema, which indicates pneumonia.

TREATMENT

Treatment is designed to maintain adequate cardiovascular and pulmonary function during resolution of the obstruction and to prevent recurrence of embolic episodes. Because most emboli resolve within 10 to 14 days, treatment consists of oxygen therapy as needed and anticoagulation with heparin to inhibit new thrombus formation, followed by oral warfarin. Heparin therapy is monitored by daily coagulation studies (partial thromboplastin time [PTT]).

Surgery is performed on patients who can't take anticoagulants, who have recurrent emboli during anticoagulant therapy, or who have been treated with thrombolytic agents or pulmonary thromboendarterectomy. This procedure (which shouldn't be performed without angiographic evidence of pulmonary embolism) consists of vena caval ligation, plication, or insertion of an inferior vena cava device to filter blood returning to the heart and lungs.

Drugs

- Anticoagulants, such as enoxaparin (Lovenox), dalteparin (Frag-

min), ardeparin (Normiflo), fondaparinux sodium (Arixtra), heparin, and warfarin (Coumadin), to prevent clot propagation and embolization
- Thrombolytic therapy with agents such as plasminogen activators (reteplase [Retavase], alteplase [Activase], urokinase [Abbokinase], streptokinase [Kabikinase, Streptase]) to enhance fibrinolysis of the pulmonary emboli and remaining thrombi
- Vasopressors to treat hypotension for emboli that cause hypotension
- Anti-infectives to treat septic emboli and endocarditis

SPECIAL CONSIDERATIONS

- Give the patient oxygen by nasal cannula or mask. Check his ABG levels if he develops fresh emboli or worsening dyspnea. Be prepared to provide endotracheal intubation with assisted ventilation if his breathing becomes severely compromised.
- Administer heparin as ordered by I.V. push or continuous drip. Monitor coagulation studies daily; effective heparin therapy raises the PTT to more than 1½ times normal. Watch closely for nosebleeds, petechiae, and other signs of abnormal bleeding and check stools for occult blood. Help protect the patient from trauma and injury; avoid I.M. injections and maintain pressure over venipuncture sites for 5 minutes or until bleeding stops to reduce hematoma.

• After the patient is stable, encourage him to move about often, and assist with isometric and range-of-motion exercises. Check his pedal pulses, temperature, and foot color to detect venostasis. Never massage his legs. Offer diversional activities to promote rest and relieve restlessness.

• Help the patient to walk as soon as possible after surgery to prevent venostasis.

• Maintain adequate nutrition and fluid balance to promote healing.

• Report frequent pleuritic chest pain so that analgesics can be prescribed. Also, provide incentive spirometry as ordered to assist in deep breathing. Provide tissues and a bag for easy disposal of expectorations.

• Warn the patient not to cross his legs because doing so promotes thrombus formation.

• To help relieve the patient's anxiety, explain procedures and treatments. Encourage the patient's family to participate in his care.

• Most patients need treatment with an oral anticoagulant such as warfarin for 3 to 6 months after a pulmonary embolism. Advise these patients to watch for signs of bleeding (bloody stools, blood in urine, and large ecchymoses), to take the prescribed medication exactly as ordered, not to change dosages without consulting their physician, and to avoid taking additional medication (including aspirin and vitamins). Stress the importance of follow-up laboratory tests (International Normalized Ratio) to monitor anticoagulant therapy.

⊠ PREVENTION

• *Encourage early ambulation for the patient predisposed to pulmonary embolism; he may also benefit from low-dose heparin given under close medical supervision.*

• *High-risk patients may receive low–molecular-weight heparin.*

Pulmonary hypertension

Pulmonary hypertension occurs when pulmonary artery pressure (PAP) rises above normal for reasons other than aging or altitude. No definitive set of values is used to diagnose pulmonary hypertension, but the National Institutes of Health defines it as a mean PAP of 25 mm Hg or more at rest. The prognosis depends on the cause of the underlying disorder.

CAUSES AND INCIDENCE

Pulmonary hypertension begins as hypertrophy of the small pulmonary arteries. The medial and intimal muscle layers of these vessels thicken, decreasing distensibility and increasing resistance. This disorder then progresses to vascular sclerosis and obliteration of small vessels. Fibrous lesions also form around the vessels, impairing distensibility and increasing vascular resistance. Pressures in the left ventricle, which receives blood from the lungs, remain normal. However, the increased pressures generated in the lungs are transmitted to the right ventricle, which supplies the pulmonary artery. Eventually, the right ventricle fails (cor pulmonale). Although oxygenation isn't severely affected initially, hypoxia and cyanosis eventually occur. Death results from cor pulmonale. (See *Changes in pulmonary hypertension,* page 148.)

In most cases, pulmonary hypertension occurs secondary to an underlying disease process. The most common cause in the United States is alveolar hypoventilation from chronic obstructive pulmonary disease. Other underlying diseases include sarcoidosis, diffuse interstitial disease, and pulmonary metastasis. In certain diseases such as scleroderma, pulmonary vascular resistance occurs secondary to hypoxemia and destruction of the alveolocapillary bed. Other disorders that cause alveolar hypoventilation without lung tissue damage include obesity, kyphoscoliosis, and obstructive sleep apnea.

Disorders that cause vascular obstruction can also result in pulmonary hypertension, including pulmonary embolism and vasculitis. Left atrial myxoma, idiopathic veno-occlusive disease, fibrosing mediastinitis, and mediastinal neoplasm cause obstruction of small or large pulmonary veins, leading to pulmonary hypertension.

Primary cardiac disease—either congenital or acquired—can also trigger the disorder. Congenital defects that cause left-to-right shunting of blood, such as patent ductus arteriosus or atrial or ventricular septal defect, increase blood flow into the lungs and, consequently, raise pulmonary vascular pressure. Acquired cardiac diseases, such as rheumatic valvular disease and mitral stenosis, increase pulmonary venous pressure by restricting blood flow returning to the heart.

Primary (or idiopathic) pulmonary hypertension is rare, occurring most commonly—and with no known cause—in women between the ages of 20 and 40. Secondary pulmonary hypertension results from existing cardiac, pulmonary, thromboembolic, or collagen vascular diseases or from the use of certain drugs.

COMPLICATIONS
- Cor pulmonale
- Cardiac failure
- Cardiac arrest

SIGNS AND SYMPTOMS
Indications of pulmonary hypertension include:
- increasing exertional dyspnea from left-sided heart failure
- fatigue and weakness from diminished tissue oxygenation
- syncope due to diminished oxygenation of brain cells
- difficulty breathing and shortness of breath from left-sided heart failure
- pain with breathing due to lactic acid buildup in the tissues
- ascites due to right-sided heart failure
- neck-vein distention from right-sided heart failure

CHANGES IN PULMONARY HYPERTENSION

The three illustrations below show the changes that occur as pulmonary hypertension progresses.

NORMAL PULMONARY ARTERY

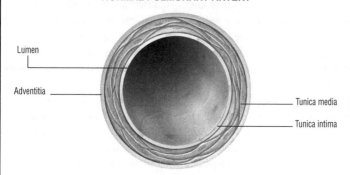

Lumen

Adventitia

Tunica media

Tunica intima

EARLY PULMONARY HYPERTENSION

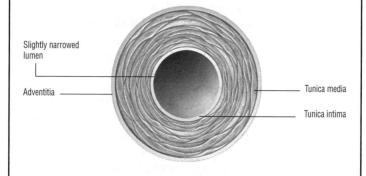

Slightly narrowed lumen

Adventitia

Tunica media

Tunica intima

LATE PULMONARY HYPERTENSION

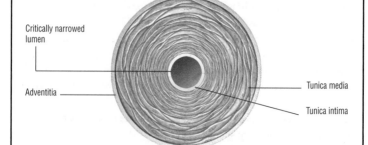

Critically narrowed lumen

Adventitia

Tunica media

Tunica intima

- restlessness, agitation, decreased level of consciousness, confusion, and memory loss due to hypoxia
- decreased diaphragmatic excursion and respiration because of hypoventilation
- possible displacement of point of maximal impulse beyond the midclavicular line due to fluid accumulation
- peripheral edema from right-sided heart failure
- easily palpable right ventricular lift due to altered cardiac output and pulmonary hypertension
- palpable and tender liver due to pulmonary hypertension
- tachycardia because of hypoxia
- systolic ejection murmur due to pulmonary hypertension and altered cardiac output
- split S2, S3, and S4 due to pulmonary hypertension and altered cardiac output
- decreased breath sounds because of fluid accumulation in the lungs
- loud, tubular breath sounds because of fluid accumulation in the lungs.

DIAGNOSIS

- Auscultation reveals abnormalities associated with the underlying disorder.
- Arterial blood gas (ABG) analysis indicates hypoxemia (decreased partial pressure of arterial oxygen).
- Electrocardiography shows right axis deviation and tall or peaked P waves in inferior leads in the patient with right ventricular hypertrophy.
- Cardiac catheterization reveals pulmonary systolic pressure above

30 mm Hg as well as increased pulmonary artery wedge pressure (PAWP) if the underlying cause is left atrial myxoma, mitral stenosis, or left-sided heart failure (otherwise normal).
- Pulmonary angiography detects filling defects in pulmonary vasculature such as those that develop in patients with pulmonary emboli.
- Pulmonary function tests may show decreased flow rates and increased residual volume in underlying obstructive disease and decreased total lung capacity in underlying restrictive disease.

TREATMENT

Treatment usually includes oxygen therapy to decrease hypoxemia and resulting pulmonary vascular resistance. It may also include vasodilator therapy (nifedipine [Procardia], diltiazem [Cardizem], or prostaglandin E). For patients with right-sided heart failure, treatment also includes fluid restriction, cardiac glycosides to increase cardiac output, and diuretics to decrease intravascular volume and extravascular fluid accumulation. Treatment also aims to correct the underlying cause.

Some patients with pulmonary hypertension may be candidates for heart-lung transplantation to improve their chances of survival.

Drugs

- Anticoagulation with warfarin (Coumadin) in those at risk for venous thromboembolism to prevent embolism formation

- Calcium channel blockers, such as nifedipine (Adalat, Procardia), diltiazem (Cardizem, Dilacor), and amlodipine (Norvasc), to produce vasodilatation in both systematic and pulmonary vascular beds
- Peripheral vasodilators, such as epoprostenol (Flolan), treprostinil (Remodulin), and iloprost (Ventavis), to dilate all vascular beds and inhibit platelet aggregation
- Diuretics such as furosemide (Lasix) to help reduce systemic congestion and edema
- Endothelin receptor antagonists, such as bosentan (Tracleer) and ambrisentan (Letairis), to reduce PAP, pulmonary vascular resistance, and mean right atrial pressure
- Phosphodiesterase type 5 enzyme inhibitors such as sildenafil (Revatio) to promote selective smooth muscle relaxation in lung vasculature, resulting in reduced pulmonary hypertension
- Cardiac glycosides such as digoxin (Lanoxin) to increase cardiac output

SPECIAL CONSIDERATIONS

- Closely observe and carefully monitor the patient and provide skilled supportive care.
- Administer oxygen therapy as ordered, and observe the patient's response. Report any signs of increasing dyspnea to the physician so he can adjust treatment accordingly.
- Monitor ABG levels for acidosis and hypoxemia. Report any change in the patient's level of consciousness at once.
- When caring for a patient with right-sided heart failure, especially one receiving diuretics, record his weight daily, carefully measure intake and output, and explain all medications and diet restrictions. Check for worsening jugular vein distention, which may indicate fluid overload.
- Monitor the patient's vital signs, especially blood pressure and heart rate. Watch for hypotension and tachycardia. If he has a pulmonary artery catheter, check PAP and PAWP as indicated. Report any changes.
- Before discharge, help the patient adjust to the limitations imposed by this disorder. Advise against overexertion, and suggest frequent rest periods between activities. Refer the patient to the social services department if he'll need special equipment such as oxygen equipment for home use. Make sure that he understands the prescribed medications and diet and the need to weigh himself daily.

Respiratory acidosis

An acid-base disturbance characterized by reduced alveolar ventilation
and manifested by hypercapnia (partial pressure of arterial carbon dioxide [$Paco_2$] greater than 45 mm
Hg), respiratory acidosis can be
acute (due to a sudden failure in
ventilation) or chronic (as in long-
term pulmonary disease). The prognosis depends on the severity of the
underlying disturbance as well as
the patient's general clinical
condition.

CAUSES AND INCIDENCE

Use of certain drugs—including
opioids, anesthetics, hypnotics,
sedatives, and some of the new de-
signer drugs such as Ecstasy—can
be a predisposing factor for respiratory acidosis because these drugs
decrease the sensitivity of the respiratory center. Other predisposing
factors include central nervous system (CNS) trauma because
medullary injury may impair ventilatory drive as well as ventilation
therapy because the use of high-flow
oxygen in chronic respiratory disorders suppresses the patient's hypoxic
drive to breathe. Neuromuscular
diseases, such as myasthenia gravis,
Guillain-Barré syndrome, and po-
liomyelitis, can result in respiratory
acidosis when the respiratory mus-

cles fail to respond properly to the
respiratory drive, decreasing alveolar ventilation.

In addition, respiratory acidosis
can result from chronic obstructive
pulmonary disease (COPD), asthma,
severe acute respiratory distress
syndrome, chronic bronchitis, a
large pneumothorax; extensive
pneumonia, pulmonary edema, and
airway obstruction or parenchymal
lung disease, which interfere with
alveolar ventilation.

A series of reactions leads to in
respiratory acidosis. When pulmonary ventilation decreases,
$Paco_2$ increases, and the CO_2 level
rises in all tissues and fluids, including the medulla and cerebrospinal
fluid. Retained CO_2 combines with
water to form carbonic acid. The
carbonic acid dissociates to release
free hydrogen and bicarbonate
(HCO_3^-) ions. Increased $Paco_2$
and free hydrogen ions stimulate the
medulla to increase respiratory
drive and expel CO_2.

As pH falls, 2, 3-diphosphoglyc-
erate accumulates in red blood cells,
where it alters hemoglobin, causing
it to release oxygen. This reduced
hemoglobin, which is strongly alkaline, picks up hydrogen ions and
CO_2 and removes them from the
serum.

As respiratory mechanisms fail,
rising $Paco_2$ stimulates the kidneys

WHAT HAPPENS IN RESPIRATORY ACIDOSIS

These illustrations explain the basic pathophysiology of respiratory acidosis.

1. Pulmonary ventilation diminishes

When pulmonary ventilation decreases, retained carbon dioxide (CO_2) in the red blood cells combines with water (H_2O) to form excess carbonic acid (H_2CO_3). The H_2CO_3 dissociates to release free hydrogen (H^+) and bicarbonate ions (HCO_3^-). In this condition, arterial blood gas (ABG) studies show increased $Paco_2$ (over 45 mm Hg) and reduced blood pH (below 7.35).

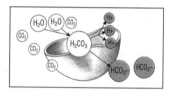

2. Oxygen saturation decreases

As pH decreases and 2,3-diphosphoglycerate (2,3-DPG) increases in red blood cells, 2,3-DPG alters hemoglobin (Hb) so it releases oxygen (O_2). This reduced Hb, which is strongly basic, picks up H^+ and CO_2, eliminating some free H^+ and excess CO_2. At this stage, arterial oxygen saturation (Sao_2) levels decrease, and the Hb dissociation curve shifts to the right.

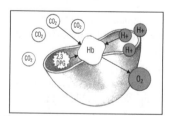

3. Respiratory rate rises

Whenever $Paco_2$ increases, CO_2 levels increase in all tissues and fluids, including the medulla and cerebrospinal fluid. CO_2 reacts with H_2O to form H_2CO_3, which dissociates into H^+ and HCO_3^-. Elevated $Paco_2$ and H^+ have a potent stimulatory effect on the medulla, increasing respirations to blow off CO_2. Look for rapid, shallow respirations and diminishing $Paco_2$ levels.

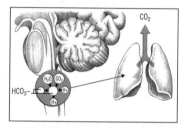

4. Blood flows to brain

The free H^+ and excess CO_2 dilate cerebral vessels and increase blood flow to the brain, causing cerebral edema and depressed central nervous system activity. At this stage, the patient experiences headache, confusion, lethargy, nausea, and vomiting.

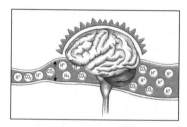

5. Kidneys compensate

As respiratory mechanisms fail, increasing $Paco_2$ stimulates the kidneys to retain HCO_3^- and sodium ions (Na^+) and to excrete H^+. As a result, more sodium bicarbonate ($NaHCO_3$) is available to buffer free H^+. Ammonium ions (NH_4^+) are also excreted to remove H^+. A patient in this condition has increased urine acidity and ammonium levels, elevated serum pH and HCO_3^- levels, and shallow, depressed respirations.

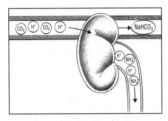

6. Acid-base balance fails

As H^+ concentration overwhelms compensatory mechanisms, H^+ ions move into the cells and potassium ions (K^+) move out. Without sufficient O_2, anaerobic metabolism produces lactic acid. Electrolyte imbalance and acidosis critically depress brain and cardiac function. ABG values in a patient in this condition show elevated $Paco_2$ and decreased Pao_2 and pH levels. The patient will experience hyperkalemia, arrhythmias, tremors, decreased level of consciousness and, possibly, coma.

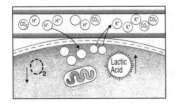

to retain HCO_3^- and sodium ions and excrete hydrogen ions. As a result, more sodium bicarbonate is available to buffer free hydrogen ions. Some hydrogen is excreted in the form of ammonium ions, neutralizing ammonia, which is an important CNS toxin.

As the hydrogen ion concentration overwhelms compensatory mechanisms, hydrogen ions move into the cells and potassium ions move out. Without enough oxygen, anaerobic metabolism produces lactic acid. Electrolyte imbalances and acidosis critically depress neurologic and cardiac functions. (See *What happens in respiratory acidosis*.)

SIGNS AND SYMPTOMS

Acute respiratory acidosis produces CNS disturbances that reflect changes in the pH of cerebrospinal fluid rather than increased CO_2 levels in cerebral circulation. Effects range from restlessness, confusion, and apprehension to somnolence, or coma and include:

• headaches resulting from cerebral vasodilation
• fine or flapping tremor (asterixis) caused by continued elevation of CO_2 levels
• dyspnea and tachypnea
• papilledema caused by increased intracranial pressure as a result of cerebral vasodilation
• depressed reflexes related to elevated CO_2 levels and CNS depression
• hypoxemia

• cardiovascular abnormalities, such as tachycardia, hypertension, and atrial and ventricular arrhythmias

• hypotension with vasodilation (bounding pulses and warm periphery).

COMPLICATIONS

• Myocardial depression leading to shock and cardiac arrest

• Profound CNS and cardiovascular deterioration due to dangerously low blood pH (less than 7.15)

• Elevated $PaCO_2$ despite optimal treatment (in chronic lung disease)

DIAGNOSIS

• Arterial blood gas (ABG) analysis confirms the diagnosis: $PaCO_2$ exceeds the normal 45 mm Hg; pH is below the normal range of 7.35 to 7.45 unless compensation has occurred; and HCO_3^- is normal in the acute stage but elevated in the chronic stage.

• Chest X-rays, computed tomography scans, and pulmonary function tests can help determine the cause.

TREATMENT

Effective treatment of respiratory acidosis requires correction of the underlying source of alveolar hypoventilation. Significantly reduced alveolar ventilation may require mechanical ventilation until the underlying condition can be treated. In COPD, this includes bronchodilators, oxygen, corticosteroids, and antibiotics for infectious conditions; drug therapy for conditions such as myasthenia gravis; removal of foreign bodies from the airway; antibiotics for pneumonia; dialysis or charcoal to remove toxic drugs; and correcting metabolic alkalosis.

Dangerously low blood pH (less than 7.15) can produce profound CNS and cardiovascular deterioration; careful administration of I.V. sodium bicarbonate may be required. In chronic lung disease, elevated CO_2 may persist despite optimal treatment.

Drugs

• Bronchodilators, such as albuterol (Proventil, Ventolin), metaproterenol (Alupent, Metaprel), ipratropium (Atrovent), theophylline (Theo-24, Theolair, Theo-Dur, Slobid), or tiotropium (Spiriva), to increase ventilation by decreasing muscle tone in both small and large airways in the lungs

• Benzodiazepine antagonists such as flumazenil (Romazicon) to reverse the CNS-depressant effects in patients with benzodiazepine overdose

• Opioid antagonists such as naloxone to reverse the effects of opiates and improve ventilation

⚠ ALERT

Opioid antagonists may precipitate withdrawal symptoms in patients who are addicted to opiates. Also, the immediate effect is short lived and the patient needs repeated doses for the drug to continue to be effective.

SPECIAL CONSIDERATIONS

• Be alert for critical changes in the patient's respiratory, CNS, and cardiovascular functions. Report such changes as well as any variations in ABG values or electrolyte status immediately. Also, maintain adequate hydration.

• Maintain a patent airway and provide adequate humidification if acidosis requires mechanical ventilation. Perform tracheal suctioning regularly and vigorous chest physiotherapy if ordered. Continuously monitor ventilator settings and respiratory status.

⚛ PREVENTION

• *To prevent respiratory acidosis, closely monitor patients with COPD and chronic CO_2 retention for signs of acidosis. Also, administer oxygen at low flow rates; closely monitor all patients who receive opioids and sedatives. Instruct patients who have received general anesthesia to turn, cough, and perform deep-breathing exercises frequently to prevent the onset of respiratory acidosis.*

Respiratory alkalosis

Respiratory alkalosis is an acid-base disturbance characterized by a decrease in the partial pressure of arterial carbon dioxide ($Paco_2$) to less than 35 mm Hg, which is due to alveolar hyperventilation. Uncomplicated respiratory alkalosis leads to a decrease in hydrogen ion concentration, which results in elevated blood pH. Hypocapnia occurs when the elimination of carbon dioxide (CO_2) by the lungs exceeds the production of CO_2 at the cellular level.

CAUSES AND INCIDENCE

Causes of respiratory alkalosis fall into two categories: pulmonary and nonpulmonary. Pulmonary causes include severe hypoxemia, pneumonia, interstitial lung disease, pulmonary vascular disease, and acute asthma. Nonpulmonary causes include anxiety, fever, aspirin toxicity, metabolic acidosis, central nervous system (CNS) disease (inflammation or tumor), sepsis, hepatic failure, and pregnancy.

Respiratory alkalosis results when pulmonary ventilation increases more than needed to maintain normal CO_2 levels, leading to the exhalation of excessive amounts of CO_2. The consequent hypocapnia leads to a chemical reduction of carbonic acid, excretion of hydrogen and bicarbonate (HCO_3^-) ions, and a rising pH. In defense against the increasing serum pH, the hydrogen-potassium buffer system pulls hydrogen ions out of the cells and into the blood in exchange for potassium ions. The hydrogen ions entering the blood combine with available HCO_3^- ions to form carbonic acid, and the pH falls.

Hypocapnia stimulates the carotid and aortic bodies as well as the medulla, increasing the heart rate (which hypokalemia can further aggravate) but not the blood pressure. At the same time, hypocapnia causes cerebral vasoconstriction and decreased cerebral blood flow. It also overexcites the medulla, pons, and other parts of the autonomic nervous system. When hypocapnia

WHAT HAPPENS IN RESPIRATORY ALKALOSIS

This series of illustrations shows how respiratory alkalosis develops at the cellular level.

1. When pulmonary ventilation increases above the amount needed to maintain normal carbon dioxide (CO_2) levels, excessive amounts of CO_2 are exhaled. This causes hypocapnia (a fall in $Paco_2$), which leads to a reduction in carbonic acid (H_2CO_3) production, a loss of hydrogen ions (H^+) and bicarbonate ions (HCO_3^-), and a subsequent rise in pH. *Look for a pH level above 7.45, a $Paco_2$ level below 35 mm Hg, and an HCO_3^- level below 22 mEq/L.*

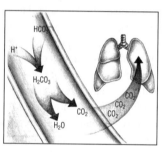

2. In defense against the rising pH, H^+ are pulled out of the cells and into the blood in exchange for potassium ions (K). The H^+ entering the blood combine with HCO_3^- to form H_2CO_3, which lowers pH. *Look for a further decrease in HCO_3^- levels, a fall in pH, and a fall in serum potassium levels (hypokalemia).*

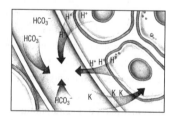

3. Hypocapnia stimulates the carotid and aortic bodies and the medulla, which causes an increase in heart rate without an increase in blood pressure. *Look for angina, electrocardiogram changes, restlessness, and anxiety.*

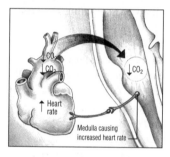

4. Simultaneously, hypocapnia produces cerebral vasoconstriction, which prompts a reduction in cerebral blood flow. Hypocapnia also overexcites the medulla, pons, and other parts of the autonomic nervous system. *Look for increasing anxiety, diaphoresis, dyspnea, alternating periods of apnea and hyperventilation, dizziness, and tingling in the fingers or toes.*

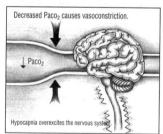

Decreased $Paco_2$ causes vasoconstriction.

$\downarrow Paco_2$

Hypocapnia overexcites the nervous system.

(continued)

WHAT HAPPENS IN RESPIRATORY ALKALOSIS *(continued)*

5. When hypocapnia lasts more than 6 hours, the kidneys increase secretion of HCO_3^- and reduce excretion of H^+. Periods of apnea may result if the pH remains high and the $Paco_2$ remains low. *Look for slowed respiratory rate, hypoventilation, and Cheyne-Stokes respirations.*

6. Continued low $Paco_2$ increases cerebral and peripheral hypoxia from vasoconstriction. Severe alkalosis inhibits calcium (Ca) ionization, which in turn causes increased nerve excitability and muscle contractions. Eventually, the alkalosis overwhelms the central nervous system and the heart. *Look for decreasing level of consciousness, hyperreflexia, carpopedal spasm, tetany, arrhythmias, seizures, and coma.*

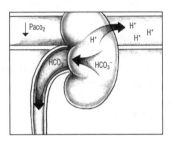
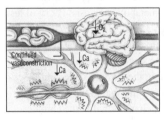

lasts more than 6 hours, the kidneys secrete more HCO_3^- and less hydrogen. Full renal adaptation to respiratory alkalosis requires normal volume status and renal function, and it may take several days.

Continued low $Paco_2$ and the vasoconstriction it causes increases cerebral and peripheral hypoxia. Severe alkalosis inhibits calcium ionization; as calcium ions become unavailable, nerves and muscles become progressively more excitable. Eventually, alkalosis overwhelms the CNS and the heart. (See *What happens in respiratory alkalosis.*)

SIGNS AND SYMPTOMS

Indications of respiratory alkalosis include:
- deep, rapid breathing, possibly exceeding 40 breaths/minute (similar to Kussmaul's respirations)
- light-headedness or dizziness (due to below-normal CO_2 levels that decrease cerebral blood flow)
- agitation
- circumoral and peripheral paresthesias
- carpopedal spasms
- twitching (possibly progressing to tetany)
- muscle weakness.
- cardiac arrhythmias that may fail to respond to conventional treatment
- seizures.

COMPLICATIONS

• Cardiac arrhythmias that may not respond to conventional treatment as the hemoglobin-oxygen buffer system becomes overwhelmed

• Hypocalcemic tetany and seizures

• Periods of apnea if pH remains high and $Paco_2$ remains low

DIAGNOSIS

• Arterial blood gas (ABG) analysis confirms respiratory alkalosis and rules out respiratory compensation for metabolic acidosis: $Paco_2$ of less than 35 mm Hg; pH elevated in proportion to the fall in $Paco_2$ in the acute stage, but falling toward normal in the chronic stage; and HCO_3^- normal in the acute stage, but below normal in the chronic stage.

• Chest X-rays or pulmonary function tests may aid in diagnosing possible lung disease.

TREATMENT

Treatment is designed to eradicate the underlying condition—for example, removing ingested toxins, treating fever or sepsis, providing oxygen for acute hypoxemia, and treating CNS disease. When hyperventilation is caused by severe anxiety, the patient may be instructed to breathe into a paper bag, which increases CO_2 levels and helps relieve anxiety.

Prevention of hyperventilation in patients receiving mechanical ventilation requires monitoring ABG levels and adjusting tidal volume and minute ventilation.

Drugs

• Benzodiazepines, such as alprazolam (Xanax) and lorazepam (Ativan), to treat hyperventilation resulting from anxiety and panic attacks; these agents bind to specific receptor sites and potentiate the effects of gamma-aminobutyrate (GABA) and facilitate inhibitory GABA neurotransmission and other inhibitory transmitters

• Selective serotonin reuptake inhibitors such as paroxetine (Paxil) to treat hyperventilation associated with anxiety

• Tricyclic antidepressants such as doxepin (Sinequan) to provide antidepressant and anxiolytic effects, thereby reducing hyperventilation

SPECIAL CONSIDERATIONS

• Watch for and report any changes in neurologic, neuromuscular, or cardiovascular functions.

• Remember that twitching and cardiac arrhythmias may be associated with alkalemia and electrolyte imbalances. Monitor ABG and serum electrolyte levels closely, reporting any variations immediately.

• Explain all diagnostic tests and procedures to reduce anxiety.

Respiratory distress syndrome

Respiratory distress syndrome (RDS), also called hyaline membrane disease, is the most common cause of neonatal mortality. In the United States alone, it occurs in approximately 20,000 to 30,000 infants each year. RDS occurs in preterm neonates and is a complication in about 1% of pregnancies. Approximately 50% of the neonates born at 26 to 28 weeks' gestation develop RDS, compared to fewer than 30% of preterm neonates born at 30 to 31 weeks. Aggressive management using mechanical ventilation can improve the prognosis, but some surviving neonates may develop some degree of bronchopulmonary dysplasia.

CAUSES AND INCIDENCE

Although the neonate's respiratory system has developed airways and alveoli by the 27th week of gestation, the neonate has weak intercostal muscles and an immature alveolar capillary system. The preterm neonate with RDS develops widespread alveolar collapse because of a lack of surfactant, a lipoprotein present in alveoli and respiratory bronchioles. Surfactant lowers surface tension and helps prevent alveolar collapse, especially at the end of expiration. This surfactant deficiency results in widespread atelectasis, which leads to inadequate alveolar ventilation with shunting of blood through collapsed areas of lung. With alveolar collapse, ventilation decreases and hypoxemia develops. The resulting pulmonary injury and inflammatory reaction lead to edema and swelling of the interstitial space, thus impeding gas exchange between the capillaries and the functional alveoli. The inflammation also stimulates pro-

duction of hyaline membranes composed of white fibrin accumulation in the alveoli. These deposits further reduce gas exchange in the lungs and decrease lung compliance, resulting in increased work of breathing.

Decreased alveolar ventilation results in a decreased ventilation-perfusion ratio and pulmonary arteriolar vasoconstriction. The pulmonary vasoconstriction can result in increased right cardiac volume and pressure, causing blood to be shunted from the right atrium, through a patent foramen ovale, and into the left atrium. Increased pulmonary resistance also results in deoxygenated blood passing through the ductus arteriosus, totally bypassing the lungs, and causing a right-to-left shunt. The shunt further increases hypoxia.

Because of the neonate's immature lungs and already increased metabolic rate, he must expend more energy to ventilate collapsed alveoli. This further increases oxygen demand and contributes to cyanosis. The infant attempts to compensate with rapid shallow breathing, causing an initial respiratory alkalosis as carbon dioxide is expelled. The increased effort at lung expansion causes respirations to slow and respiratory acidosis to occur, leading to respiratory failure.

RDS occurs almost exclusively in neonates born before 37 weeks' gestation. The incidence is greatest in those with birth weights of 500 to 750 grams, occurring in about 71%

of these infants. Infants of diabetic mothers, those born by cesarean birth, second-born twins, infants with perinatal asphyxia, and those delivered suddenly after antepartum hemorrhage are more commonly affected.

SIGNS AND SYMPTOMS

Although a neonate with RDS may breathe normally at first, he usually develops rapid, shallow respirations within minutes or hours of birth, with intercostal, subcostal, or sternal retractions; nasal flaring; and audible expiratory grunting. This grunting is a natural compensatory mechanism designed to produce positive end-expiratory pressure (PEEP) and prevent further alveolar collapse.

Severe disease is marked by apnea, bradycardia, and cyanosis (from hypoxemia, left-to-right shunting through the foramen ovale, or right-to-left intrapulmonary shunting through atelectatic regions of the lung). Other clinical features include:

- pallor
- frothy sputum
- low body temperature as a result of an immature nervous system and the absence of subcutaneous fat.

⚠ ALERT

Suspect RDS in a pregnant mother who might give birth to a neonate with RDS if the mother has a history that includes preterm birth (before 28 weeks gestation), cesarean birth, diabetes, or antepartum hemorrhage.

COMPLICATIONS

- Pneumothorax
- Pneumomediastinum
- Pneumopericardium
- Bronchopulmonary dysplasia
- Intraventricular bleed
- Hemorrhage into lungs after surfactant use
- Retinopathy of prematurity
- Delayed mental development or mental retardation

DIAGNOSIS

- Signs of respiratory distress in a preterm neonate during the first few hours of life strongly suggest RDS but chest X-rays and arterial blood gas (ABG) analysis are required for confirmation.
- A chest X-ray may be normal for the first 6 to 12 hours (in 50% of neonates with RDS), but 24 hours after birth, it will show characteristic ground-glass appearance and air bronchograms.
- ABG analysis shows decreased partial pressure of arterial oxygen; normal, decreased, or increased partial pressure of arterial carbon dioxide; and decreased pH (from respiratory or metabolic acidosis or both).
- Chest auscultation reveals normal or diminished air entry and crackles (rare in early stages).
- When a cesarean birth is necessary before 36 weeks' gestation, amniocentesis allows determination of the lecithin/sphingomyelin (L/S) ratio and the presence of phosphatidylglycerol; an L/S ratio of more than 2:1 and the presence of

phosphatidylglycerol indicate a lower likelihood of RDS.

TREATMENT

An infant with RDS requires vigorous respiratory support. Warm, humidified, oxygen-enriched gases are administered by oxygen hood or, if such treatment fails, by mechanical ventilation. Severe cases may require mechanical ventilation with PEEP or continuous positive airway pressure (CPAP) administered by nasal prongs or, when necessary, endotracheal (ET) intubation. Special ventilation techniques, including high-frequency jet ventilation and high-frequency oscillatory ventilation, can be used on patients resistant to conventional mechanical ventilation. Extracorporeal membrane oxygenation, the last choice for ventilation, is only available in certain specialized facilities.

Treatment also includes use of a radiant warmer or Isolette for thermoregulation, administration of I.V. fluids and sodium bicarbonate to control acidosis and maintain fluid and electrolyte balance, and tube feedings or total parenteral nutrition if the neonate is too weak to eat. In addition, studies show that administration of surfactant by an ET tube can improve the course of RDS and reduce mortality or prevent RDS in a neonate who is at high risk but hasn't yet developed signs of the disorder.

Drugs

● Adrenal corticosteroids such as methylprednisolone (Medrol, Solu-Medrol), which have anti-inflammatory effects, to help dampen the fibrotic response and allow for salvage of viable lung tissue

● Surfactants such as calfactant (Infasurf) to reduce surface tension and stabilize alveoli, decreasing the work of breathing and increasing lung compliance

SPECIAL CONSIDERATIONS

● Provide continual assessment and monitoring in an intensive care nursery for the neonate.

● Closely monitor arterial blood gas levels as well as fluid intake and output. If the neonate has an umbilical catheter (arterial or venous), check for arterial hypotension or abnormal central venous pressure. Watch for complications, such as infection, thrombosis, or decreased circulation to the legs. If the neonate has a transcutaneous oxygen monitor, change the site of the lead placement every 2 to 4 hours.

● To evaluate his progress, assess skin color, rate and depth of respirations, severity of retractions, nostril flaring, frequency of expiratory grunting, frothing at the lips, and restlessness.

● Regularly assess the effectiveness of oxygen or ventilator therapy. Evaluate every change in fraction of inspired oxygen and PEEP or CPAP by monitoring arterial oxygen saturation or ABG levels. Adjust the PEEP or CPAP as indicated, based on findings.

● Keep in mind that neonates receive mechanical ventilation in a pressure-limited mode rather than the volume-limited mode used in adults.

• When the neonate is on mechanical ventilation, watch carefully for signs of barotrauma (an increase in respiratory distress and subcutaneous emphysema) and accidental disconnection from the ventilator. Check ventilator settings frequently. Be alert for signs of complications of PEEP or CPAP therapy, such as decreased cardiac output, pneumothorax, and pneumomediastinum. Mechanical ventilation increases the risk of infection in the preterm neonate, so preventive measures are essential.

• As needed, arrange for follow-up care with a neonatal ophthalmologist to check for retinal damage. Preterm neonates in an oxygen-rich environment are at increased risk for developing retinopathy of prematurity.

• Monitor the infant for bronchopulmonary dysplasia, which may occur in those treated with oxygen and positive-pressure ventilation.

• Teach the parents about their neonate's condition and, if possible, let them participate in his care (using sterile technique) to encourage normal parent-infant bonding. Advise parents that full recovery may take up to 12 months. When the prognosis is poor, prepare the parents for the neonate's impending death and offer emotional support.

• Help reduce mortality in the neonate with RDS by detecting respiratory distress early. Recognize intercostal retractions and grunting, especially in a preterm neonate, as signs of RDS; make sure the neonate receives immediate treatment.

⊠ PREVENTION

• *Prenatal care can help prevent prematurity.*

• *Corticosteroids may be administered to the mother to stimulate surfactant production in a fetus at high risk for preterm deliveries.*

• *Delaying birth as much as possible of a mother in preterm labor may prevent RDS.*

Respiratory syncytial virus infection

Respiratory syncytial virus (RSV) infection results from a subgroup of the myxoviruses that resemble paramyxovirus. RSV infection is the leading cause of lower respiratory tract infections in infants and young children. It's the major cause of pneumonia, tracheobronchitis, and bronchiolitis in this age group and a suspected cause of the fatal respiratory diseases of infancy.

CAUSES AND INCIDENCE

The organism that causes RSV is transmitted from person to person by respiratory secretions and has an incubation period of 4 to 5 days. Inoculation of the virus occurs in the upper respiratory tract in respiratory epithelial cells. The virus spreads down the respiratory tract by cell-to-cell transfer of the virus. The illness may begin with upper respiratory signs and symptoms and progress rapidly over 1 to 2 days to the development of diffuse small airway disease, characterized by cough, runny nose, wheezing and crackles, low-grade fever, and decreased oral intake. Antibody titers seem to indicate that few children younger than age 4 escape contracting some form of RSV, even if it's mild. In fact, RSV is the only viral disease that has its maximum impact during the first few months of life (incidence of RSV bronchiolitis peaks at age 2 months). School-age children, adolescents, and young adults with mild reinfections are probably the source of infection for infants and young children. Reinfection is common, producing milder symptoms than the primary infection.

This virus occurs in annual epidemics during the late winter and early spring in temperate climates and during the rainy season in the tropics. It can also be seen in immunocompromised adults, especially patients with bone marrow transplants. RSV has also been identified in patients with a variety of central nervous system disorders, such as meningitis and myelitis.

SIGNS AND SYMPTOMS

Clinical features of RSV infection vary in severity from mild, coldlike signs and symptoms to bronchiolitis or bronchopneumonia and, in a few patients, severe, life-threatening lower respiratory tract infections. Other signs and symptoms include:
- coughing
- wheezing
- malaise
- pharyngitis
- dyspnea
- inflamed mucous membranes in the nose and throat.

COMPLICATIONS
- Pneumonia
- Bronchiolitis
- Tracheobronchitis
- Otitis media (in infants)
- Apnea
- Respiratory failure

DIAGNOSIS
- Clinical findings and epidemiologic information provide a diagnosis.
- Many facilities use fluid obtained from the nose to perform rapid tests to detect the virus.
- Cultures of nasal and pharyngeal secretions may show RSV; however, the virus is labile, so cultures aren't always reliable.
- Serum antibody titers may be elevated.
- Indirect immunofluorescent and ELISA methods, recently developed serologic techniques, to show the presence of the virus in nasal secretions.
- Chest X-rays help detect pneumonia.

TREATMENT

Treatment aims to support respiratory function, maintain fluid balance, and relieve symptoms.

Drugs

- Ribavirin (Virazole) in aerosol form for severely ill patients or those at high risk for complications, initiated promptly at the onset of the infection to inhibit the virus from replicating
- Bronchodilators, such as albuterol (Salbutamol, Proventil, Ventolin) or racemic epinephrine (microNefrin, Nephron, S-2), to decrease muscle tone in the small and large airways, increasing ventilation
- Antibody immunoglobulins such as palivizumab (Synagis) for high-risk patients as prophylaxis against RSV infection

SPECIAL CONSIDERATIONS

- Monitor respiratory status, including rate and pattern. Watch for nasal flaring or retraction, cyanosis, pallor, and dyspnea; auscultate for wheezing, rhonchi, or other signs of respiratory distress. Monitor arterial blood gas levels and oxygen saturation.
- Maintain a patent airway, and be especially watchful when the patient has periods of acute dyspnea. Perform percussion and provide drainage and suction when necessary. Provide a high-humidity atmosphere. Semi-Fowler's position may help prevent aspiration of secretions.
- Monitor intake and output carefully. Observe for signs of dehydration such as decreased skin turgor. Encourage the patient to drink plenty of high-calorie fluids. Administer I.V. fluids as needed.

- Promote bed rest. Plan your nursing care to allow uninterrupted rest.
- Hold and cuddle infants; talk to and play with toddlers. Offer diversionary activities that are appropriate for the child's condition and age. Encourage parental visits and cuddling. Restrain the child only as necessary.
- Impose droplet precautions. Enforce strict hand hygiene because RSV may be transmitted from contaminated surfaces. Avoid hand contact with the nose or eyes; wear a surgical mask and eye protection.

❯ PREVENTION

- *Make sure that staff members with respiratory illnesses don't care for infants.*
- *Hand washing and cleaning of environmental surfaces help prevent RSV transmission; in the hospital setting, isolating patients and wearing a mask and gown during close contact with infected children help control nosocomial spread.*

Rotavirus

Rotavirus is the most common cause of severe diarrhea among children. The disease is characterized by vomiting and watery diarrhea, commonly accompanied by fever and abdominal pain, that lasts for 3 to 8 days.

In the United States and other countries with a temperate climate, the disease has a winter seasonal pattern, with annual epidemics occurring from November to May. The illness occurs most often in infants and young children; the disease occurs most commonly in children younger than age 5.

CAUSES AND INCIDENCE

The primary mode of transmission is fecal-oral, although some have reported low titers of virus in respiratory tract secretions and other body fluids. Because of the endurance of the virus in the environment, transmission may occur through ingestion of contaminated water or food or contact with contaminated surfaces.

Rotavirus infections lead to malabsorption as a result of impaired hydrolysis of carbohydrates and excessive fluid loss from the intestine. Increased motility further exacerbates the illness, which may be secondary to virus-induced functional changes in the epithelium of the villus. In immunocompromised patients, infection may occur in another organ system, although this rarely happens in patients who aren't immunocompromised.

Even before signs and symptoms appear, the virus is shed in high titers in stool, and billions of rotavirus particles continue to be passed in stool for up to 10 days after signs and symptoms appear. Small numbers of the rotavirus may lead to infection, which can occur if a baby puts contaminated fingers or other objects into its mouth; young children can also pass the virus on to siblings and parents.

Immunity after infection is incomplete, but recurrent infections tend to be less severe than the original infection. Rotavirus is responsible for the hospitalization of about 80,000 children each year in the United States and for the deaths of between 352,000 and 592,000 children annually worldwide.

Rotavirus is the most common diagnosis for young children with acute diarrhea, but other causes of diarrhea include bacteria (*Salmonella, Shigella,* and *Campylobacter* are the most common), parasites (*Giardia* and *Cryptosporidium* are the most common), localized infection elsewhere, antibiotic-associated adverse effects (such as those related to treatment for *Clostridium difficile*), and food poisoning. Noninfectious causes include overfeeding (particularly of fruit juices), irritable bowel syndrome, celiac disease, milk protein intolerance, lactose intolerance, cystic fibrosis, and inflammatory bowel syndrome.

SIGNS AND SYMPTOMS

Signs and symptoms of infection with rotavirus include:
- fever
- nausea
- vomiting
- diarrhea.

COMPLICATIONS
- Severe dehydration
- Shock
- Skin breakdown

DIAGNOSIS
- Rapid antigen testing reveals the rotavirus in stool specimens.

TREATMENT

For a person with a healthy immune system, rotavirus gastroenteritis is a self-limited illness, lasting only days. Treatment is nonspecific and consists of oral rehydration therapy to prevent dehydration.

Drugs

• Rotavirus vaccine (RotaTeq), a live, oral vaccine given in three doses at ages 2, 4, and 6 months, to prevent infection with rotavirus

SPECIAL CONSIDERATIONS

• Enforce strict hand-washing and careful cleaning of all equipment, including the child's toys, to prevent the spread of rotavirus.

• Implement contact precautions.

• Help the patient maintain adequate hydration. Remember that dehydration occurs rapidly in infants and young children. Include ice pops, gelatin, and ice chips in the patient's diet to help maintain hydration.

• Breast-fed infants should continue to nurse without restrictions. Lactose-free soybean formulas may be used for bottle-fed infants.

• Carefully monitor intake and output (including stools).

• Clean the perineum thoroughly to prevent skin breakdown.

• Instruct the parents about proper hand-washing techniques for themselves and the infant. Provide instructions about diaper changing and cleaning all affected surfaces.

• Teach parents and caregivers how to measure intake and output. Tell them to notify their practitioner about any increased diarrhea or dehydration.

⊵ PREVENTION

• *Because rotavirus is contagious, explain the importance of good hand-washing technique to caregivers. Tell them not to allow asymptomatic children to play with symptomatic children during the diarrheal phase of the illness.*

• *Daycare centers should keep symptomatic children together and separated from asymptomatic children; staff members who take care of symptomatic children should also be segregated if possible. Objects that have been in contact with the virus should be disinfected to prevent viral spread.*

• *Health care workers need to be extra vigilant about hand washing during outbreaks.*

S

Sarcoidosis

Sarcoidosis is a multisystem, granulomatous disorder that characteristically produces lymphadenopathy, pulmonary infiltration, and skeletal, liver, eye, or skin lesions. Acute sarcoidosis usually resolves within 2 years. Chronic, progressive sarcoidosis, which is uncommon (occurring in 10% of cases), is associated with pulmonary fibrosis and progressive pulmonary disability.

CAUSES AND INCIDENCE

The cause of sarcoidosis is unknown, but several factors may play a role, including a hypersensitivity response (possibly from T-cell imbalance) to such agents as atypical mycobacteria, fungi, and pine pollen; a genetic predisposition (suggested by a slightly higher incidence of sarcoidosis within the same family); and an extreme immune response to infection.

Organ dysfunction results from an accumulation of T lymphocytes, mononuclear phagocytes, and nonsecreting epithelial granulomas, which distort normal tissue architecture. Evidence suggests that the disease is a result of exaggerated cellular immune response to a limited class of antigens.

The disease's true prevalence isn't known because of underreporting in younger populations. It occurs at an annual incidence in adults of 10.9 per cases 100,000 people in whites and 35.5 cases per 100,000 people in blacks. In both children and adult, sarcoidosis may be asymptomatic and remain undiagnosed.

More than 70% of childhood cases in the United States occur in Virginia, North Carolina, South Carolina, and Arkansas, suggesting the southeastern and south central states are endemic for childhood sarcoidosis. Most reported childhood cases occur in patients ages 13 to 15 years; in adults, the majority of cases are reported in patients ages 20 to 30 years. (See *Lung changes in sarcoidosis,* page 168.)

SIGNS AND SYMPTOMS

Initial indications of sarcoidosis include arthralgia (in the wrists, ankles, and elbows), fatigue, malaise, and weight loss. Other clinical features vary according to the extent and location of the fibrosis:
• Respiratory sarcoidosis is marked by breathlessness, cough (usually nonproductive), and substernal pain.
• Cutaneous involvement can cause erythema nodosum, subcutaneous skin nodules with maculopapular eruptions, and extensive nasal mucosal lesions.

LUNG CHANGES IN SARCOIDOSIS

NORMAL LUNGS AND ALVEOLI

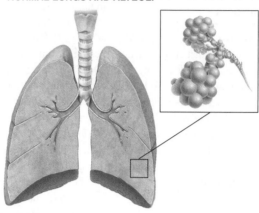

GRANULOMATOUS TISSUE FORMATION

ALVEOLITIS

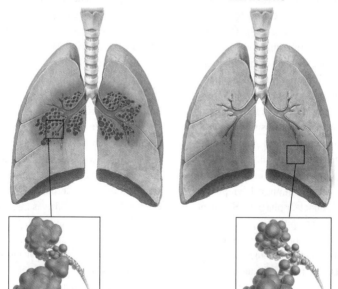

- Ophthalmic involvement can cause anterior uveitis and glaucoma.
- Lymphatic sarcoidosis can result in bilateral hilar and right paratracheal lymphadenopathy and splenomegaly.
- Musculoskeletal signs and symptoms include muscle weakness, polyarthralgia, pain, and punched-out lesions on phalanges.
- Hepatic involvement causes granulomatous hepatitis.
- Genitourinary involvement can cause hypercalciuria.
- Cardiovascular involvement can result in arrhythmias.
- Central nervous system signs and symptoms include cranial or peripheral nerve palsies, basilar meningitis, seizures, and diabetes insipidus.

COMPLICATIONS

- Pulmonary fibrosis
- Pulmonary hypertension
- Cor pulmonale

DIAGNOSIS

- Typical clinical features with appropriate laboratory data and X-ray findings suggest sarcoidosis.
- A positive skin lesion biopsy supports the initial diagnosis.
- Chest X-rays reveal bilateral hilar and right paratracheal adenopathy with or without diffuse interstitial infiltrates; occasionally, large nodular lesions present in lung parenchyma.
- Lymph node or lung biopsy reveals noncaseating granulomas with negative cultures for mycobacteria and fungi.

- Pulmonary function tests show decreased total lung capacity and compliance as well as decreased diffusing capacity.
- Arterial blood gas (ABG) analysis reveals decreased arterial oxygen tension.
- A negative tuberculin skin test, fungal serologies, and sputum cultures for mycobacteria and fungi as well as negative biopsy cultures help rule out infection.

TREATMENT

Sarcoidosis that produces no symptoms requires no treatment. Because sarcoidosis can cause varied signs and symptoms, pulmonologists, rheumatologists, and ophthalmologists may need to be consulted to provide specific care for those areas affected. Those severely affected with sarcoidosis require treatment with corticosteroids. Such therapy is usually continued for 1 to 2 years, but some patients may need lifelong therapy. If organ failure occurs (although this is rare), transplantation may be required. Patients with hypercalcemia should maintain a low-calcium diet and avoid direct exposure to sunlight.

Drugs

- Corticosteroids such as prednisone (Deltasone, Orasone) to deter granuloma formation and reduce inflammation
- Azathioprine (Imuran, Azasan) to act as a steroid-sparing agent, which affects the autoimmune process, to prevent inflammation caused by the infection

- Chlorambucil (Leukeran) used to act as a steroid-sparing agent and, at high doses, as an alkalizing agent
- Cyclosporine (Neoral, Gengraf), a fungus-derived cyclic peptide, to suppress activated T-cells in the lungs
- Immunosuppressive agents such as methotrexate (Folex PFS, Rheumatrex) for persistent active or progressive disease unresponsive to corticosteroids to deter granuloma formation and reduce inflammation
- Pentoxifylline (Trental) to inhibit formation and maintenance of granulomas
- Infliximab (Remicade) monoclonal antibody to neutralize tumor necrosis factor antagonists, which are thought to accelerate the inflammatory process in sarcoidosis

SPECIAL CONSIDERATIONS

- Watch for and report any complications. Be aware of abnormal laboratory results (anemia, for example) that could alter patient care.
- For the patient with arthralgia, administer analgesics as ordered. Record signs of progressive muscle weakness.
- Provide a nutritious, high-calorie diet and plenty of fluids. If the patient has hypercalcemia, suggest a low-calcium diet. Weigh the patient regularly to detect weight loss.
- Monitor respiratory function. Check chest X-rays for the extent of lung involvement; note and record any bloody sputum or increase in sputum. If the patient has pulmonary hypertension or end-stage cor pulmonale, check ABG levels, observe for arrhythmias, and administer oxygen, as needed. Also monitor spirometry and the diffusing capacity of carbon dioxide.
- Because steroids may induce or worsen diabetes mellitus, perform fingerstick glucose tests at least every 12 hours at the beginning of steroid therapy. Also, watch for other steroid adverse effects, such as fluid retention, electrolyte imbalance (especially hypokalemia), moon face, hypertension, and personality change. During or after steroid withdrawal (particularly in association with infection or other types of stress), watch for and report vomiting, orthostatic hypotension, hypoglycemia, restlessness, anorexia, malaise, and fatigue. Remember that the patient on long-term or high-dose steroid therapy is vulnerable to infection.
- When preparing the patient for discharge, stress the need for compliance with prescribed steroid therapy and regular, careful follow-up examinations and treatment. Refer the patient with failing vision to community support and resource groups as well as the American Foundation for the Blind if necessary.

Severe acute respiratory syndrome

Severe acute respiratory syndrome (SARS) is a viral respiratory infection that can progress to pneumonia and, eventually, death. The disease was first recognized in 2003 with outbreaks in China, Canada, Singapore, Taiwan, and Vietnam, with other countries—including the United States—reporting smaller numbers of cases.

CAUSES AND INCIDENCE

SARS is caused by the SARS-associated coronavirus (SARS-CoV). Coronaviruses are a common cause of mild respiratory illnesses in humans, but researchers believe that a virus may have mutated, allowing it to cause this potentially life-threatening disease.

Close contact with a person who's infected with SARS, including contact with infectious aerosolized droplets or body secretions, is the method of transmission. The disease can be acquired after the skin, respiratory system, or mucous membranes come into contact with infectious droplets propelled into the air by a coughing or sneezing patient with SARS. SARS may also be spread when a person touches infectious secretions or a contaminated surface or object and then directly contacts his or her own eyes, nose, or mouth.

Most people who contracted the disease during the 2003 outbreak contracted it during travel to endemic areas. However, the virus has been found to live on hands, tissues, and other surfaces for up to 6 hours in its droplet form. It has also been found to live in the stool of people with SARS for up to 4 days. The virus may be able to live for months

or years in below-freezing temperatures. (See *Lungs and alveoli in SARS,* page 172.)

The overall mortality rate of SARS is 10%. However individuals older than 65 years have a mortality rate above 50%, according to the Centers for Disease Control and World Health Organization.

SIGNS AND SYMPTOMS

The incubation period for SARS is typically 3 to 5 days but may last as long as 14 days. Initial signs and symptoms include:
- fever
- shortness of breath and other minor respiratory symptoms
- general discomfort
- headache
- rigors
- chills
- myalgia
- sore throat
- dry cough
- diarrhea or rash (in some individuals).

COMPLICATIONS
- Respiratory failure
- Liver failure
- Heart failure
- Myelodysplastic syndromes
- Death

DIAGNOSIS
- Diagnosis of severe respiratory illness is made when the patient has a fever greater than 100.4° F (38° C) or upon clinical findings of lower respiratory illness.

LUNGS AND ALVEOLI IN SARS

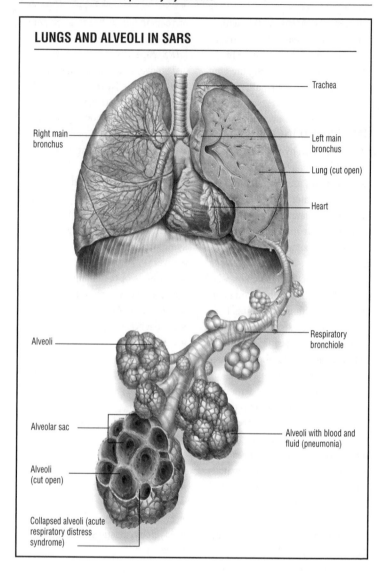

- Trachea
- Left main bronchus
- Lung (cut open)
- Heart
- Respiratory bronchiole
- Right main bronchus
- Alveoli
- Alveolar sac
- Alveoli (cut open)
- Collapsed alveoli (acute respiratory distress syndrome)
- Alveoli with blood and fluid (pneumonia)

- Chest X-rays demonstrate pneumonia or acute respiratory distress syndrome.
- Laboratory validation for the virus includes cell culture of SARS-CoV, detection of SARS-CoV ribonucleic acid by the reverse transcription polymerase chain reaction (PCR) test, or detection of serum antibodies to SARS-CoV. Detectable levels of antibodies may not be present until 21 days after the

onset of illness, but some individuals develop antibodies within 14 days. A negative PCR, antibody test, or cell culture doesn't rule out the diagnosis.

TREATMENT

Treatment is symptomatic and supportive and includes maintenance of a patent airway and adequate nutrition. Other treatment measures include supplemental oxygen, chest physiotherapy, and mechanical ventilation. The recommended precautions for hospitalized patients include standard precautions, contact precautions requiring gowns and gloves for all patient contacts, and airborne precautions using a negative-pressure isolation room and properly fitted N-95 respirators. Quarantine can help prevent the spread of infection.

Patients who develop bacterial atypical pneumonia can receive antibiotics. Antiviral medications have also been used. High doses of corticosteroids may reduce lung inflammation. In some serious cases, patients have received serum from individuals who have already recovered from SARS (convalescent serum). The general benefit of convalescent serum treatment hasn't been determined conclusively.

Drugs

● Beta-agonists such as albuterol (Proventil) for bronchospasm to relax bronchial smooth muscle
● Because SARS mimics bronchiolitis obliterans, steroids to reduce inflammation until diagnosis is differentiated (use is controversial)
● Combination of antiviral drugs normally used to treat acquired immunodeficiency syndrome—lopinavir plus ritonavir (Kaletra) along with ribavirin (Copegus)—to prevent serious complications and death (shown in clinical studies to be effective)

SPECIAL CONSIDERATIONS

● Report suspected cases of SARS to local and national health organizations.
● Frequently monitor the patient's vital signs and respiratory status.
● Maintain isolation as recommended. The patient will need emotional support to deal with anxiety and fear related to the diagnosis of SARS and as a result of isolation.
● Provide patient and family teaching, including the importance of frequent hand washing, covering the mouth and nose when coughing or sneezing, and avoiding close personal contact while infected or potentially infected. Instruct the patient and his family that such items as eating utensils, towels, and bedding shouldn't be shared until they have been washed with soap and hot water and that disposable gloves and household disinfectant should be used to clean any surface that may have been exposed to the patient's body fluids.
● Emphasize the importance of the patient not going to work, school, or other public places, as recommended by the health care provider.

Silicosis

Silicosis is the term used for a lung disease that results from inorganic (minerals) and organic (small dust silica) crystal inhalation that's not related to an allergic reaction. It's a progressive disease characterized by nodular lesions that commonly progress to fibrosis. The most common form of pneumoconiosis, silicosis can be classified according to the severity of pulmonary disease and the rapidity of its onset and progression. It usually begins with breathlessness and sometimes weight loss; as it advances, the airways become obstructed and lungs become distorted by large, hard (calcified), nodular collagen masses.

Acute silicosis develops after 1 to 3 years in workers exposed to very high concentrations of respirable silica, such as sand blasters and tunnel workers. Accelerated silicosis appears after an average of 10 years of exposure to lower concentrations of free silica. Chronic silicosis develops after 20 or more years of exposure to still lower concentrations of free silica; chronic silicosis is further subdivided into simple and complicated forms.

The prognosis is generally good, unless the disease has progressed over the years into the complicated fibrotic form that involves all lobes and upper lung fields and produces such complications as hypoxemia, pulmonary hypertension, respiratory insufficiency, and cor pulmonale.

Lung destruction is related to restriction, obstruction, and infections. Pulmonary disease may be malignant or nonmalignant; however, unlike asbestosis, silicosis doesn't predispose a patient to cancer.

CAUSES AND INCIDENCE

Silicosis results from the inhalation and pulmonary deposition of respirable crystalline silica dust, mostly from quartz, stone, sand, or flint. Silicosis can also develop from talc, vermiculites, and mica. The danger to the worker depends on the concentration of dust in the atmosphere, the percentage of respirable free silica particles in the dust, and the duration of exposure. Respirable particles are less than 10 microns in diameter, but the disease-causing particles deposited in the alveolar space are usually 1 to 3 microns in diameter. Silicosis severity is graded on the International Organization Scale based on size, shape, location, and profusion of the opacities. Confluent silicotic nodules destroy lung parenchyma, so the severest grading results in massive pulmonary fibrosis, which is indistinguishable from other forms of fibrotic lung disease.

Industrial sources of silica in its pure form include the manufacture of ceramics (flint) and building materials (sandstone). Silica occurs in mixed form in the production of construction materials (cement). It's found in powder form (silica flour) in paints, porcelain, scouring soaps, and wood fillers as well as in the mining of gold, coal, lead, zinc, and iron. Foundry workers, boiler scalers, and stonecutters are all exposed to silica dust and, therefore, are at high risk for developing silicosis.

Nodules result when alveolar macrophages ingest silica particles, which they're unable to process. As a result, the macrophages release cytokines, proteolytic enzymes, tumor necrosing factor, and growth factor into surrounding tissue, stimulating the inflammatory response. The subsequent inflammation attracts other macrophages and fibroblasts into the region to produce fibrous tissue and wall off the reaction. The resulting nodule has an onionskin appearance when viewed under a microscope. Nodules develop adjacent to terminal and respiratory bronchioles, concentrate in the upper lobes, and are commonly accompanied by bullous changes in both lobes. If the disease process doesn't progress, minimal physiologic disturbances and no disability occur. Occasionally, however, the fibrotic response accelerates, engulfing and destroying large areas of the lung (progressive massive fibrosis or conglomerate lesions). Fibrosis may continue even after exposure to dust has ended. Patients exposed to silica, even without silicosis, have three times the risk of developing tuberculosis (TB).

The incidence of silicosis has decreased since the Occupational Safety and Health Administration (OSHA) instituted regulations requiring the use of protective equipment that limits the amount of silica dust inhaled.

SIGNS AND SYMPTOMS

Initially, silicosis may be either asymptomatic or produce dyspnea on exertion, usually attributed to being "out of shape" or "slowing down." As the disorder progresses, signs and symptoms may include:
- tachypnea
- an insidious dry cough that's most pronounced in the morning
- dyspnea on minimal exertion
- worsening cough
- pulmonary hypertension
- right-sided heart failure and cor pulmonale
- confusion
- lethargy
- a decrease in the rate and depth of respiration
- malaise
- disturbed sleep
- hoarseness.

COMPLICATIONS
- Tracheobronchial obstruction
- Spontaneous pneumothorax
- Pulmonary fibrosis
- Emphysema
- Broncholithiasis
- Pulmonary hypertension
- Ventricular or respiratory failure
- Cor pulmonale
- Tuberculosis

DIAGNOSIS
- Patient history reveals occupational exposure to silica dust.

• Physical examination is normal in simple silicosis; in chronic silicosis with conglomerate lesions, it may reveal decreased chest expansion, diminished intensity of breath sounds, areas of hyperresonance, fine to medium crackles, and tachypnea.

• Chest X-rays show small, discrete, nodular lesions distributed throughout both lung fields but typically concentrated in the upper lung zones; the hilar lung nodes may be enlarged and exhibit "eggshell" calcification (in simple silicosis) or more conglomerate masses of dense tissue (complicated silicosis).

• Pulmonary function tests show reduced forced vital capacity (FVC) in complicated silicosis; reduced forced expiratory volume in 1 second (FEV_1) in obstructive disease (emphysematous areas of silicosis) and complicated silicosis (although the ratio of FEV_1 to FVC is normal or high in silicosis); reduced maximal voluntary ventilation in restrictive and obstructive diseases; and reduced carbon dioxide diffusing capacity when fibrosis destroys alveolar walls and obliterates pulmonary capillaries or when fibrosis thickens the alveolocapillary membrane.

TREATMENT

The first treatment is to remove workers from further exposure or use respiratory masks. No other effective treatment exists outside of supportive care. Supportive care includes relieving respiratory symptoms, managing hypoxemia and cor pulmonale, and preventing respiratory tract irritation and infections. Treatment also includes careful observation for the development of TB. Daily use of inhaled bronchodilators and increased fluid intake (at least 3 qt [3 L] daily) can help relieve respiratory symptoms. Steam inhalation and chest physiotherapy techniques, such as controlled coughing and segmental bronchial drainage with chest percussion and vibration, help clear secretions. In severe cases, the patient with chronic hypoxemia may require oxygen administered by cannula or mask (at 1 to 2 L/minute) or by mechanical ventilation if arterial oxygen levels can't be maintained above 40 mm Hg. Respiratory infections require prompt administration of antibiotics.

Whole lung lavage may be used in some cases of acute silicosis as well as corticosteroid administration. As a last resort for severe cases, lung transplantation may be considered.

Drugs

• Antitubercular medications, such as isoniazid (Nydrazid), rifampin (Rifadin), pyrazinamide (PZA), streptomycin, or ethambutol (Myambutol) for patients who test positive for *Mycobacterium tuberculosis* to treat TB

SPECIAL CONSIDERATIONS

• Teach the patient to prevent infections by avoiding crowds and persons with respiratory infections and by receiving influenza and pneumococcal vaccines.

● Increase exercise tolerance by encouraging regular activity. Advise the patient to plan his daily activities to decrease the work of breathing. Instruct the patient to pace himself, rest often, and generally move slowly through his daily routine.

▷ PREVENTION

● *Monitoring air quality and dust concentrations in the workplace can help prevent silicosis and other pneumoconioses. Other prevention measures include limiting exposure to harmful dusts by suppressing dust generation, filtering or capturing dust particles, diluting the concentration of dust with fresh air, and using personal protective respiratory equipment.*

● *Following the permissible exposure limits set for silica by OSHA (10 mg/m³) and the National Institute for Occupational Safety and Health (0.05 mg/m³) helps prevent the disorder. Workers in high-risk occupations should be monitored with chest radiography and incentive spirometry to identify early disease and stop further exposure.*

Sinusitis

Sinusitis—inflammation of the paranasal sinuses—may be acute (lasting less than 4 weeks), subacute (lasting from 4 to 12 weeks), chronic (lasting more than 12 weeks and recurring four or more times per year), allergic, or hyperplastic.

Acute sinusitis usually results from the common cold and lingers in subacute form in only about 10% of patients. The acute form may be bacterial or viral, with viral being the most common. Chronic sinusitis follows persistent bacterial infection and allergic sinusitis accompanies allergic rhinitis; hyperplastic sinusitis is a combination of purulent acute sinusitis and allergic sinusitis or rhinitis. The prognosis is good for all types.

CAUSES AND INCIDENCE

The majority of cases of acute rhinosinusitis result from viral infections; acute bacterial infections cause the disorder in only 0.5% to 2% of episodes. The most common viral agents are rhinovirus, influenza virus, and parainfluenza virus. Viral sinusitis usually follows an upper respiratory infection in which the virus penetrates the normal mucous membrane, decreasing ciliary transport and impairing mucociliary clearance and leading to mucosal edema, copious and thick secretions, and ciliary dyskinesia.

Acute bacterial sinusitis typically results from *Streptococcus pneumoniae*, *Moraxella catarrhalis,* and *Haemophilus influenzae*. Predisposing factors include any condition that interferes with sinus drainage and ventilation, such as allergy, mechanical obstruction of the nose, swimming, odontogenic infection, intranasal cocaine, impaired mucociliary clearance, immunodeficiency, chronic nasal edema,

LOOKING AT SINUSITIS

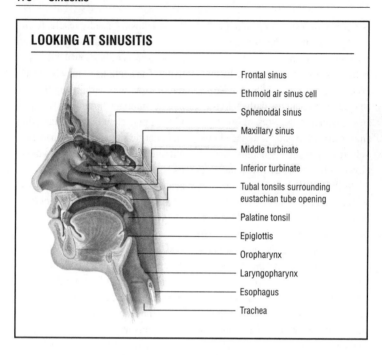

- Frontal sinus
- Ethmoid air sinus cell
- Sphenoidal sinus
- Maxillary sinus
- Middle turbinate
- Inferior turbinate
- Tubal tonsils surrounding eustachian tube opening
- Palatine tonsil
- Epiglottis
- Oropharynx
- Laryngopharynx
- Esophagus
- Trachea

deviated nasal septum, and viscous mucus. Bacterial invasion may also result from swimming in contaminated water. Generalized debilitating conditions, including chemotherapy, malnutrition, diabetes, blood dyscrasias, long-term steroid use, and immunodeficiency, may also predispose an individual to sinusitis. (See *Looking at sinusitis*.)

⚠ ALERT

The incidence of both acute and chronic sinusitis increases in later childhood. Sinusitis may be more prevalent in children who have had tonsils and adenoids removed.

SIGNS AND SYMPTOMS

Signs and symptoms of acute sinusitis include:

- nasal congestion that precedes a gradual buildup of pressure in the affected sinus
- edematous nasal mucosa
- fatigue
- nonproductive cough
- sore throat
- localized headache
- a general feeling of malaise
- pain specific to the affected sinus: cheeks and upper teeth for maxillary sinusitis; over the eyes for ethmoid sinusitis; and over the eyebrows for frontal sinusitis
- purulent nasal drainage that continues longer than 3 weeks after an acute infection subsides
- low-grade fever of 99° to 99.5° F (37.2° to 37.5° C)
- swollen areas over the sinuses

- enlarged turbinates
- thickening of the mucosal lining
- mucosal polyps (hyperplastic sinusitis).

Chronic sinusitis can cause continuous mucopurulent discharge.

COMPLICATIONS

- Meningitis
- Cavernous and sinus thrombosis
- Bacteremia or septicemia
- Brain abscess
- Osteomyelitis
- Mucocele
- Orbital cellulitis abscess

DIAGNOSIS

- Nasal examination reveals inflammation and pus.
- Sinus X-rays (not routinely performed) reveal cloudiness in the affected sinus, air, fluid, and possibly thickening of the mucosal lining.
- Transillumination, a simple diagnostic tool that involves shining a light into the patient's mouth with his lips closed around the light, shows darkness if the sinuses are infected (normal sinuses transilluminate).
- Ultrasonography, computed tomography scanning, magnetic resonance imaging, and X-rays help diagnose suspected complications.

TREATMENT

Antibiotics are the primary treatment for acute bacterial sinusitis. An analgesic may be prescribed for pain; however, mechanical irrigation with a filtered hypotonic saline solution may reduce the need for pain medication.

Other appropriate measures include vasoconstrictors, such as epinephrine and phenylephrine, to decrease nasal secretions and steam inhalation to promote vasoconstriction and encourage drainage. Treatment of acute viral sinusitis aims to reduce nasal obstruction and rhinorrhea but can't shorten the duration of the illness.

Antibiotic therapy—usually with amoxicillin or ampicillin—combats chronic infection. Local heat application may help to relieve pain and congestion. In patients with subacute sinusitis, antibiotic therapy is also the primary treatment. As in those with acute sinusitis, a vasoconstrictor may reduce nasal secretions.

Treatment for allergic sinusitis must include treatment for allergic rhinitis—administration of antihistamines, identification of allergens by skin testing, and desensitization by immunotherapy. Severe allergic symptoms may require treatment with corticosteroids and epinephrine.

Drugs

- Alpha-adrenergic vasoconstrictors, including pseudoephedrine and phenylephrine, given for 10 to 14 days to allow for restoration of normal mucociliary function and drainage
- Mucolytic agents such as guaifenesin (Mucinex) to thin mucous secretions and help improve drainage
- Topical glucocorticoids, such as mometasone (Nasonex), budesonide (Rhinocort), triamcinolone

(Nasacort), fluticasone (Flonase), beclomethasone (Beconase), flunisolide (Nasarel), or fluticasone (Veramyst), to reduce mucous membrane swelling
• Intranasal steroids to help decrease inflammation in acute sinusitis
• Antihistamines, such as loratadine (Claritin), cetirizine (Zyrtec), fexofenadine (Allegra), or diphenhydramine (Benadryl), to reduce ostiomeatal obstruction in patients with allergies and acute sinusitis; however, these drugs can also thicken secretions and cause complications
• Antibiotic therapy—usually with amoxicillin, ampicillin, trimethoprim, erythromycin, or azithromycin—to combat persistent infection

SPECIAL CONSIDERATIONS
• Enforce bed rest, and encourage the patient to drink plenty of fluids to promote drainage. Don't elevate the head of the bed more than 30 degrees.
• To relieve pain and promote drainage, apply warm compresses continuously or four times daily for 2-hour intervals. Also, give analgesics and antihistamines as needed.
• Watch for and report complications, such as vomiting, chills, fever, edema of the forehead or eyelids, blurred or double vision, and mental status changes.
• If surgery is necessary, tell the patient what to expect postoperatively: He'll have nasal packing in place for

12 to 24 hours following surgery and he'll have to breathe through his mouth and won't be able to blow his nose. After surgery, monitor for excessive drainage or bleeding and watch for complications.
• To prevent edema and promote drainage, place the patient in semi-Fowler's position. To relieve edema and pain and to minimize bleeding, apply ice compresses over the nose, and iced saline gauze over the eyes. Continue these measures for 24 hours.
• Frequently change the mustache dressing or drip pad, and record the consistency, amount, and color of drainage (expect scant, bright red, and clotty drainage).
• Because the patient will be breathing through his mouth, provide meticulous mouth care.
• Tell the patient that even after the packing is removed, nose blowing may cause bleeding and swelling. If the patient is a smoker, instruct him not to smoke for at least 2 days after surgery.
• Tell the patient to finish the prescribed antibiotics, even if his symptoms disappear.

Sleep apnea

Sleep apnea is a disruption in breathing during sleep. An episode generally lasts at least 10 seconds and typically occurs more than five times in 1 hour.

CAUSES AND INCIDENCE
Sleep apnea is most commonly related to a type of respiratory

obstruction in which the soft palate or tongue obstructs the upper airway. Factors that contribute to sleep apnea include obesity, family history, large neck circumference, and abnormal anatomy (recessed chin, abnormal upper airway, large tonsils or adenoids, nasal obstruction, or craniofacial anomalies); it also occurs more frequently in those over 40, in men, and in menopausal or postmenopausal women.

Conditions that can cause or be exacerbated by sleep apnea include hypertension, atrial fibrillation, hypothyroidism, atherosclerosis, and diabetes. Using central nervous system (CNS) depressants, such as muscle relaxants, sedatives, analgesics, or alcohol, may also worsen or cause sleep apnea by further relaxing the airway muscles and reducing the respiratory drive. Smoking can cause swelling, inflammation, and narrowing of the upper airway. The supine position may also be a factor because gravity increases the likelihood that the tongue will occlude the airway or that muscles and tissues will collapse.

Sleep apnea occurs when the skeletal muscles relax during sleep, displacing the tongue and other anatomic structures of the head and neck. The displacement can result in obstruction of the upper airway, even though the chest wall continues to move. Absence of breathing causes an increase in arterial carbon dioxide levels and lowers the pH level. These changes stimulate the nervous system, and the sleeping person responds after 10 or more seconds of apnea. This arousal episode corrects the obstruction, and breathing resumes. The cycle repeats itself as often as every 5 minutes during sleep, affecting the patient's ability to get a restful night of sleep. (See *Understanding obstructive sleep apnea,* page 182.)

SIGNS AND SYMPTOMS

Indications of sleep apnea include:
- snoring
- excessive daytime sleepiness
- intellectual impairment
- memory loss
- morning headache
- daytime fatigue
- gastroesophageal reflux
- impotence
- tossing and turning or a fitful sleep
- chest pain
- decreased libido
- depression
- personality changes
- concentration changes
- weight gain
- poor judgment.

COMPLICATIONS
- Hypertension
- Heart failure
- Stroke

DIAGNOSIS
- Polysomnography performed during an overnight sleep study records eye movement, muscle activity, heart rate, respiration, blood oxygen levels, air flow, and brain activity,

UNDERSTANDING OBSTRUCTIVE SLEEP APNEA

When breathing is unobstructed, air flows normally. During an apneic event, the airway becames blocked and air ceases to flow.

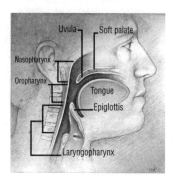
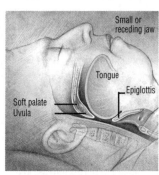

which may show abnormality in sleep patterns.

• A multiple sleep latency test measures the time it takes for a patient to fall asleep and can also measures the amount of daytime sleepiness a patient has.

TREATMENT

Mild cases of sleep apnea may be resolved by weight loss or a change in sleeping position. Elevating the head of the bed 30 degrees tends to bring the tongue forward, which helps maintain the airway. Side sleeping also prevents the tongue from falling to the back of the throat.

Because CNS depressants relax the pharyngeal muscles, avoiding alcohol and other CNS depressants for 6 hours before bed can help prevent sleep apnea. Using devices that prevent obstruction by the tongue or

nonsurgical neck structures to eliminate displacement of these structures can also prevent sleep apnea, although severe cases commonly require surgical intervention. For moderate to severe sleep apnea, continuous positive airway pressure (CPAP) is the first line of treatment.

If other treatments aren't effective, surgery can correct abnormalities of the soft tissue or bone structure that obstruct the patient's airway. Uvulopalatopharyngoplasty, a laser-assisted procedure, removes part of the uvular and excess soft tissue on the palate and posterior pharyngeal wall. Nasal surgery to remove polyps or correct such abnormalities as a deviated septum can improve airway patency. Maxillomandibular advancement enlarges the entire upper airway by expanding the bones that surround the airway. Genioglossus advancement places tension on the tongue, preventing it from displacing backward during sleep, and hyoid advancement repositions the hyoid bone to expand the airway.

Drugs

• Protriptyline (Vivactil) to decrease the amount of rapid eye movement cycles
• Modafinil (Provigil) for narcolepsy and hypopnea to improve daytime sleepiness
• Medroxyprogesterone, acetazolamide (Diamox), clomipramine, and theophylline to stimulate the respiratory drive

SPECIAL CONSIDERATIONS

• Educate the patient and his family about the disorder and its possible causes.
• Perform an assessment and collect a health history to determine contributing causes for the condition.
• Using the health history, assess the patient's sleep patterns, including the degree of fatigue during the day and interference in his ability to function because of interrupted sleep patterns.
• Encourage a smoking-cessation program if the patient smokes.
• Encourage a weight-loss program for the obese patient.
• Provide information and teaching on the use of a CPAP device, and make sure the nasal or full face mask that is used with the CPAP device fits properly to ensure optimal functioning.

• If the patient requires surgery, provide preoperative and postoperative teaching for the patient and his partner.
• Administer medications as ordered, and explain possible adverse reactions and what to do if they occur.

Submersion injury

In a submersion injury, the victim survives (at least temporarily) the physiologic effects of suffocation by submersion in a fluid medium. Hypoxemia and acidosis are the primary problems in victims of submersion injury.

CAUSES AND INCIDENCE

A submersion injury occurs in three forms. In dry submersion injury, the victim doesn't aspirate fluid but suffers respiratory obstruction secondary to laryngospasm or asphyxia (10% to 15% of patients). In wet submersion injury, the victim aspirates fluid and suffers from asphyxia or secondary changes from fluid aspiration (about 85% of patients). In secondary submersion injury, the victim suffers recurrence of respiratory distress (usually aspiration pneumonia or pulmonary edema) within minutes or 1 to 2 days after a near-drowning incident.

Regardless of the tonicity of the fluid aspirated, hypoxemia is the most serious consequence of submersion injury, followed by metabolic acidosis, hypothermia, and bradycardia. Other consequences depend on the kind of fluid aspirated. After freshwater aspiration, changes in the character of lung surfactant result in exudation of protein-rich plasma into the alveoli. Aspiration of hypotonic fluid results in fluid rapidly passing through lungs, leading to volume overload and dilution of serum electrolytes. This, plus increased capillary permeability, leads to pulmonary edema and hypoxemia.

After saltwater aspiration, the hypertonicity of salt water exerts an osmotic force, which pulls fluid from pulmonary capillaries into the alveoli and pulmonary interstitium. The resulting intrapulmonary shunt causes hypoxemia. The pulmonary capillary membrane may be injured and may induce pulmonary edema. In wet and secondary submersion injury, pulmonary edema and hypoxemia occur secondary to aspiration.

Regardless of the type of submersion injury (freshwater or salt water), aspiration of contaminants can occur. The victim may aspirate chlorine, mud, algae, weeds, and other foreign material. Saltwater aspiration is considered more dangerous than freshwater because salt water contains more types of disease-causing bacteria. These contaminants may lead to obstruction, aspiration pneumonia, and pulmonary fibrosis.

A protective effect may occur in cold-water submersion (exposure to temperatures below 69.8° F [21° C]) because rapid body cooling results in cardiac arrest and decreased tissue oxygen demand. The protective effect is most pronounced in children, possibly because of the large ration of body surface area to mass. Because water rapidly conducts heat away from the body, even people who experience a submersion injury in warm water may suffer from hypothermia. (See *Physiologic changes in submersion injury*.)

SIGNS AND SYMPTOMS

On initial observation, the patient may be unconscious, semiconscious, or awake. If he's conscious, he may complain of a headache or substernal chest pain. He may appear apprehensive, irritable, restless, or lethargic, and he may vomit. Your initial assessment of vital signs may detect fever; rapid, slow, or absent pulse; shallow, gasping, or absent respirations; confusion; and seizures. If he was exposed to cold temperatures, he may experience hypothermia. Other signs and symptoms may include:

- cyanosis or pink, frothy sputum (indicating pulmonary edema)
- abdominal distention
- crackles, rhonchi, wheezing, or apnea
- tachycardia, arrhythmias, or cardiac arrest
- hypotension
- weak pulses (in hypothermia).

COMPLICATIONS

- Neurologic impairment
- Cerebral edema

PHYSIOLOGIC CHANGES IN SUBMERSION INJURY

The flowchart below shows the primary cellular alterations that occur during submersion injury. Separate pathways are shown for saltwater and freshwater incidents. Hypothermia presents a separate pathway that may preserve neurologic function by decreasing the metabolic rate. All pathways lead to diffuse pulmonary edema.

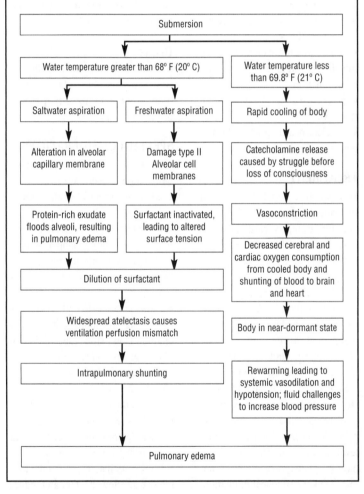

- Increased intracranial pressure
- Pulmonary edema
- Acute respiratory distress
- Hypoxia
- Acute tubular necrosis
- Bacterial aspiration
- Arrhythmias
- Decreased blood pressure

DIAGNOSIS

• Arterial blood gas (ABG) analysis indicates the degree of hypoxia, intrapulmonary shunting, and acid-base balance.
• Serum electrolyte levels allow monitoring of the patient's electrolyte balance.
• A complete blood count determines hemolysis.
• Blood urea nitrogen and creatinine levels and urinalysis evaluate renal function.
• A cervical spine X-ray rules out fractures.
• An electrocardiogram (ECG) detects myocardial ischemia.

TREATMENT

Prehospital care includes stabilizing the patient's neck and spine to prevent further injury, cardiopulmonary resuscitation (CPR) as needed, and administration of supplemental oxygen.

After the patient reaches the hospital, resuscitation continues. His oxygenation and circulation are maintained. X-rays confirm cervical spine integrity, and the patient's blood pH and electrolyte imbalances are corrected. If he's hypothermic, steps are taken to rewarm him.

If the patient can't maintain an open airway, has abnormal ABG levels and pH values, or doesn't have spontaneous respirations, he may need endotracheal intubation and mechanical ventilation. If he develops bronchospasm, he may need bronchodilators. Central venous pressure or pulmonary artery wedge pressure (PAWP) indicates the need for fluid replacement and cardiac drug therapy. The patient may also require standard treatment for pulmonary edema. Nasogastric (NG) tube drainage prevents vomiting, and an indwelling urinary catheter allows monitoring of urine output.

Drugs

• Bronchodilators, such as albuterol (Proventil), levalbuterol (Xopenex), or ipratropium (Atrovent), to treat bronchospasm

SPECIAL CONSIDERATIONS

• Continue CPR as indicated. Assist with endotracheal intubation if needed, and administer supplemental oxygen.
• If the patient has been submerged in cold water, use a bladder probe or a pulmonary artery line thermistor to determine his core body temperature.
• If the patient is hypothermic, start rewarming procedures during resuscitation. Don't stop resuscitation until the patient's body temperature ranges between 86° and 90.3° F (30° to 32.4° C).
• Protect the cervical spine until fracture is ruled out.
• Ensure peripheral I.V. access, and administer I.V. fluids as needed.
• If ordered, insert an NG tube to remove swallowed water and reduce the risk of vomiting and aspiration.
• Insert an indwelling urinary catheter to monitor urine output. Metabolic acidosis may develop to

compensate for impaired renal function.

• Assess ABG levels and obtain an ECG; the patient will most likely need continuous cardiac monitoring.

• Continually monitor the patient's vital signs and neurologic status. He may have central nervous system damage despite treatment for hypoxia and shock.

• Obtain baseline serum electrolyte levels; continue monitoring these levels.

• If the patient has a central line in place, closely monitor all hemodynamic parameters: cardiac output, central venous pressure, PAWP, heart rate, and arterial blood pressure.

• Administer bronchodilators to the patient as ordered.

Sudden infant death syndrome

A medical mystery of early infancy, sudden infant death syndrome (SIDS), also called *crib death,* is the unexpected, sudden death of an infant or child younger than age 1 year. Reasons for the death remain unexplained even after an autopsy. Typically, parents put the infant to bed and later find him dead, commonly with no indications of a struggle or distress of any kind.

CAUSES AND INCIDENCE

SIDS is the third leading cause of death in infants between age 1 month and 1 year. It occurs more commonly in winter months. The incidence is higher in males, preterm neonates, and those who sleep on their stomachs or in cribs with soft bedding; the incidence has dropped with the practice of teaching parents to place infants on their backs to sleep. Incidence is also higher among neonates born in conditions of poverty or who were one of a single multiple birth, such as twins and triplets. Neonates whose mothers smoke, take drugs, or didn't seek prenatal care until late in the pregnancy also have a higher incidence.

SIDS may result from an abnormality in the control of ventilation that allows carbon dioxide to build up in the blood, causing prolonged apneic periods with profound hypoxemia and serious cardiac arrhythmias. It's also thought to be associated with problems in sleep arousal.

SIGNS AND SYMPTOMS

Although the parents may find the infant wedged in a crib corner or with blankets wrapped around his head, and autopsy rules out suffocation as the cause of death. Autopsy also shows a patent airway, ruling out aspiration of vomitus as the cause of death. Typically, SIDS babies don't cry out and show no signs of having been disturbed in their sleep. However, their positions or tangled blankets may suggest movement just before death, perhaps due to terminal spasm.

Depending on how long the infant has been dead, he may have a mottled complexion with extreme cyanosis of the lips and fingertips or pooling of blood in the legs and feet that may be mistaken for bruises. Pulses and respirations are absent, and the diaper is wet and full of stool. The infant's mouth and nostrils are frequently filled with blood-tinged sputum

DIAGNOSIS

An autopsy is needed to rule out other causes of death. Characteristic histologic findings on autopsy include small or normal adrenal glands and petechiae over the visceral surfaces of the pleura, within the thymus, and in the epicardium. Autopsy also reveals extremely well-preserved lymphoid structures and certain pathologic characteristics such as increased pulmonary artery smooth muscle that suggest chronic hypoxemia. Examination also shows edematous, congestive lungs fully expanded in the pleural cavities, liquid (not clotted) blood in the heart, and curd from the stomach inside the trachea.

TREATMENT

If the parents bring the infant to the emergency department (ED), the physician will decide whether to try to resuscitate him. An "aborted SIDS" infant is one who's found apneic and is successfully resuscitated. Such an infant, or any infant who had a sibling stricken by SIDS, should be tested for infantile apnea. If tests are positive, a home apnea monitor may be recommended.

However, because the infant usually can't be resuscitated, treatment focuses on providing emotional support for the family.

Drugs
● No specific drug exists to treat SIDS

SPECIAL CONSIDERATIONS
● Make sure that parents are present when the child's death is announced. They may lash out at ED personnel, the babysitter, or anyone else involved in the child's care, even each other. Stay calm and let them express their feelings. Reassure them that they weren't to blame.
● Let the parents see the baby in a private room. Allow them to express their grief in their own way. Stay in the room with them if appropriate. Offer to call clergy, friends, or relatives.
● After the parents and family have recovered from their initial shock, explain the necessity for an autopsy to confirm the diagnosis of SIDS (in some states, this is mandatory). At this time, provide the family with some basic facts about SIDS, and encourage them to give their consent for the autopsy. Make sure that they receive the autopsy report promptly.
● Find out whether your community has a local counseling and information program for SIDS parents. Participants in such a program will contact the parents, ensure that they receive the autopsy report promptly, put them in touch with a professional

counselor, and maintain supportive telephone contact. Also, find out whether there's a local SIDS parent group; such a group can provide significant emotional support. Contact the National Sudden Infant Death Foundation for information about such local groups.

● If your facility's policy is to assign a public health nurse to the family, she will provide the continuing reassurance and assistance the parents will need.

● If the parents decide to have another child, they'll need information and counseling to help them through the pregnancy and the first year of the new infant's life.

● Infants at high risk for SIDS may be placed on apnea monitoring at home.

● All new parents should be informed of the American Academy of Pediatrics' recommendation that an infant be positioned on his back—not his stomach or side—for sleeping.

▷ PREVENTION

● *Tell parents to place infants on their backs to sleep.*

● *Tell parents that infants should sleep on a firm mattress and shouldn't have soft objects, such as stuffed toys and blankets, in the crib.*

● *Tell parents that infants shouldn't sleep in the same bed as their parents.*

● *Tell parents to give infants pacifiers at bedtime.*

● *Tell parents that infants shouldn't be exposed to secondhand smoke.*

Tonsillitis

Tonsillitis—inflammation of the tonsils—can be acute or chronic. The uncomplicated acute form usually lasts 2 to 5 days. The presence of proven chronic tonsillitis justifies tonsillectomy, the only effective treatment. Tonsils tend to hypertrophy during childhood and atrophy after puberty.

CAUSES AND INCIDENCE

Viral or bacterial infections and immunologic factors can lead to tonsillitis and its complications. Tonsillitis generally results from infection with beta-hemolytic streptococci but can result from other bacteria or viruses or from oral anaerobes. It commonly affects children between ages 5 and 10.

SIGNS AND SYMPTOMS

Signs and symptoms of tonsillitis include:
- mild to severe sore throat (parents of a child too young to complain of throat pain may report that the child has stopped eating)
- muscle and joint pain
- chills
- malaise
- headache
- pain that's frequently referred to the ears

- a constant urge to swallow
- a constricted feeling in the back of the throat
- fever of 100° F (37.8° F) or higher
- swollen, tender lymph nodes in the submandibular area
- inflammation of the pharyngeal wall
- swollen tonsils that project from between the pillars of the fauces and exude white or yellow follicles (see *Looking at tonsillitis*)
- purulent drainage that becomes apparent when you apply pressure to the tonsillar pillars
- edematous and inflamed uvula
- purulent drainage in the tonsillar crypts.

COMPLICATIONS

- Chronic upper airway obstruction
- Sleep apnea or sleep disturbances
- Cor pulmonale
- Failure to thrive
- Eating or swallowing disorders
- Febrile seizures
- Otitis media
- Cardiac valvular disease
- Peritonsillar abscesses
- Subacute bacterial endocarditis
- Cervical lymph node abscesses
- Streptococcal toxic shock syndrome
- Pediatric autoimmune neuropsychiatric disorder associated with streptococcal infections (PANDAS)

LOOKING AT TONSILLITIS

The illustration below shows inflammation of the pharyngeal wall with swollen tonsils.

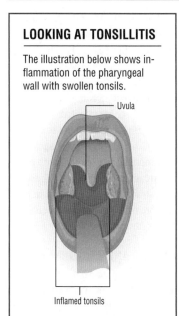

Uvula

Inflamed tonsils

DIAGNOSIS

• A throat culture may determine the infecting organism and indicate appropriate antibiotic therapy; the culture may also show leukocytosis.
• Differential diagnosis rules out infectious mononucleosis and diphtheria.

TREATMENT

Treatment for acute tonsillitis requires rest, adequate fluid intake, analgesics and, for bacterial infection, antibiotics. When the causative organism is group A beta-hemolytic streptococcus, penicillin is the drug of choice (another broad-spectrum antibiotic may be substituted). Most oral anaerobes also respond to penicillin. To prevent complications, antibiotic therapy should continue for 10 to 14 days.

Chronic tonsillitis (six infections per year or four infections each year for 2 years) or the development of complications (obstructions from tonsillar hypertrophy or peritonsillar abscess) may require a tonsillectomy, but only after the patient has been free from tonsillar or respiratory tract infections for 3 to 4 weeks.

Drugs

• Anti-infectives, such as erythromycin, clarithromycin (Biaxin), azithromycin (Zithromax), and clindamycin (Cleocin), to combat infection
• Analgesics for pain

SPECIAL CONSIDERATIONS

• Despite dysphagia, urge the patient to drink plenty of fluids, especially if he has a fever. Offer a child flavored drinks and ices. Suggest gargling with warm salt water to soothe the throat, unless it exacerbates pain. Make sure the patient and his parents understand the importance of completing the prescribed course of antibiotic therapy.
• Before tonsillectomy, explain to the adult patient that a local anesthetic prevents pain but allows a sensation of pressure during surgery. Warn the patient to expect considerable throat discomfort and some bleeding postoperatively. Watch for continuous swallowing, a sign of heavy bleeding.

- For the pediatric patient, keep your explanation simple and non-threatening. Show him the operating and recovery areas, and briefly explain the facility routine. Most facilities allow one parent to stay with the child.

- Postoperatively, maintain a patent airway. To prevent aspiration, place the patient on his side. Monitor vital signs frequently, and check for bleeding. Immediately report excessive bleeding, increased pulse rate, or dropping blood pressure. After the patient is fully alert and the gag reflex has returned, allow him to drink water. Later, urge him to drink plenty of nonirritating fluids, to ambulate, and to take frequent deep breaths to prevent pulmonary complications. Give pain medication as needed.

- Before discharge, provide the patient or his parents with written instructions on home care. Tell them to expect a white scab to form in the throat between 5 and 10 days postoperatively, and to report bleeding, ear discomfort, or a fever that lasts longer than 3 days.

⧉ **PREVENTION**

- *The use of the antipneumococcal vaccine may help prevent acute tonsillitis, although there's not yet sufficient evidence to confirm that the vaccine will prevent infection.*

Tuberculosis

An acute or chronic infection caused by *Mycobacterium tuberculosis*, tuberculosis (TB) is characterized by pulmonary infiltrates, formation of granulomas with caseation, fibrosis, and cavitation. People who live in crowded, poorly ventilated conditions and those who are immunocompromised are most likely to become infected. In patients with strains that are sensitive to the usual antitubercular agents, the prognosis is excellent with correct treatment. However, in those with strains that are resistant to two or more of the major antitubercular agents, mortality is 50%.

CAUSES AND INCIDENCE

After exposure to *M. tuberculosis*, roughly 5% of infected people develop active TB within 1 year; in the remainder, microorganisms cause a latent infection. The host's immune system usually controls the tubercle bacillus by enclosing it in a tiny nodule (tubercle). The bacillus may lie dormant within the tubercle for years and later reactivate and spread.

Although the primary infection site is the lungs, mycobacteria commonly exist in other parts of the body. Several factors increase the risk of infection reactivation: gastrectomy, uncontrolled diabetes mellitus, Hodgkin's lymphoma, leukemia, silicosis, acquired immunodeficiency syndrome, treatment with corticosteroids or immunosuppressants, and advanced age.

Transmission is by droplet nuclei, which is produced when infected persons cough or sneeze. People with cavitary lesions are particularly infectious because their sputum typically contains anywhere from 1 to 100 million bacilli per ml. If an inhaled tubercle bacillus settles in an alveolus, infection occurs, leading to alveolocapillary dilation and endothelial cell swelling. Alveolitis results, with replication of tubercle bacilli and influx of polymorphonuclear leukocytes. These organisms spread through the lymph system to the circulatory system and then throughout the body.

Cell-mediated immunity to the mycobacteria, which develops 3 to 6 weeks later, usually contains the infection and arrests the disease. If the infection reactivates, the body's response characteristically leads to caseation—the conversion of necrotic tissue to a cheeselike material. The caseum may localize, undergo fibrosis, or excavate and form cavities, the walls of which are studded with multiplying tubercle bacilli. If this happens, infected caseous debris may spread throughout the lungs by the tracheobronchial tree. Sites of extrapulmonary TB include the pleurae, meninges, joints, lymph nodes, peritoneum, genitourinary tract, and bowel. (See *Appearance of tuberculosis on lung tissue,* page 194.)

The incidence of TB has been increasing in the United States secondary to homelessness, drug abuse, crowded living conditions, drug-resistant strains, and human immunodeficiency virus infection. Globally, TB is the leading infectious cause of morbidity and mortality, generating 8 to 10 million new cases each year.

SIGNS AND SYMPTOMS

After an incubation period of 4 to 8 weeks, TB is usually asymptomatic in primary infection but may produce nonspecific symptoms, such as:

- fatigue
- weakness
- anorexia
- weight loss
- night sweats
- low-grade fever
- chills
- loss of appetite
- painful breathing or coughing
- crepitant crackles
- bronchial breath sounds
- wheezing
- whispered pectoriloquy
- dullness over the affected area.

⚠ ALERT

Fever and night sweats, the typical hallmarks of TB, may not be present in elderly patients, who instead may exhibit a change in activity or weight. Assess older patients carefully.

In reactivation, signs and symptoms may include a cough that produces mucopurulent sputum, occasional hemoptysis, and chest pain.

COMPLICATIONS

- Respiratory failure
- Bronchopleural fistulas
- Pneumothorax
- Hemorrhage
- Pleural effusion
- Pneumonia

APPEARANCE OF TUBERCULOSIS ON LUNG TISSUE

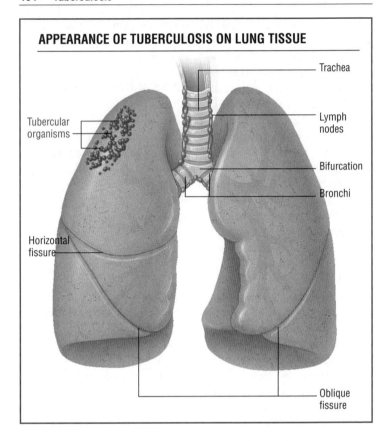

DIAGNOSIS

• A chest X-ray shows nodular lesions, patchy infiltrates (mainly in upper lobes), cavity formation, scar tissue, and calcium deposits; however, it may not be able to distinguish active from inactive TB.

• A tuberculin skin test detects TB infection. Intermediate-strength purified protein derivative of five tuberculin units (0.1 ml) are injected intracutaneously on the forearm. The test results are read in 48 to 72 hours; a positive reaction (induration of 5 to 15 mm or more, depend-

ing on risk factors) develops 2 to 10 weeks after infection in active and inactive TB. However, severely immunosuppressed patients may never develop a positive reaction.

• Stains and cultures of sputum, cerebrospinal fluid, urine, drainage from abscess, or pleural fluid show heat-sensitive, nonmotile, aerobic, acid-fast bacilli.

TREATMENT

Drug therapy must be selected according to the patient's condition and organism susceptibility. Interruption of drug therapy may require initiation of therapy from the beginning of the regimen or additional treatment. Directly observed therapy (DOT) may be selected or required. In this therapy, an assigned caregiver directly observes the administration of the drug. The goal of DOT is to monitor the treatment regimen and reduce the development of resistant organisms.

Drugs

- Antitubercular medications, including isoniazid (Laniazid, Nydrazid), rifampin (Rifadin, Rifadin IV, Rimactane), pyrazinamide, ethambutol (Myambutol), streptomycin sulfate, capreomycin (Capastat), clofazimine (Lamprene), cycloserine (Seromycin), ethionamide (Trecator), dapsone (Avlosulfon), ciprofloxacin (Cipro), and levofloxacin (Levaquin), often used in various combinations, to combat *M. tuberculosis*

SPECIAL CONSIDERATIONS

- Initiate acid-fast bacillus (AFB) isolation precautions immediately for all patients suspected or confirmed of having TB. AFB isolation precautions include the use of a private room with negative pressure in relation to surrounding areas and a minimum of six air exchanges per hour (air exhausted should be exhausted directly to the outside).
- Continue AFB isolation until there's clinical evidence of reduced infectiousness (substantially decreased cough, fewer organisms on sequential sputum smears, and three consecutive negative sputum culture smears).
- Teach the infectious patient to cough and sneeze into tissues and to dispose of all secretions properly. Place a covered trash can nearby, or tape a lined bag to the side of the bed to dispose of used tissues.
- Instruct the patient to wear a mask when outside his room.
- Ensure that visitors and staff members wear particulate respirators that fit closely around the face when they're in the patient's room.
- Remind the patient to get plenty of rest. Stress the importance of eating balanced meals to promote recovery. If the patient is anorexic, urge him to eat small meals frequently. Record weight weekly.
- Be alert for adverse effects of medications. Because isoniazid sometimes leads to hepatitis or peripheral neuritis, monitor aspartate aminotransferase and alanine aminotransferase levels. To prevent or treat peripheral neuritis, give pyridoxine (vitamin B_6) as ordered. If the patient receives ethambutol, watch for optic neuritis; if it develops, discontinue the drug. If he receives rifampin, watch for hepatitis and purpura. Also watch for other complications such as hemoptysis.
- Before discharge, advise the patient to watch for adverse effects from the medication and to report them immediately. Emphasize the importance of regular follow-up examinations. Teach the patient and his

⊒ PREVENTION
PREVENTING TUBERCULOSIS

The best way to prevent tuberculosis (TB) is early detection to prevent it from becoming active. Hospitalized patients with TB should be isolated from other patients using airborne precautions. Staff members should also use disposable HEPA filter masks which serve as adequate respiratory protection when caring for patients who are in airborne isolation.

Other ways to prevent the spread of TB include:
■ If a patient has a weakened immune system or has human immunodeficiency virus, it is recommended that he receive annual TB testing. Annual testing is also recommended for health care workers, those who work in a prison or a long-term care facility, and those with a substantially increased risk of exposure to the disease.
■ If a patient tests positive for latent TB infection but has no evidence of active TB, he may be able to reduce his risk of developing active TB by taking a course of therapy with isoniazid.

To prevent the spread of disease from those with active TB or from those who are receiving treatment, the following recommendations should be followed:
■ Stress the need to maintain the treatment regimen and to not stop or skip doses. When the treatment regimen is stopped, the TB bacteria can mutate and become drug resistant.
■ The patient who is on a treatment regimen is still contagious until he has been taking the medications for two to three weeks. Encouraging the patient to stay indoors and home from school or work is recommended. If he must leave his home, a mask is recommended during this initial treatment time to lessen the risk of transmission.

---

family the signs and symptoms of recurring TB. Stress the need to follow long-term treatment faithfully.

● Emphasize the importance of taking the medication daily as pre-scribed. He may enroll in a supervised administration program to avoid the development of drug-resistant organisms. (See *Preventing tuberculosis*.)

Part

2

Drugs

acetazolamide
ah-set-a-ZOLE-ah-mide

Acetazolam†, Diamox Sequels

acetazolamide sodium

Pharmacologic class: carbonic
anhydrase inhibitor
Pregnancy risk category C

AVAILABLE FORMS
acetazolamide
Capsules (extended-release): 500 mg
Tablets: 125 mg, 250 mg
acetazolamide sodium
Powder for injection: 500-mg vial

INDICATIONS & DOSAGES
➤ **Secondary glaucoma; preoperative treatment of acute angle-closure glaucoma**
Adults: 250 mg P.O. every 4 hours or
250 mg P.O. b.i.d. for short-term therapy.
In acute cases, 500 mg P.O.; then 125 to
250 mg P.O. every 4 hours. To rapidly
lower intraocular pressure (IOP), initially, 500 mg I.V.; may repeat in 2 to
4 hours, if needed, followed by 125 to
250 mg P.O. every 4 to 6 hours.
Children: 10 to 15 mg/kg P.O. daily in
divided doses every 6 to 8 hours. For acute
angle-closure glaucoma, 5 to 10 mg/kg I.V.
every 6 hours.
➤ **Chronic open-angle glaucoma**
Adults: 250 mg to 1 g P.O. daily in divided
doses q.i.d., or 500 mg extended-release
P.O. b.i.d.
➤ **To prevent or treat acute mountain sickness (high-altitude sickness)**
Adults: 500 mg to 1 g (regular or extended-
release) P.O. daily in divided doses every
12 hours. Start 24 to 48 hours before
ascent and continue for 48 hours while
at high altitude. When rapid ascent is
required, start with 1,000 mg P.O. daily.
➤ **Adjunct for epilepsy and myoclonic, refractory, generalized tonic-clonic, absence, or mixed seizures**

Adults and children: 8 to 30 mg/kg P.O.
daily in divided doses. For adults, 375 mg
to 1 g daily is ideal. If given with other
anticonvulsants, start at 250 mg P.O. once
daily, and increase to 375 mg to 1 g daily.
➤ **Edema caused by heart failure;
drug-induced edema**
Adults: 250 mg to 375 mg (5 mg/kg) P.O.
daily in the morning. For best results, use
every other day or 2 days on followed by 1
to 2 days off.
Children: 5 mg/kg or 150 mg/m² P.O. or
I.V. daily in the morning.

ADMINISTRATION
P.O.
● Give drug with food to minimize GI
upset.
● Don't crush or open extended-release
capsules.
● If patient can't swallow oral form, pharmacist may make a suspension using
crushed tablets in a highly flavored syrup,
such as cherry, raspberry, or chocolate to
mask the bitter flavor. Although concentrations up to 500 mg/5 ml are possible,
concentrations of 250 mg/5 ml are more
palatable.
● Refrigeration improves palatability but
doesn't improve stability. Suspensions are
stable for 1 week.
I.V.
● Reconstitute drug in 500-mg vial with at
least 5 ml of sterile water for injection. Use
within 12 hours of reconstitution.
● Inject 100 to 500 mg/minute into a large
vein using a 21G or 23G needle.
● Direct I.V. injection is the preferred
route.
● Intermittent and continuous infusions
aren't recommended.
● **Incompatibilities:** Multivitamins.

ACTION
Promotes renal excretion of sodium,
potassium, bicarbonate, and water. As
anticonvulsant, drug normalizes neuronal discharge. In mountain sickness,
drug stimulates ventilation and increases

cerebral blood flow. In glaucoma, drug reduces intraocular pressure (IOP).

Route	Onset	Peak	Duration
P.O.	60–90 min	1–4 hr	8–12 hr
P.O. (extended-release)	2 hr	3–6 hr	18–24 hr
I.V.	2 min	15 min	4–5 hr

Half-life: 10 to 15 hours.

ADVERSE REACTIONS

CNS: *seizures,* drowsiness, paresthesia, confusion, depression, weakness, ataxia.
EENT: transient myopia, hearing dysfunction, tinnitus.
GI: nausea, vomiting, anorexia, metallic taste, diarrhea, black tarry stools, constipation.
GU: polyuria, hematuria, crystalluria, glycosuria, phosphaturia, renal calculus.
Hematologic: *aplastic anemia, leukopenia, thrombocytopenia,* hemolytic anemia.
Metabolic: hypokalemia, asymptomatic hyperuricemia, hyperchloremic acidosis.
Skin: *pain at injection site, Stevens-Johnson syndrome,* rash, urticaria.
Other: sterile abscesses.

INTERACTIONS

Drug-drug. *Amphetamines, anticholinergics, mecamylamine, procainamide, quinidine:* May decrease renal clearance of these drugs, increasing toxicity. Monitor patient for toxicity.
Cyclosporine: May increase cyclosporine level, causing nephrotoxicity and neurotoxicity. Monitor patient for toxicity.
Diflunisal: May increase acetazolamide adverse effects; may significantly decrease IOP. Use together cautiously.
Lithium: May increase lithium excretion, decreasing its effect. Monitor lithium level.
Methenamine: May reduce methenamine effect. Avoid using together.
Primidone: May decrease serum and urine primidone levels. Monitor patient closely.
Salicylates: May cause accumulation and toxicity of acetazolamide, including CNS depression and metabolic acidosis. Monitor patient for toxicity.
Drug-lifestyle. *Sun exposure:* May increase risk of photosensitivity reactions.

Advise patient to avoid excessive sunlight exposure.

EFFECTS ON LAB TEST RESULTS

• May increase uric acid level. May decrease potassium and hemoglobin levels and hematocrit.
• May decrease WBC and platelet counts.
• May decrease iodine uptake by the thyroid in hyperthyroid and euthyroid patients. May cause false-positive urine protein test result.

CONTRAINDICATIONS & CAUTIONS

• Contraindicated in patients hypersensitive to drug and in those with hyponatremia or hypokalemia, renal or hepatic disease or dysfunction, renal calculi, adrenal gland failure, hyperchloremic acidosis, or severe pulmonary obstruction.
• Contraindicated in those receiving long-term treatment for chronic noncongestive angle-closure glaucoma.
• Use cautiously in patients receiving other diuretics and in those with respiratory acidosis or COPD.

NURSING CONSIDERATIONS

• Cross-sensitivity between antibacterial sulfonamides and sulfonamide-derivative diuretics such as acetazolamide has been reported.
• Monitor fluid intake and output, glucose, and electrolytes, especially potassium, bicarbonate, and chloride. When drug is used in diuretic therapy, consult prescriber and dietitian about providing a high-potassium diet.
• Monitor elderly patients closely because they are especially susceptible to excessive diuresis.
• Weigh patient daily. Rapid or excessive fluid loss may cause weight loss and hypotension.
• Diuretic effect decreases when acidosis occurs but can be reestablished by using intermittent administration schedules.
• Monitor patient for signs of hemolytic anemia (pallor, weakness, and palpitations).
• Drug may increase glucose level and cause glycosuria.
• *Look alike–sound alike:* Don't confuse acetazolamide with acetaminophen or acyclovir.

Reactions may be *common,* uncommon, *life-threatening,* or COMMON AND LIFE-THREATENING.
Interaction may have a *rapid onset* or *delayed onset.*

PATIENT TEACHING
- Tell patient to take oral form with food to minimize GI upset.
- Tell patient not to crush, chew, or open capsules.
- Caution patient not to perform hazardous activities if adverse CNS reactions occur.
- Instruct patient to avoid prolonged exposure to sunlight because drug may cause phototoxicity.
- Instruct patient to notify prescriber of any unusual bleeding, bruising, tingling, or tremors.

---

acetylcysteine
a-se-teel-SIS-tay-een

Acetadote, Mucomyst

Pharmacologic class: L-cysteine derivative
Pregnancy risk category B

AVAILABLE FORMS
Solution: 10%, 20%
I.V. injection: 200 mg/ml

INDICATIONS & DOSAGES
➤ **Adjunct therapy for abnormal viscid or thickened mucous secretions in patients with pneumonia, bronchitis, bronchiectasis, primary amyloidosis of the lung, tuberculosis, cystic fibrosis, emphysema, atelectasis, pulmonary complications of thoracic surgery, or CV surgery**
Adults and children: 1 to 2 ml 10% or 20% solution by direct instillation into trachea as often as every hour. Or, 1 to 10 ml of 20% solution or 2 to 20 ml of 10% solution by nebulization every 2 to 6 hours, p.r.n.
➤ **Acetaminophen toxicity**
Adults and children: Initially, 140 mg/kg P.O.; then 70 mg/kg P.O. every 4 hours for 17 doses (total). Or, a loading dose of 150 mg/kg I.V. over 60 minutes; then I.V. maintenance dose of 50 mg/kg infused over 4 hours, followed by 100 mg/kg infused over 16 hours.

ADMINISTRATION
P.O.
- Dilute oral dose (used for acetaminophen overdose) with cola, fruit juice, or water.

Dilute 20% solution to 5% (add 3 ml of diluent to each milliliter of drug). If patient vomits within 1 hour of receiving loading or maintenance dose, repeat dose. Use diluted solution within 1 hour.
- Drug smells strongly of sulfur. Mixing oral form with juice or cola improves its taste.
- Drug delivered through nasogastric tube may be diluted with water.
- Store opened, undiluted oral solution in the refrigerator for up to 96 hours.
I.V.
- Drug may turn from a colorless liquid to a slight pink or purple color once the stopper is punctured. This color change doesn't affect the drug.
- Drug is hyperosmolar and is compatible with D_5W, half-normal saline, and sterile water for injection.
- Adjust total volume given for patients who weigh less than 40 kg or who are fluid restricted.
- For patients who weigh 40 kg (88 lb) or more, dilute loading dose in 200 ml of D_5W, second dose in 500 ml, and third dose in 1,000 ml.
- For patients who weigh 25 to 40 kg (55 to 88 lb), dilute loading dose in 100 ml, second dose in 250 ml, and third dose in 500 ml.
- For patients who weigh 20 kg (44 lb), dilute loading dose in 60 ml, second dose in 140 ml, and third dose in 280 ml.
- For patients who weigh 15 kg (33 lb), dilute loading dose in 45 ml, second dose in 105 ml, and third dose in 210 ml.
- For patients who weigh 10 kg (22 lb), dilute loading dose in 30 ml, second dose in 70 ml, and third dose in 140 ml.
- Reconstituted solution is stable for 24 hours at room temperature.
- Vials contain no preservatives; discard after opening.
- **Incompatibilities:** Incompatible with rubber and metals, especially iron, copper, and nickel.
Inhalational
- Use plastic, glass, stainless steel, or another nonreactive metal when giving by nebulization. Hand-bulb nebulizers aren't recommended because output is too small and particle size too large.
- **Incompatibilities:** Physically or chemically incompatible with inhaled

tetracyclines, erythromycin lactobionate, amphotericin B, and ampicillin sodium. If given by aerosol inhalation, nebulize these drugs separately. Iodized oil, trypsin, and hydrogen peroxide are physically incompatible with acetylcysteine; don't add to nebulizer.

ACTION
Reduces the viscosity of pulmonary secretions by splitting disulfide linkages between mucoprotein molecular complexes. Also, restores liver stores of glutathione to treat acetaminophen toxicity.

Route	Onset	Peak	Duration
P.O., I.V., inhalation	Unknown	Unknown	Unknown

Half-life: 6¼ hours.

ADVERSE REACTIONS
CNS: abnormal thinking, fever, drowsiness, gait disturbances.
CV: chest tightness, flushing, hypertension, hypotension, tachycardia.
EENT: *rhinorrhea,* ear pain, eye pain, pharyngitis, throat tightness.
GI: *nausea, stomatitis, vomiting.*
Respiratory: *bronchospasm,* cough, dyspnea, rhonchi.
Skin: clamminess, diaphoresis, pruritus, rash, urticaria.
Other: *anaphylactoid reaction, angioedema,* chills.

INTERACTIONS
Drug-drug. *Activated charcoal:* May limit acetylcysteine's effectiveness. Avoid using activated charcoal before or with acetylcysteine.

EFFECTS ON LAB TEST RESULTS
None reported.

CONTRAINDICATIONS & CAUTIONS
• Contraindicated in patients hypersensitive to drug.

• Use cautiously in elderly or debilitated patients with severe respiratory insufficiency. Use I.V. form cautiously in patients with asthma or a history of bronchospasm.

NURSING CONSIDERATIONS
• Monitor cough type and frequency.
• *Alert:* Monitor patient for bronchospasm, especially if he has asthma.
• Ingestion of more than 150 mg/kg of acetaminophen may cause liver toxicity. Measure acetaminophen level 4 hours after ingestion to determine risk of liver toxicity.
• *Alert:* Drug is used for acetaminophen overdose within 24 hours of ingestion. Start drug immediately; don't wait for results of acetaminophen level. Give within 10 hours of acetaminophen ingestion to minimize hepatic injury.
• If you suspect acetaminophen overdose, obtain baseline AST, ALT, bilirubin, PT, BUN, creatinine, glucose, and electrolyte levels.
• *Alert:* Monitor patient receiving I.V. form for anaphylactoid reactions. If anaphylactoid reaction occurs, stop infusion and treat anaphylaxis. Once anaphylaxis treatment starts, restart infusion. If anaphylactoid symptoms return, stop drug. Contact the Poison Control Center at (800) 222-1222 for more information.
• Facial erythema may occur within 30 to 60 minutes of start of I.V. infusion and usually resolves without stopping infusion.
• When acetaminophen level is below toxic level according to nomogram, stop therapy.
• *Look alike–sound alike:* Don't confuse acetylcysteine with acetylcholine.
• The vial stopper doesn't contain natural rubber latex, dry natural rubber, or blends of natural rubber.

PATIENT TEACHING
• Warn patient that drug may have a foul taste or smell that may be distressing.
• For maximum effect, instruct patient to cough to clear his airway before aerosol administration.

acyclovir
ay-SYE-kloe-ver

Zovirax

acyclovir sodium
Zovirax

Pharmacologic class: synthetic
purine nucleoside
Pregnancy risk category B

AVAILABLE FORMS
Capsules: 200 mg
Injection: 500 mg/vial, 1 g/vial
Suspension: 200 mg/5 ml
Tablets: 400 mg, 800 mg

INDICATIONS & DOSAGES
➤ **First and recurrent episodes of
mucocutaneous herpes simplex
virus (HSV-1 and HSV-2) infections
in immunocompromised patients;
severe first episodes of genital herpes
in patients who aren't immunocompromised**
Adults and children age 12 and older:
5 mg/kg given I.V. over 1 hour every
8 hours for 7 days. Give for 5 to 7 days for
severe first episode of genital herpes.
Children younger than age 12: Give
10 mg/kg I.V. over 1 hour every 8 hours for
7 days.
➤ **First genital herpes episode**
Adults: 200 mg P.O. every 4 hours while
awake, five times daily; or 400 mg P.O.
every 8 hours. Continue for 7 to 10 days.
➤ **Intermittent therapy for recurrent genital herpes**
Adults: 200 mg P.O. every 4 hours while
awake, five times daily. Continue for
5 days. Begin therapy at first sign of recurrence.
➤ **Long-term suppressive therapy
for recurrent genital herpes**
Adults: 400 mg P.O. b.i.d. for up to
12 months. Or, 200 mg P.O. three to five
times daily for up to 12 months.
➤ **Varicella (chickenpox) infections
in immunocompromised patients**
Adults and children age 12 and older:
10 mg/kg I.V. over 1 hour every 8 hours
for 7 days. Dosage for obese patients is
10 mg/kg based on ideal body weight

every 8 hours for 7 days. Don't exceed
maximum dosage equivalent of 20 mg/kg
every 8 hours.
Children younger than age 12: Give
20 mg/kg I.V. over 1 hour every 8 hours for
7 days.
➤ **Varicella infection in immunocompetent patients**
*Adults and children who weigh more than
40 kg (88 lb):* 800 mg P.O. q.i.d. for 5 days.
*Children age 2 and older, who weigh
less than 40 kg:* 20 mg/kg (maximum
800 mg/dose) P.O. q.i.d. for 5 days. Start
therapy as soon as symptoms appear.
➤ **Acute herpes zoster infection in
immunocompetent patients**
Adults and children age 12 and older:
800 mg P.O. every 4 hours five times daily
for 7 to 10 days.
➤ **Herpes simplex encephalitis**
Adults and children age 12 and older:
10 mg/kg I.V. over 1 hour every 8 hours for
10 days.
Children ages 3 months to 12 years:
20 mg/kg I.V. over 1 hour every 8 hours for
10 days.
➤ **Neonatal herpes simplex virus
infection**
Neonates to 3 months old: 10 mg/kg I.V.
over 1 hour every 8 hours for 10 days.
Adjust-a-dose: For patients receiving the
I.V. form, if creatinine clearance is 25 to
50 ml/minute, give 100% of dose every
12 hours; if clearance is 10 to
24 ml/minute, give 100% of dose every
24 hours; if clearance is less than
10 ml/minute, give 50% of dose every
24 hours.

For patients receiving the P.O. form,
if normal dose is 200 mg every 4 hours
five times daily and creatinine clearance
is less than 10 ml/minute, give 200 mg
P.O. every 12 hours. If normal dose is
400 mg every 12 hours and clearance
is less than 10 ml/minute, give 200 mg
every 12 hours. If normal dose is
800 mg every 4 hours five times daily
and clearance is 10 to 25 ml/minute, give
800 mg every 8 hours; if clearance is less
than 10 ml/minute, give 800 mg every
12 hours.

ADMINISTRATION

P.O.
• Give drug without regard for meals, but give with food if stomach irritation occurs.
• Patient should take drug as prescribed, even after he feels better.

I.V.
• Solutions concentrated at 7 mg/ml or more may cause a higher risk of phlebitis.
• Encourage fluid intake because patient must be adequately hydrated during infusion.
• Bolus injection, dehydration (decreased urine output), renal disease, and use with other nephrotoxic drugs increase the risk of renal toxicity. Don't give by bolus injection.
• Give I.V. infusion over at least 1 hour to prevent renal tubular damage.
• Monitor intake and output, especially during the first 2 hours after administration.
• *Alert:* Don't give I.M. or subcutaneously.
• **Incompatibilities:** Amifostine, aztreonam, biological or colloidal solutions, cefepime, cisatracurium besylate, diltiazem hydrochloride, dobutamine hydrochloride, dopamine hydrochloride, fludarabine phosphate, foscarnet sodium, gemcitabine hydrochloride, idarubicin hydrochloride, levofloxacin, meperidine hydrochloride, meropenem, morphine sulfate, ondansetron hydrochloride, parabens, piperacillin sodium and tazobactam sodium, sargramostim, tacrolimus, vinorelbine tartrate.

ACTION
Interferes with DNA synthesis and inhibits viral multiplication.

Route	Onset	Peak	Duration
P.O.	Unknown	2½ hr	Unknown
I.V.	Immediate	Immediate	Unknown

Half-life: 2 to 3½ hours with normal renal function; up to 19 hours with renal impairment.

ADVERSE REACTIONS
CNS: *headache, malaise, encephalopathic changes (including lethargy, obtundation, tremor, confusion, hallucinations, agitation, seizures, coma).*
GI: *nausea, vomiting,* diarrhea.
GU: *acute renal failure,* hematuria.

Hematologic: *leukopenia, thrombocytopenia,* thrombocytosis.
Skin: *inflammation or phlebitis at injection site,* itching, rash, urticaria.

INTERACTIONS
Drug-drug. *Interferon:* May have synergistic effect. Monitor patient closely.
Probenecid: May increase acyclovir level. Monitor patient for possible toxicity.
Zidovudine: May cause drowsiness or lethargy. Use together cautiously.

EFFECTS ON LAB TEST RESULTS
• May increase BUN and creatinine levels.
• May decrease WBC count. May increase or decrease platelet count.

CONTRAINDICATIONS & CAUTIONS
• Contraindicated in patients hypersensitive to drug.
• Use cautiously in patients with neurologic problems, renal disease, or dehydration, and in those receiving other nephrotoxic drugs.
• Adequate studies haven't been done in pregnant women; use only if potential benefits outweigh risks to fetus.

NURSING CONSIDERATIONS
• In patients with renal disease or dehydration and in those taking other nephrotoxic drugs, monitor renal function.
• Encephalopathic changes are more likely to occur in patients with neurologic disorders and in those who have had neurologic reactions to cytotoxic drugs.
• *Look alike–sound alike:* Don't confuse acyclovir sodium (Zovirax) with acetazolamide sodium (Diamox) vials, which may look alike.
• *Look alike–sound alike:* Don't confuse Zovirax with Zyvox.

PATIENT TEACHING
• Tell patient to take drug as prescribed, even after he feels better.
• Tell patient drug is effective in managing herpes infection but doesn't eliminate or cure it. Warn patient that drug won't prevent spread of infection to others.
• Tell patient to avoid sexual contact while visible lesions are present.
• Teach patient about early signs and symptoms of herpes infection (such as

tingling, itching, or pain). Tell him to notify prescriber and get a prescription for drug before the infection fully develops. Early treatment is most effective.

adefovir dipivoxil
ah-DEF-oh-veer

Hepsera

Pharmacologic class: acyclic nucleotide analogue
Pregnancy risk category C

AVAILABLE FORMS
Tablets: 10 mg

INDICATIONS & DOSAGES
➤ **Chronic hepatitis B infection**
Adults: 10 mg P.O. once daily.
Adjust-a-dose: In patients with creatinine clearance of 20 to 49 ml/minute, give 10 mg P.O. every 48 hours. In patients with clearance of 10 to 19 ml/minute, give 10 mg P.O. every 72 hours. In patients receiving hemodialysis, give 10 mg P.O. every 7 days, after dialysis session.

ADMINISTRATION
P.O.
● Give drug without regard for meals.

ACTION
An acyclic nucleotide analogue that inhibits hepatitis B virus reverse transcription via viral DNA chain termination.

Route	Onset	Peak	Duration
P.O.	Unknown	1–4 hr	Unknown

Half-life: Unknown.

ADVERSE REACTIONS
CNS: *asthenia,* fever, headache.
EENT: pharyngitis, sinusitis.
GI: abdominal pain, diarrhea, dyspepsia, flatulence, nausea, vomiting.
GU: *renal failure, renal insufficiency, hematuria,* glycosuria.
Hepatic: *hepatic failure,* hepatomegaly with steatosis.
Metabolic: *lactic acidosis.*
Respiratory: cough.
Skin: pruritus, rash.

INTERACTIONS
Drug-drug. *Ibuprofen:* May increase adefovir bioavailability. Monitor patient for adverse effects.
Nephrotoxic drugs (aminoglycosides, cyclosporine, NSAIDs, tacrolimus, vancomycin): May increase risk of nephrotoxicity. Use together cautiously.

EFFECTS ON LAB TEST RESULTS
● May increase ALT, amylase, AST, CK, creatinine, and lactate levels.

CONTRAINDICATIONS & CAUTIONS
● Contraindicated in patients hypersensitive to any component of the drug.
● Use cautiously in patients with renal dysfunction, in those receiving nephrotoxic drugs, and in those with known risk factors for hepatic disease.
● In elderly patients, use cautiously because they're more likely to have decreased renal and cardiac function.
● Safety and effectiveness in children haven't been established.

NURSING CONSIDERATIONS
● Monitor renal function, especially in patients with renal dysfunction or those taking nephrotoxic drugs.
● *Alert:* Patients may develop lactic acidosis and severe hepatomegaly with steatosis during treatment. Women, obese patients, and those taking antiretrovirals are at higher risk.
● Monitor hepatic function. Notify prescriber if patient develops signs or symptoms of lactic acidosis and severe hepatomegaly with steatosis. Stop drug, if needed.
● Stopping adefovir may cause severe worsening of hepatitis. Monitor hepatic function closely in patients who stop antihepatitis B therapy.
● The ideal length of treatment hasn't been established.
● Offer patients HIV antibody testing; drug may promote resistance to antiretrovirals in patients with unrecognized or untreated HIV infection.
● For pregnant women, call the Antiretroviral Pregnancy Registry at 1-800-258-4263 to monitor fetal outcome.

PATIENT TEACHING
• Inform the patient that drug may be taken without regard to meals.
• Tell patient to immediately report weakness, muscle pain, trouble breathing, stomach pain with nausea and vomiting, dizziness, light-headedness, fast or irregular heartbeat, and feeling cold, especially in arms and legs.
• Warn patient not to stop taking this drug unless directed because it could cause hepatitis to become worse.
• Instruct woman to tell her prescriber if she becomes pregnant or is breast-feeding. It's unknown if drug appears in breast milk. Use cautiously in breast-feeding women.

---

albuterol sulfate
al-BYOO-ter-ole

AccuNeb, ProAir HFA, Proventil, Proventil HFA, Ventolin, Ventolin HFA, VoSpire ER

Pharmacologic class: adrenergic
Pregnancy risk category C

AVAILABLE FORMS
Inhalation aerosol: 90 mcg/metered spray
Solution for inhalation: 0.083% (2.5 mg/ 3 ml), 0.5% (5 mg/ml), 0.042% (1.25 mg/ 3 ml), 0.021% (0.63 mg/3 ml)
Syrup: 2 mg/5 ml
Tablets: 2 mg, 4 mg
Tablets (extended-release): 4 mg, 8 mg

INDICATIONS & DOSAGES
➤ **To prevent or treat bronchospasm in patients with reversible obstructive airway disease**
Tablets (extended-release)
Adults and children age 12 and older: 4 to 8 mg P.O. every 12 hours. Maximum, 32 mg daily.
Children ages 6 to 11: 4 mg P.O. every 12 hours. Maximum, 24 mg daily.
Tablets
Adults and children age 12 and older: 2 to 4 mg P.O. t.i.d. or q.i.d. Maximum, 32 mg daily.
Children ages 6 to 11: 2 mg P.O. t.i.d. or q.i.d. Maximum, 24 mg daily.

Solution for inhalation
Adults and children age 12 and older: 2.5 mg t.i.d. or q.i.d. by nebulizer, given over 5 to 15 minutes. To prepare solution, use 0.5 ml of 0.5% solution diluted with 2.5 ml of normal saline solution. Or, use 3 ml of 0.083% solution.
Children ages 2 to 12 weighing more than 15 kg (33 lb): 2.5 mg by nebulizer given over 5 to 15 minutes t.i.d. or q.i.d., with subsequent doses adjusted to response. Don't exceed 2.5 mg t.i.d. or q.i.d.
Children ages 2 to 12 weighing 15 kg or less: 0.63 mg or 1.25 mg by nebulizer given over 5 to 15 minutes t.i.d. or q.i.d. with subsequent doses adjusted to response. Don't exceed 2.5 mg t.i.d. or q.i.d.
Syrup
Adults and children older than age 14: 2 to 4 mg (1 to 2 tsp) P.O. t.i.d. or q.i.d. Maximum, 32 mg daily.
Children ages 6 to 13: 2 mg (1 tsp) P.O. t.i.d. or q.i.d. Maximum, 24 mg daily.
Children ages 2 to 5: Initially, 0.1 mg/kg P.O. t.i.d. Starting dose shouldn't exceed 2 mg (1 tsp) t.i.d. Maximum, 12 mg daily.
Adjust-a-dose: For elderly patients and those sensitive to sympathomimetic amines, 2 mg P.O. t.i.d. or q.i.d. as oral tablets or syrup. Maximum, 32 mg daily
Inhalation aerosol
Adults and children age 4 and older: 1 to 2 inhalations every 4 to 6 hours as needed. Regular use for maintenance therapy to control asthma symptoms isn't recommended.
➤ **To prevent exercise-induced bronchospasm**
Adults and children age 4 and older: 2 inhalations using the inhalation aerosol 15 minutes before exercise; up to 12 inhalations may be taken in 24 hours.

ADMINISTRATION
P.O.
• When switching patient from regular to extended-release tablets, remember that a regular 2-mg tablet every 6 hours is equivalent to an extended-release 4-mg tablet every 12 hours.
• Give drug whole; don't break or crush extended-release tablets or mix them with food.

Inhalational
- If more than 1 inhalation is ordered, wait at least 2 minutes between inhalations.
- Use spacer device to improve drug delivery, if appropriate.
- Shake the inhaler before use.

ACTION
Relaxes bronchial, uterine, and vascular smooth muscle by stimulating beta$_2$ receptors.

Route	Onset	Peak	Duration
P.O.	15–30 min	2–3 hr	4–8 hr
P.O. (extended)	Unknown	6 hr	12 hr
Inhalation	5–15 min	30–120 min	2–6 hr

Half-life: About 4 hours.

ADVERSE REACTIONS
CNS: *tremor, nervousness, headache, hyperactivity,* insomnia, dizziness, weakness, CNS stimulation, malaise.
CV: *tachycardia, palpitations,* hypertension.
EENT: dry and irritated nose and throat with inhaled form, nasal congestion, epistaxis, hoarseness.
GI: *nausea, vomiting,* heartburn, anorexia, altered taste, increased appetite.
Metabolic: hypokalemia.
Musculoskeletal: muscle cramps.
Respiratory: *bronchospasm,* cough, wheezing, dyspnea, bronchitis, increased sputum.
Other: hypersensitivity reactions.

INTERACTIONS
Drug-drug. *CNS stimulants:* May increase CNS stimulation. Avoid using together.
Digoxin: May decrease digoxin level. Monitor digoxin level closely.
MAO inhibitors, tricyclic antidepressants: May increase adverse CV effects. Monitor patient closely.
Propranolol and other beta blockers: May cause mutual antagonism. Monitor patient carefully.

EFFECTS ON LAB TEST RESULTS
- May decrease potassium level.

CONTRAINDICATIONS & CAUTIONS
- Contraindicated in patients hypersensitive to drug or its ingredients.
- Use cautiously in patients with CV disorders (including coronary insufficiency and hypertension), hyperthyroidism, or diabetes mellitus and in those who are unusually responsive to adrenergics.
- Use extended-release tablets cautiously in patients with GI narrowing.

NURSING CONSIDERATIONS
- Drug may decrease sensitivity of spirometry used for diagnosis of asthma.
- Syrup contains no alcohol or sugar and may be taken by children as young as age 2.
- In children, syrup may rarely cause erythema multiforme or Stevens-Johnson syndrome.
- The HFA form uses the propellant hydrofluoroalkane (HFA) instead of chlorofluorocarbons.
- **Alert:** Patient may use tablets and aerosol together. Monitor these patients closely for signs and symptoms of toxicity.
- **Look alike–sound alike:** Don't confuse albuterol with atenolol or Albutein.

PATIENT TEACHING
- Warn patient about risk of paradoxical bronchospasm and to stop drug immediately if it occurs.
- Teach patient to perform oral inhalation correctly. Give the following instructions for using the MDI:
  – Shake the inhaler.
  – Clear nasal passages and throat.
  – Breathe out, expelling as much air from lungs as possible.
  – Place mouthpiece well into mouth, seal lips around mouthpiece, and inhale deeply as you release a dose from inhaler. Or, hold inhaler about 1 inch (two fingerwidths) from open mouth; inhale while dose is released.
  – Hold breath for several seconds, remove mouthpiece, and exhale slowly.
- If prescriber orders more than 1 inhalation, tell patient to wait at least 2 minutes before repeating procedure.
- Tell patient that use of a spacer device may improve drug delivery to lungs.
- If patient is also using a corticosteroid inhaler, instruct him to use the

bronchodilator first and then to wait about 5 minutes before using the corticosteroid. This lets the bronchodilator open the air passages for maximal effectiveness of the corticosteroid.
• Tell patient to remove canister and wash inhaler with warm, soapy water at least once a week.
• Advise patient to contact prescriber if using more than 4 inhalations per day for 2 or more days or more than one canister in 8 weeks.
• Advise patient not to chew or crush extended-release tablets or mix them with food.

SAFETY ALERT!

alprazolam
al-PRAH-zoe-lam

Apo-Alpraz†, Apo-Alpraz TS†, Niravam, Novo-Alprazol†, Xanax, Xanax XR

Pharmacologic class: benzodi-azepine
Pregnancy risk category D
Controlled substance schedule IV

AVAILABLE FORMS
Oral solution: 1 mg/ml (concentrate)
Orally disintegrating tablets (ODTs):
0.25 mg, 0.5 mg, 1 mg, 2 mg
Tablets: 0.25 mg, 0.5 mg, 1 mg, 2 mg
Tablets (extended-release): 0.5 mg, 1 mg, 2 mg, 3 mg

INDICATIONS & DOSAGES
➤ **Anxiety**
Adults: Usual first dose, 0.25 to 0.5 mg P.O. t.i.d. Maximum, 4 mg daily in divided doses.
Elderly patients: Usual first dose, 0.25 mg P.O. b.i.d. or t.i.d. Maximum, 4 mg daily in divided doses.
➤ **Panic disorders**
Adults: 0.5 mg P.O. t.i.d., increased at intervals of 3 to 4 days in increments of no more than 1 mg. Maximum, 10 mg daily in divided doses. If using extended-release tablets, start with 0.5 to 1 mg P.O. once daily. Increase by no more than 1 mg every 3 to 4 days. Maximum daily dose is 10 mg.

Adjust-a-dose: For debilitated patients or those with advanced hepatic disease, usual first dose is 0.25 mg P.O. b.i.d. or t.i.d. Maximum, 4 mg daily in divided doses.

ADMINISTRATION
P.O.
• Don't break or crush extended-release tablets.
• Mix oral solution with liquids or semisolid food, such as water, juices, carbonated beverages, applesauce, and puddings. Use only calibrated dropper provided with this product.
• Use dry hands to remove ODTs from bottle. Discard cotton from inside bottle.
• Discard unused portion if breaking scored ODT.

ACTION
Unknown. Probably potentiates the effects of GABA, depresses the CNS, and suppresses the spread of seizure activity.

Route	Onset	Peak	Duration
P.O.	Unknown	1–2 hr	Unknown
P.O. (extended-release)	Unknown	Unknown	Unknown

Half-life: Immediate-release, 12 to 15 hours; extended-release, 11 to 16 hours.

ADVERSE REACTIONS
CNS: *insomnia, irritability, dizziness, headache, anxiety, confusion, drowsiness, light-headedness, sedation, somnolence, difficulty speaking, impaired coordination, memory impairment, fatigue, depression, suicide,* mental impairment, ataxia, paresthesia, dyskinesia, hypoesthesia, lethargy, decreased or increased libido, vertigo, malaise, tremor, nervousness, restlessness, agitation, nightmare, syncope, akathisia, mania.
CV: palpitations, chest pain, hypotension.
EENT: sore throat, allergic rhinitis, blurred vision, nasal congestion.
GI: *diarrhea, dry mouth, constipation,* nausea, increased or decreased appetite, anorexia, vomiting, dyspepsia, abdominal pain.
GU: dysmenorrhea, sexual dysfunction, premenstrual syndrome, difficulty urinating.

Reactions may be *common*, uncommon, *life-threatening*, or COMMON AND LIFE-THREATENING.
Interaction may have a *rapid onset* or *delayed onset*.

Metabolic: increased or decreased weight.
Musculoskeletal: arthralgia, myalgia, arm or leg pain, back pain, muscle rigidity, muscle cramps, muscle twitch.
Respiratory: upper respiratory tract infection, dyspnea, hyperventilation.
Skin: pruritus, increased sweating, dermatitis.
Other: influenza, injury, emergence of anxiety between doses, dependence, feeling warm.

INTERACTIONS
Drug-drug. *Anticonvulsants, antidepressants, antihistamines, barbiturates, benzodiazepines, general anesthetics, narcotics, phenothiazines:* May increase CNS depressant effects. Avoid using together.
Azole antifungals (including fluconazole, itraconazole, ketoconazole, miconazole): May increase and prolong alprazolam level, CNS depression, and psychomotor impairment. Avoid using together.
Carbamazepine, *propoxyphene:* May induce alprazolam metabolism and may reduce therapeutic effects. May need to increase dose.
Cimetidine, fluoxetine, fluvoxamine, hormonal contraceptives, nefazodone: May increase alprazolam level. Use cautiously together, and consider alprazolam dosage reduction.
Tricyclic antidepressants: May increase levels of these drugs. Monitor patient closely.
Drug-herb. *Kava, valerian root:* May increase sedation. Discourage use together.
St. John's wort: May decrease drug level. Discourage use together.
Drug-food. *Grapefruit juice:* May increase drug level. Discourage use together.
Drug-lifestyle. *Alcohol use:* May cause additive CNS effects. Discourage use together.
Smoking: May decrease effectiveness of drug. Monitor patient closely.

EFFECTS ON LAB TEST RESULTS
● May increase ALT and AST levels.

CONTRAINDICATIONS & CAUTIONS
● Contraindicated in patients hypersensitive to drug or other benzodiazepines and in those with acute angle-closure glaucoma.

● Use cautiously in patients with hepatic, renal, or pulmonary disease.

NURSING CONSIDERATIONS
● The optimum duration of therapy is unknown.
● *Alert:* Don't withdraw drug abruptly; withdrawal symptoms, including seizures, may occur. Abuse or addiction is possible.
● Monitor hepatic, renal, and hematopoietic function periodically in patients receiving repeated or prolonged therapy.
● *Look alike–sound alike:* Don't confuse alprazolam with alprostadil. Don't confuse Xanax with Zantac or Tenex.

PATIENT TEACHING
● Warn patient to avoid hazardous activities that require alertness and good coordination until effects of drug are known.
● Tell patient to avoid use of alcohol while taking drug.
● Advise patient that smoking may decrease drug's effectiveness.
● Warn patient not to stop drug abruptly because withdrawal symptoms or seizures may occur.
● Tell patient to swallow extended-release tablets whole.
● Tell patient using ODT to remove it from bottle using dry hands and to immediately place it on his tongue where it will dissolve and can be swallowed with saliva.
● Tell patient taking half a scored ODT to discard the unused half.
● Advise patient to discard the cotton from the bottle of ODTs and keep it tightly sealed to prevent moisture from dissolving the tablets.

SAFETY ALERT!

alteplase (tissue plasminogen activator, recombinant; t-PA)
al-ti-PLAZE

Activase, Cathflo Activase

Pharmacologic class: enzyme
Pregnancy risk category C

AVAILABLE FORMS
Cathflo Activase injection: 2-mg single-patient vials

Injection: 50-mg (29 million international units), 100-mg (58 million international units) vials

INDICATIONS & DOSAGES
➤ **Lysis of thrombi obstructing coronary arteries in acute MI**
3-hour infusion
Adults who weigh 65 kg (143 lb) or more: 100 mg by I.V. infusion over 3 hours, as follows: 60 mg in first hour, 6 to 10 mg of which is given as a bolus over first 1 to 2 minutes. Then 20 mg/hour infused for 2 hours.
Adults who weigh less than 65 kg: Give 1.25 mg/kg in a similar fashion (60% in first hour, 10% of which is given as a bolus; then 20% of total dose per hour for 2 hours. Don't exceed total dose of 100 mg.
Accelerated infusion
Adults who weigh more than 67 kg (147 lb): 100 mg maximum total dose. Give 15 mg I.V. bolus over 1 to 2 minutes, followed by 50 mg infused over the next 30 minutes; then 35 mg infused over the next hour.
Adults who weigh 67 kg or less: 15 mg I.V. bolus over 1 to 2 minutes, followed by 0.75 mg/kg (not to exceed 50 mg) infused over the next 30 minutes; then 0.5 mg/kg (not to exceed 35 mg) infused over the next hour. Don't exceed total dose of 100 mg.
➤ **To manage acute massive pulmonary embolism**
Adults: 100 mg by I.V. infusion over 2 hours. Begin heparin at end of infusion when PTT or thrombin time returns to twice normal or less. Don't exceed 100-mg dose. Higher doses may increase risk of intracranial bleeding.
➤ **Acute ischemic stroke**
Adults: 0.9 mg/kg by I.V. infusion over 1 hour with 10% of total dose given as an initial I.V. bolus over 1 minute. Maximum total dose is 90 mg.
➤ **To restore function to central venous access devices**
Cathflo Activase
Adults and children older than age 2: For patients who weigh more than 30 kg (66 lb), instill 2 mg in 2 ml sterile water into catheter. For patients who weigh 10 kg (22 lb) to 30 kg, instill 110% of the internal lumen volume of the catheter, not

to exceed 2 mg in 2 ml sterile water. After 30 minutes of dwell time, assess catheter function by aspirating blood. If function is restored, aspirate 4 ml to 5 ml of blood to remove drug and residual clot, and gently irrigate the catheter with normal saline solution. If catheter function isn't restored after 120 minutes, instill a second dose.
➤ **Lysis of arterial occlusion in a peripheral vessel or bypass graft ♦**
Adults: 0.05 to 0.1 mg/kg/hour infused intra-arterially for 1 to 8 hours.

ADMINISTRATION
I.V.
• Immediately before use, reconstitute solution with unpreserved sterile water for injection. Check manufacturer's labeling for specific information.
• Don't use 50-mg vial if vacuum isn't present; 100-mg vials don't have a vacuum.
• Using an 18G needle, direct stream of sterile water at lyophilized cake. Don't shake.
• Slight foaming is common. Let it settle before giving drug. Solution should be colorless or pale yellow.
• Drug may be given reconstituted (at 1 mg/ml) or diluted with an equal volume of normal saline solution or D_5W to yield 0.5 mg/ml.
• Give drug using a controlled infusion device.
• Discard any unused drug after 8 hours.
Cathflo Activase
• Assess the cause of catheter dysfunction before using drug. Possible causes of occlusion include catheter malposition, mechanical failure, constriction by a suture, and lipid deposits or drug precipitates in the catheter lumen. Don't try to suction the catheter because you risk damaging the vessel wall or collapsing a soft-walled catheter.
• Reconstitute Cathflo Activase with 2.2 ml sterile water to yield 1 mg/ml. Dissolve completely to produce a colorless to pale yellow solution.
• Don't use excessive pressure while instilling drug into catheter; doing so could rupture the catheter or expel a clot into circulation.
• Solution is stable up to 8 hours at room temperature.

• **Incompatibilities:** None reported, but don't mix with other drugs.

ACTION

Converts plasminogen to plasmin by directly cleaving peptide bonds at two sites, causing fibrinolysis.

Route	Onset	Peak	Duration
I.V.	Unknown	Unknown	Unknown

Half-life: Less than 10 minutes.

ADVERSE REACTIONS

CNS: *cerebral hemorrhage,* fever.
CV: *arrhythmias,* hypotension, edema, *cholesterol embolization, venous thrombosis.*
GI: *bleeding (Cathflo Activase),* nausea, vomiting.
GU: *bleeding.*
Hematologic: *spontaneous bleeding.*
Skin: ecchymosis.
Other: *anaphylaxis, sepsis (Cathflo Activase),* bleeding at puncture sites, hypersensitivity reactions.

INTERACTIONS

Drug-drug. *Aspirin, clopidogrel, dipyridamole, drugs affecting platelet activity (abciximab), heparin, warfarin anticoagulants:* May increase risk of bleeding. Monitor patient carefully.
Nitroglycerin: May decrease alteplase antigen level. Avoid using together. If use together is unavoidable, use the lowest effective dose of nitroglycerin.

EFFECTS ON LAB TEST RESULTS

• May alter coagulation and fibrinolytic test results.

CONTRAINDICATIONS & CAUTIONS

• Contraindicated in patients with active internal bleeding, intracranial neoplasm, arteriovenous malformation, aneurysm, severe uncontrolled hypertension, or history or current evidence of intracranial hemorrhage, suspicion of subarachnoid hemorrhage, or seizure at onset of stroke when used for acute ischemic stroke.
• Contraindicated in patients with history of stroke, intraspinal or intracranial trauma or surgery within 2 months, or known bleeding diathesis.

• Use cautiously in patients having major surgery within 10 days (when bleeding is difficult to control because of its location); organ biopsy; trauma (including cardiopulmonary resuscitation); GI or GU bleeding; cerebrovascular disease; systolic pressure of 180 mm Hg or higher or diastolic pressure of 110 mm Hg or higher; mitral stenosis, atrial fibrillation, or other conditions that may lead to left heart thrombus; acute pericarditis or subacute bacterial endocarditis; hemostatic defects caused by hepatic or renal impairment; septic thrombophlebitis; or diabetic hemorrhagic retinopathy.
• Use cautiously in patients receiving anticoagulants, in patients age 75 and older, and during pregnancy and the first 10 days postpartum.

NURSING CONSIDERATIONS

• *Alert:* When used for acute ischemic stroke, give drug within 3 hours after symptoms occur and only when intracranial bleeding has been ruled out.
• Drug may be given to menstruating women.
• To recanalize occluded coronary arteries and to improve heart function, begin treatment as soon as possible after symptoms start.
• Anticoagulant and antiplatelet therapy is commonly started during or after treatment, to decrease risk of another thrombosis.
• Monitor vital signs and neurologic status carefully. Keep patient on strict bed rest.
• Coronary thrombolysis is linked with arrhythmias caused by reperfusion of ischemic myocardium. Such arrhythmias don't differ from those commonly linked with MI. Have antiarrhythmics readily available, and carefully monitor ECG.
• Avoid invasive procedures during thrombolytic therapy. Closely monitor patient for signs of internal bleeding, and frequently check all puncture sites. Bleeding is the most common adverse effect and may occur internally and at external puncture sites.
• If uncontrollable bleeding occurs, stop infusion (and heparin) and notify prescriber.
• Avoid I.M. injections.

PATIENT TEACHING
● Explain use and administration of drug to patient and family.
● Tell patient to report adverse reactions promptly.

---

amantadine hydrochloride
a-MAN-ta-deen

Symmetrel

Pharmacologic class: synthetic cyclic primary amine
Pregnancy risk category C

AVAILABLE FORMS
Capsules: 100 mg
Syrup: 50 mg/5 ml
Tablets: 100 mg

INDICATIONS & DOSAGES
➤ **Parkinson disease**
Adults: Initially, if used as monotherapy, 100 mg P.O. b.i.d. In patients with serious illness or in those already receiving high doses of other antiparkinsonians, begin dose at 100 mg P.O. once daily. Increase to 100 mg b.i.d. if needed after at least 1 week. Some patients may benefit from 400 mg daily in divided doses.
➤ **To prevent or treat symptoms of influenza type A virus and respiratory tract illnesses**
Children age 13 or older and adults up to age 65: 200 mg P.O. daily in a single dose or 100 mg P.O. b.i.d.
Children ages 9 to 12: 100 mg P.O. b.i.d.
Children ages 1 to 8 or who weigh less than 45 kg (99 lb): 4.4 to 8.8 mg/kg P.O. as a total daily dose given once daily or divided equally b.i.d. Maximum daily dose is 150 mg.
Elderly patients: 100 mg P.O. once daily in patients older than age 65 with normal renal function.

Begin treatment within 24 to 48 hours after symptoms appear and continue for 24 to 48 hours after symptoms disappear (usually 2 to 7 days). Start prophylaxis as soon as possible after exposure and continue for at least 10 days after exposure. May continue prophylactic treatment up to 90 days for repeated or suspected exposures if influenza vaccine is unavailable. If used with influenza vaccine, continue dose for 2 to 3 weeks until antibody response to vaccine has developed.
Adjust-a-dose: For patients with creatinine clearance of 30 to 50 ml/minute, 200 mg the first day and 100 mg thereafter; if clearance is 15 to 29 ml/minute, 200 mg the first day and then 100 mg on alternate days; if clearance is less than 15 ml/minute or if patient is receiving hemodialysis, 200 mg every 7 days.
➤ **Drug-induced extrapyramidal reactions**
Adults: 100 mg P.O. b.i.d. May increase to 300 mg daily in divided doses.

ADMINISTRATION
P.O.
● Give drug without regard for food.

ACTION
May exert its antiparkinsonian effect by causing the release of dopamine in the substantia nigra. As an antiviral, may prevent release of viral nucleic acid into the host cell, reducing duration of fever and other systemic symptoms.

Route	Onset	Peak	Duration
P.O.	Unknown	1–4 hr	Unknown

Half-life: About 24 hours; with renal dysfunction, as long as 10 days.

ADVERSE REACTIONS
CNS: *dizziness, insomnia, irritability, light-headedness,* depression, fatigue, confusion, hallucinations, anxiety, ataxia, headache.
CV: *heart failure,* peripheral edema, orthostatic hypotension.
EENT: blurred vision.
GI: *nausea,* anorexia, constipation, vomiting, dry mouth.
Skin: livedo reticularis.

INTERACTIONS
Drug-drug. *Anticholinergics:* May increase anticholinergic effects. Use together cautiously; reduce dosage of anticholinergic before starting amantadine.
CNS stimulants: May increase CNS stimulation. Use together cautiously.
Co-trimoxazole, quinidine, thiazide diuretics, triamterene: May increase amantadine

---

level, increasing the risk of toxicity. Use together cautiously.
Thioridazine: May worsen Parkinson disease tremor. Monitor patient closely.
Drug-herb. *Jimsonweed:* May adversely affect CV function. Discourage use together.
Drug-lifestyle. *Alcohol use:* May increase CNS effects, including dizziness, confusion, and orthostatic hypotension. Discourage use together.

EFFECTS ON LAB TEST RESULTS
• May increase CK, BUN, creatinine, alkaline phosphatase, LDH, bilirubin, GGT, AST, and ALT levels.

CONTRAINDICATIONS & CAUTIONS
• Contraindicated in patients hypersensitive to drug.
• Use cautiously in elderly patients and in patients with seizure disorders, heart failure, peripheral edema, hepatic disease, mental illness, eczematoid rash, renal impairment, orthostatic hypotension, and CV disease. Monitor renal and liver function tests.

NURSING CONSIDERATIONS
• Patients with Parkinson disease who don't respond to anticholinergics may respond to this drug.
• Begin treatment for influenza within 24 to 48 hours after symptoms appear and continue for 24 to 48 hours after symptoms disappear (usually 2 to 7 days of therapy).
• Start influenza prophylaxis as soon as possible after first exposure and continue for at least 10 days after exposure. For repeated or suspected exposures, if influenza vaccine is unavailable, may continue prophylaxis for up to 90 days. If used with influenza vaccine, continue dose for 2 to 3 weeks until antibody response to vaccine has developed.
• **Alert:** Elderly patients are more susceptible to adverse neurologic effects. Monitor patient for mental status changes.
• Suicidal ideation and attempts may occur in any patient, regardless of psychiatric history.
• Drug can worsen mental problems in patients with a history of psychiatric disorders or substance abuse.

• *Look alike–sound alike:* Don't confuse amantadine with rimantadine.

PATIENT TEACHING
• **Alert:** Tell patient to take drug exactly as prescribed because not doing so may result in serious adverse reactions or death.
• If insomnia occurs, tell patient to take drug several hours before bedtime.
• If patient gets dizzy when he stands up, instruct him not to stand or change positions too quickly.
• Instruct patient to notify prescriber of adverse reactions, especially dizziness, depression, anxiety, nausea, and urine retention.
• Caution patient to avoid activities that require mental alertness until effects of drug are known.
• Encourage patient with Parkinson disease to gradually increase his physical activity as his symptoms improve.
• Advise patient to avoid alcohol while taking drug.

SAFETY ALERT!
✳ NEW DRUG

ambrisentan
am-bree-SEN-tan

Pharmacologic class: endothelin-receptor antagonist
Pregnancy risk category X

AVAILABLE FORMS
Tablets: 5 mg, 10 mg

INDICATIONS & DOSAGES
➤ **Pulmonary arterial hypertension in patients with World Health Organization class II (with significant exertion) or III (with mild exertion) symptoms to improve exercise tolerance and decrease rate of clinical worsening**
Adults: 5 mg P.O. once daily; may increase to 10 mg P.O. once daily if tolerated.
Adjust-a-dose: Don't start therapy in patients with elevated aminotransferase levels (ALT and AST) of more than three times the upper limit of normal (ULN) at baseline. If ALT elevations during therapy are between three and five times the ULN, remeasure. If confirmed level is in the

same range, reduce dose or stop therapy and remeasure every 2 weeks until levels are less than three times ULN. If ALT and AST are between five and eight times the ULN, stop therapy and monitor until the levels are less than three times ULN. Restart therapy with more frequent monitoring. If ALT and AST exceed eight times the ULN, stop therapy and don't restart.

ADMINISTRATION

P.O.
- Give drug without regard for food.
- Give drug whole; don't crush or split tablets.

ACTION

Blocks endothelin-1 receptors on vascular endothelin and smooth muscle. Stimulation of these receptors in smooth muscle cells is associated with vasoconstriction and PAH.

Route	Onset	Peak	Duration
P.O.	Rapid	2 hr	Unknown

Half-life: 9 hours.

ADVERSE REACTIONS

CNS: *headache.*
CV: *peripheral edema,* flushing, palpitations.
EENT: nasal congestion, sinusitis, nasopharyngitis.
GI: abdominal pain, constipation.
Hematologic: anemia.
Hepatic: hepatic impairment.
Respiratory: dyspnea.

INTERACTIONS

Drug-drug. *CYP enzyme inducers, such as carbamazepine, phenobarbital, phenytoin, and rifampin:* May decrease effects of ambrisentan. Use together cautiously.
CYP enzyme inhibitors, such as atanazavir, clarithromycin, fluvoxamine, fluconazole, indinavir, itraconazole, ketoconazole, nefazodone, nelfinavir, omeprazole, ritonavir, saquinavir, telithromycin, and ticlopidine: May increase the effects of ambrisentan. Use together cautiously.

Cyclosporine: May increase ambrisentan levels. Use together cautiously and monitor patient for increased adverse effects.

EFFECTS ON LAB TEST RESULTS

- May increase AST, ALT, and bilirubin levels. May decrease hemoglobin level and hematocrit.

CONTRAINDICATIONS & CAUTIONS

- Contraindicated in patients hypersensitive to drug or its components.
- Contraindicated in pregnant women because it may harm the fetus.
- Contraindicated in those with moderate to severe hepatic impairment; don't begin therapy in those with elevated baseline ALT and AST levels of more than three times the ULN.
- Use cautiously in those with mild hepatic impairment.
- Use cautiously in those with renal impairment; drug hasn't been studied in those with severe renal impairment.

PATIENT TEACHING

- Inform female patient that she'll need to have a pregnancy test done monthly and to report suspected pregnancy to her prescriber immediately.
- *Alert:* Teach woman of childbearing age to use two reliable birth control methods unless she has had tubal sterilization or has a Copper T 380A intrauterine device (IUD) or an LNg 20 IUD inserted.
- Tell patient that monthly blood tests will be done to monitor for adverse effects.
- Advise patient to take the pill whole and not to split, crush, or chew the tablet.
- *Alert:* Teach patient to notify prescriber immediately of signs or symptoms of liver injury, including anorexia, nausea, vomiting, fever, malaise, fatigue, right upper quadrant abdominal discomfort, itching, and jaundice.
- Tell the patient to report edema and weight gain.

amikacin sulfate
am-i-KAY-sin

Amikin

Pharmacologic class: aminoglycoside
Pregnancy risk category D

AVAILABLE FORMS
Injection: 50 mg/ml (pediatric) vial,
250 mg/ml vial, 250 mg/ml disposable
syringe

INDICATIONS & DOSAGES
➤ **Serious infections caused by
sensitive strains of** *Pseudomonas
aeruginosa, Escherichia coli, Proteus,
Klebsiella,* **or** *Staphylococcus*
Adults and children: 15 mg/kg/day I.M. or
I.V. infusion, in divided doses every 8 to
12 hours for 7 to 10 days.
Neonates: Initially, loading dose of
10 mg/kg I.V.; then 7.5 mg/kg every
12 hours for 7 to 10 days.
➤ **Uncomplicated UTI caused by
organisms not susceptible to less
toxic drugs**
Adults: 250 mg I.M. or I.V. b.i.d.
➤ **Active tuberculosis, with other
antituberculotics ♦**
Adults and children age 15 and older:
15 mg/kg (up to 1 g) I.M. or I.V. once
daily five to seven times per week for 2 to
4 months or until culture conversion. Then
reduce dose to 15 mg/kg daily given two
or three times weekly depending on other
drugs in regimen. Patients older than age
59 may receive a reduced dose of 10 mg/kg
(up to 750 mg) daily.
Children younger than age 15: Give 15 to
30 mg/kg (up to 1 g) I.M. or I.V. once daily
or twice weekly.
➤ *Mycobacterium avium* **complex
(MAC) infection ♦**
Adults: 15 mg/kg/day I.V. in divided doses
every 8 to 12 hours as part of a multiple-
drug regimen.
Adjust-a-dose: For adults with impaired
renal function, initially, 7.5 mg/kg I.M.
or I.V. Subsequent doses and frequency
determined by amikacin levels and renal
function studies. For adults receiving
hemodialysis, give supplemental doses

of 50% to 75% of initial loading dose at
end of each dialysis session. Monitor drug
levels and adjust dosage accordingly.

ADMINISTRATION
I.V.
● Obtain specimen for culture and sensitivity tests before giving first dose. Begin
therapy while awaiting results.
● For adults, dilute I.V. drug in 100 to
200 ml of D_5W or normal saline solution.
For children, the amount of fluid will
depend on the ordered dose.
● In adults and children, infuse over 30
to 60 minutes. In infants, infuse over 1 to
2 hours.
● After infusion, flush line with normal
saline solution or D_5W.
● **Incompatibilities:** Allopurinol, aminophylline, amphotericin B, ampicillin,
azithromycin, bacitracin, cefazolin, ceftazidime, chlorothiazide sodium, cisplatin,
heparin sodium, hetastarch in 0.9% sodium
chloride, oxacillin, phenytoin, propofol,
thiopental, vancomycin, vitamin B complex with C.
I.M.
● Obtain specimen for culture and sensitivity tests before giving first dose. Begin
therapy while awaiting results.
● Obtain blood for peak level 1 hour after
I.M. injection and 30 minutes to 1 hour
after I.V. infusion ends; for trough levels,
draw blood just before next dose. Don't
collect blood in a heparinized tube; heparin
is incompatible with aminoglycosides.

ACTION
Inhibits protein synthesis by binding
directly to the 30S ribosomal subunit;
bactericidal.

Route	Onset	Peak	Duration
I.V.	Immediate	30 min	8–12 hr
I.M.	Unknown	1 hr	8–12 hr

Half-life: Adults, 2 to 3 hours. Patients with
severe renal damage, 30 to 86 hours.

ADVERSE REACTIONS
CNS: *neuromuscular blockade.*
EENT: *ototoxicity.*
GU: *azotemia,* **nephrotoxicity,** increase in
urinary excretion of casts.
Musculoskeletal: arthralgia.
Respiratory: *apnea.*

INTERACTIONS
Drug-drug. *Acyclovir, amphotericin B, bacitracin, cephalosporins, cidofovir, cisplatin, methoxyflurane, vancomycin, other aminoglycosides:* May increase nephrotoxicity. Use together cautiously, and monitor renal function test results.
Atracurium, pancuronium, rocuronium, vecuronium: May increase effects of non-depolarizing muscle relaxants, including prolonged respiratory depression. Use together only when necessary, and expect to reduce dosage of nondepolarizing muscle relaxant.
Dimenhydrinate: May mask ototoxicity symptoms. Monitor patient's hearing.
General anesthetics: May increase neuromuscular blockade. Monitor patient for increased effects.
Indomethacin: May increase trough and peak amikacin levels. Monitor amikacin level.
I.V. loop diuretics such as furosemide: May increase ototoxicity. Use together cautiously, and monitor patient's hearing.
Parenteral penicillins: May inactivate amikacin in vitro. Don't mix.

EFFECTS ON LAB TEST RESULTS
• May increase BUN, creatinine, nonprotein nitrogen, and urine urea levels.

CONTRAINDICATIONS & CAUTIONS
• Contraindicated in patients hypersensitive to drug or other aminoglycosides.
• Use cautiously in patients with impaired renal function or neuromuscular disorders, in neonates and infants, and in elderly patients.

NURSING CONSIDERATIONS
• *Alert:* Evaluate patient's hearing before and during therapy if he'll be receiving the drug for longer than 2 weeks. Notify prescriber if patient has tinnitus, vertigo, or hearing loss.
• Weigh patient and review renal function studies before therapy begins.
• Correct dehydration before therapy because of increased risk of toxicity.
• Peak drug levels more than 35 mcg/ml and trough levels more than 10 mcg/ml may be linked to a higher risk of toxicity.
• *Alert:* Monitor renal function: urine output, specific gravity, urinalysis, BUN and

creatinine levels, and creatinine clearance. Report to prescriber evidence of declining renal function.
• Watch for signs and symptoms of super-infection (especially of upper respiratory tract), such as continued fever, chills, and increased pulse rate.
• *Alert:* Neuromuscular blockage and respiratory paralysis have been reported after aminoglycoside administration. Monitor patient closely.
• Therapy usually continues for 7 to 10 days. If no response occurs after 3 to 5 days, stop therapy and obtain new specimens for culture and sensitivity testing.
• *Look alike–sound alike:* Don't confuse Amikin with Amicar. Don't confuse amikacin with anakinra.

PATIENT TEACHING
• Instruct patient to promptly report adverse reactions to prescriber.
• Encourage patient to maintain adequate fluid intake.

amlodipine besylate
am-LOE-di-peen

Norvasc

Pharmacologic class: calcium channel blocker
Pregnancy risk category C

AVAILABLE FORMS
Tablets: 2.5 mg, 5 mg, 10 mg

INDICATIONS & DOSAGES
➤ **Chronic stable angina, vasospastic angina (Prinzmetal's or variant angina)**
Adults: Initially, 5 to 10 mg P.O. daily. Most patients need 10 mg daily.
Elderly patients: Initially, 5 mg P.O. daily.
Adjust-a-dose: For patients who are small or frail or have hepatic insufficiency, initially, 5 mg P.O. daily.
➤ **Hypertension**
Adults: Initially, 2.5 to 5 mg P.O. daily. Dosage adjusted according to patient response and tolerance. Maximum daily dose is 10 mg.

Elderly patients: Initially, 2.5 mg P.O. daily.
Adjust-a-dose: For patients who are small or frail, are taking other antihypertensives, or have hepatic insufficiency, initially, 2.5 mg P.O. daily.

ADMINISTRATION
P.O.
● Give drug without regard for food.

ACTION
Inhibits calcium ion influx across cardiac and smooth-muscle cells, dilates coronary arteries and arterioles, and decreases blood pressure and myocardial oxygen demand.

Route	Onset	Peak	Duration
P.O.	Unknown	6–12 hr	24 hr

Half-life: 30 to 50 hours.

ADVERSE REACTIONS
CNS: headache, somnolence, fatigue, dizziness, light-headedness, paresthesia.
CV: *edema,* flushing, palpitations.
GI: nausea, abdominal pain.
GU: sexual difficulties.
Musculoskeletal: muscle pain.
Respiratory: dyspnea.
Skin: rash, pruritus.

INTERACTIONS
None reported.

EFFECTS ON LAB TEST RESULTS
None reported.

CONTRAINDICATIONS & CAUTIONS
● Contraindicated in patients hypersensitive to drug.
● Use cautiously in patients receiving other peripheral vasodilators, especially those with severe aortic stenosis, and in those with heart failure. Because drug is metabolized by the liver, use cautiously and in reduced dosage in patients with severe hepatic disease.

NURSING CONSIDERATIONS
● ***Alert:*** Monitor patient carefully. Some patients, especially those with severe obstructive coronary artery disease, have developed increased frequency, duration, or severity of angina or acute MI after initiation of calcium channel blocker therapy or at time of dosage increase.
● Monitor blood pressure frequently during initiation of therapy. Because drug-induced vasodilation has a gradual onset, acute hypotension is rare.
● Notify prescriber if signs of heart failure occur, such as swelling of hands and feet or shortness of breath.
● ***Alert:*** Abrupt withdrawal of drug may increase frequency and duration of chest pain. Taper dose gradually under medical supervision.
● ***Look alike–sound alike:*** Don't confuse amlodipine with amiloride.

PATIENT TEACHING
● Caution patient to continue taking drug, even when he feels better.
● Tell patient S.L. nitroglycerin may be taken as needed when angina symptoms are acute. If patient continues nitrate therapy during adjustment of amlodipine dosage, urge continued compliance.

amoxicillin and clavulanate potassium (amoxycillin and clavulanate potassium)
a-mox-i-SILL-in

Aclavulanate†, Amoxiclav†, Augmentin, Augmentin ES-600, Augmentin XR, Clavamoxin†, Clavulin†

Pharmacologic class: aminopenicillin and beta-lactamase inhibitor
Pregnancy risk category B

AVAILABLE FORMS
Oral suspension: 125 mg amoxicillin trihydrate and 31.25 mg clavulanic acid/5 ml (after reconstitution); 200 mg amoxicillin trihydrate and 28.5 mg clavulanic acid/5 ml (after reconstitution); 250 mg amoxicillin trihydrate and 62.5 mg clavulanic acid/5 ml (after reconstitution); 400 mg amoxicillin trihydrate and 57 mg clavulanic acid/5 ml (after reconstitution); 600 mg amoxicillin trihydrate and 42.9 mg clavulanic acid/5 ml (after reconstitution)
Tablets (chewable): 125 mg amoxicillin trihydrate, 31.25 mg clavulanic acid;

200 mg amoxicillin trihydrate, 28.5 mg clavulanic acid; 250 mg amoxicillin trihydrate, 62.5 mg clavulanic acid; 400 mg amoxicillin trihydrate, 57 mg clavulanic acid
Tablets (extended-release): 1,000 mg amoxicillin trihydrate, 62.5 mg clavulanic acid
Tablets (film-coated): 250 mg amoxicillin trihydrate, 125 mg clavulanic acid; 500 mg amoxicillin trihydrate, 125 mg clavulanic acid; 875 mg amoxicillin trihydrate, 125 mg clavulanic acid

INDICATIONS & DOSAGES
➤ **Recurrent or persistent acute otitis media caused by** *Streptococcus pneumoniae, Haemophilus influenzae,* **or** *Moraxella catarrhalis* **in patients exposed to antibiotics within the previous 3 months, who are 2 years old or younger or in day care facilities**
Children age 3 months and older:
90 mg/kg/day Augmentin ES-600 P.O., based on amoxicillin component, every 12 hours for 10 days.
➤ **Lower respiratory tract infections, otitis media, sinusitis, skin and skin-structure infections, and UTIs caused by susceptible strains of gram-positive and gram-negative organisms**
Adults and children weighing 40 kg (88 lb) or more: 250 mg P.O., based on amoxicillin component, every 8 hours; or 500 mg every 12 hours. For more severe infections, 500 mg every 8 hours or 875 mg every 12 hours.
Children age 3 months and older and weighing less than 40 kg: 20 to 45 mg/kg P.O., based on amoxicillin component and severity of infection, daily in divided doses every 8 to 12 hours.
Children younger than age 3 months:
30 mg/kg/day P.O., based on amoxicillin component of the 125-mg/5-ml oral suspension, in divided doses every 12 hours.
Adjust-a-dose: Don't give the 875-mg tablet to patients with creatinine clearance less than 30 ml/minute. If clearance is 10 to 30 ml/minute, give 250 to 500 mg P.O. every 12 hours. If clearance is less than 10 ml/minute, give 250 to 500 mg P.O. every 24 hours. Give hemodialysis patients

250 to 500 mg P.O. every 24 hours with an additional dose both during and after dialysis.
➤ **Community-acquired pneumonia or acute bacterial sinusitis caused by** *H. influenzae, M. catarrhalis, H. parainfluenzae, Klebsiella pneumoniae,* **methicillin-susceptible** *Staphylococcus aureus,* **or** *S. pneumoniae* **with reduced susceptibility to penicillin**
Adults and children age 16 and older:
2,000 mg/125 mg Augmentin XR tablets every 12 hours for 7 to 10 days for pneumonia; 10 days for sinusitis.
Adjust-a-dose: In patients with creatinine clearance less than 30 ml/minute and patients receiving hemodialysis, don't use Augmentin XR.

ADMINISTRATION
P.O.
● Before giving drug, ask patient about allergic reactions to penicillin. A negative history of penicillin allergy is no guarantee against an allergic reaction.
● Obtain specimen for culture and sensitivity tests before giving first dose. Begin therapy while awaiting results.
● Give drug at least 1 hour before a bacteriostatic antibiotic.
● Avoid use of 250-mg tablet in children weighing less than 40 kg (88 lb). Use chewable form instead.
● After reconstitution, refrigerate the oral suspension; discard after 10 days.

ACTION
Prevents bacterial cell-wall synthesis during replication. Increases amoxicillin's effectiveness by inactivating beta-lactamases, which destroy amoxicillin.

Route	Onset	Peak	Duration
P.O.	Unknown	1–2½ hr	6–8 hr
P.O. (Augmentin ES-600)	Unknown	1–4 hr	Unknown
P.O. (Augmentin XR)	Unknown	1–6 hr	Unknown

Half-life: 1 to 1½ hours. For patients with severe renal impairment, 7½ hours for amoxicillin and 4½ hours for clavulanate.

ADVERSE REACTIONS

CNS: agitation, anxiety, behavioral changes, confusion, dizziness, insomnia.
GI: nausea, vomiting, *diarrhea,* indigestion, gastritis, stomatitis, glossitis, black hairy tongue, enterocolitis, *pseudomembranous colitis,* mucocutaneous candidiasis, abdominal pain.
GU: vaginal candidiasis, vaginitis.
Hematologic: anemia, *thrombocytopenia, thrombocytopenic purpura,* eosinophilia, *leukopenia, agranulocytosis.*
Other: hypersensitivity reactions, *anaphylaxis,* pruritus, rash, urticaria, *angioedema,* overgrowth of nonsusceptible organisms, serum sickness–like reaction.

INTERACTIONS

Drug-drug. *Allopurinol:* May increase risk of rash. Monitor patient for rash.
Hormonal contraceptives: May decrease hormonal contraceptive effectiveness. Advise use of additional form of contraception during penicillin therapy.
Probenecid: May increase levels of amoxicillin and other penicillins. Probenecid may be used for this purpose.
Drug-herb. *Khat:* May decrease antimicrobial effect of certain penicillins. Discourage khat chewing, or tell patient to take amoxicillin 2 hours after khat chewing.

EFFECTS ON LAB TEST RESULTS

● May increase eosinophil count.
● May falsely decrease aminoglycoside level. May alter results of urine glucose tests that use cupric sulfate, such as Benedict's reagent and Clinitest.

CONTRAINDICATIONS & CAUTIONS

● Contraindicated in patients hypersensitive to drug or other penicillins and in those with a history of amoxicillin-related cholestatic jaundice or hepatic dysfunction.
● Augmentin XR is contraindicated in patients receiving hemodialysis and those with creatinine clearance less than 30 ml/minute.
● Use cautiously in patients with other drug allergies (especially to cephalosporins) because of possible cross-sensitivity and in those with mononucleosis because of high risk of maculopapular rash.
● Use cautiously in breast-feeding women; it's unknown if drug appears in breast milk.
● Use cautiously in hepatically impaired patients, and monitor the hepatic function of these patients.

NURSING CONSIDERATIONS

● Each Augmentin XR tablet contains 29.3 mg (1.27 mEq) of sodium.
● Augmentin XR isn't indicated for treating infections caused by *S. pneumoniae* with penicillin minimum inhibitory concentration, or MIC, of 4 mcg/ml or greater.
● If large doses are given or therapy is prolonged, bacterial or fungal superinfection may occur, especially in elderly, debilitated, or immunosuppressed patients.
● *Alert:* Don't interchange the oral suspensions because of varying clavulanic acid contents.
● Augmentin ES-600 is intended only for children ages 3 months to 12 years with persistent or recurrent acute otitis media.
● *Alert:* Both 250- and 500-mg film-coated tablets contain the same amount of clavulanic acid (125 mg). Therefore, two 250-mg tablets aren't equivalent to one 500-mg tablet. Regular tablets aren't equivalent to Augmentin XR.
● This drug combination is particularly useful in clinical settings with a high prevalence of amoxicillin-resistant organisms.
● *Look alike–sound alike:* Don't confuse amoxicillin with amoxapine.

PATIENT TEACHING

● Tell patient to take entire quantity of drug exactly as prescribed, even after feeling better.
● Instruct patient to take drug with food to prevent GI upset. If he's taking the oral suspension, tell him to keep drug refrigerated, to shake it well before taking it, and to discard remaining drug after 10 days.
● Tell patient to call prescriber if a rash occurs because rash is a sign of an allergic reaction.

amoxicillin trihydrate
(amoxycillin trihydrate)
a-mox-i-SILL-in

Amoxil, Apo-Amoxi†, DisperMox,
Novamoxin†, Nu-Amoxi†, Trimox

Pharmacologic class: aminopenicillin
Pregnancy risk category B

AVAILABLE FORMS
Capsules: 250 mg, 500 mg
Oral suspension: 50 mg/ml (pediatric drops), 125 mg/5 ml, 200 mg/5 ml, 250 mg/5 ml, 400 mg/5 ml (after reconstitution)
Tablets (chewable): 125 mg, 200 mg, 250 mg, 400 mg
Tablets (film-coated): 500 mg, 875 mg
Tablets for oral suspension: 200 mg, 400 mg

INDICATIONS & DOSAGES
➤ **Mild to moderate infections of the ear, nose, and throat; skin and skin structure; or GU tract**
Adults and children who weigh 40 kg (88 lb) or more: 500 mg P.O. every 12 hours or 250 mg P.O. every 8 hours.
Children older than age 3 months who weigh less than 40 kg: 25 mg/kg/day P.O. divided every 12 hours or 20 mg/kg/day P.O. divided every 8 hours.
Neonates and infants up to age 3 months: Up to 30 mg/kg/day P.O. divided every 12 hours.
➤ **Mild to severe infections of the lower respiratory tract and severe infections of the ear, nose, and throat; skin and skin structure; or genitourinary tract**
Adults and children who weigh 40 kg or more: 875 mg P.O. every 12 hours or 500 mg P.O. every 8 hours.
Children older than age 3 months weighing less than 40 kg: 45 mg/kg/day P.O. divided every 12 hours or 40 mg/kg/day P.O. divided every 8 hours.
➤ **Uncomplicated gonorrhea**
Adults and children who weigh more than 45 kg (99 lb): 3 g P.O. with 1 g probenecid given as a single dose.
Children age 2 and older who weigh less than 45 kg: 50 mg/kg to a maximum of 3 g P.O. with 25 mg/kg, to a maximum of 1 g of probenecid as a single dose. Don't give probenecid to children younger than age 2.
➤ **To prevent endocarditis in patients having dental, oral, or respiratory tract procedures and in moderate-risk patients undergoing GI and GU procedures ♦**
Adults: 2 g P.O. 1 hour before procedure.
Children: 50 mg/kg P.O. 1 hour before procedure.
➤ **To prevent penicillin-susceptible anthrax after exposure ♦**
Adults and children older than age 9: 500 mg P.O. t.i.d. for 60 days.
Children younger than age 9: 80 mg/kg daily P.O., divided b.i.d. or t.i.d. for 60 days.
➤ **Early Lyme disease, localized or disseminated, associated with erythema migrans, without neurologic involvement or third-degree AV heart block ♦**
Adults: 500 mg P.O. t.i.d. for 14 to 21 days.

ADMINISTRATION
P.O.
• Before giving, ask patient about allergic reactions to penicillin. A negative history of penicillin allergy is no guarantee against allergic reaction.
• Obtain specimen for culture and sensitivity tests before giving first dose. Begin therapy while awaiting results.
• Give drug with or without food.
• For a child, place drops directly on child's tongue for swallowing or add to formula, milk, fruit juice, water, ginger ale, or a cold drink for immediate and complete consumption.
• For a child taking DisperMox, mix one tablet in about 10 ml of water, have the child drink the resulting solution, rinse container with a small amount of water, and have the child drink again to ensure the whole dose is taken. Mix tablet only in water. Don't let child chew tablets, swallow them whole, or let them dissolve in mouth.
• Store Trimox oral suspension in refrigerator, if possible. It also may be stored at room temperature for up to 2 weeks. Be sure to check individual product labels for storage information.

ACTION
Inhibits cell-wall synthesis during bacterial multiplication.

Route	Onset	Peak	Duration
P.O.	Unknown	1–2 hr	6–8 hr

Half-life: 1 to 1½ hours (7½ hours in severe renal impairment).

ADVERSE REACTIONS
CNS: *seizures,* lethargy, hallucinations, anxiety, confusion, agitation, depression, dizziness, fatigue.
GI: *diarrhea, nausea, pseudomembranous colitis,* vomiting, glossitis, stomatitis, gastritis, enterocolitis, abdominal pain, black hairy tongue.
GU: interstitial nephritis, nephropathy, vaginitis.
Hematologic: *agranulocytosis, leukopenia, thrombocytopenia, thrombocytopenic purpura,* anemia, eosinophilia, hemolytic anemia.
Other: *anaphylaxis,* hypersensitivity reactions, overgrowth of nonsusceptible organisms.

INTERACTIONS
Drug-drug. *Allopurinol:* May increase risk of rash. Monitor patient for rash.
Hormonal contraceptives: May decrease contraceptive effectiveness. Advise use of additional form of contraception during penicillin therapy.
Probenecid: May increase levels of amoxicillin and other penicillins. Probenecid may be used for this purpose.
Drug-herb. *Khat:* May decrease antimicrobial effect of certain penicillins. Discourage herb use, or tell patient to take drug 2 hours after herb use.

EFFECTS ON LAB TEST RESULTS
● May decrease hemoglobin level.
● May increase eosinophil count. May decrease granulocyte, platelet, and WBC counts.
● May falsely decrease aminoglycoside level. May alter results of urine glucose tests that use cupric sulfate, such as Benedict's reagent and Clinitest.

CONTRAINDICATIONS & CAUTIONS
● Contraindicated in patients hypersensitive to drug or other penicillins.
● Use cautiously in patients with other drug allergies (especially to cephalosporins) because of possible cross-sensitivity.
● Use cautiously in those with mononucleosis because of high risk of maculopapular rash.

NURSING CONSIDERATIONS
● If large doses are given or if therapy is prolonged, bacterial or fungal superinfection may occur, especially in elderly, debilitated, or immunosuppressed patients.
● Amoxicillin usually causes fewer cases of diarrhea than ampicillin.
● *Look alike–sound alike:* Don't confuse amoxicillin with amoxapine.

PATIENT TEACHING
● Tell patient to take entire quantity of drug exactly as prescribed, even after he feels better.
● Instruct patient to take drug with or without food.
● Tell patient to notify prescriber if rash, fever, or chills develop. A rash is the most common allergic reaction, especially if allopurinol is also being taken.
● Tell parent to place drops directly on child's tongue for swallowing or add to formula, milk, fruit juice, water, ginger ale, or a cold drink for immediate and complete consumption.
● If child takes DisperMox, tell parent to mix one tablet in about 10 ml of water, to have the child drink the resulting solution, to rinse container with a small amount of water, and to have the child drink again to ensure the whole dose is taken. Parent should mix tablet only in water. Caution parent against allowing child to chew tablets, to swallow them whole, or to let them dissolve in mouth.

ampicillin
am-pi-SILL-in

Apo-Ampi†, Nu-Ampi†

ampicillin sodium

ampicillin trihydrate
Principen

Pharmacologic class: aminopenicillin
Pregnancy risk category B

AVAILABLE FORMS
Capsules: 250 mg, 500 mg
Injection: 250 mg, 500 mg, 1 g, 2 g
Oral suspension: 125 mg/5 ml,
250 mg/5 ml

INDICATIONS & DOSAGES
➤ **Respiratory tract or skin and skin-structure infections**
Adults and children who weigh 40 kg (88 lb) or more: 250 to 500 mg P.O. every 6 hours.
Children who weigh less than 40 kg: 25 to 50 mg/kg/day P.O. in equally divided doses every 6 to 8 hours. Pediatric dosages shouldn't exceed recommended adult dosages.
➤ **GI infections or UTIs**
Adults and children who weigh 40 kg (88 lb) or more: 500 mg P.O. every 6 hours. For severe infections, larger doses may be needed.
Children who weigh less than 40 kg: 50 to 100 mg/kg/day P.O. in equally divided doses every 6 hours.
➤ **Bacterial meningitis or septicemia**
Adults: 150 to 200 mg/kg/day I.V. in divided doses every 3 to 4 hours. May be given I.M. after 3 days of I.V. therapy. Maximum recommended daily dose is 14 g.
Children: 150 to 200 mg/kg I.V. daily in divided doses every 3 to 4 hours. Give I.V. for 3 days; then give I.M.
➤ **Uncomplicated gonorrhea**
Adults and children who weigh more than 45 kg (99 lb): 3.5 g P.O. with 1 g probenecid given as a single dose.

➤ **To prevent endocarditis in patients having dental, GI, and GU procedures ♦**
Adults: 2 g I.M. or I.V. within 30 minutes before procedure. For high-risk patients, also give 1.5 mg/kg gentamicin 30 minutes before the procedure; 6 hours later, give 1 g ampicillin I.M. or I.V. or 1 g amoxicillin P.O.
Children: 50 mg/kg I.M. or I.V. within 30 minutes before procedure. For high-risk patients, also give 1.5 mg/kg gentamicin 30 minutes before the procedure; 6 hours later, give 25 mg/kg ampicillin I.M. or I.V. or 25 mg/kg amoxicillin P.O.
Adjust-a-dose: In patients with creatinine clearance of 10 to 50 ml/minute, use same dose but increase dosing interval to 6 to 12 hours; for those with a clearance less than 10 ml/minute, increase dosing interval to 12 to 24 hours.

ADMINISTRATION
P.O.
● Before giving drug, ask patient about allergic reactions to penicillin. A negative history of penicillin allergy is no guarantee against a future allergic reaction.
● Obtain specimen for culture and sensitivity tests before giving. Begin therapy while awaiting results.
● Give drug 1 to 2 hours before or 2 to 3 hours after meals. When given orally, drug may cause GI disturbances. Food may interfere with absorption.
● Give drug I.M. or I.V. if infection is severe or if patient can't take oral dose.
I.V.
● Before giving drug, ask patient about allergic reactions to penicillin. A negative history of penicillin allergy is no guarantee against a future allergic reaction.
● Obtain specimen for culture and sensitivity tests before giving. Begin therapy while awaiting results.
● Give drug I.M. or I.V. only if infection is severe or if patient can't take oral dose.
● Give drug intermittently to prevent vein irritation. Change site every 48 hours.
● For direct injection, reconstitute with bacteriostatic water for injection. Use 5 ml for 250-mg or 500-mg vials, 7.4 ml for 1-g vials, and 14.8 ml for 2-g vials. Give drug over 10 to 15 minutes to avoid seizures. Don't exceed 100 mg/minute.

• For intermittent infusion, dilute in 50 to 100 ml of normal saline solution for injection. Give drug over 15 to 30 minutes.
• Use first dilution within 1 hour. Follow manufacturer's directions for stability data when drug is further diluted for I.V. infusion.
• **Incompatibilities:** Amikacin, amino acid solutions, chlorpromazine, dextran solutions, dextrose solutions, dopamine, erythromycin lactobionate, 10% fat emulsions, fructose, gentamicin, heparin sodium, hetastarch, hydrocortisone sodium succinate, hydromorphone, kanamycin, lidocaine, lincomycin, polymyxin B, prochlorperazine edisylate, sodium bicarbonate, streptomycin, tobramycin.

I.M.
• Before giving drug, ask patient about allergic reactions to penicillin. A negative history of penicillin allergy is no guarantee against a future allergic reaction.
• Obtain specimen for culture and sensitivity tests before giving. Begin therapy while awaiting results.
• Give drug I.M. or I.V. only if infection is severe or if patient can't take oral dose.

ACTION
Inhibits cell-wall synthesis during bacterial multiplication.

Route	Onset	Peak	Duration
P.O.	Unknown	2 hr	6–8 hr
I.V.	Immediate	Immediate	Unknown
I.M.	Unknown	1 hr	Unknown

Half-life: 1 to 1½ hours (10 to 24 hours in severe renal impairment).

ADVERSE REACTIONS
CNS: *seizures,* agitation, anxiety, confusion, depression, dizziness, hallucinations, lethargy, fatigue.
CV: thrombophlebitis, vein irritation.
GI: *diarrhea, nausea, pseudomembranous colitis,* abdominal pain, black hairy tongue, enterocolitis, gastritis, glossitis, stomatitis, vomiting.
GU: interstitial nephritis, nephropathy, vaginitis.
Hematologic: *leukopenia, thrombocytopenia, thrombocytopenic purpura,* anemia, eosinophilia, hemolytic anemia, *agranulocytosis.*

Skin: pain at injection site.
Other: hypersensitivity reactions, overgrowth of nonsusceptible organisms.

INTERACTIONS
Drug-drug. *Allopurinol:* May increase risk of rash. Monitor patient for rash.
H_2 antagonists, proton pump inhibitors: May decrease ampicillin absorption and level. Separate administration times. Monitor patient for continued antibiotic effectiveness.
Hormonal contraceptives: May decrease hormonal contraceptive effectiveness. Advise use of another form of contraception during therapy.
Oral anticoagulants: May increase risk of bleeding. Monitor PT and INR.
Probenecid: May increase levels of ampicillin and other penicillins. Probenecid may be used for this purpose.

EFFECTS ON LAB TEST RESULTS
• May decrease hemoglobin level.
• May increase eosinophil count. May decrease granulocyte, platelet, and WBC counts.
• May falsely decrease aminoglycoside level. May alter results of urine glucose tests that use cupric sulfate, such as Benedict reagent and Clinitest.

CONTRAINDICATIONS & CAUTIONS
• Contraindicated in patients hypersensitive to drug or other penicillins.
• Use cautiously in patients with other drug allergies (especially to cephalosporins) because of possible cross-sensitivity, and in those with mononucleosis because of high risk of maculopapular rash.

NURSING CONSIDERATIONS
• Monitor sodium level because each gram of ampicillin contains 2.9 mEq of sodium.
• If large doses are given or if therapy is prolonged, bacterial or fungal superinfection may occur, especially in elderly, debilitated, or immunosuppressed patients.
• Watch for signs and symptoms of hypersensitivity, such as erythematous maculopapular rash, urticaria, and anaphylaxis.
• In patients with impaired renal function, decrease dosage.

• In pediatric meningitis, drug may be given with parenteral chloramphenicol for 24 hours, pending cultures.
• To prevent bacterial endocarditis in patients at high risk, give drug with gentamicin.

PATIENT TEACHING
• Tell patient to take entire quantity of drug exactly as prescribed, even after he feels better.
• Instruct patient to take oral form on an empty stomach 1 hour before or 2 hours after meals.
• Inform patient to notify prescriber if rash, fever, or chills develop. A rash is the most common allergic reaction, especially if allopurinol is also being taken.
• Advise patient to report discomfort at I.V. injection site.

---

arformoterol tartrate
arr-fohr-MOH-tur-ahl

Brovana

Pharmacologic class: long-acting selective beta₂ agonist
Pregnancy risk category C

AVAILABLE FORMS
Solution for inhalation: 15 mcg/2-ml vials

INDICATIONS & DOSAGES
➤ **Long-term maintenance treatment of bronchoconstriction in patients with COPD, including chronic bronchitis and emphysema**
Adults: 15 mcg, inhaled b.i.d. (morning and evening) via nebulizer. Maximum dose is 30 mcg daily.

ADMINISTRATION
Inhalational
• Use only the recommended nebulizer and compressor for treatment.
• Don't mix drugs with other drugs or solutions in the nebulizer.
• Store vials in the foil pouches in the refrigerator and use immediately after opening.

ACTION
Relaxes bronchial and cardiac smooth muscle by acting on beta₂-adrenergic receptors; stimulates the enzyme adenyl cyclase, which catalyzes the conversion from ATP to cAMP. This further relaxes bronchial smooth muscle and inhibits release of mediators (like histamine and leukotrienes) from mast cells.

Route	Onset	Peak	Duration
Inhalation	Rapid	30 min	Unknown

Half-life: 26 hours.

ADVERSE REACTIONS
CV: *chest pain, AV block,* atrial flutter, *heart failure, MI, prolonged QT interval, supraventricular tachycardia,* inverted T wave, peripheral edema.
EENT: sinusitis.
GI: diarrhea.
Metabolic: *hypoglycemia,* hypokalemia.
Musculoskeletal: back pain, leg cramps.
Respiratory: dyspnea, pulmonary or congestion, *bronchospasm.*
Skin: rash.
Other: hypersensitivity reaction, *pain,* flu syndrome.

INTERACTIONS
Drug-drug. *Aminophylline, corticosteroids (such as dexamethasone, prednisone), theophylline:* May increase the risk of hypokalemia. Monitor patient's potassium level.
Beta blockers (such as metoprolol, atenolol): May decrease effectiveness of arformoterol and increase risk of bronchospasm. Avoid using together, if possible; otherwise, use with extreme caution.
Non–potassium-sparing diuretics (such as furosemide, hydrochlorothiazide): May increase the risk of hypokalemia and ECG changes. Use cautiously together and monitor patient's ECG and potassium level.
Other beta₂ adrenergics (such as albuterol, formoterol): May cause additive effects. Avoid using together.
QT interval-prolonging drugs (such as MAO inhibitors, tricyclic antidepressants): May increase risk of ventricular arrhythmias. Use cautiously together.

EFFECTS ON LAB TEST RESULTS
• May increase PSA levels. May decrease potassium levels. May increase or decrease glucose levels.

CONTRAINDICATIONS & CAUTIONS
• Contraindicated in patients hypersensitive to drug, formoterol, or any other components of this drug.
• Don't use in patients with acutely deteriorating COPD.
• Use cautiously in patients with seizure disorder; thyrotoxicosis; hepatic insufficiency; preexisting cardiovascular disease, including coronary insufficiency, arrhythmias and hypertension; or in those unresponsive to sympathomimetic amines.

NURSING CONSIDERATIONS
• Drug may increase the risk of asthma-related death.
• Drug is twice as potent as formoterol inhaler.
• *Alert:* Make sure patient has a rescue inhaler, such as albuterol, to treat an acute asthma attack or bronchospasm.
• *Alert:* Notify prescriber if patient experiences decreasing control of symptoms or begins using his short-acting beta$_2$ agonist more often.
• If paradoxical bronchospasm occurs, stop drug immediately.
• Monitor blood pressure, pulse, and ECG, as indicated.
• *Look alike–sound alike:* Don't confuse Brovana (arformoterol tartrate) with Boniva (ibandronate sodium).

PATIENT TEACHING
• Tell patient to store vials in the foil pouches in the refrigerator and use immediately after opening.
• Tell patient to use only the recommended nebulizer and compressor for treatment and not to mix drug with other inhaled drugs or solutions.
• *Alert:* Warn patient that drug is for maintenance treatment only and shouldn't be used to stop an asthma attack or bronchospasm. For emergency treatment, use a short-acting rescue inhaler such as albuterol.
• Educate patient using a short-acting bronchodilator on a scheduled basis, to stop scheduled use and use only for rescue therapy.
• *Alert:* Warn patient that serious adverse effects, including death, can occur at higher than recommended doses and not to take more inhalations than prescribed.
• Tell patient to stop drug immediately and obtain medical help if life-threatening bronchospasm, severe rash, or swelling in throat occurs.
• Inform patient that he may experience palpitations, chest pain, rapid heartbeat, tremors, or nervousness.
• Tell patient not to swallow the inhalation solution.
• Caution patient to notify prescriber if he notices a decrease in symptom control or more frequent use of his rescue inhaler.

---

azathioprine
ay-za-THYE-oh-preen

Azasan, Imuran

Pharmacologic class: purine antagonist
Pregnancy risk category D

AVAILABLE FORMS
Powder for injection: 100 mg
Tablets: 25 mg, 50 mg, 75 mg, 100 mg

INDICATIONS & DOSAGES
➤ **Immunosuppression in kidney transplantation**
Adults: Initially, 3 to 5 mg/kg P.O. or I.V. daily, usually beginning on day of transplantation. Maintained at 1 to 3 mg/kg daily based on patient response and tolerance.
Adjust-a-dose: Give drug in lower doses to patients with oliguria in the posttransplant period and in those with impaired renal function. In patients receiving allopurinol, decrease azathioprine dose to one-fourth to one-third of the usual dose.
➤ **Severe, refractory rheumatoid arthritis**
Adults: Initially, 1 mg/kg P.O. as single dose or divided into two doses. Usual dose is 50 to 100 mg. If patient response isn't satisfactory after 6 to 8 weeks, dosage may be increased by 0.5 mg/kg daily to maximum of 2.5 mg/kg daily at

4-week intervals. Maintenance therapy should be at lowest effective dose. Attempt gradual dose reduction once the patient is stable. Reduce dosage by 0.5 mg/kg (about 25 mg daily) every 4 weeks.

ADMINISTRATION
P.O.
● Give drug after meals to minimize adverse GI effects.
I.V.
● Use only in patients who can't tolerate oral drugs.
● Reconstitute drug in 100-mg vial with 10 ml of sterile water for injection.
● Inspect for particles before use.
● Give by direct I.V. injection, or further dilute in normal saline solution for injection or D$_5$W solution and infuse over 30 to 60 minutes.
● **Incompatibilities:** None reported.

ACTION
May cause variable alterations in antibody production.

Route	Onset	Peak	Duration
P.O., I.V.	Unknown	Unknown	Unknown

Half-life: About 5 hours.

ADVERSE REACTIONS
CNS: fever.
GI: *nausea, vomiting,* anorexia, *pancreatitis,* steatorrhea, diarrhea, abdominal pain.
Hematologic: LEUKOPENIA, *myelosuppression,* macrocytic anemia, anemia, *pancytopenia,* THROMBOCYTOPENIA, *immunosuppression.*
Hepatic: *hepatotoxicity,* jaundice.
Musculoskeletal: arthralgia, myalgia.
Skin: rash, alopecia.
Other: *infections, increased risk of neoplasia.*

INTERACTIONS
Drug-drug. *ACE inhibitors:* May cause severe leukopenia. Monitor patient closely.
Allopurinol: May impair inactivation of azathioprine. Avoid using if possible; decrease azathioprine to one-third to one-fourth usual dose.
Co-trimoxazole and other drugs that interfere with myelopoiesis: May cause severe

leukopenia, especially in renal transplant patients. Use cautiously together.
Cyclosporine: May decrease cyclosporine level. Monitor cyclosporine level closely.
Warfarin: May decrease action of warfarin. Monitor patient closely.

EFFECTS ON LAB TEST RESULTS
● May increase alkaline phosphatase, ALT, AST, and bilirubin levels. May decrease hemoglobin and uric acid levels.
● May decrease platelet, RBC, and WBC counts.

CONTRAINDICATIONS & CAUTIONS
● Contraindicated in patients hypersensitive to drug or its components.
● Use cautiously in patients with hepatic or renal dysfunction.
● Benefits must be weighed against risk when giving to patient with systemic viral infection, such as chickenpox or herpes zoster.
● Patients with rheumatoid arthritis previously treated with alkylating drugs, such as cyclophosphamide, chlorambucil, or melphalan, may be at risk for tumor development if treated with this drug.

NURSING CONSIDERATIONS
● To prevent bleeding, avoid all I.M. injections when platelet count is below 100,000/mm^3.
● Monitor CBC and platelet counts weekly for 1 month and then twice monthly. Notify prescriber if counts drop suddenly or become dangerously low. Drug may need to be temporarily withheld.
● Watch for early signs and symptoms of hepatotoxicity (such as clay-colored stools, dark urine, pruritus, and yellow skin and sclera) and for increased alkaline phosphatase, bilirubin, AST, and ALT levels.
● Therapeutic response usually occurs within 8 weeks. Patients not improved after 12 weeks can be considered refractory to treatment.
● *Look alike–sound alike:* Don't confuse azathioprine with Azulfidine or azatadine. Don't confuse Imuran with Inderal.

PATIENT TEACHING
● Warn patient to report even mild infections (colds, fever, sore throat, malaise),

---

Reactions may be *common,* uncommon, *life-threatening,* or COMMON AND LIFE-THREATENING.
Interaction may have a *rapid onset* or *delayed onset.*

because drug is a potent immunosuppressant.

● Instruct patient to avoid conception during therapy and for 4 months after therapy stops.

● Warn patient that some hair thinning is possible.

● Tell patient taking drug for refractory rheumatoid arthritis that it may take up to 12 weeks to be effective.

● Advise patient to report unusual bleeding or bruising.

● Tell patient that drug may be taken with food to decrease nausea.

● Advise patient to use soft toothbrush and perform oral care cautiously.

---

aztreonam
AZ-tree-oh-nam

Azactam

Pharmacologic class: monobactam
Pregnancy risk category B

AVAILABLE FORMS
Injection: 500-mg vials, 1-g vials, 2-g vials

INDICATIONS & DOSAGES
➤ **UTI; septicemia; infections of lower respiratory tract, skin, and skin structures; intra-abdominal infections, surgical infections, and gynecologic infections caused by susceptible** *Escherichia coli, Klebsiella pneumoniae, Proteus mirabilis, Pseudomonas aeruginosa, Enterobacter cloacae, K. oxytoca, Citrobacter* **species, and** *Serratia marcescens;* **respiratory infections caused by** *Haemophilus influenzae*
Adults: 500 mg to 2 g I.V. or I.M. every 8 to 12 hours. For severe systemic or life-threatening infections, 2 g every 6 to 8 hours. Maximum dose is 8 g daily.
Children ages 9 months to 15 years: 30 mg/kg every 6 to 8 hours I.V. Maximum dose is 120 mg/kg/day.
Neonates age 1 to 4 weeks who weigh more than 2 kg (4.4 lb) ◆: 30 mg/kg I.V. every 6 hours.
Neonates age 1 to 4 weeks who weigh 2 kg or less ◆: 30 mg/kg I.V. every 8 hours.

Neonates younger than 7 days who weigh more than 2 kg ◆: 30 mg/kg I.V. every 8 hours.
Neonates younger than 7 days who weigh 2 kg or less ◆: 30 mg/kg I.V. every 12 hours.
Adjust-a-dose: For adults with a creatinine clearance of 10 to 30 ml/minute, give 1 to 2 g; then give 50% of the usual dose at usual interval. If clearance is less than 10 ml/minute, give 500 mg to 2 g; then give 25% of the usual dose at usual interval. For serious infections, add 12½% of the initial dose to maintenance doses after each hemodialysis session. For adults with alcoholic cirrhosis, decrease dose by 20% to 25%.

ADMINISTRATION
I.V.
● Obtain specimen for culture and sensitivity tests before giving first dose. Begin therapy while awaiting results.

● For direct injection, reconstitute with 6 to 10 ml of sterile water for injection and immediately shake vial vigorously.

● To give a bolus, inject drug over 3 to 5 minutes, directly into a vein or I.V. tubing.

● For infusion, reconstitute with a compatible I.V. solution to yield 20 mg/ml or less.

● Give infusions over 20 minutes to 1 hour.

● Give thawed solutions only by I.V. infusion.

● **Incompatibilities:** Acyclovir, amphotericin B, ampicillin sodium, azithromycin, cephradine, chlorpromazine, daunorubicin, ganciclovir, lorazepam, metronidazole, mitomycin, mitoxantrone, nafcillin, prochlorperazine, streptozocin, vancomycin.
I.M.
● To prepare I.M. injection, add at least 3 ml of one of the following solutions per gram of aztreonam: sterile water for injection, bacteriostatic water for injection, normal saline solution, or bacteriostatic normal saline solution.

● Give I.M. injections deep into a large muscle, such as the upper outer quadrant of the gluteus maximus or the side of the thigh. Give doses more than 1 g by I.V. route.

• *Alert:* Don't give I.M. injection to children.
• Pain and swelling may occur at injection site.

ACTION

Inhibits bacterial cell-wall synthesis, ultimately causing cell-wall destruction; bactericidal.

Route	Onset	Peak	Duration
I.V.	Unknown	Immediate	Unknown
I.M.	Unknown	< 1 hr	Unknown

Half-life: 2 hours.

ADVERSE REACTIONS

CNS: *seizures,* confusion, headache, insomnia.
CV: hypotension, thrombophlebitis.
GI: *pseudomembranous colitis,* diarrhea, nausea, vomiting.
Hematologic: *neutropenia, pancytopenia, thrombocytopenia,* anemia, leukocytosis, thrombocytosis.
Skin: discomfort and swelling at I.M. injection site, rash.
Other: hypersensitivity reactions.

INTERACTIONS

Drug-drug. *Aminoglycosides:* May have synergistic nephrotoxic effects. Monitor renal function.
Cefoxitin, imipenem: May have antagonistic effect. Avoid using together.
Probenecid: May increase aztreonam level. Avoid using together.

EFFECTS ON LAB TEST RESULTS

• May increase ALT, AST, BUN, creatinine, and LDH levels. May decrease hemoglobin level.
• May increase PT, PTT, and INR. May decrease neutrophil and RBC counts. May increase or decrease platelet and WBC counts.
• May cause false-positive Coombs' test result. May alter urine glucose determinations using cupric sulfate (Clinitest or Benedict reagent).

CONTRAINDICATIONS & CAUTIONS

• Contraindicated in patients hypersensitive to drug or any of its components.

• Use cautiously in elderly patients and in those with impaired renal or hepatic function. Dosage adjustment may be needed. Monitor renal function test results.

NURSING CONSIDERATIONS

• Observe patient for signs and symptoms of superinfection.
• *Alert:* Because drug is ineffective against gram-positive and anaerobic organisms, combine it with other antibiotics for immediate treatment of life-threatening illnesses.
• *Alert:* Patients allergic to penicillins or cephalosporins may not be allergic to this drug. Monitor closely those who have had an immediate hypersensitivity reaction to these antibiotics, especially to ceftazidime.

PATIENT TEACHING

• Warn patient receiving I.M. drug that pain and swelling may occur at injection site.
• Tell patient to report discomfort at I.V. insertion site.
• Instruct patient to report adverse reactions and signs and symptoms of superinfection promptly.

beclomethasone dipropionate
be-kloe-METH-a-sone

QVAR

Pharmacologic class: glucocorticoid
Pregnancy risk category C

AVAILABLE FORMS

Oral inhalation aerosol: 40 mcg/metered spray, 80 mcg/metered spray

INDICATIONS & DOSAGES

➤ **Chronic asthma**
Adults and children age 12 and older: Starting dose, 40 to 80 mcg b.i.d. when previously used bronchodilators alone, or 40 to 160 mcg b.i.d. when previously used inhaled corticosteroids. Maximum, 320 mcg b.i.d.
Children ages 5 to 12: Give 40 mcg b.i.d., up to 80 mcg b.i.d.

ADMINISTRATION
Inhalational
• Prime the inhaler before first use by depressing canister twice into the air.
• Allow 1 minute to elapse between inhalations.

ACTION
May decrease inflammation by decreasing the number and activity of inflammatory cells, inhibiting bronchoconstrictor mechanisms producing direct smooth-muscle relaxation, and decreasing airway hyperresponsiveness.

Route	Onset	Peak	Duration
Inhalation	1–4 wk	Unknown	Unknown

Half-life: 2.8 hours.

ADVERSE REACTIONS
EENT: *hoarseness, throat irritation,* fungal infection of throat.
GI: *fungal infection of mouth,* dry mouth.
Respiratory: *bronchospasm,* cough, wheezing.
Other: *angioedema,* facial edema, hypersensitivity reactions, *adrenal insufficiency,* suppression of hypothalamic-pituitary-adrenal function.

INTERACTIONS
None significant.

EFFECTS ON LAB TEST RESULTS
None reported.

CONTRAINDICATIONS & CAUTIONS
• Contraindicated in patients hypersensitive to drug or its ingredients and in those with status asthmaticus, nonasthmatic bronchial diseases, or asthma controlled by bronchodilators or other noncorticosteroids alone.
• Use cautiously, if at all, in patients with tuberculosis, fungal or bacterial infections, ocular herpes simplex, or systemic viral infections.
• Use cautiously in patients receiving systemic corticosteroid therapy.

NURSING CONSIDERATIONS
• Check mucous membranes frequently for signs and symptoms of fungal infection.

• During times of stress (trauma, surgery, or infection), systemic corticosteroids may be needed to prevent adrenal insufficiency in previously corticosteroid-dependent patients.
• Periodic measurement of growth and development may be needed during high-dose or prolonged therapy in children.
• *Alert:* Taper oral corticosteroid therapy slowly. Acute adrenal insufficiency and death may occur in patients with asthma who change abruptly from oral corticosteroids to beclomethasone.

PATIENT TEACHING
• Tell patient to prime the inhaler before first use, or after 10 days of not using it, by depressing canister twice into the air.
• Inform patient that drug doesn't relieve acute asthma attacks.
• Tell patient who needs a bronchodilator to use it several minutes before beclomethasone.
• Instruct patient to carry or wear medical identification indicating his need for supplemental systemic corticosteroids during stress.
• Advise patient to allow 1 minute to elapse between inhalations of drug and to hold his breath for a few seconds to enhance drug action.
• Tell patient it may take up to 4 weeks to feel the full benefit of the drug.
• Tell patient to keep inhaler clean by wiping it weekly with a dry tissue or cloth; don't get it wet.
• Advise patient to prevent oral fungal infections by gargling or rinsing his mouth with water after each use. Caution him not to swallow the water.
• Tell patient to report evidence of corticosteroid withdrawal, including fatigue, weakness, arthralgia, orthostatic hypotension, and dyspnea.
• Instruct patient to store drug at 77° F (25° C). Advise patient to ensure delivery of proper dose by gently warming canister to room temperature before using.

benzonatate
ben-ZOE-na-tate

Tessalon, Tessalon Perles

Pharmacologic class: local anesthetic
Pregnancy risk category C

AVAILABLE FORMS
Capsules: 100 mg, 200 mg

INDICATIONS & DOSAGES
➤ **Symptomatic relief of cough**
Adults and children older than age 10:
Give 100 to 200 mg P.O. t.i.d.; up to 600 mg daily.

ADMINISTRATION
P.O.
• Protect drug from light and moisture.

ACTION
Chemical relative of tetracaine that suppresses the cough reflex by direct action on the cough center in the medulla and through an anesthetic action on stretch receptors of vagal afferent fibers in the respiratory passages, lungs, and pleura.

Route	Onset	Peak	Duration
P.O.	15–20 min	Unknown	3–8 hr

Half-life: Unknown.

ADVERSE REACTIONS
CNS: dizziness, headache, sedation.
EENT: nasal congestion, burning sensation in eyes.
GI: nausea, constipation, GI upset.
Other: chills, hypersensitivity reactions.

INTERACTIONS
None significant.

EFFECTS ON LAB TEST RESULTS
None reported.

CONTRAINDICATIONS & CAUTIONS
• Contraindicated in patients hypersensitive to drug or related compounds.
• Use cautiously in patients hypersensitive to PABA anesthetics (procaine, tetracaine) because cross-sensitivity reactions may occur.

NURSING CONSIDERATIONS
• Don't use drug when cough is a valuable diagnostic sign or is beneficial (such as after thoracic surgery).
• Monitor cough type and frequency.
• Use with percussion and chest vibration.

PATIENT TEACHING
• Warn patient not to chew capsules or dissolve in mouth, which produces either local anesthesia that may result in aspiration, or CNS stimulation that may cause restlessness, tremor, and seizures.
• Instruct patient to report adverse reactions.
• Instruct patient to protect drug from light and moisture.
• Tell patient to contact his prescriber if cough lasts longer than 1 week, recurs frequently, or is accompanied by high fever, rash, or severe headache.

beractant (natural lung surfactant)
ber-AK-tant

Survanta

Pharmacologic class: bovine lung extract
Pregnancy risk category NR

AVAILABLE FORMS
Suspension for intratracheal instillation: 25 mg/ml

INDICATIONS & DOSAGES
➤ **To prevent respiratory distress syndrome (RDS), also known as hyaline membrane disease, in premature neonates weighing 1,250 g (2 lb, 12 ounces) or less at birth, or having symptoms consistent with surfactant deficiency**
Neonates: 4 ml/kg intratracheally. Divide each dose into four quarter-doses and give each quarter-dose with infant in a different position to ensure even distribution of drug; between quarter-doses, use a hand-held resuscitation bag at 60 breaths/minute and sufficient oxygen to prevent cyanosis.

Give drug as soon as possible, preferably within 15 minutes of birth. Repeat in 6 hours if respiratory distress continues. Give no more than four doses in 48 hours.

➤ **Rescue treatment of RDS in premature infants**

Neonates: 4 ml/kg intratracheally; before giving, increase ventilator rate to 60 breaths/minute with an inspiratory time of 0.5 second and a fraction of inspired oxygen of 1. Divide each dose into four quarter-doses and give each quarter-dose with infant in a different position to ensure even distribution of drug; between quarter-doses, continue mechanical ventilation for at least 30 seconds or until stable. Give dose as soon as RDS is confirmed by X-ray, preferably within 8 hours of birth. Repeat in 6 hours if respiratory distress continues. Give no more than four doses in 48 hours.

ADMINISTRATION

Inhalational

● Refrigerate at 36° to 46° F (2° to 8° C). Warm before use by allowing drug to stand at room temperature for at least 20 minutes or by holding in hand for at least 8 minutes. Don't use artificial warming methods. Unopened vials that have been warmed to room temperature may be returned to the refrigerator within 24 hours; however, warm and return drug to the refrigerator only once. Vials are for single use only; discard unused drug.

● Beractant doesn't need sonication or reconstitution before use. Inspect contents before giving; make sure color is off-white to light brown and that contents are uniform. If settling occurs, swirl vial gently; don't shake. Some foaming is normal.

● Use a 20G or larger needle to draw up drug; don't use a filter. Give drug using a #5 French end-hole catheter. Premeasure and shorten catheter before use. Fill catheter with beractant and discard excess drug so that only total dose to be given remains in the syringe. Insert catheter into neonate's endotracheal tube; make sure catheter tip protrudes just beyond end of tube above neonate's carina. Don't instill drug into a mainstream bronchus.

● Even distribution of drug is important. Give each dose in four quarter-doses, with each quarter-dose being given over 2 to 3 seconds and with the patient positioned differently after each use. Between giving quarter-doses, remove the catheter and ventilate the patient. Give the first quarter-dose with the patient's head and body inclined slightly downward, and the head turned to the right. Give the second quarter-dose with the head turned to the left. Then, incline the head and body slightly upward with the head turned to the right to give the third quarter-dose. Turn the head to the left for the fourth quarter-dose.

ACTION

Lowers alveolar surface tension during respiration and stabilizes alveoli against collapse. Drug contains neutral lipids, fatty acids, surfactant-related proteins, and phospholipids that mimic naturally occurring surfactant.

Route	Onset	Peak	Duration
Intratracheal	30–120 min	Unknown	2–3 days

Half-life: Unknown.

ADVERSE REACTIONS

CV: TRANSIENT BRADYCARDIA, hypotension, vasoconstriction.
Respiratory: *apnea, endotracheal tube reflux or blockage, decreased oxygen saturation, hypercapnia, hypocapnia.*
Skin: pallor.

INTERACTIONS

None significant.

EFFECTS ON LAB TEST RESULTS

None reported.

CONTRAINDICATIONS & CAUTIONS

● In infants who weigh less than 600 g at birth or more than 1,750 g at birth, use hasn't been studied.

NURSING CONSIDERATIONS

● Only staff experienced in treating clinically unstable premature neonates, including neonatal intubation and airway management, should give drug.
● Accurate weight determination is essential for proper measurement of dosage.

• Continuously monitor neonate before, during, and after giving beractant. The endotracheal tube may be suctioned before giving drug; allow neonate to stabilize before proceeding with administration.
• Immediately after giving, moist breath sounds and crackles can occur. Don't suction the neonate for 1 hour unless he has other signs or symptoms of airway obstruction.
• Continuous monitoring of ECG and transcutaneous oxygen saturation are essential; frequent arterial blood pressure monitoring and frequent arterial blood gas sampling are highly desirable.
• Transient bradycardia and oxygen desaturation are common after dosing.
• *Alert:* Drug can rapidly affect oxygenation and lung compliance. Peak ventilator inspiratory pressures may need to be adjusted if chest expansion improves substantially after drug administration. Notify prescriber and adjust immediately as directed because failing to do so may cause lung overdistention and fatal pulmonary air leakage.
• Review manufacturer's audiovisual materials that describe dosage and usage procedures.
• *Look alike–sound alike:* Don't confuse Survanta with Sufenta.

PATIENT TEACHING
• Inform parents of neonate's need for drug, and explain drug action and use.
• Encourage parents to ask questions, and address their concerns.

SAFETY ALERT!

bevacizumab
beh-vah-SIZZ-yoo-mab

Avastin

Pharmacologic class: monoclonal antibody
Pregnancy risk category C

AVAILABLE FORMS
Solution: 25 mg/ml in 4-ml and 16-ml vials

INDICATIONS & DOSAGES
➤ **First- or second-line treatment, with fluorouracil-based chemotherapy, for metastatic colon or rectal cancer**
Adults: If used with bolus irinotecan, fluorouracil, and leucovorin (IFL) regimen, give 5 mg/kg I.V. every 14 days. If used with oxaliplatin, fluorouracil, and leucovorin (known as FOLFOX 4) regimen, give 10 mg/kg I.V. every 14 days. Infusion rate varies by patient tolerance and number of infusions.
➤ **With carboplatin and paclitaxel as first-line treatment of unresectable, locally advanced, recurrent, or metastatic nonsquamous, non–small cell lung cancer**
Adults: 15 mg/kg I.V. infusion once every 3 weeks.

ADMINISTRATION
I.V.
• Don't freeze or shake vials.
• Dilute drug using aseptic technique. Withdraw proper dose and mix in a total volume of 100 ml normal saline solution in an I.V. bag.
• Don't give by I.V. push or bolus.
• Give the first infusion over 90 minutes and, if tolerated, the second infusion over 60 minutes. Later infusions can be given over 30 minutes if previous infusions were tolerated.
• Discard unused portion; drug is preservative-free.
• Drug is stable 8 hours if refrigerated at 36° to 46° F (2° to 8° C) and protected from light.
• **Incompatibilities:** Dextrose solutions.

ACTION
A recombinant humanized vascular endothelial growth factor (VEGF) inhibitor. Because VEGF promotes angiogenesis to tumors, it may contribute to metastatic tumor growth.

Route	Onset	Peak	Duration
I.V.	Unknown	Unknown	Unknown

Half-life: About 20 days.

ADVERSE REACTIONS

CNS: *asthenia, dizziness, headache,* abnormal gait, confusion, pain, syncope.

CV: INTRA-ABDOMINAL THROMBOSIS, *hypertension, **thromboembolism, deep vein thrombosis,*** heart failure, hypotension.

EENT: *epistaxis,* excess lacrimation, gum bleeding, nasal septum perforation, taste disorder, voice alteration.

GI: *anorexia, constipation, diarrhea, dyspepsia, flatulence, stomatitis, vomiting, **GI hemorrhage,*** abdominal pain, colitis, dry mouth, nausea.

GU: ***vaginal hemorrhage,*** proteinuria, urinary urgency.

Hematologic: ***leukopenia, neutropenia, thrombocytopenia.***

Metabolic: *hypokalemia, weight loss,* bilirubinemia.

Musculoskeletal: *myalgia.*

Respiratory: HEMOPTYSIS, *dyspnea, upper respiratory tract infection.*

Skin: *alopecia, dermatitis, discoloration, dry skin, exfoliative dermatitis,* nail disorder, skin ulcer.

Other: decreased wound healing, hypersensitivity.

INTERACTIONS

Drug-drug. *Irinotecan:* May increase level of irinotecan metabolite. Monitor patient.

EFFECTS ON LAB TEST RESULTS

● May increase bilirubin and urine protein levels. May decrease potassium level.
● May decrease neutrophil, platelet, and WBC counts.

CONTRAINDICATIONS & CAUTIONS

● Contraindicated in patients with recent hemoptysis or within 28 days after major surgery.
● Use cautiously in patients hypersensitive to drug or its components, in those who need surgery, are taking anticoagulants, or have significant CV disease.

NURSING CONSIDERATIONS

● *Alert:* Reversible posterior leukoencephalopathy syndrome (RPLS)-associated symptoms (hypertension, headache, visual disturbances, altered mental function, and seizures) may occur 16 hours to 1 year after starting the drug. Monitor patient closely. If syndrome occurs, stop drug and provide supportive care.
● RPLS can be confirmed only by MRI.
● Hypersensitivity reactions can occur during infusion. Monitor the patient closely.
● In patients who develop nephrotic syndrome, severe hypertension, hypertensive crisis, serious hemorrhage, GI perforation, or wound dehiscence that needs intervention, stop drug.
● Before elective surgery, stop drug, considering drug's half-life is about 20 days. Don't resume therapy until incision is fully healed.
● *Alert:* Drug may increase risk of serious arterial thromboembolic events including MI, TIAs, stroke, and angina. Those patients at highest risk are age 65 or older, have a history of arterial thromboembolism, and have taken the drug before. If patient has an arterial thrombotic event, permanently stop drug.
● *Alert:* Drug may cause fatal GI perforation. Monitor patient closely.
● Monitor urinalysis for worsening proteinuria. Patients with 2+ or greater urine dipstick test should undergo 24-hour urine collection.
● Monitor patient's blood pressure every 2 to 3 weeks.
● It's unknown whether drug appears in breast milk. Women shouldn't breast-feed during therapy and for about 3 weeks after therapy ends.
● Adverse reactions occur more often in older patients.

PATIENT TEACHING

● Inform patient about potential adverse reactions.
● Tell patient to report adverse reactions immediately, especially abdominal pain, constipation, and vomiting.
● Advise patient that blood pressure and urinalysis will be monitored during treatment.
● Caution woman of childbearing age to avoid pregnancy during treatment.
● Urge patient to alert other health care providers about treatment and to avoid elective surgery during treatment.

bleomycin sulfate
blee-oh-MYE-sin

Blenoxane

Pharmacologic class: cytotoxic
glycopeptide antibiotic
Pregnancy risk category D

AVAILABLE FORMS
Injection: 15-unit vials, 30-unit vials

INDICATIONS & DOSAGES
➤ **Squamous cell carcinoma (head,
neck, skin, penis, cervix, and vulva),
non-Hodgkin lymphoma, testicular
carcinoma**
Adults: 2 units or less of bleomycin for
injection for the first two doses. If no acute
reaction occurs, then 10 to 20 units/m^2
I.V., I.M., or subcutaneously once or twice
weekly to total of 400 units.
➤ **Hodgkin lymphoma**
Adults: 2 units or less of bleomycin for
injection for the first two doses. If no acute
reaction occurs, then 10 to 20 units/m^2 I.V.,
I.M., or subcutaneously one or two times
weekly. After 50% response, maintenance
dose is 1 unit I.V. or I.M. daily or 5 units
I.V. or I.M. weekly. Total cumulative dose
is 400 units.
➤ **Malignant pleural effusion**
Adults: 60 units given as single-dose bolus
intrapleural injection.

ADMINISTRATION
I.V.
● Preparing and giving parenteral form
of drug may be mutagenic, teratogenic,
and carcinogenic. Follow facility policy to
reduce risks.
● Drug may adsorb to plastic I.V. bags. For
prolonged infusions, use glass containers.
● Reconstitute drug with 5 or 10 ml of
normal saline solution for injection to
equal 3 units/ml solution.
● Use reconstituted solution within
24 hours.
● Refrigerate unopened vials containing
dry powder.
● **Incompatibilities:** Amino acids; aminophylline; ascorbic acid injection; cefazolin;
diazepam; drugs containing sulfhydryl
groups; fluids containing dextrose;

furosemide; hydrocortisone; methotrexate; mitomycin; nafcillin; penicillin G;
riboflavin; solutions containing divalent
and trivalent cations, especially calcium
salts and copper; terbutaline sulfate.
I.M.
● Dilute drug in 1 to 5 ml of sterile water
for injection, bacteriostatic water for injection, or normal saline solution for injection.
● Monitor injection site for irritation.
Subcutaneous
● Dilute drug in 1 to 5 ml of sterile water
for injection, bacteriostatic water for
injection, or normal saline solution for
injection.
● Monitor injection site for irritation.

ACTION
May inhibit DNA synthesis and cause
scission of single- and double-stranded
DNA; also inhibits RNA and protein
synthesis.

Route	Onset	Peak	Duration
I.V., Subcut	Unknown	Unknown	Unknown
I.M.	Unknown	30–60 min	Unknown

Half-life: 2 hours.

ADVERSE REACTIONS
CNS: fever.
GI: *stomatitis, anorexia, nausea, vomiting,*
diarrhea.
Metabolic: weight loss, hyperuricemia.
Respiratory: PNEUMONITIS, *pulmonary
fibrosis.*
Skin: *erythema, hyperpigmentation, acne,
rash, striae, skin tenderness, pruritus,
reversible alopecia,* hyperkeratosis, nail
changes.
Other: *chills, anaphylactoid reactions.*

INTERACTIONS
Drug-drug. *Anesthesia:* May increase
oxygen requirements. Monitor patient
closely.
Cardiac glycosides: May decrease digoxin
level. Monitor digoxin level closely.
Fosphenytoin, phenytoin: May decrease
phenytoin and fosphenytoin levels.
Monitor drug levels closely.

EFFECTS ON LAB TEST RESULTS
● May increase uric acid level.

CONTRAINDICATIONS & CAUTIONS
• Contraindicated in patients hypersensitive to drug.
• Use cautiously in patients with renal or pulmonary impairment.

NURSING CONSIDERATIONS
• Obtain pulmonary function tests. If tests show a marked decline, stop drug.
• *Alert:* Pulmonary toxicity appears to be dose-related, with an increase when total dose is more than 400 units. Give total doses of more than 400 units with caution.
• *Alert:* Adverse pulmonary reactions are more common in patients older than age 70. Pulmonary fibrosis is fatal in 1% of patients, especially when cumulative dosage exceeds 400 units. Also, in patients receiving radiation therapy, patients with lung disease, and patients who need oxygen therapy, pulmonary toxic adverse effects may be increased.
• Monitor chest X-ray and listen to lungs regularly.
• Obtain pulmonary function tests and chest X-rays before each course of therapy.
• Watch for fever, which may be treated with antipyretics. Fever usually occurs within 3 to 6 hours of administration.
• *Alert:* Watch for hypersensitivity reactions, which may be delayed for several hours, especially in patients with lymphoma. (Give test dose of 1 to 2 units before first two doses in these patients. If no reaction occurs, follow regular dosage schedule.)
• For intrapleural use, dilute 60 units of drug in 50 to 100 ml normal saline solution for injection; give drug through a thoracotomy tube.
• If patient's condition requires sclerosis, instill drug when chest tube drainage is 100 to 300 ml/24 hours; ideally, drainage should be less than 100 ml. After instillation, clamp thoracotomy tube and move patient from his back to his left then right side for the next 4 hours. Remove clamp and reestablish suction. Amount of time chest tube is left in place after sclerosis depends on patient's condition.
• Don't use adhesive dressings.

PATIENT TEACHING
• Warn patient that hair loss may occur but is usually reversible.

• Tell patient to report adverse reactions promptly and to take infection-control and bleeding precautions.
• For patient who's to receive anesthesia, tell him to inform anesthesiologist that he has taken this drug. High oxygen levels inhaled during surgery may enhance pulmonary toxicity of drug.

---

bosentan
bow-SEN-tan

Tracleer

Pharmacologic class: endothelin-receptor antagonist
Pregnancy risk category X

AVAILABLE FORMS
Tablets: 62.5 mg, 125 mg

INDICATIONS & DOSAGES
➤ **Pulmonary arterial hypertension in patients with World Health Organization class III (with mild exertion) or IV (at rest) symptoms, to improve exercise ability and decrease rate of clinical worsening**
Adults: 62.5 mg P.O. b.i.d. in the morning and evening for 4 weeks. Increase to maintenance dosage of 125 mg P.O. b.i.d. in the morning and evening.
Adjust-a-dose: For patients who develop ALT and AST abnormalities, the dose may need to be decreased or the therapy stopped until ALT and AST levels return to normal. If therapy is resumed, begin with initial dose. Test levels within 3 days; then give using the following table. If liver function abnormalities are accompanied by symptoms of liver injury or if bilirubin level is at least twice the upper limit of normal (ULN), stop treatment and don't restart. In patients who weigh less than 40 kg (88 lb), the initial and maintenance dosage is 62.5 mg b.i.d.

ADMINISTRATION
P.O.
• Give drug in morning and evening without regard for meals.

ALT and AST levels	Treatment and monitoring recommendations
> 3 and < 5 times upper limit of normal (ULN)	Confirm with repeat test; if confirmed, reduce dose or interrupt treatment and retest every 2 wk. Once ALT and AST return to pretreatment levels, continue or reintroduce treatment at starting dose.
> 5 and < 8 times ULN	Confirm with repeat test; if confirmed, stop treatment and retest at least every 2 wk. Once levels return to pretreatment levels, consider reintroduction of treatment.
> 8 times ULN	Stop treatment; don't consider restarting drug.

ACTION

Specific and competitive antagonist for endothelin-1 (ET-1). ET-1 levels are elevated in patients with pulmonary arterial hypertension, suggesting a pathogenic role for ET-1 in this disease.

Route	Onset	Peak	Duration
P.O.	Unknown	3–5 hr	Unknown

Half-life: About 5 hours.

ADVERSE REACTIONS

CNS: *headache,* fatigue.
CV: edema, flushing, hypotension, palpitations.
EENT: *nasopharyngitis.*
GI: dyspepsia.
Hematologic: *anemia.*
Hepatic: HEPATOTOXICITY.
Skin: pruritus.
Other: leg edema.

INTERACTIONS

Drug-drug. *Cyclosporine A:* May increase bosentan level and decrease cyclosporine level. Use together is contraindicated.
Glyburide: May increase risk of elevated liver function test values and decrease levels of both drugs. Use together is contraindicated.

Hormonal contraceptives: May cause contraceptive failure. Advise use of an additional method of birth control.
Ketoconazole: May increase bosentan effect. Watch for adverse effects.
Simvastatin, other statins: May decrease levels of these drugs. Monitor cholesterol levels to assess need to adjust statin dose.
Tacrolimus: May increase bosentan levels. Use together cautiously.

EFFECTS ON LAB TEST RESULTS

• May increase liver aminotransferase level. May decrease hemoglobin level and hematocrit.

CONTRAINDICATIONS & CAUTIONS

• Contraindicated in patients hypersensitive to drug, in pregnant patients, and in those taking cyclosporine A or glyburide.
• Generally avoid using in patients with moderate to severe liver impairment or in those with elevated aminotransferase levels greater than three times the ULN.
• Use cautiously in patients with mild liver impairment.
• Drug may harm fetus. Be sure woman isn't pregnant before starting treatment.
• Because it's unknown whether drug appears in breast milk, drug isn't recommended for breast-feeding women.
• Safety and efficacy in children haven't been established.

NURSING CONSIDERATIONS

• Use of this drug can cause serious liver injury. AST and ALT level elevations may be dose dependent and reversible, so measure these levels before treatment and monthly thereafter, adjusting dosage accordingly. If elevations are accompanied by symptoms of liver injury (nausea, vomiting, fever, abdominal pain, jaundice, or unusual lethargy or fatigue) or if bilirubin level increases by greater than twice the ULN, notify prescriber immediately.
• Fluid retention and heart failure may occur. Patient may require diuretics, fluid management, or hospitalization for decompensating heart failure.
• Monitor hemoglobin level after 1 and 3 months of therapy; then every 3 months.
• Gradually reduce dose before stopping drug.

PATIENT TEACHING
● Advise patient to take doses in the morning and evening, with or without food.
● Warn patient to avoid becoming pregnant while taking this drug. Hormonal contraceptives, including oral, implantable, and injectable methods, may not be effective when used with this drug. Advise patient to use a backup method of contraception. A monthly pregnancy test must be performed.
● Advise patient to have liver function tests and blood counts performed regularly.

---

budesonide
byoo-DES-oh-nide

Pulmicort Respules, Pulmicort Turbuhaler

Pharmacologic class: corticosteroid
Pregnancy risk category B

AVAILABLE FORMS
Dry powder inhaler: 200 mcg/dose
Inhalation suspension: 0.25 mg, 0.5 mg

INDICATIONS & DOSAGES
➤ **As a preventative in maintenance of asthma**
All patients: Use lowest effective dose after stabilizing asthma.
Adults previously taking bronchodilator alone: Initially, inhaled dose of 200 to 400 mcg b.i.d. to maximum of 400 mcg b.i.d.
Adults previously taking inhaled corticosteroid: Initially, inhaled dose of 200 to 400 mcg b.i.d. to maximum of 800 mcg b.i.d.
Adults previously taking oral corticosteroid: Initially, inhaled dose of 400 to 800 mcg b.i.d. to maximum of 800 mcg b.i.d.
Children older than age 6 previously taking bronchodilator alone or inhaled corticosteroid: Initially, inhaled dose of 200 mcg b.i.d. to maximum of 400 mcg b.i.d.
Children older than age 6 previously taking oral corticosteroid: 400 mcg b.i.d., maximum.
Children ages 1 to 8: Give 0.25 mg Respules via jet nebulizer with compressor once daily. Increase to 0.5 mg daily or 0.25 mg b.i.d. in child not receiving systemic or inhaled corticosteroid or 1 mg daily or 0.5 mg b.i.d. in child receiving oral corticosteroid.

ADMINISTRATION
Inhalational
● Give inhalation suspension at regular intervals once a day or b.i.d., as directed.
● Give suspension with a jet nebulizer connected to a compressor with adequate airflow. Make sure that it's equipped with a mouthpiece or suitable face mask.
● When aluminum foil envelope has been opened, the shelf-life of unused ampules is 2 weeks when protected from light.

ACTION
Exhibits potent glucocorticoid activity and weak mineralocorticoid activity. Drug inhibits mast cells, macrophages, and mediators (such as leukotrienes) involved in inflammation.

Route	Onset	Peak	Duration
Inhalation, powder	24 hr	1–2 wk	Unknown
Inhalation, Respules	2–8 days	4–6 wk	Unknown

Half-life: 2 to 3 hours.

ADVERSE REACTIONS
CNS: *headache,* asthenia, fever, hypertonia, insomnia, pain, syncope.
EENT: *sinusitis, pharyngitis,* rhinitis, voice alteration.
GI: abdominal pain, dry mouth, dyspepsia, gastroenteritis, nausea, oral candidiasis, taste perversion, vomiting.
Metabolic: weight gain.
Musculoskeletal: back pain, fractures, myalgia.
Respiratory: *respiratory tract infection, bronchospasm,* increased cough.
Skin: ecchymoses.
Other: flulike symptoms, hypersensitivity reactions.

INTERACTIONS
Drug-drug. *Ketoconazole:* May inhibit metabolism and increase level of budesonide. Monitor patient.

EFFECTS ON LAB TEST RESULTS
None reported.

CONTRAINDICATIONS & CAUTIONS
• Contraindicated in patients hypersensitive to drug and in those with status asthmaticus or other acute asthma episodes.
• Use cautiously, if at all, in patients with active or inactive tuberculosis, ocular herpes simplex, or untreated systemic fungal, bacterial, viral, or parasitic infections.

NURSING CONSIDERATIONS
• When transferring from systemic corticosteroid to this drug, use caution and gradually decrease corticosteroid dose to prevent adrenal insufficiency.
• Drug doesn't remove the need for systemic corticosteroid therapy in some situations.
• If bronchospasm occurs after use, stop therapy and treat with a bronchodilator.
• Lung function may improve within 24 hours of starting therapy, but maximum benefit may not be achieved for 1 to 2 weeks or longer.
• For Pulmicort Respules, lung function improves in 2 to 8 days, but maximum benefit may not be seen for 4 to 6 weeks.
• Watch for *Candida* infections of the mouth or pharynx.
• *Alert:* Corticosteroids may increase risk of developing serious or fatal infections in patients exposed to viral illnesses, such as chickenpox or measles.
• In rare cases, inhaled corticosteroids have been linked to increased intraocular pressure and cataract development. Stop drug if local irritation occurs.

PATIENT TEACHING
• Tell patient that budesonide inhaler isn't a bronchodilator and isn't intended to treat acute episodes of asthma.
• Instruct patient to use the inhaler at regular intervals because effectiveness depends on twice-daily use on a regular basis, by following these instructions:
– Keep Pulmicort Turbuhaler upright (mouthpiece on top) during loading, to provide the correct dose.
– Prime Turbuhaler when using it for the first time. To prime, hold unit upright and turn brown grip fully to the right, then fully to the left until it clicks. Repeat priming.
– Load first dose by holding unit upright and turning brown grip to the right and then to the left until it clicks.
– Turn your head away from the inhaler and breathe out.
– During inhalation, Turbuhaler must be in the upright or horizontal position.
– Don't shake inhaler.
– Place mouthpiece between lips and inhale forcefully and deeply.
– You may not taste the drug or sense it entering your lungs, but this doesn't mean it isn't effective.
– Don't exhale through the Turbuhaler. If more than one dose is required, repeat steps.
– Rinse your mouth with water and then spit out the water after each dose to decrease the risk of developing oral candidiasis.
– When 20 doses remain in the Turbuhaler, a red mark appears in the indicator window. When red mark reaches the bottom, the unit's empty.
– Don't use Turbuhaler with a spacer device and don't chew or bite the mouthpiece.
– Replace mouthpiece cover after use and always keep it clean and dry.
• Tell patient that improvement in asthma control may be seen within 24 hours, although the maximum benefit may not appear for 1 to 2 weeks. If signs or symptoms worsen during this time, instruct patient to contact prescriber.
• Advise patient to avoid exposure to chickenpox or measles and to contact prescriber if exposure occurs.
• Instruct patient to carry or wear medical identification indicating need for supplementary corticosteroids during periods of stress or an asthma attack.
• Advise patient that unused Respules are good for 2 weeks after the foil envelope has been opened; however, unused Respules should be returned to the envelope to protect them from light.
• Tell patient to read and follow the patient information leaflet contained in the package.

bumetanide
byoo-MET-a-nide

Bumex

Pharmacologic class: loop diuretic
Pregnancy risk category C

AVAILABLE FORMS
Injection: 0.25 mg/ml
Tablets: 0.5 mg, 1 mg, 2 mg

INDICATIONS & DOSAGES
➤ **Edema caused by heart failure or hepatic or renal disease**
Adults: 0.5 to 2 mg P.O. once daily. If diuretic response isn't adequate, a second or third dose may be given at 4- to 5-hour intervals. Maximum dose is 10 mg daily. May be given parenterally if oral route isn't possible. Usual first dose is 0.5 to 1 mg given I.V. or I.M. If response isn't adequate, a second or third dose may be given at 2- to 3-hour intervals. Maximum, 10 mg daily.

ADMINISTRATION
P.O.
• Give drug with food to minimize GI upset.
• To prevent nocturia, give drug in morning. If second dose is needed, give in early afternoon.
I.V.
• For direct injection, give drug over 1 or 2 minutes using a 21G or 23G needle.
• For intermittent infusion, give diluted drug through an intermittent infusion device or piggyback into an I.V. line containing a free-flowing, compatible solution.
• **Incompatibilities:** Dobutamine, fenoldopam, midazolam.
I.M.
• Document injection site.

ACTION
Inhibits sodium and chloride reabsorption in the ascending loop of Henle.

Route	Onset	Peak	Duration
P.O.	30–60 min	1–2 hr	4–6 hr
I.V.	Within min	15–30 min	30–60 min
I.M.	40 min	Unknown	5–6 hr

Half-life: 1 to 1½ hours.

ADVERSE REACTIONS
CNS: *weakness,* dizziness, headache, vertigo.
CV: orthostatic hypotension, ECG changes, chest pain.
EENT: transient deafness.
GI: nausea, vomiting, upset stomach, dry mouth, diarrhea.
GU: premature ejaculation, difficulty maintaining erection, oliguria.
Hematologic: *thrombocytopenia,* azotemia.
Metabolic: volume depletion and dehydration, hypokalemia, hypochloremic alkalosis, *hypomagnesemia,* asymptomatic hyperuricemia.
Musculoskeletal: arthritic pain, muscle cramps and pain.
Skin: rash, pruritus, diaphoresis.

INTERACTIONS
Drug-drug. *Aminoglycoside antibiotics:* May increase ototoxicity. Avoid using together if possible.
Antidiabetics: May decrease hypoglycemic effects. Monitor glucose level.
Antihypertensives: May increase hypotensive effects. Consider dosage adjustment.
Cardiac glycosides: May increase risk of digoxin toxicity from bumetanide-induced hypokalemia. Monitor potassium and digoxin levels.
Chlorothiazide, chlorthalidone, hydrochlorothiazide, indapamide, metolazone: May cause excessive diuretic response, causing serious electrolyte abnormalities or dehydration. Adjust doses carefully, and monitor patient closely for signs and symptoms of excessive diuretic response.
Cisplatin: May increase risk of ototoxicity. Monitor patient closely.
Lithium: May decrease lithium clearance, increasing risk of lithium toxicity. Monitor lithium level.

Neuromuscular blockers: May prolong neuromuscular blockade. Monitor patient closely.

NSAIDs, probenecid: May inhibit diuretic response. Use together cautiously.

Other potassium-wasting drugs (such as amphotericin B, corticosteroids): May increase risk of hypokalemia. Use together cautiously.

Warfarin: May increase anticoagulant effect. Use together cautiously.

Drug-herb. *Dandelion:* May interfere with drug activity. Discourage use together.

Licorice: May cause unexpected, rapid potassium loss. Discourage use together.

EFFECTS ON LAB TEST RESULTS

• May increase alkaline phosphatase, ALT, AST, bilirubin, cholesterol, creatinine, glucose, LDH, and urine urea levels. May decrease calcium, magnesium, potassium, sodium, and chloride levels.

• May decrease platelet count.

CONTRAINDICATIONS & CAUTIONS

• Contraindicated in patients hypersensitive to drug or sulfonamides (possible cross-sensitivity) and in patients with anuria, hepatic coma, or severe electrolyte depletion.

• Use cautiously in patients with hepatic cirrhosis and ascites, in elderly patients, and in those with decreased renal function.

NURSING CONSIDERATIONS

• Safest and most effective dosage schedule is alternate days or 3 or 4 consecutive days with 1 or 2 days off between cycles.

• Monitor fluid intake and output, weight, and electrolyte, BUN, creatinine, and carbon dioxide levels frequently.

• Watch for evidence of hypokalemia, such as muscle weakness and cramps. Instruct patient to report these symptoms.

• Consult prescriber and dietitian about a high-potassium diet. Foods rich in potassium include citrus fruits, tomatoes, bananas, dates, and apricots.

• Monitor glucose level in diabetic patients.

• Monitor uric acid level, especially in patients with history of gout.

• Monitor blood pressure and pulse rate during rapid diuresis. Profound water and electrolyte depletion may occur.

• If oliguria or azotemia develops or increases, prescriber may stop drug.

• Drug can be safely used in patients allergic to furosemide; 1 mg of bumetanide equals about 40 mg of furosemide.

• *Look alike–sound alike:* Don't confuse Bumex with Buprenex.

PATIENT TEACHING

• Instruct patient to take drug with food to minimize GI upset.

• Advise patient to take drug in morning to avoid need to urinate at night; if patient needs second dose, have him take it in early afternoon.

• Advise patient to avoid sudden posture changes and to rise slowly to avoid dizziness upon standing quickly.

• Instruct patient to notify prescriber about extreme thirst, muscle weakness, cramps, nausea, or dizziness.

• Instruct patient to weigh himself daily to monitor fluid status.

---

calfactant
kal-FAK-tant

Infasurf

Pharmacologic class: bovine lung extract
Pregnancy risk category NR

AVAILABLE FORMS

Intratracheal suspension: 35 mg phospholipids and 0.65 mg proteins/ml; 6-ml vial

INDICATIONS & DOSAGES

➤ **To prevent respiratory distress syndrome (RDS) in premature infants younger than 29 weeks' gestational age at high risk for RDS; to treat infants younger than 72 hours of age, who develop RDS (confirmed by clinical and radiologic findings) and need an endotracheal tube (ETT)**

Neonates: 3 ml/kg of body weight at birth intratracheally, given in two aliquots of 1.5 ml/kg each, every 12 hours for total of three doses.

ADMINISTRATION
Inhalational
• Suspension settles during storage. Gentle swirling or agitation of the vial is commonly needed for redispersion. Don't shake vial. Visible flecks in the suspension and foaming at the surface are normal.
• Withdraw dose into a syringe from single-use vial using a 20G or larger needle; avoid excessive foaming.
• Give through a side-port adapter into the ETT. Make sure two medical staff are present while giving dose. Give dose in two aliquots of 1.5 ml/kg each. Place infant on one side after first aliquot and other side after second aliquot. Give while ventilation is continued over 20 to 30 breaths for each aliquot, with small bursts timed only during the inspiratory cycles. Evaluate respiratory status and reposition infant between each aliquot.
• Enter each single-use vial only once; discard unused material.
• Unopened, unused vials that have warmed to room temperature can be rerefrigerated within 24 hours for future use. Avoid repeated warming to room temperature.
• Store drug at 36° to 46° F (2° to 8° C). It isn't necessary to warm drug before use.

ACTION
Modifies alveolar surface tension, which stabilizes the alveoli.

Route	Onset	Peak	Duration
Intratracheal	Unknown	Unknown	Unknown

Half-life: Unknown.

ADVERSE REACTIONS
CV: BRADYCARDIA.
Respiratory: AIRWAY OBSTRUCTION, APNEA, *cyanosis, hypoventilation.*
Other: *reflux of drug into ETT, dislodgment of ETT.*

INTERACTIONS
None significant.

EFFECTS ON LAB TEST RESULTS
None reported

CONTRAINDICATIONS & CAUTIONS
• None known

NURSING CONSIDERATIONS
• Give drug under supervision of medical staff experienced in the acute care of neonates with respiratory failure who need intubation.
• *Alert:* Drug intended only for intratracheal use; to prevent RDS, give to infant as soon as possible after birth, preferably within 30 minutes.
• Monitor patient for reflux of drug into ETT, cyanosis, bradycardia, or airway obstruction during the procedure. If these occur, stop drug and take appropriate measures to stabilize infant. After infant is stable, resume drug with appropriate monitoring.
• After giving drug, carefully monitor infant so that oxygen therapy and ventilatory support can be modified in response to improvements in oxygenation and lung compliance.

PATIENT TEACHING
• Explain to parents the function of drug in preventing and treating RDS.
• Notify parents that, although infant may improve rapidly after treatment, he may continue to need intubation and mechanical ventilation.
• Notify parents of possible adverse effects of drug, including bradycardia, reflux into ETT, airway obstruction, cyanosis, dislodgment of ETT, and hypoventilation.
• Reassure parents that infant will be carefully monitored.

captopril
KAP-toe-pril

Capoten

Pharmacologic class: ACE inhibitor
Pregnancy risk category C; D in 2nd and 3rd trimesters

AVAILABLE FORMS
Tablets: 12.5 mg, 25 mg, 50 mg, 100 mg

INDICATIONS & DOSAGES
➤ Hypertension
Adults: Initially, 25 mg P.O. b.i.d. or t.i.d. If dosage doesn't control blood pressure satisfactorily in 1 or 2 weeks, increase it to 50 mg b.i.d. or t.i.d. If that dosage doesn't

control blood pressure satisfactorily after another 1 or 2 weeks, expect to add a diuretic. If patient needs further blood pressure reduction, dosage may be raised to 150 mg t.i.d. while continuing diuretic. Maximum daily dose is 450 mg.

➤ **Diabetic nephropathy**
Adults: 25 mg P.O. t.i.d.

➤ **Heart failure**
Adults: Initially, 25 mg P.O. t.i.d. Patients with normal or low blood pressure who have been vigorously treated with diuretics and who may be hyponatremic or hypovolemic may start with 6.25 or 12.5 mg P.O. t.i.d.; starting dosage may be adjusted over several days. Gradually increase dosage to 50 mg P.O. t.i.d.; once patient reaches this dosage, delay further dosage increases for at least 2 weeks. Maximum dosage is 450 mg daily.
Elderly patients: Initially, 6.25 mg P.O. b.i.d. Increase gradually as needed.

➤ **Left ventricular dysfunction after acute MI**
Adults: Start therapy as early as 3 days after MI with 6.25 mg P.O. for one dose, followed by 12.5 mg P.O. t.i.d. Increase over several days to 25 mg P.O. t.i.d.; then increase to 50 mg P.O. t.i.d. over several weeks.

ADMINISTRATION
P.O.
● Give 1 hour before meals to enhance drug absorption.

ACTION
Inhibits ACE, preventing conversion of angiotensin I to angiotensin II, a potent vasoconstrictor. Less angiotensin II decreases peripheral arterial resistance, decreasing aldosterone secretion, which reduces sodium and water retention and lowers blood pressure.

Route	Onset	Peak	Duration
P.O.	15–60 min	60–90 min	6–12 hr

Half-life: Less than 2 hours.

ADVERSE REACTIONS
CNS: dizziness, fainting, headache, malaise, fatigue, fever.
CV: tachycardia, hypotension, angina pectoris.

GI: abdominal pain, anorexia, constipation, diarrhea, dry mouth, dysgeusia, nausea, vomiting.
Hematologic: *leukopenia, agranulocytosis, thrombocytopenia, pancytopenia,* anemia.
Metabolic: hyperkalemia.
Respiratory: *dry, persistent, nonproductive cough,* dyspnea.
Skin: *urticarial rash, maculopapular rash,* pruritus, alopecia.
Other: *angioedema.*

INTERACTIONS
Drug-drug. *Antacids:* May decrease captopril effect. Separate dosage times.
Digoxin: May increase digoxin level by 15% to 30%. Monitor digoxin level, and observe patient for signs of digoxin toxicity.
Diuretics, other antihypertensives: May cause excessive hypotension. May need to stop diuretic or reduce captopril dosage.
Insulin, oral antidiabetics: May cause hypoglycemia when captopril therapy is started. Monitor patient closely.
Lithium: May increase lithium level; symptoms of toxicity possible. Monitor patient closely.
NSAIDs: May reduce antihypertensive effect. Monitor blood pressure.
Potassium-sparing diuretics, potassium supplements: May cause hyperkalemia. Avoid using together unless hypokalemia is confirmed.
Drug-herb. *Black catechu:* May cause additional hypotensive effect. Discourage use together.
Capsaicin: May worsen cough. Discourage use together.
Drug-food. *Salt substitutes containing potassium:* May cause hyperkalemia. Monitor patient closely.

EFFECTS ON LAB TEST RESULTS
● May increase alkaline phosphatase, bilirubin, and potassium levels. May decrease hemoglobin level and hematocrit.
● May decrease granulocyte, platelet, RBC, and WBC counts.
● May cause false-positive urine acetone test results.

CONTRAINDICATIONS & CAUTIONS
• Contraindicated in patients hypersensitive to drug or other ACE inhibitors.
• Use cautiously in patients with impaired renal function or serious autoimmune disease, especially systemic lupus erythematosus, and in those who have been exposed to other drugs that affect WBC counts or immune response.

NURSING CONSIDERATIONS
• Monitor patient's blood pressure and pulse rate frequently.
• *Alert:* Elderly patients may be more sensitive to drug's hypotensive effects.
• Assess patient for signs of angioedema.
• Drug causes the most frequent occurrence of cough, compared with other ACE inhibitors.
• In patients with impaired renal function or collagen vascular disease, monitor WBC and differential counts before starting treatment, every 2 weeks for the first 3 months of therapy, and periodically thereafter.
• *Look alike–sound alike:* Don't confuse captopril with Capitrol.

PATIENT TEACHING
• Instruct patient to take drug 1 hour before meals; food in the GI tract may reduce absorption.
• Inform patient that light-headedness is possible, especially during first few days of therapy. Tell him to rise slowly to minimize this effect and to report occurrence to prescriber. If fainting occurs, he should stop drug and call prescriber immediately.
• Tell patient to use caution in hot weather and during exercise. Lack of fluids, vomiting, diarrhea, and excessive perspiration can lead to light-headedness and syncope.
• Advise patient to report signs and symptoms of infection, such as fever and sore throat.
• Tell women to notify prescriber if pregnancy occurs. Drug will need to be stopped.
• Urge patient to promptly report swelling of the face, lips, or mouth; or difficulty breathing.

cefaclor
SEF-ah-klor

Ceclor, Ceclor CD, Raniclor

Pharmacologic class: second-generation cephalosporin
Pregnancy risk category B

AVAILABLE FORMS
Capsules: 250 mg, 500 mg
Oral suspension: 125 mg/5 ml, 187 mg/5 ml, 250 mg/5 ml, 375 mg/5 ml
Tablets (chewable): 125 mg, 187 mg, 250 mg, 375 mg
Tablets (extended-release): 375 mg, 500 mg

INDICATIONS & DOSAGES
➤ **Respiratory tract infections, UTIs, skin and soft-tissue infections, and otitis media caused by** *Haemophilus influenzae, Streptococcus pneumoniae, S. pyogenes, Escherichia coli, Proteus mirabilis, Klebsiella* **species, and staphylococci**
Adults: 250 to 500 mg P.O. every 8 hours. For pharyngitis or otitis media, daily dose may be given in two equally divided doses every 12 hours. For extended-release forms in bronchitis, 500 mg P.O. every 12 hours for 7 days; for extended-release forms in pharyngitis or skin and skin-structure infections, 375 mg P.O. every 12 hours for 10 days and 7 to 10 days, respectively.
Children: 20 mg/kg daily P.O. in divided doses every 8 hours. For pharyngitis or otitis media, daily dose may be given in two equally divided doses every 12 hours. In more serious infections, 40 mg/kg daily is recommended, not to exceed 1 g daily.

ADMINISTRATION
P.O.
• Before giving, ask patient if he's allergic to penicillins or cephalosporins.
• Obtain specimen for culture and sensitivity tests before giving. Begin therapy while awaiting results.
• Give drug with meals.
• Extended-release tablets shouldn't be crushed, cut, or chewed.

● Store reconstituted suspension in refrigerator. Suspension is stable for 14 days if refrigerated. Shake well before use.

ACTION
Inhibits cell-wall synthesis, promoting osmotic instability; usually bactericidal.

Route	Onset	Peak	Duration
P.O.	Unknown	30–60 min	Unknown
P.O. (extended)	Unknown	1½–2½ hr	Unknown

Half-life: ½ to 1 hour.

ADVERSE REACTIONS
CNS: fever, dizziness, headache, somnolence, malaise.
GI: *diarrhea, nausea, **pseudomembranous colitis,** vomiting, anorexia, dyspepsia, abdominal cramps, oral candidiasis.
GU: vaginal candidiasis, vaginitis.
Hematologic: *thrombocytopenia, transient leukopenia,* anemia, eosinophilia, lymphocytosis.
Skin: *maculopapular rash,* dermatitis, pruritus.
Other: *anaphylaxis,* hypersensitivity reactions, serum sickness.

INTERACTIONS
Drug-drug. *Aminoglycosides:* May increase risk of nephrotoxicity. Avoid using together.
Antacids: May decrease absorption of extended-release cefaclor if taken within 1 hour. Separate doses by 1 hour.
Anticoagulants: May increase anticoagulant effects. Monitor PT and INR.
Chloramphenicol: May cause antagonistic effect. Avoid using together.
Probenecid: May inhibit excretion and increase cefaclor level. Monitor patient for increased adverse reactions.

EFFECTS ON LAB TEST RESULTS
● May increase alkaline phosphatase, ALT, AST, bilirubin, GGT, and LDH levels. May decrease hemoglobin level.
● May increase eosinophil count. May decrease platelet and WBC counts.
● May falsely increase serum or urine creatinine level in tests using Jaffe reaction. May cause false-positive results of Coombs' test and urine glucose tests that use cupric sulfate, such as Benedict's reagent and Clinitest.

CONTRAINDICATIONS & CAUTIONS
● Contraindicated in patients hypersensitive to drug or other cephalosporins.
● Use cautiously in patients hypersensitive to penicillin because of the possibility of cross-sensitivity with other beta-lactam antibiotics.
● Use cautiously in breast-feeding women and in patients with a history of colitis or renal insufficiency.

NURSING CONSIDERATIONS
● If large doses are given, therapy is prolonged, or patient is at high risk, monitor patient for signs and symptoms of superinfection.
● *Look alike–sound alike:* Don't confuse drug with other cephalosporins that sound alike.

PATIENT TEACHING
● Tell patient to take entire amount of drug exactly as prescribed, even after he feels better.
● Tell patient that drug may be taken with meals. If suspension is used, instruct him to shake container well before measuring dose and to keep the drug refrigerated.
● Advise patient to notify prescriber if rash develops or signs and symptoms of superinfection appear.
● Inform patient not to crush, cut, or chew extended-release tablets.

---

cefadroxil
sef-a-DROX-ill

Duricef

Pharmacologic class: first-generation cephalosporin
Pregnancy risk category B

AVAILABLE FORMS
Capsules: 500 mg
Oral suspension: 125 mg/5 ml, 250 mg/5 ml, 500 mg/5 ml
Tablets: 1 g

INDICATIONS & DOSAGES

➤ **UTIs caused by *Escherichia coli*, *Proteus mirabilis*, and *Klebsiella* species; skin and soft-tissue infections caused by staphylococci and streptococci; pharyngitis or tonsillitis caused by group A beta-hemolytic streptococci**

Adults: 1 to 2 g P.O. daily, depending on infection being treated. Usually given once daily or in two divided doses.

Children: 30 mg/kg P.O. daily in two divided doses every 12 hours.

Adjust-a-dose: In patients with renal impairment, give first dose of 1 g. Reduce additional doses based on creatinine clearance. If clearance is 25 to 50 ml/minute, give 500 mg P.O. every 12 hours. If clearance is 10 to 25 ml/minute, give 500 mg P.O. every 24 hours; if clearance is less than 10 ml/minute, give 500 mg P.O. every 36 hours.

ADMINISTRATION
P.O.
● Before administration, ask patient if he's allergic to penicillins or cephalosporins.
● Obtain specimen for culture and sensitivity tests before giving first dose. Begin therapy while awaiting results.
● Give drug with food or milk to lessen GI discomfort.

ACTION
Inhibits cell-wall synthesis, promoting osmotic instability; usually bactericidal.

Route	Onset	Peak	Duration
P.O.	Unknown	1–2 hr	Unknown

Half-life: About 1 to 2 hours.

ADVERSE REACTIONS
CNS: *seizures,* fever, dizziness, headache.
GI: *diarrhea, nausea, pseudomembranous colitis,* vomiting, glossitis, abdominal cramps, oral candidiasis.
GU: genital pruritus, candidiasis, vaginitis, renal dysfunction.
Hematologic: *transient neutropenia, leukopenia, agranulocytosis, thrombocytopenia,* anemia, eosinophilia.
Respiratory: dyspnea.
Skin: *maculopapular and erythematous rashes,* urticaria.

Other: *anaphylaxis, angioedema,* hypersensitivity reactions.

INTERACTIONS
Drug-drug. *Aminoglycosides:* May increase risk of nephrotoxicity. Avoid using together.
Probenecid: May inhibit excretion and increase cefadroxil level. Use together cautiously.

EFFECTS ON LAB TEST RESULTS
● May increase alkaline phosphatase, ALT, AST, bilirubin, GGT, and LDH levels. May decrease hemoglobin level.
● May increase eosinophil count. May decrease granulocyte, neutrophil, platelet, and WBC counts.
● May falsely increase serum or urine creatinine level in tests using Jaffe reaction. May cause false-positive results of Coombs' test and urine glucose tests that use cupric sulfate, such as Benedict's reagent and Clinitest.

CONTRAINDICATIONS & CAUTIONS
● Contraindicated in patients hypersensitive to drug or other cephalosporins.
● Use cautiously in patients with a history of sensitivity to penicillin and in breast-feeding women.
● Use cautiously in patients with impaired renal function; adjust dosage as needed.

NURSING CONSIDERATIONS
● If creatinine clearance is less than 50 ml/minute, lengthen dosage interval so drug doesn't accumulate. Monitor renal function in patients with renal dysfunction.
● If large doses are given, therapy is prolonged, or patient is high risk, monitor patient for superinfection.
● *Look alike–sound alike:* Don't confuse drug with other cephalosporins that sound alike.

PATIENT TEACHING
● Instruct patient to take drug with food or milk to lessen GI discomfort.
● Tell patient to take entire amount of drug exactly as prescribed, even after he feels better.

• Advise patient to notify prescriber if rash develops or if signs and symptoms of superinfection appear, such as recurring fever, chills, and malaise.

---

cefazolin sodium
sef-AH-zoe-lin

Ancef

Pharmacologic class: first-generation cephalosporin
Pregnancy risk category B

AVAILABLE FORMS
Infusion: 500 mg/50-ml bag,
1 g/50-ml bag
Injection (parenteral): 500 mg, 1 g

INDICATIONS & DOSAGES
➤ **Perioperative prevention in contaminated surgery**
Adults: 1 g I.M. or I.V. 30 to 60 minutes before surgery; then 0.5 to 1 g I.M. or I.V. every 6 to 8 hours for 24 hours. In operations lasting longer than 2 hours, give another 0.5- to 1-g dose I.M. or I.V. intraoperatively. Continue treatment for 3 to 5 days if life-threatening infection is likely.
➤ **Infections of respiratory, biliary, and GU tracts; skin, soft-tissue, bone, and joint infections; septicemia; endocarditis caused by** *Escherichia coli, Enterobacteriaceae,* **gonococci,** *Haemophilus influenzae, Klebsiella* **species,** *Proteus mirabilis, Staphylococcus aureus, Streptococcus pneumoniae,* **and group A beta-hemolytic streptococci**
Adults: 250 mg to 500 mg I.M. or I.V. every 8 hours for mild infections or 500 mg to 1.5 g I.M. or I.V. every 6 to 8 hours for moderate to severe or life-threatening infections. Maximum 12 g/day in life-threatening situations.
Children older than age 1 month: 25 to 50 mg/kg/day I.M. or I.V. in three or four divided doses. In severe infections, dose may be increased to 100 mg/kg/day.
Adjust-a-dose: For patients with creatinine clearance of 35 to 54 ml/minute, give full dose every 8 hours; if clearance is 11 to 34 ml/minute, give 50% of usual dose every 12 hours; if clearance is below 10 ml/minute, give 50% of usual dose every 18 to 24 hours.

ADMINISTRATION
I.V.
• Before giving first dose, obtain specimen for culture and sensitivity tests. Begin therapy while awaiting results.
• Before giving drug, ask patient if he's allergic to penicillins or cephalosporins.
• Give commercially available frozen solutions in D_5W only by intermittent or continuous I.V. infusion.
• Reconstitute drug with sterile water, bacteriostatic water, or normal saline solution as follows: Add 2 ml to 500-mg vial or 2.5 ml to 1-g vial, yielding 225 mg/ml or 330 mg/ml, respectively.
• Shake well until dissolved.
• For direct injection, further dilute with 5 ml of sterile water for injection.
• Inject into a large vein or into the tubing of a free-flowing I.V. solution over 3 to 5 minutes.
• For intermittent infusion, add reconstituted drug to 50 to 100 ml of compatible solution or use premixed solution.
• If I.V. therapy lasts longer than 3 days, alternate injection sites. Use of small I.V. needles in larger available veins may be preferable.
• Reconstituted drug is stable 24 hours at room temperature or 96 hours refrigerated.
• **Incompatibilities:** Aminoglycosides, amiodarone, amobarbital, ascorbic acid injection, bleomycin, calcium gluconate, cimetidine, colistimethate, hydrocortisone, idarubicin, lidocaine, norepinephrine, oxytetracycline, pentobarbital sodium, polymyxin B, ranitidine, tetracycline, theophylline, vitamin B complex with C.
I.M.
• Before giving first dose, obtain specimen for culture and sensitivity tests. Begin therapy while awaiting results.
• After reconstitution, inject drug I.M. without further dilution. This drug isn't as painful as other cephalosporins. Give injection deep into a large muscle, such as the gluteus maximus or the side of the thigh.

ACTION
Inhibits cell-wall synthesis, promoting osmotic instability; usually bactericidal.

Route	Onset	Peak	Duration
I.V.	Immediate	Immediate	Unknown
I.M.	Unknown	1–2 hr	Unknown

Half-life: About 1 to 2 hours.

ADVERSE REACTIONS
CNS: *seizures,* headache, confusion.
CV: *phlebitis, thrombophlebitis with I.V. injection.*
GI: *diarrhea, pseudomembranous colitis,* nausea, anorexia, vomiting, glossitis, dyspepsia, abdominal cramps, anal pruritus, oral candidiasis.
GU: genital pruritus, candidiasis, vaginitis.
Hematologic: *neutropenia, leukopenia, thrombocytopenia,* eosinophilia.
Skin: *maculopapular and erythematous rashes, urticaria, pruritus, pain, induration, sterile abscesses, tissue sloughing at injection site,* **Stevens-Johnson syndrome.**
Other: *anaphylaxis,* hypersensitivity reactions, serum sickness, drug fever.

INTERACTIONS
Drug-drug. *Aminoglycosides:* May increase risk of nephrotoxicity. Avoid using together.
Anticoagulants: May increase anticoagulant effects. Monitor PT and INR.
Probenecid: May inhibit excretion and increase cefazolin level. Use together cautiously.

EFFECTS ON LAB TEST RESULTS
● May increase alkaline phosphatase, ALT, AST, bilirubin, GGT, and LDH levels.
● May increase eosinophil count. May decrease neutrophil, platelet, and WBC counts.
● May falsely increase serum or urine creatinine level in tests using Jaffe reaction. May cause false-positive results of Coombs' test and urine glucose tests that use cupric sulfate, such as Benedict's reagent and Clinitest.

CONTRAINDICATIONS & CAUTIONS
● Contraindicated in patients hypersensitive to drug or other cephalosporins.
● Use cautiously in patients hypersensitive to penicillin because of the possibility of cross-sensitivity with other beta-lactam antibiotics.
● Use cautiously in breast-feeding women and in patients with a history of colitis or renal insufficiency.

NURSING CONSIDERATIONS
● If creatinine clearance falls below 55 ml/minute, adjust dosage.
● If large doses are given, therapy is prolonged, or patient is at high risk, monitor patient for signs and symptoms of superinfection.
● **Look alike–sound alike:** Don't confuse drug with other cephalosporins that sound alike.

PATIENT TEACHING
● Instruct patient to report adverse reactions promptly.
● Tell patient to report discomfort at I.V. injection site.
● Advise patient to notify prescriber if a rash develops or if signs and symptoms of superinfection appear, such as recurring fever, chills, and malaise.

---

cefdinir
sef-DIN-er

Omnicef

Pharmacologic class: third-generation cephalosporin
Pregnancy risk category B

AVAILABLE FORMS
Capsules: 300 mg
Suspension: 125 mg/5 ml, 250 mg/5 ml

INDICATIONS & DOSAGES
➤ **Mild to moderate infections caused by susceptible strains of microorganisms in community-acquired pneumonia, acute worsening of chronic bronchitis, acute maxillary sinusitis, acute bacterial otitis media, and uncomplicated skin and skin-structure infections**
Adults and children age 12 and older: 300 mg P.O. every 12 hours or 600 mg P.O. every 24 hours for 10 days. Give every

12 hours for pneumonia and skin infections.

Children ages 6 months to 12 years:
7 mg/kg P.O. every 12 hours or 14 mg/kg P.O. every 24 hours, for 10 days, up to maximum dose of 600 mg daily. Give every 12 hours for skin infections.

➤ **Pharyngitis, tonsillitis**
Adults and children age 12 and older:
300 mg P.O. every 12 hours for 5 to 10 days or 600 mg P.O. every 24 hours for 10 days.
Children ages 6 months to 12 years:
7 mg/kg P.O. every 12 hours for 5 to 10 days; or 14 mg/kg P.O. every 24 hours, for 10 days.
Adjust-a-dose: If creatinine clearance is less than 30 ml/minute, reduce dosage to 300 mg P.O. once daily for adults and 7 mg/kg up to 300 mg P.O. once daily for children. In patients receiving long-term hemodialysis, give 300 mg or 7 mg/kg P.O. at end of each dialysis session and then every other day.

ADMINISTRATION
P.O.
• Before administration, ask patient if he's allergic to penicillins or cephalosporins.
• Give antacids and iron supplements 2 hours before or after a dose of cefdinir.
• Give drug without regard for meals.

ACTION
Inhibits cell-wall synthesis, promoting osmotic instability; usually bactericidal. Some microorganisms resistant to penicillins and cephalosporins are susceptible to cefdinir. Active against a broad range of gram-positive and gram-negative aerobic microorganisms.

Route	Onset	Peak	Duration
P.O.	Unknown	2–4 hr	Unknown

Half-life: 1¾ hours.

ADVERSE REACTIONS
CNS: headache.
GI: *diarrhea, pseudomembranous colitis,* abdominal pain, nausea, vomiting.
GU: vaginal candidiasis, vaginitis, increased urine proteins, WBCs, and RBCs.
Skin: rash, cutaneous candidiasis.
Other: hypersensitivity reactions, *anaphylaxis.*

INTERACTIONS
Drug-drug. *Aminoglycosides:* May increase risk of nephrotoxicity. Avoid using together.
Antacids containing aluminum and magnesium, iron supplements, multivitamins containing iron: May decrease rate of absorption and bioavailability of cefdinir. Give such preparations 2 hours before or after cefdinir.
Probenecid: May inhibit renal excretion of cefdinir. Monitor patient for adverse reactions.

EFFECTS ON LAB TEST RESULTS
• May increase alkaline phosphatase, GGT, and LDH levels. May decrease bicarbonate levels.
• May increase eosinophil, lymphocyte, and platelet counts.
• May falsely increase serum or urine creatinine level in tests using Jaffe reaction. May cause false-positive results of Coombs' test and urine glucose tests that use cupric sulfate, such as Benedict's reagent and Clinitest.

CONTRAINDICATIONS & CAUTIONS
• Contraindicated in patients hypersensitive to drug or other cephalosporins.
• Use cautiously in patients hypersensitive to penicillin because of the possibility of cross-sensitivity with other beta-lactam antibiotics.
• Use cautiously in patients with history of colitis or renal insufficiency.

NURSING CONSIDERATIONS
• Prolonged drug treatment may result in emergence and overgrowth of resistant organisms. Monitor patient for signs and symptoms of superinfection.
• Pseudomembranous colitis has been reported with cefdinir and should be considered in patients with diarrhea after antibiotic therapy and in those with history of colitis.
• *Look alike–sound alike:* Don't confuse drug with other cephalosporins that sound alike.

PATIENT TEACHING
• Instruct patient to take antacids and iron supplements 2 hours before or after a dose of cefdinir.

Reactions may be *common,* uncommon, *life-threatening,* or COMMON AND LIFE-THREATENING.
Interaction may have a *rapid onset* or *delayed onset.*

• Inform diabetic patient that each tea-spoon of suspension contains 2.86 g of sucrose.
• Tell patient that drug may be taken without regard to meals.
• Tell patient to take drug as prescribed, even after he feels better.
• Advise patient to report severe diarrhea or diarrhea with abdominal pain.
• Tell patient to report adverse reactions or signs and symptoms of superinfection promptly.

cefditoren pivoxil
SEF-di-tore-en

Spectracef

Pharmacologic class: third-generation cephalosporin
Pregnancy risk category B

AVAILABLE FORMS
Tablets: 200 mg

INDICATIONS & DOSAGES
➤ **Acute bacterial worsening of chronic bronchitis or community-acquired pneumonia caused by *Haemophilus influenzae, H. parainfluenzae, Streptococcus pneumoniae,* or *Moraxella catarrhalis***
Adults and adolescents age 12 and older: 400 mg P.O. b.i.d. with meals for 10 days (chronic bronchitis) or 14 days (community-acquired pneumonia).
➤ **Pharyngitis or tonsillitis caused by *Streptococcus pyogenes;* uncomplicated skin and skin-structure infections caused by *S. pyogenes* or *Staphylococcus aureus***
Adults and adolescents age 12 and older: 200 mg P.O. b.i.d. with meals for 10 days.
Adjust-a-dose: For patients with creatinine clearance of 30 to 49 ml/minute, don't exceed 200 mg b.i.d. For patients with clearance less than 30 ml/minute, give 200 mg daily.

ADMINISTRATION
P.O.
• Before administration, ask patient if he's allergic to penicillins or cephalosporins.

• Obtain specimen for culture and sensitivity tests before giving. Begin therapy while awaiting results.
• Give drug with a fatty meal to increase its bioavailability.

ACTION
Adheres to bacterial penicillin-binding proteins, inhibiting cell-wall synthesis. Drug is active against many gram-positive and gram-negative organisms.

Route	Onset	Peak	Duration
P.O.	Unknown	1½–3 hr	Unknown

Half-life: 1¼ to 2 hours.

ADVERSE REACTIONS
CNS: headache.
GI: *diarrhea,* abdominal pain, dyspepsia, nausea, vomiting.
GU: vaginal candidiasis, hematuria.
Metabolic: hyperglycemia.

INTERACTIONS
Drug-drug. *H₂-receptor antagonists, magnesium, and aluminum antacids:* May decrease cefditoren absorption. Avoid using together.
Probenecid: May increase cefditoren level. Avoid using together.
Drug-food. *Moderate- or high-fat meal:* May increase drug bioavailability. Advise patient to take drug with meals.

EFFECTS ON LAB TEST RESULTS
• May decrease glucose and hemoglobin level and hematocrit.
• May increase WBC count in urine.
• May cause a false-positive direct Coombs' test result and a false-positive reaction for urine glucose in copper reduction tests (using Benedict's or Fehling's solution or Clinitest tablets).

CONTRAINDICATIONS & CAUTIONS
• Contraindicated in patients hypersensitive to drug or other cephalosporins.
• Contraindicated in patients with carnitine deficiency or inborn errors of metabolism that may result in significant carnitine deficiency.
• Because tablets contain sodium caseinate, a milk protein, don't give drug to patients hypersensitive to milk protein (not lactose intolerance).

- Use cautiously in breast-feeding women because cephalosporins appear in breast milk, and safe use hasn't been established.
- Use cautiously in patients with impaired renal function or penicillin allergy.

NURSING CONSIDERATIONS
- If patient develops diarrhea, keep in mind that this drug may cause pseudomembranous colitis.
- Don't use this drug if patient needs prolonged treatment.
- Monitor patient for overgrowth of resistant organisms.
- Patients with renal or hepatic impairment, in poor nutritional state, receiving a protracted course of antibiotics, or previously stabilized on anticoagulants may be at risk for decreased prothrombin activity. Monitor PT in these patients.

PATIENT TEACHING
- Instruct patient to take drug exactly as prescribed.
- Tell patient to take drug with food to increase its absorption.
- Caution patient not to take drug with an H_2-receptor antagonist or an antacid because either may reduce cefditoren absorption.
- Instruct patient not to stop drug before completing course and to call prescriber immediately if he experiences any unpleasant adverse reactions.
- Instruct patient to contact prescriber if signs and symptoms of infection don't improve after several days of therapy.
- Inform patient of potential adverse reactions.
- Urge patient not to miss any doses. However, if he does, tell him to take the missed dose as soon as possible unless it's within 4 hours of the next scheduled dose. In that case, tell him to skip the missed dose and go back to the regular dosing schedule. Tell him not to double the dose.

cefepime hydrochloride
SEF-ah-peem

Maxipime

Pharmacologic class: fourth-generation cephalosporin
Pregnancy risk category B

AVAILABLE FORMS
Injection: 500-mg vial, 1-g/100-ml piggyback bottle, 1-g ADD-Vantage vial, 1-g vial, 2-g/100-ml piggyback bottle, 2-g ADD-Vantage vial, 2-g vial

INDICATIONS & DOSAGES
➤ **Mild to moderate UTI caused by** *Escherichia coli, Klebsiella pneumoniae,* **or** *Proteus mirabilis,* **including concurrent bacteremia with these microorganisms**
Adults and children age 12 and older: 0.5 to 1 g I.M. or I.V. over 30 minutes every 12 hours for 7 to 10 days. Use I.M. only for *E. coli* infection.
➤ **Severe UTI, including pyelonephritis, caused by** *E. coli* **or** *K. pneumoniae*
Adults and children age 12 and older: 2 g I.V. over 30 minutes every 12 hours for 10 days.
➤ **Moderate to severe pneumonia caused by** *Streptococcus pneumoniae, Pseudomonas aeruginosa, K. pneumoniae,* **or** *Enterobacter* **species**
Adults and children age 12 and older: 1 to 2 g I.V. over 30 minutes every 12 hours for 10 days.
➤ **Moderate to severe skin infection, uncomplicated skin infection, and skin-structure infection caused by** *Streptococcus pyogenes* **or methicillin-susceptible strains of** *Staphylococcus aureus*
Adults and children age 12 and older: 2 g I.V. over 30 minutes every 12 hours for 10 days.
➤ **Complicated intra-abdominal infection caused by** *E. coli,* **viridans group streptococci,** *P. aeruginosa, K. pneumoniae, Enterobacter* **species, or** *Bacteroides fragilis*

Adults: 2 g I.V. over 30 minutes every 12 hours for 7 to 10 days. Give with metronidazole.

➤ **Empiric therapy for febrile neutropenia**
Adults: 2 g I.V. every 8 hours for 7 days or until neutropenia resolves.

➤ **Uncomplicated and complicated UTI (including pyelonephritis), uncomplicated skin and skin-structure infection, pneumonia, empiric therapy for febrile neutropenic children**
Children ages 2 months to 16 years who weigh up to 40 kg (88 lb): 50 mg/kg/dose I.V. over 30 minutes every 12 hours, or every 8 hours for febrile neutropenia, for 7 to 10 days. Don't exceed 2 g/dose.

Adjust-a-dose: Adjust dosage based on creatinine clearance, as shown in the table. For patients receiving hemodialysis, about 68% of drug is removed after a 3-hour dialysis session. Give a repeat dose, equivalent to the first dose, at the completion of dialysis. For patients receiving continuous ambulatory peritoneal dialysis, give normal dose every 48 hours.

ADMINISTRATION
I.V.
● Before giving drug, ask patient if he's allergic to penicillins or cephalosporins.
● Obtain specimen for culture and sensitivity tests before giving. Begin therapy while awaiting results.
● Follow manufacturer's guidelines closely when reconstituting drug. They vary with concentration of drug ordered and how drug is packaged (piggyback vial, ADD-Vantage vial, or regular vial).
● The type of diluent varies with the product used. Use only solutions recommended by the manufacturer.
● Give intermittent I.V. infusion with a Y-type administration and compatible solutions.
● Stop the main I.V. fluid while infusing.
● Infuse over about 30 minutes.
● **Incompatibilities:** Aminophylline, amphotericin B, amphotericin B cholesteryl sulfate complex, ciprofloxacin, gentamicin, metronidazole, tobramycin, vancomycin.

I.M.
● Before giving drug, ask patient if he's allergic to penicillins or cephalosporins.
● Obtain specimen for culture and sensitivity tests before giving. Begin therapy while awaiting results.
● Reconstitute drug using sterile water for injection, normal saline solution for injection, D_5W injection, 0.5% or 1% lidocaine hydrochloride, or bacteriostatic water for injection with parabens or benzyl alcohol. Follow manufacturer's guidelines for quantity of diluent to use.
● Inspect solution for particulate matter before use. The powder and its solutions tend to darken, depending on storage conditions. If stored as recommended, potency isn't adversely affected.
● Pain may occur at injection site.

ACTION
Inhibits bacterial cell-wall synthesis, promotes osmotic instability, and destroys bacteria.

Route	Onset	Peak	Duration
I.V., I.M.	30 min	1–2 hr	Unknown

Half-life: Adults: 2 to 2½ hours. Children: 1½ to 2 hours.

ADVERSE REACTIONS
CNS: fever, headache.
CV: phlebitis.
GI: colitis, diarrhea, nausea, vomiting, oral candidiasis.
GU: vaginitis.
Skin: rash, pruritus, urticaria.
Other: *anaphylaxis,* pain, inflammation, hypersensitivity reactions.

INTERACTIONS
Drug-drug. *Aminoglycosides:* May increase risk of nephrotoxicity. Monitor renal function closely.
Potent diuretics: May increase risk of nephrotoxicity. Monitor renal function closely.
Probenecid: May inhibit renal excretion of cefepime. Monitor patient for adverse reactions.

Dosage adjustments for renal impairment

Creatinine clearance (ml/min)	500 mg every 12 hr	If normal dosage would be		
		1 g every 12 hr	2 g every 12 hr	2 g every 8 hr
30–60	500 mg every 24 hr	1 g every 24 hr	2 g every 24 hr	2 g every 12 hr
11–29	500 mg every 24 hr	500 mg every 24 hr	1 g every 24 hr	2 g every 24 hr
< 11	250 mg every 24 hr	250 mg every 24 hr	500 mg every 24 hr	1 g every 24 hr

EFFECTS ON LAB TEST RESULTS
• May increase ALT and AST levels. May decrease phosphorus level.
• May increase eosinophil count. May alter PT and PTT.
• May falsely increase serum or urine creatinine level in tests using Jaffe reaction. May cause false-positive results of Coombs' test and urine glucose tests that use cupric sulfate, such as Benedict's reagent and Clinitest.

CONTRAINDICATIONS & CAUTIONS
• Contraindicated in patients hypersensitive to drug, cephalosporins, beta-lactam antibiotics, or penicillins.
• Use cautiously in patients hypersensitive to penicillin because of possibility of cross-sensitivity with other beta-lactam antibiotics.
• Use cautiously in breast-feeding women and in patients with history of colitis or renal insufficiency.

NURSING CONSIDERATIONS
• Adjust dosage in patients with impaired renal function. If dosage isn't adjusted, serious adverse reactions, including encephalopathy, myoclonus, seizures, and renal failure may occur.
• Monitor patient for superinfection. Drug may cause overgrowth of nonsusceptible bacteria or fungi.
• Drug may reduce PT activity. Patients at risk include those with renal or hepatic impairment or poor nutrition and those receiving prolonged therapy. Monitor PT and INR in these patients. Give vitamin K, as indicated.

• *Look alike–sound alike:* Don't confuse drug with other cephalosporins that sound alike.

PATIENT TEACHING
• Warn patient receiving drug I.M. that pain may occur at injection site.
• Advise patient to notify prescriber if a rash develops or if signs and symptoms of superinfection appear, such as recurring fever, chills, and malaise.
• Instruct patient to report adverse reactions promptly.

cefotaxime sodium
sef-oh-TAKS-eem

Claforan

Pharmacologic class: third-generation cephalosporin
Pregnancy risk category B

AVAILABLE FORMS
Infusion: 1-g, 2-g premixed package
Injection: 500-mg, 1-g, 2-g vials

INDICATIONS & DOSAGES
➤ **Perioperative prevention in contaminated surgery**
Adults: 1 g I.M. or I.V. 30 to 90 minutes before surgery. In patients undergoing bowel surgery, provide preoperative mechanical bowel cleansing and give a nonabsorbable anti-infective, such as neomycin. In patients undergoing cesarean delivery, give 1 g I.M. or I.V. as soon as the umbilical cord is clamped; then 1 g I.M. or I.V. 6 and 12 hours later.

➤ **Uncomplicated gonorrhea caused by penicillinase-producing strains or non–penicillinase-producing strains of** *Neisseria gonorrhoeae*
Adults and adolescents: 500 mg I.M. as a single dose.

➤ **Rectal gonorrhea**
Men: 1 g I.M. as a single dose.
Women: 500 mg I.M. as a single dose.

➤ **Serious infection of the lower respiratory and urinary tract, CNS, skin, bone, and joints; gynecologic and intra-abdominal infection; bacteremia; septicemia caused by susceptible microorganisms, such as streptococci (including** *Streptococcus pneumoniae* **and** *S. pyogenes,* *Staphylococcus aureus* **[penicillinase- and non–penicillinase-producing] and** *S. epidermidis), Escherichia coli, Klebsiella, Haemophilus influenzae, Serratia marcescens,* **and species of** *Pseudomonas* **(including** *P. aeruginosa),* *Enterobacter, Proteus,* **and** *Peptostreptococcus*
Adults and children who weigh 50 kg (110 lb) or more: 1 to 2 g I.V. or I.M. every 6 to 8 hours. Up to 12 g daily can be given for life-threatening infections.
Children ages 1 month to 12 years who weigh less than 50 kg: 50 to 180 mg/kg/day I.M. or I.V. in four to six divided doses.
Neonates ages 1 to 4 weeks: 50 mg/kg I.V. every 8 hours.
Neonates to age 1 week: 50 mg/kg I.V. every 12 hours.
Adjust-a-dose: For patients with creatinine clearance less than 20 ml/minute, give half usual dose at usual interval.

ADMINISTRATION
I.V.
● Before giving drug, ask patient if he's allergic to penicillins or cephalosporins.
● Obtain specimen for culture and sensitivity tests before giving. Begin therapy while awaiting results.
● For direct injection, reconstitute drug in 500-mg, 1-g, or 2-g vials with 10 ml of sterile water for injection. Solutions containing 1 g/14 ml are isotonic.
● Inject drug over 3 to 5 minutes into a large vein or into the tubing of a free-flowing I.V. solution.

● For infusion, reconstitute drug in infusion vials with 50 to 100 ml of D_5W or normal saline solution.
● Interrupt flow of primary I.V. solution, and infuse this drug over 20 to 30 minutes.
● **Incompatibilities:** Allopurinol, aminoglycosides, aminophylline, azithromycin, doxapram, filgrastim, fluconazole, hetastarch, pentamidine isethionate, sodium bicarbonate injection, vancomycin.
I.M.
● Before giving drug, ask patient if he's allergic to penicillins or cephalosporins.
● Obtain specimen for culture and sensitivity tests before giving. Begin therapy while awaiting results.
● For doses of 2 g, divide the dose and give at different sites.
● Inject deep into a large muscle, such as the gluteus maximus or the side of the thigh.

ACTION
Inhibits cell-wall synthesis, promoting osmotic instability; usually bactericidal.

Route	Onset	Peak	Duration
I.V.	Immediate	Immediate	Unknown
I.M.	Unknown	30 min	Unknown

Half-life: 1 to 2 hours.

ADVERSE REACTIONS
CNS: fever, headache, dizziness.
CV: *phlebitis, thrombophlebitis.*
GI: *diarrhea, **pseudomembranous colitis,*** nausea, vomiting.
GU: vaginitis, candidiasis, interstitial nephritis.
Hematologic: *agranulocytosis, thrombocytopenia, transient neutropenia,* eosinophilia, hemolytic anemia.
Skin: *maculopapular and erythematous rashes, urticaria, pain, induration, sterile abscesses, temperature elevation, tissue sloughing at I.M. injection site.*
Other: *anaphylaxis,* hypersensitivity reactions, serum sickness.

INTERACTIONS
Drug-drug. *Aminoglycosides:* May increase risk of nephrotoxicity. Monitor patient's renal function tests.
Probenecid: May inhibit excretion and increase cefotaxime. Use together cautiously.

EFFECTS ON LAB TEST RESULTS
• May increase alkaline phosphatase, ALT, AST, bilirubin, GGT, and LDH levels. May decrease hemoglobin level.
• May increase eosinophil count. May decrease granulocyte, neutrophil, and platelet counts.
• May cause positive Coombs' test results.

CONTRAINDICATIONS & CAUTIONS
• Contraindicated in patients hypersensitive to drug or other cephalosporins.
• Use cautiously in patients hypersensitive to penicillin because of possibility of cross-sensitivity with other beta-lactam antibiotics.
• Use cautiously in breast-feeding women and in patients with history of colitis or renal insufficiency.

NURSING CONSIDERATIONS
• If large doses are given, therapy is prolonged, or patient is at high risk, monitor patient for superinfection.
• *Look alike–sound alike:* Don't confuse drug with other cephalosporins that sound alike.

PATIENT TEACHING
• Tell patient to report adverse reactions and signs and symptoms of superinfection promptly.
• Instruct patient to report discomfort at I.V. insertion site.

---

cefoxitin sodium
se-FOX-i-tin

Mefoxin

Pharmacologic class: second-generation cephalosporin
Pregnancy risk category B

AVAILABLE FORMS
Infusion: 1 g, 2 g in 50-ml or 100-ml container
Injection: 1 g, 2 g

INDICATIONS & DOSAGES
➤ **Serious infection of the respiratory and GU tracts; skin, soft-tissue, bone, or joint infection; bloodstream or intra-abdominal infection caused by susceptible organisms (such as *Escherichia coli* and other coliform bacteria, penicillinase- and non–penicillinase-producing *Staphylococcus aureus, S. epidermidis,* streptococci, *Klebsiella, Haemophilus influenzae,* and *Bacteroides,* including *B. fragilis*)**
Adults: 1 to 2 g I.V. or I.M. every 6 to 8 hours for uncomplicated infections. Up to 12 g daily may be used in life-threatening infections.
Children older than age 3 months: 80 to 160 mg/kg daily I.V. or I.M., given in four to six equally divided doses. Maximum daily dose is 12 g.
➤ **Uncomplicated gonorrhea**
Adults: 2 g I.M. with 1 g probenecid P.O. as a single dose. Give probenecid within 30 minutes before cefoxitin dose.
➤ **Perioperative prevention**
Adults: 2 g I.M. or I.V. 30 to 60 minutes before surgery; then 2 g I.M. or I.V. every 6 hours for up to 24 hours. For transurethral prostatectomy, 1 g I.M. or I.V. before surgery; then continue giving 1 g every 8 hours for up to 5 days.
Children age 3 months and older: 30 to 40 mg/kg I.M. or I.V. 30 to 60 minutes before surgery; then 30 to 40 mg/kg every 6 hours for up to 24 hours.
Adjust-a-dose: For patients with creatinine clearance of 30 to 50 ml/minute, 1 to 2 g every 8 to 12 hours; if clearance is 10 to 29 ml/minute, 1 to 2 g every 12 to 24 hours; if clearance is 5 to 9 ml/minute, 0.5 to 1 g every 12 to 24 hours; and if clearance is less than 5 ml/minute, 0.5 to 1 g every 24 to 48 hours. For patients receiving hemodialysis, give a loading dose of 1 to 2 g after each hemodialysis session; then give the maintenance dose based on creatinine level.

ADMINISTRATION
I.V.
• Before giving drug, ask patient if he's allergic to penicillins or cephalosporins.
• Obtain specimen for culture and sensitivity tests before giving. Begin therapy while awaiting results.
• Reconstitute 1 g with at least 10 ml of sterile water for injection and 2 g with 10 to 20 ml of sterile water for injection.

Solutions of D_5W and normal saline
solution for injection also may be used.
• For direct injection, give drug over 3 to
5 minutes into a large vein or into the
tubing of a free-flowing I.V. solution.
• For intermittent infusion, add reconstituted drug to 50 or 100 ml of D_5W or
normal saline solution for injection.
• Interrupt flow of primary solution during
infusion.
• Assess site often to detect evidence of
thrombophlebitis.
• **Incompatibilities:** Aminoglycosides,
filgrastim, hetastarch, pentamidine isethionate, ranitidine.
I.M.
• Before giving drug, ask patient if he's
allergic to penicillins or cephalosporins.
• Obtain specimen for culture and sensitivity tests before giving. Begin therapy while
awaiting results.
• Reconstitute each 1 g of drug with 2 ml
of sterile water for injection or 0.5% or
1% lidocaine hydrochloride (without
epinephrine) to minimize pain. Inject deep
into a large muscle, such as the gluteus
maximus or the lateral aspect of the thigh.
• After reconstitution, drug may be stored
for 24 hours at room temperature or
1 week under refrigeration.

ACTION

Inhibits cell-wall synthesis, promoting
osmotic instability; usually bactericidal.

Route	Onset	Peak	Duration
I.V.	Immediate	Immediate	Unknown
I.M.	Unknown	20–30 min	Unknown

Half-life: About ½ to 1 hours.

ADVERSE REACTIONS

CNS: fever.
CV: *phlebitis, thrombophlebitis,* hypoten-
sion.
GI: *diarrhea, pseudomembranous colitis,*
nausea, vomiting.
GU: *acute renal failure.*
Hematologic: *thrombocytopenia, tran-
sient neutropenia,* eosinophilia, hemolytic
anemia, anemia.
Respiratory: dyspnea.
Skin: *maculopapular and erythematous
rashes, urticaria, pain, induration, sterile*

*abscesses, tissue sloughing at injection
site,* exfoliative dermatitis.
Other: *anaphylaxis,* hypersensitivity
reactions, serum sickness.

INTERACTIONS

Drug-drug. *Aminoglycosides:* May increase risk of nephrotoxicity. Monitor
patient's renal function tests.
Probenecid: May inhibit excretion and
increase cefoxitin level. Probenecid may
be used for this effect.

EFFECTS ON LAB TEST RESULTS

• May increase alkaline phosphatase,
ALT, AST, bilirubin, and LDH levels. May
decrease hemoglobin level.
• May increase eosinophil count. May
decrease neutrophil and platelet counts.
• May falsely increase serum or urine
creatinine level in tests using Jaffe reaction. May cause false-positive results
of Coombs' test and urine glucose tests
that use cupric sulfate, such as Benedict's
reagent and Clinitest.

CONTRAINDICATIONS & CAUTIONS

• Contraindicated in patients hypersensitive to drug or other cephalosporins.
• Use cautiously in patients hypersensitive
to penicillin because of possibility of
cross-sensitivity with other beta-lactam
antibiotics.
• Use cautiously in breast-feeding women
and in patients with history of colitis or
renal insufficiency.

NURSING CONSIDERATIONS

• *Alert:* The premixed frozen product is for
I.V. use only.
• If large doses are given, therapy is prolonged, or patient is at high risk, monitor
patient for signs and symptoms of superinfection.
• *Look alike–sound alike:* Don't confuse
drug with other cephalosporins that sound
alike.

PATIENT TEACHING

• Tell patient to report adverse reactions
and signs and symptoms of superinfection
promptly.
• Instruct patient to report discomfort at
I.V. site.

• Advise patient to notify prescriber about loose stools or diarrhea.

---

cefpodoxime proxetil
SEF-pod-OX-eem

Vantin

Pharmacologic class: third-generation cephalosporin
Pregnancy risk category B

AVAILABLE FORMS
Oral suspension: 50 mg/5 ml or 100 mg/5 ml in 50-, 75-, or 100-ml bottles
Tablets (film-coated): 100 mg, 200 mg

INDICATIONS & DOSAGES
➤ **Acute, community-acquired pneumonia caused by strains of** *Haemophilus influenzae* **or** *Streptococcus pneumoniae*
Adults and children age 12 and older: 200 mg P.O. every 12 hours for 14 days.
➤ **Acute bacterial worsening of chronic bronchitis caused by** *S. pneumoniae* **or** *H. influenzae* **(strains that don't produce beta-lactamase only), or** *Moraxella catarrhalis*
Adults and children age 12 and older: 200 mg P.O. every 12 hours for 10 days.
➤ **Uncomplicated gonorrhea in men and women; rectal gonococcal infections in women**
Adults and children age 12 and older: 200 mg P.O. as a single dose. Follow with doxycycline 100 mg P.O. b.i.d. for 7 days.
➤ **Uncomplicated skin and skin-structure infections caused by** *Staphylococcus aureus* **or** *S. pyogenes*
Adults and children age 12 and older: 400 mg P.O. every 12 hours for 7 to 14 days.
➤ **Acute otitis media caused by** *S. pneumoniae* **(penicillin-susceptible strains only),** *S. pyogenes,* *H. influenzae,* **or** *M. catarrhalis*
Children age 2 months to 12 years: 5 mg/kg P.O. every 12 hours for 5 days. Don't exceed 200 mg per dose.
➤ **Pharyngitis or tonsillitis caused by** *S. pyogenes*

Adults: 100 mg P.O. every 12 hours for 5 to 10 days.
Children ages 2 months to 12 years: 5 mg/kg P.O. every 12 hours for 5 to 10 days. Don't exceed 100 mg per dose.
➤ **Uncomplicated UTIs caused by** *Escherichia coli, Klebsiella pneumoniae, Proteus mirabilis,* **or** *Staphylococcus saprophyticus*
Adults: 100 mg P.O. every 12 hours for 7 days.
➤ **Mild to moderate acute maxillary sinusitis caused by** *H. influenzae,* *S. pneumoniae,* **or** *M. catarrhalis*
Adults and adolescents age 12 and older: 200 mg P.O. every 12 hours for 10 days.
Children ages 2 months to 12 years: 5 mg/kg P.O. every 12 hours for 10 days; maximum is 200 mg/dose.
Adjust-a-dose: For patients with creatinine clearance less than 30 ml/minute, increase dosage interval to every 24 hours. Give to dialysis patients three times weekly after dialysis.

ADMINISTRATION
P.O.
• Before administration, ask patient if he's allergic to penicillins or cephalosporins.
• Obtain specimen for culture and sensitivity tests before giving. Begin therapy while awaiting results.
• Give drug with food to enhance absorption. Shake suspension well before using.
• Store suspension in the refrigerator (36° to 46° F [2° to 8° C]). Discard unused portion after 14 days.

ACTION
Inhibits cell-wall synthesis, promoting osmotic instability; usually bactericidal.

Route	Onset	Peak	Duration
P.O.	Unknown	2–3 hr	Unknown

Half-life: 2 to 3 hours.

ADVERSE REACTIONS
CNS: headache.
GI: *diarrhea, pseudomembranous colitis,* nausea, vomiting, abdominal pain.
GU: vaginal fungal infections.
Skin: rash.
Other: *anaphylaxis,* hypersensitivity reactions.

INTERACTIONS

Drug-drug. *Aminoglycosides:* May increase risk of nephrotoxicity. Monitor renal function tests closely.

Antacids, H_2-receptor antagonists: May decrease absorption of cefpodoxime. Avoid using together.

Probenecid: May decrease excretion of cefpodoxime. Monitor patient for toxicity.

Drug-food. *Any food:* May increase absorption. Give tablets with food to enhance absorption. Oral suspension may be given without regard to food.

EFFECTS ON LAB TEST RESULTS

• May falsely increase serum or urine creatinine level in tests using Jaffe reaction. May cause false-positive results of Coombs' test and urine glucose tests that use cupric sulfate, such as Benedict's reagent and Clinitest.

CONTRAINDICATIONS & CAUTIONS

• Contraindicated in patients hypersensitive to drug or other cephalosporins.

• Use cautiously in patients with a history of penicillin hypersensitivity because of risk of cross-sensitivity.

• Use cautiously in patients receiving nephrotoxic drugs because other cephalosporins have been shown to have nephrotoxic potential.

• Use cautiously in breast-feeding women because drug appears in breast milk.

NURSING CONSIDERATIONS

• Monitor renal function and compare with baseline.

• Monitor patient for superinfection. Drug may cause overgrowth of nonsusceptible bacteria or fungi.

• *Look alike–sound alike:* Don't confuse drug with other cephalosporins that sound alike.

PATIENT TEACHING

• Tell patient to take drug as prescribed, even after he feels better.

• Instruct patient to take drug with food. If patient is using suspension, tell him to shake container before measuring dose and to keep container refrigerated.

• Tell patient to call prescriber if rash or signs and symptoms of superinfection occur.

• Instruct patient to notify prescriber about loose stools or diarrhea.

---

cefprozil
sef-PRO-zil

Cefzil

Pharmacologic class: second-generation cephalosporin
Pregnancy risk category B

AVAILABLE FORMS

Oral suspension: 125 mg/5 ml, 250 mg/5 ml
Tablets: 250 mg, 500 mg

INDICATIONS & DOSAGES

➤ **Pharyngitis or tonsillitis caused by** *Streptococcus pyogenes*
Adults and children age 13 and older: 500 mg P.O. daily for at least 10 days.

➤ **Otitis media caused by** *Streptococcus pneumoniae, Haemophilus influenzae,* **and** *Moraxella catarrhalis*
Infants and children ages 6 months to 12 years: 15 mg/kg P.O. every 12 hours for 10 days.

➤ **Secondary bacterial infections of acute bronchitis and acute bacterial worsening of chronic bronchitis caused by** *S. pneumoniae, H. influenzae,* **and** *M. catarrhalis*
Adults and children age 13 and older: 500 mg P.O. every 12 hours for 10 days.

➤ **Uncomplicated skin and skin-structure infections caused by** *Staphylococcus aureus* **and** *S. pyogenes*
Adults and children age 13 and older: 250 or 500 mg P.O. every 12 hours or 500 mg daily for 10 days.

➤ **Acute sinusitis caused by** *S. pneumoniae, H. influenzae* **(beta-lactamase–positive and –negative strains), and** *M. catarrhalis* **(including strains that produce beta-lactamase)**
Adults and children age 13 and older: 250 mg P.O. every 12 hours for 10 days; for moderate to severe infection, 500 mg P.O. every 12 hours for 10 days.
Children ages 6 months to 12 years: 7.5 mg/kg P.O. every 12 hours for 10 days; for moderate to severe infections, 15 mg/kg P.O. every 12 hours for 10 days.

Adjust-a-dose: If creatinine clearance is less than 30 ml/minute, give 50% of standard dose at standard intervals. If patient is receiving dialysis, give dose after hemodialysis is completed; drug is removed by hemodialysis.

ADMINISTRATION
P.O.
• Obtain specimen for culture and sensitivity tests before giving first dose. Start therapy while awaiting results.
• Before giving, ask patient if he's allergic to penicillins or cephalosporins.
• Shake suspension well before using.

ACTION
Inhibits cell-wall synthesis, promoting osmotic instability; usually bactericidal.

Route	Onset	Peak	Duration
P.O.	Unknown	1½ hr	Unknown

Half-life: 1¼ hours in patients with normal renal function; 2 hours in patients with impaired hepatic function; and 5¼ to 6 hours in patients with end-stage renal disease.

ADVERSE REACTIONS
CNS: dizziness, hyperactivity, headache, nervousness, insomnia, confusion, somnolence.
GI: diarrhea, nausea, vomiting, abdominal pain.
GU: genital pruritus, vaginitis.
Hematologic: eosinophilia.
Skin: rash, urticaria, diaper rash.
Other: *anaphylaxis,* superinfection, hypersensitivity reactions, serum sickness.

INTERACTIONS
Drug-drug. *Aminoglycosides:* May increase risk of nephrotoxicity. Monitor renal function tests closely.
Probenecid: May inhibit excretion and increase cefprozil level. Use together cautiously.

EFFECTS ON LAB TEST RESULTS
• May increase alkaline phosphatase, ALT, AST, bilirubin, BUN, creatinine, and LDH levels.

• May increase eosinophil count. May decrease leukocyte, platelet, and WBC counts.
• May falsely increase serum or urine creatinine level in tests using Jaffe reaction. May cause false-positive results of Coombs' test and urine glucose tests that use cupric sulfate, such as Benedict's reagent and Clinitest.

CONTRAINDICATIONS & CAUTIONS
• Contraindicated in patients hypersensitive to drug or other cephalosporins.
• Use cautiously in patients hypersensitive to penicillin because of possibility of cross-sensitivity with other beta-lactam antibiotics.
• Use cautiously in breast-feeding women and in patients with history of colitis and renal insufficiency.

NURSING CONSIDERATIONS
• Monitor renal function and liver function test results.
• Monitor patient for superinfection. May cause overgrowth of nonsusceptible bacteria or fungi.
• ***Look alike–sound alike:*** Don't confuse drug with other cephalosporins that sound alike.

PATIENT TEACHING
• Advise patient to take drug as prescribed, even after he feels better.
• Tell patient to shake suspension well before measuring dose.
• Inform patient or parent that oral suspension is bubble gum–flavored to improve palatability and promote compliance in children. Tell him to refrigerate reconstituted suspension and to discard unused drug after 14 days.
• Instruct patient to notify prescriber if rash or signs and symptoms of superinfection occur.

ceftazidime
sef-TAZ-i-deem

Ceptaz, Fortaz, Tazicef

Pharmacologic class: third-generation cephalosporin
Pregnancy risk category B

AVAILABLE FORMS
Infusion: 1 g, 2 g in 50-ml and 100-ml vials (premixed)
Injection (with arginine): 500 mg, 1 g, 2 g
Injection (with sodium carbonate): 500 mg, 1 g, 2 g

INDICATIONS & DOSAGES
➤ **Serious UTI and lower respiratory tract infection; skin, gynecologic, intra-abdominal, and CNS infection; bacteremia; and septicemia caused by susceptible microorganisms, such as streptococci (including** *Streptococcus pneumoniae* **and** *S. pyogenes*), **penicillinase- and non–penicillinase-producing** *Staphylococcus aureus, Escherichia coli, Klebsiella, Proteus, Enterobacter, Haemophilus influenzae, Pseudomonas,* **and some strains of** *Bacteroides*
Adults and children age 12 and older: 1 to 2 g I.V. or I.M. every 8 to 12 hours; up to 6 g daily in life-threatening infections.
Children ages 1 month to 12 years: 30 to 50 mg/kg I.V. every 8 hours. Maximum dose is 6 g/day. Use sodium carbonate formulation.
Neonates up to age 4 weeks: 30 mg/kg I.V. every 12 hours. Use sodium carbonate formulation.
➤ **Uncomplicated UTI**
Adults: 250 mg I.V. or I.M. every 12 hours.
➤ **Complicated UTI**
Adults and children age 12 and older: 500 mg to 1 g I.V. or I.M. every 8 to 12 hours.
Adjust-a-dose: If creatinine clearance is 31 to 50 ml/minute, give 1 g every 12 hours; if clearance is 16 to 30 ml/minute, give 1 g every 24 hours; if clearance is 6 to 15 ml/minute, give 500 mg every 24 hours; if clearance is less than 5 ml/minute, give 500 mg every 48 hours. Ceftazidime is removed by hemodialysis;

give a loading dose of 1 g, followed by 1 g after each hemodialysis period.

ADMINISTRATION
I.V.
● Before administration, ask patient if he's allergic to penicillins or cephalosporins.
● Obtain specimen for culture and sensitivity tests before giving. Begin therapy while awaiting results.
● Each brand of drug includes specific instructions for reconstitution. Read and follow them carefully.
● To reconstitute solution that contains sodium carbonate, add 5 ml sterile water for injection to a 500-mg vial, or add 10 ml to a 1-g or 2-g vial. Shake well to dissolve drug. Because carbon dioxide is released during dissolution, positive pressure will develop in vial.
● To reconstitute solution that contains arginine, use 10 ml of sterile water for injection. This product won't release gas bubbles.
● Infuse drug over 15 to 30 minutes.
● **Incompatibilities:** Aminoglycosides, aminophylline, amiodarone, amphotericin B cholesteryl sulfate complex, azithromycin, clarithromycin, fluconazole, idarubicin, midazolam, pentamidine isethionate, ranitidine hydrochloride, sargramostim, sodium bicarbonate solutions, vancomycin.
I.M.
● Before administration, ask patient if he's allergic to penicillins or cephalosporins.
● Obtain specimen for culture and sensitivity tests before giving. Begin therapy while awaiting results.
● Inject deep into a large muscle, such as the gluteus maximus or the side of the thigh.

ACTION
Inhibits cell-wall synthesis, promoting osmotic instability; usually bactericidal.

Route	Onset	Peak	Duration
I.V.	Immediate	Immediate	Unknown
I.M.	Unknown	1 hr	Unknown

Half-life: 1½ to 2 hours.

ADVERSE REACTIONS

CNS: *seizures,* headache, dizziness, paresthesia.
CV: *phlebitis, thrombophlebitis.*
GI: *pseudomembranous colitis,* nausea, vomiting, diarrhea, abdominal cramps.
GU: vaginitis, candidiasis.
Hematologic: *agranulocytosis, leukopenia, thrombocytopenia,* eosinophilia, thrombocytosis, hemolytic anemia.
Skin: *maculopapular and erythematous rashes, urticaria, pain, induration, sterile abscesses, tissue sloughing at injection site.*
Other: *anaphylaxis,* hypersensitivity reactions, serum sickness.

INTERACTIONS

Drug-drug. *Aminoglycosides:* May cause additive or synergistic effect against some strains of *Pseudomonas aeruginosa* and *Enterobacteriaceae;* may increase risk of nephrotoxicity. Monitor patient for effects and monitor renal function.
Chloramphenicol: May cause antagonistic effect. Avoid using together.

EFFECTS ON LAB TEST RESULTS

● May increase alkaline phosphatase, ALT, AST, bilirubin, and LDH levels. May decrease hemoglobin level.
● May increase eosinophil count. May decrease granulocyte and WBC counts. May increase or decrease platelet count.
● May falsely increase serum or urine creatinine level in tests using Jaffe reaction. May cause false-positive results of Coombs' test and urine glucose tests that use cupric sulfate, such as Benedict's reagent and Clinitest.

CONTRAINDICATIONS & CAUTIONS

● Contraindicated in patients hypersensitive to drug or other cephalosporins.
● Use cautiously in patients hypersensitive to penicillin because of possibility of cross-sensitivity with other beta-lactam antibiotics.
● Use cautiously in breast-feeding women and in patients with history of colitis or renal insufficiency.

NURSING CONSIDERATIONS

● If large doses are given, therapy is prolonged, or patient is at high risk, monitor patient for signs and symptoms of superinfection.
● *Alert:* Drug contains either sodium carbonate (Fortaz or Tazicef) or arginine (Ceptaz) to facilitate dissolution of drug. Safety and effectiveness of solutions containing arginine in children younger than age 12 haven't been established.
● *Look alike–sound alike:* Don't confuse drug with other cephalosporins that sound alike.

PATIENT TEACHING

● Tell patient to report adverse reactions or signs and symptoms of superinfection promptly.
● Instruct patient to report discomfort at I.V. insertion site.
● Advise patient to notify prescriber about loose stools or diarrhea.

---

ceftizoxime sodium
sef-ti-ZOX-eem

Cefizox

Pharmacologic class: third-generation cephalosporin
Pregnancy risk category B

AVAILABLE FORMS

Infusion: 1 g, 2 g in 100-ml vials or in 50-ml containers
Injection: 500 mg, 1 g, 2 g

INDICATIONS & DOSAGES

➤ **Serious UTI, lower respiratory tract infection, gynecologic infection, bacteremia, septicemia, meningitis, intra-abdominal infection, bone or joint infection, and skin infection caused by susceptible microorganisms, such as streptococci (including *Streptococcus pneumoniae* and *S. pyogenes*), *Staphylococcus aureus, S. epidermidis, Escherichia coli, Haemophilus influenzae,* and *Klebsiella, Enterobacter, Proteus, Peptostreptococcus,* and some *Pseudomonas* species**
Adults: 1 to 2 g I.V. or I.M. every 8 to 12 hours. For life-threatening infections, give up to 2 g I.V. every 4 hours, or 3 to 4 g I.V. every 8 hours.

Children older than age 6 months:
50 mg/kg I.V. every 6 to 8 hours. For serious infections, up to 200 mg/kg/day in divided doses may be used. Don't exceed 12 g/day.

➤ **Uncomplicated gonorrhea**
Adults: 1 g I.M. as a single dose.

Adjust-a-dose: If creatinine clearance is 50 to 79 ml/minute, give 500 mg to 1.5 g every 8 hours; if clearance is 5 to 49 ml/minute, give 250 mg to 1 g every 12 hours; if clearance is less than 5 ml/minute or patient undergoes hemodialysis, give 500 mg to 1 g every 48 hours, or 250 to 500 mg every 24 hours.

ADMINISTRATION
I.V.
- Before giving drug, ask patient if he's allergic to penicillins or cephalosporins.
- Obtain specimen for culture and sensitivity tests before giving. Begin therapy while awaiting results.
- To reconstitute powder, add 5 ml of sterile water to a 500-mg vial, 10 ml to a 1-g vial, or 20 ml to a 2-g vial.
- Reconstitute drug in piggyback vials with 50 to 100 ml of normal saline solution or D_5W. Shake well.
- For direct injection, give drug over 3 to 5 minutes or slowly into I.V. tubing of free-flowing compatible solution.
- For infusion, give drug over 15 to 30 minutes.
- **Incompatibilities:** Aminoglycosides, cisatracurium besylate, filgrastim; possibly promethazine hydrochloride and vancomycin hydrochloride.

I.M.
- Before giving drug, ask patient if he's allergic to penicillins or cephalosporins.
- Obtain specimen for culture and sensitivity tests before giving. Begin therapy while awaiting results.
- Mix 1.5 ml of diluent per 500 mg of drug. Inject deep into a large muscle, such as the gluteus maximus or the side of the thigh. Divide doses of more than 2 g and give at two separate sites.

ACTION
Inhibits cell-wall synthesis, promoting osmotic instability; usually bactericidal.

Route	Onset	Peak	Duration
I.V.	Immediate	Immediate	Unknown
I.M.	Unknown	30–90 min	Unknown

Half-life: 1½ to 2 hours.

ADVERSE REACTIONS
CNS: fever.
CV: *phlebitis, thrombophlebitis.*
GI: *diarrhea, pseudomembranous colitis,* nausea, anorexia, vomiting.
GU: vaginitis.
Hematologic: *thrombocytopenia, thrombocytosis, transient neutropenia,* eosinophilia, hemolytic anemia, anemia.
Respiratory: dyspnea.
Skin: *maculopapular and erythematous rashes, urticaria, pain, induration, sterile abscesses, tissue sloughing at injection site.*
Other: *anaphylaxis,* hypersensitivity reactions, serum sickness.

INTERACTIONS
Drug-drug. *Aminoglycosides:* May increase nephrotoxicity. Monitor renal function.
Probenecid: May inhibit excretion and increase ceftizoxime level. Use probenecid for this effect.

EFFECTS ON LAB TEST RESULTS
- May increase alkaline phosphatase, ALT, AST, bilirubin, BUN, creatinine, GGT, and LDH levels. May decrease albumin, hemoglobin, and protein levels.
- May decrease PT and granulocyte, neutrophil, platelet, RBC, and WBC counts.
- May falsely increase serum or urine creatinine level in tests using Jaffe reaction. May cause false-positive results of Coombs' test and urine glucose tests that use cupric sulfate, such as Benedict's reagent and Clinitest.

CONTRAINDICATIONS & CAUTIONS
- Contraindicated in patients hypersensitive to drug or other cephalosporins.
- Use cautiously in patients hypersensitive to penicillin because of possible cross-sensitivity with other beta-lactam antibiotics.

• Use cautiously in breast-feeding women and in patients with history of colitis or renal insufficiency.

NURSING CONSIDERATIONS
• If large doses are given, therapy is prolonged, or patient is at high risk, monitor patient for signs or symptoms of superinfection.
• *Look alike–sound alike:* Don't confuse drug with other cephalosporins that sound alike.

PATIENT TEACHING
• Tell patient to report adverse reactions and signs and symptoms of superinfection promptly.
• Instruct patient to report discomfort at I.V. site.
• Tell patient to notify prescriber about loose stools or diarrhea.

---

ceftriaxone sodium
sef-try-AX-ohn

Rocephin

Pharmacologic class: third-generation cephalosporin
Pregnancy risk category B

AVAILABLE FORMS
Infusion: 1 g, 2–g piggyback; 1 g, 2 g/50 ml premixed
Injection: 250 mg, 500 mg, 1 g, 2 g

INDICATIONS & DOSAGES
➤ **Uncomplicated gonococcal vulvovaginitis**
Adults: 125 mg I.M. as a single dose, plus azithromycin 1 g P.O. as a single dose or doxycycline 100 mg P.O. b.i.d. for 7 days.
➤ **UTI; lower respiratory tract, gynecologic, bone or joint, intraabdominal, skin, or skin structure infection; septicemia**
Adults and children older than age 12 years: 1 to 2 g I.M. or I.V. daily or in equally divided doses every 12 hours. Total daily dose shouldn't exceed 4 g.
Children age 12 and younger: 50 to 75 mg/kg I.M. or I.V., not to exceed 2 g/day, given in divided doses every 12 hours.

➤ **Meningitis**
Adults and children: Initially, 100 mg/kg I.M. or I.V. Don't exceed 4 g; then 100 mg/kg I.M. or I.V., given once daily or in divided doses every 12 hours, not to exceed 4 g, for 7 to 14 days.
➤ **Perioperative prevention**
Adults: 1 g I.V. as a single dose 30 minutes to 2 hours before surgery.
➤ **Acute bacterial otitis media**
Children: 50 mg/kg I.M. as a single dose. Don't exceed 1 g.
➤ **Neurologic complications, carditis, and arthritis from penicillin G–refractory Lyme disease ◆**
Adults: 2 g I.V. daily for 14 to 28 days.

ADMINISTRATION
I.V.
• Before giving drug, ask patient if he's allergic to penicillins or cephalosporins.
• Obtain specimen for culture and sensitivity tests before giving first dose. Begin therapy while awaiting results.
• Reconstitute drug with sterile water for injection, normal saline solution for injection, D_5W, or a combination of normal saline solution and dextrose injection and other compatible solutions.
• Add 2.4 ml of diluent to the 250-mg vial, 4.8 ml to the 500-mg vial, 9.6 ml to the 1-g vial, and 19.2 ml to the 2-g vial. All reconstituted solutions average 100 mg/ml.
• For intermittent infusion, dilute further to achieve desired concentration.
• Diluted I.V. preparation is stable 24 hours at room temperature or 10 days if refrigerated.
• *Alert:* Don't mix or coadminister ceftriaxone with calcium-containung I.V. solutions, including parenteral nutrition. This includes the use of different infusion lines at different sites. Don't administer within 48 hours of each other in any patient.
• **Incompatibilities:** Aminoglycosides, aminophylline, amphotericin B cholesteryl sulfate complex, azithromycin, calcium, clindamycin phosphate, filgrastim, fluconazole, gentamicin, labetalol, lidocaine hydrochloride, linezolid, metronidazole, pentamidine isethionate, theophylline, vancomycin, vinorelbine tartrate.

I.M.
- Before giving drug, ask patient if he's allergic to penicillins or cephalosporins.
- Obtain specimen for culture and sensitivity tests before giving first dose. Begin therapy while awaiting results.
- Inject deep into a large muscle, such as the gluteus maximus or the lateral aspect of the thigh.

ACTION
Inhibits cell-wall synthesis, promoting osmotic instability; usually bactericidal.

Route	Onset	Peak	Duration
I.V.	Immediate	Immediate	Unknown
I.M.	Unknown	1½–4 hr	Unknown

Half-life: 5½ to 11 hours.

ADVERSE REACTIONS
CNS: fever, headache, dizziness.
CV: phlebitis.
GI: *pseudomembranous colitis,* diarrhea.
GU: genital pruritus, candidiasis.
Hematologic: eosinophilia, thrombocytosis, *leukopenia.*
Skin: pain, induration, tenderness at injection site, *rash,* pruritus.
Other: hypersensitivity reactions, serum sickness, *anaphylaxis,* chills.

INTERACTIONS
Drug-drug. *Aminoglycosides:* May cause synergistic effect against some strains of *P. aeruginosa* and *Enterobacteriaceae* species. Monitor patient.
Probenecid: High doses (1 g or 2 g daily) may enhance hepatic clearance of ceftriaxone and shorten its half-life. Avoid using together.

EFFECTS ON LAB TEST RESULTS
- May increase alkaline phosphatase, ALT, AST, bilirubin, BUN, and LDH levels.
- May increase eosinophil and platelet counts. May decrease WBC count.

- May falsely increase serum or urine creatinine level in tests using Jaffe reaction. May cause false-positive results of Coombs' test and urine glucose tests that use cupric sulfate, such as Benedict's reagent and Clinitest.

CONTRAINDICATIONS & CAUTIONS
- Contraindicated in patients hypersensitive to drug or other cephalosporins.
- Use cautiously in patients hypersensitive to penicillin because of possibility of cross-sensitivity with other beta-lactam antibiotics.
- Use cautiously in breast-feeding women and in patients with history of colitis and renal insufficiency.

NURSING CONSIDERATIONS
- If large doses are given, therapy is prolonged, or patient is at high risk, monitor patient for signs and symptoms of superinfection.
- Monitor PT and INR in patients with impaired vitamin K synthesis or low vitamin K stores. Vitamin K therapy may be needed.
- Drug is commonly used in home antibiotic programs for outpatient treatment of serious infections, such as osteomyelitis and community-acquired pneumonia.
- *Look alike–sound alike:* Don't confuse drug with other cephalosporins that sound alike.

PATIENT TEACHING
- Tell patient to report adverse reactions promptly.
- Instruct patient to report discomfort at I.V. insertion site.
- Teach patient and family receiving home care how to prepare and give drug.
- If home care patient is diabetic and is testing his urine for glucose, tell him drug may affect results of cupric sulfate tests; he should use an enzymatic test instead.
- Tell patient to notify prescriber about loose stools or diarrhea.

cefuroxime axetil
se-fyoor-OX-eem

Ceftin

cefuroxime sodium
Zinacef

Pharmacologic class: second-generation cephalosporin
Pregnancy risk category B

AVAILABLE FORMS
cefuroxime axetil
Suspension: 125 mg/5 ml, 250 mg/5 ml
Tablets: 125 mg, 250 mg, 500 mg
cefuroxime sodium
Infusion: 750–mg, 1.5–g vials, infusion packs, and ADD-Vantage vials
Injection: 750 mg, 1.5 g

INDICATIONS & DOSAGES
➤ **Serious lower respiratory tract infection, UTI, skin or skin-structure infections, bone or joint infection, septicemia, meningitis, and gonorrhea**
Adults and children age 13 and older:
750 mg to 1.5 g cefuroxime sodium I.V. or I.M. every 8 hours for 5 to 10 days. For life-threatening infections and infections caused by less susceptible organisms, 1.5 g I.V. or I.M. every 6 hours; for bacterial meningitis, up to 3 g I.V. every 8 hours.
Children age 3 months to 12 years: 50 to 100 mg/kg/day cefuroxime sodium I.V. or I.M. in equally divided doses every 6 to 8 hours. Use higher dosage of 100 mg/kg/day, not to exceed maximum adult dosage, for more severe or serious infections. For bacterial meningitis, 200 to 240 mg/kg/day cefuroxime sodium I.V. in divided doses every 6 to 8 hours.
➤ **Perioperative prevention**
Adults: 1.5 g I.V. 30 to 60 minutes before surgery; in lengthy operations, 750 mg I.V. or I.M. every 8 hours. For open-heart surgery, 1.5 g I.V. at induction of anesthesia and then every 12 hours for a total dose of 6 g.
➤ **Bacterial exacerbations of chronic bronchitis or secondary bacterial infection of acute bronchitis**
Adults and children age 13 and older:
250 or 500 mg P.O. b.i.d. for 10 days (chronic bronchitis) or 5 to 10 days (acute bronchitis).
➤ **Acute bacterial maxillary sinusitis**
Adults and children age 13 and older:
250 mg P.O. b.i.d. for 10 days.
Children ages 3 months to 12 years:
250 mg b.i.d. for 10 days. For children who can't swallow tablets whole, 30 mg/kg/day oral suspension divided b.i.d. for 10 days.
➤ **Pharyngitis and tonsillitis**
Adults and children age 13 and older:
250 mg P.O. b.i.d. for 10 days.
Children ages 3 months to 12 years:
125 mg P.O. b.i.d. for 10 days. For children who can't swallow tablets whole, give 20 mg/kg daily of oral suspension divided b.i.d. for 10 days. Maximum daily dose for suspension is 500 mg.
➤ **Otitis media**
Children ages 3 months to 12 years:
250 mg P.O. b.i.d. for 10 days. For children who can't swallow tablets whole, give 30 mg/kg/day of oral suspension divided b.i.d. for 10 days. Maximum daily dose for suspension is 1,000 mg.
➤ **Uncomplicated skin and skin structure infection**
Adults and children age 13 and older:
250 or 500 mg P.O. b.i.d. for 10 days.
➤ **Uncomplicated UTI**
Adults: 125 or 250 mg P.O. b.i.d. for 7 to 10 days.
➤ **Uncomplicated gonorrhea**
Adults: 1.5 g I.M. with 1 g probenecid P.O. for one dose. Or, 1 g P.O. as a single dose.
➤ **Early Lyme disease**
Adults and children age 13 and older:
500 mg P.O. b.i.d. for 20 days.
➤ **Impetigo**
Children ages 3 months to 12 years:
30 mg/kg/day of oral suspension divided b.i.d. for 10 days. Maximum daily dose, 1,000 mg.
Adjust-a-dose: In adults with creatinine clearance of 10 to 20 ml/minute, give 750 mg I.V. or I.M. every 12 hours; if clearance is less than 10 ml/min, give 750 mg I.V. or I.M. every 24 hours.

ADMINISTRATION

P.O.
• Before giving drug, ask patient if he's allergic to penicillins or cephalosporins.
• Obtain specimen for culture and sensitivity tests before giving first dose. Therapy may begin while awaiting results.
• Give tablets without regard for meals; give oral suspension with food.
• Crush tablets, if absolutely necessary, for patients who can't swallow tablets. Tablets may be dissolved in small amounts of apple, orange, or grape juice or chocolate milk. However, the drug has a bitter taste that is difficult to mask, even with food.

I.V.
• Before giving drug, ask patient if he's allergic to penicillins or cephalosporins.
• Obtain specimen for culture and sensitivity tests before giving first dose. Therapy may begin while awaiting results.
• Reconstitute each 750-mg vial with 8 ml and each 1.5-g vial with 16 ml of sterile water for injection.
• Withdraw entire contents of vial for a dose.
• For direct injection, inject over 3 to 5 minutes into a large vein or into the tubing of a free-flowing I.V. solution.
• For intermittent infusion, add reconstituted drug to 100 ml D₅W, normal saline solution for injection, or other compatible I.V. solution.
• Infuse over 15 to 60 minutes.
• **Incompatibilities:** Aminoglycosides, azithromycin, ciprofloxacin, cisatracurium, clarithromycin, cyclophosphamide, doxapram, filgrastim, fluconazole, gentamicin, midazolam, ranitidine, sodium bicarbonate injection, vancomycin, vinorelbine tartrate.

I.M.
• Before giving drug, ask patient if he's allergic to penicillins or cephalosporins.
• Obtain specimen for culture and sensitivity tests before giving first dose. Therapy may begin while awaiting results.
• Inject deep into a large muscle, such as the gluteus maximus or the side of the thigh.

ACTION
Inhibits cell-wall synthesis, promoting osmotic instability; usually bactericidal.

Route	Onset	Peak	Duration
P.O.	Unknown	15–60 min	Unknown
I.V.	Immediate	Immediate	Unknown
I.M.	Unknown	2 hr	Unknown

Half-life: 1 to 2 hours.

ADVERSE REACTIONS
CV: *phlebitis, thrombophlebitis.*
GI: *diarrhea, **pseudomembranous colitis,*** nausea, anorexia, vomiting.
Hematologic: *hemolytic anemia, **thrombocytopenia, transient neutropenia,*** eosinophilia.
Skin: *maculopapular and erythematous rashes, urticaria, pain, induration, sterile abscesses, temperature elevation, tissue sloughing at I.M. injection site.*
Other: ***anaphylaxis,*** hypersensitivity reactions, serum sickness.

INTERACTIONS
Drug-drug. *Aminoglycosides:* May cause synergistic activity against some organisms; may increase nephrotoxicity. Monitor patient's renal function closely.
Loop diuretics: May increase risk of adverse renal reactions. Monitor renal function test results closely.
Probenecid: May inhibit excretion and increase cefuroxime level. Probenecid may be used for this effect.
Drug-food. *Any food:* May increase absorption. Give drug with food.

EFFECTS ON LAB TEST RESULTS
• May increase alkaline phosphatase, ALT, AST, bilirubin, and LDH levels. May decrease hemoglobin level and hematocrit.
• May increase PT and INR and eosinophil count. May decrease neutrophil and platelet counts.
• May falsely increase serum or urine creatinine level in tests using Jaffe reaction. May cause false-positive results of Coombs' test and urine glucose tests that use cupric sulfate, such as Benedict's reagent and Clinitest.

CONTRAINDICATIONS & CAUTIONS
• Contraindicated in patients hypersensitive to drug or other cephalosporins.
• Use cautiously in patients hypersensitive to penicillin because of possibility of

cross-sensitivity with other beta-lactam antibiotics.
• Use cautiously in breast-feeding women and in patients with history of colitis or renal insufficiency.

NURSING CONSIDERATIONS
• *Alert:* Tablets and suspension aren't bioequivalent and can't be substituted milligram-for-milligram.
• Monitor patient for signs and symptoms of superinfection.
• *Look alike–sound alike:* Don't confuse drug with other cephalosporins that sound alike.

PATIENT TEACHING
• Tell patient to take drug as prescribed, even after he feels better.
• If patient has difficulty swallowing tablets, show him how to dissolve or crush tablets, but warn him that the bitter taste is hard to mask, even with food.
• Tell parent to shake suspension well before measuring dose. Suspension may be stored at room temperature or refrigerated, but must be discarded after 10 days.
• Instruct caregiver to give oral suspension with food.
• Instruct patient to notify prescriber about rash, loose stools, diarrhea, or evidence of superinfection.
• Advise patient receiving drug I.V. to report discomfort at I.V. insertion site.

---

cephalexin
sef-a-LEX-in

Apo-Cephalex†, Keflex, Novo-Lexin†, Nu-Cephalex†

Pharmacologic class: first-generation cephalosporin
Pregnancy risk category B

AVAILABLE FORMS
Capsules: 250 mg, 333 mg, 500 mg, 750 mg
Oral suspension: 125 mg/5 ml, 250 mg/5 ml
Tablets: 250 mg, 500 mg

INDICATIONS & DOSAGES
➤ **Respiratory tract, GI tract, skin, soft-tissue, bone, and joint infections and otitis media caused by** *Escherichia coli* **and other coliform bacteria, group A beta-hemolytic streptococci,** *Klebsiella* **species,** *Proteus mirabilis, Streptococcus pneumoniae,* **and staphylococci**
Adults: 250 mg to 1 g P.O. every 6 hours or 500 mg every 12 hours. Maximum 4 g daily.
Children: 25 to 50 mg/kg/day P.O. in two to four equally divided doses. In severe infections, dose can be doubled.
Adjust-a-dose: For adults with impaired renal function, initial dose is the same. Then, for those with creatinine clearance of 11 to 40 ml/minute, give 500 mg P.O. every 8 to 12 hours; for clearance of 5 to 10 ml/minute, give 250 mg P.O. every 12 hours; and for clearance of less than 5 ml/minute, give 250 mg P.O. every 12 to 24 hours.

ADMINISTRATION
P.O.
• Before giving, ask patient if he's allergic to penicillins or cephalosporins.
• Obtain specimen for culture and sensitivity tests before giving. Begin therapy while awaiting results.
• To prepare oral suspension, add required amount of water to powder in two portions. Shake well after each addition. After mixing, store in refrigerator. Mixture will remain stable for 14 days. Keep tightly closed and shake well before using.
• Give drug with food or milk to lessen GI discomfort.

ACTION
Inhibits cell-wall synthesis, promoting osmotic instability; usually bactericidal.

Route	Onset	Peak	Duration
P.O.	Unknown	1 hr	Unknown

Half-life: 30 minutes to 1 hour.

ADVERSE REACTIONS
CNS: dizziness, headache, fatigue, agitation, confusion, hallucinations.
GI: *anorexia, diarrhea, nausea,* ***pseudomembranous colitis,*** vomiting, gastritis,

---

glossitis, dyspepsia, abdominal pain, anal pruritus, tenesmus, oral candidiasis.

GU: genital pruritus, candidiasis, vaginitis, interstitial nephritis.

Hematologic: *neutropenia, thrombocytopenia,* eosinophilia, anemia.

Musculoskeletal: arthritis, arthralgia, joint pain.

Skin: *maculopapular and erythematous rashes, urticaria.*

Other: *anaphylaxis,* hypersensitivity reactions, serum sickness.

INTERACTIONS

Drug-drug. *Aminoglycosides:* May increase risk of nephrotoxicity. Avoid using together.

Probenecid: May increase cephalosporin level. Use probenecid for this effect.

EFFECTS ON LAB TEST RESULTS

• May increase alkaline phosphatase, ALT, AST, bilirubin, and LDH levels. May decrease hemoglobin level.

• May increase eosinophil count. May decrease neutrophil and platelet counts.

• May falsely increase serum or urine creatinine level in tests using Jaffe reaction. May cause false-positive results of Coombs' test and urine glucose tests that use cupric sulfate, such as Benedict's reagent and Clinitest.

CONTRAINDICATIONS & CAUTIONS

• Contraindicated in patients hypersensitive to cephalosporins.

• Use cautiously in patients hypersensitive to penicillin because of possibility of cross-sensitivity with other beta-lactam antibiotics.

• Use cautiously in breast-feeding women and in patients with history of colitis or renal insufficiency.

NURSING CONSIDERATIONS

• If large doses are given or if therapy is prolonged, monitor patient for superinfection, especially if patient is high risk.

• Treat group A beta-hemolytic streptococcal infections for a minimum of 10 days.

• *Look alike–sound alike:* Don't confuse drug with other cephalosporins that sound alike.

PATIENT TEACHING

• Tell patient to take drug exactly as prescribed, even after he feels better.

• Instruct patient to take drug with food or milk to lessen GI discomfort. If patient is taking suspension form, instruct him to shake container well before measuring dose and to store in refrigerator.

• Tell patient to notify prescriber if rash or signs and symptoms of superinfection develop.

---

cetirizine hydrochloride
se-TEER-i-zeen

Zyrtec ◊

Pharmacologic class: piperazine derivative
Pregnancy risk category B

AVAILABLE FORMS

Oral solution: 5 mg/5 ml ◊
Tablets: 5 mg, 10 mg ◊
Tablets (chewable): 5 mg ◊, 10 mg ◊

INDICATIONS & DOSAGES

➤ **Seasonal allergic rhinitis**

Adults and children age 6 and older: 5 to 10 mg P.O. once daily.

Children ages 2 to 5: 2.5 mg P.O. once daily. Maximum daily dose is 5 mg.

➤ **Perennial allergic rhinitis, chronic urticaria**

Adults and children age 6 and older: 5 to 10 mg P.O. once daily.

Children ages 6 months to 5 years: 2.5 mg P.O. once daily; in children ages 1 to 5, increase to maximum of 5 mg daily. Children ages 12 to 23 months should receive the 5-mg dose as two divided doses.

Adjust-a-dose: In adults and children age 6 and older receiving hemodialysis, those with hepatic impairment, and those with creatinine clearance less than 31 ml/minute, give 5 mg P.O. daily. Don't use in children younger than age 6 with renal or hepatic impairment.

ADMINISTRATION

P.O.

• Give drug without regard for food.

ACTION

A long-acting, nonsedating antihistamine that selectively inhibits peripheral H_1 receptors.

Route	Onset	Peak	Duration
P.O.	Rapid	60 min	24 hr

Half-life: About 8 hours.

ADVERSE REACTIONS

CNS: *somnolence,* fatigue, dizziness, headache.
EENT: pharyngitis.
GI: dry mouth, nausea, vomiting, abdominal distress.

INTERACTIONS

Drug-drug. *CNS depressants:* May cause additive effect. Monitor patient closely for excessive sedation or other adverse effects.
Theophylline: May decrease cetirizine clearance. Monitor patient closely.
Drug-lifestyle. *Alcohol use:* May cause additive effects. Discourage use together.

EFFECTS ON LAB TEST RESULTS

• May prevent, reduce, or mask positive result in diagnostic skin test.

CONTRAINDICATIONS & CAUTIONS

• Contraindicated in patients hypersensitive to drug or to hydroxyzine and in breast-feeding women.
• Use cautiously in patients with renal or hepatic impairment.

NURSING CONSIDERATIONS

• Stop drug 4 days before diagnostic skin testing because antihistamines can prevent, reduce, or mask positive skin test response.
• *Look alike–sound alike:* Don't confuse Zyrtec with Zyprexa or Zantac.

PATIENT TEACHING

• Warn patient not to perform hazardous activities until CNS effects of drug are known. Somnolence is a common adverse reaction.
• Advise patient not to use alcohol or other CNS depressants while taking drug.
• Inform patient that sugarless gum, hard candy, or ice chips may relieve dry mouth.

chlorambucil
klor-AM-byoo-sill

Leukeran

Pharmacologic class: nitrogen mustard
Pregnancy risk category D

AVAILABLE FORMS

Tablets: 2 mg

INDICATIONS & DOSAGES

➤ **Chronic lymphocytic leukemia; malignant lymphomas, including lymphosarcoma, giant follicular lymphoma, and Hodgkin lymphoma**
Adults: 0.1 to 0.2 mg/kg P.O. daily for 3 to 6 weeks; then adjust for maintenance (usually 4 to 10 mg daily); or, 3 to 6 mg/m² P.O. daily.
Children: 0.1 to 0.2 mg/kg P.O. or 4.5 mg/m² P.O. daily for 3 to 6 weeks.
Adjust-a-dose: Reduce first dose if given within 4 weeks after a full course of radiation therapy or myelosuppressive drugs, or if pretreatment leukocyte or platelet counts are depressed from bone marrow disease.
➤ **Macroglobulinemia** ♦
Adults: 2 to 10 mg P.O. daily for up to 9 years. Or, 8 mg/m² P.O. daily with prednisone for 10 days; repeat every 6 to 8 weeks as needed.
➤ **Nephrotic syndrome** ♦
Children: 0.1 to 0.2 mg/kg P.O. daily with prednisone for 8 to 12 weeks.
➤ **Intractable idiopathic uveitis, Behçet syndrome** ♦
Adults: 6 to 12 mg or 0.1 to 0.2 mg/kg P.O. daily for at least 1 year.

ADMINISTRATION

P.O.
• For initial therapy and short courses of therapy, give entire daily dose at one time.

ACTION

Cross-links strands of cellular DNA and interferes with RNA transcription, causing an imbalance of growth that leads to cell death. Not specific to cell cycle.

Reactions may be **common**, uncommon, *life-threatening*, or COMMON AND LIFE-THREATENING.
Interaction may have a *rapid onset* or **delayed onset**.

Route	Onset	Peak	Duration
P.O.	Unknown	1 hr	Unknown

Half-life: 2 hours for parent compound; 2½ hours for phenylacetic acid metabolite.

ADVERSE REACTIONS

CNS: *seizures,* peripheral neuropathy, tremor, muscle twitching, confusion, agitation, ataxia, flaccid paresis.
GI: *nausea, vomiting,* stomatitis, diarrhea.
GU: *azoospermia, infertility,* sterile cystitis.
Hematologic: *neutropenia, bone marrow suppression, thrombocytopenia,* anemia, *myelosuppression.*
Hepatic: *hepatotoxicity.*
Respiratory: interstitial pneumonitis, *pulmonary fibrosis.*
Skin: rash, *erythema multiforme, epidermal necrolysis, Stevens-Johnson syndrome.*
Other: drug fever, hypersensitivity reactions, *secondary malignancies.*

INTERACTIONS

Drug-drug. *Anticoagulants, aspirin:* May increase risk of bleeding. Avoid using together.
Myelosuppressives: May increase myelosuppression. Monitor patient.

EFFECTS ON LAB TEST RESULTS

• May increase alkaline phosphatase, AST, and blood and urine uric acid levels. May decrease hemoglobin level.
• May decrease granulocyte, neutrophil, platelet, RBC, and WBC counts.

CONTRAINDICATIONS & CAUTIONS

• Contraindicated in patients with hypersensitivity or resistance to previous therapy. Patients hypersensitive to other alkylating drugs may also be hypersensitive to this drug.
• Use cautiously in patients with history of head trauma or seizures and in patients receiving other drugs that lower the seizure threshold.
• Use cautiously within 4 weeks of a full course of radiation or chemotherapy.

NURSING CONSIDERATIONS

• Monitor CBC with differential.
• Monitor patient for neutropenia, which may not appear until after the 3rd week of treatment. The absolute neutrophil count (ANC) may continue to decrease for up to 10 days after treatment ends.
• Use the ANC to calculate the patient's immunosuppression.
• Monitor uric acid level. To prevent hyperuricemia with resulting uric acid nephropathy, allopurinol may be used with adequate hydration.
• If WBC count falls below 2,000/mm³ or granulocyte count falls below 1,000/mm³, follow institutional policy for infection control in immunocompromised patients. Patients may receive injections of WBC colony-stimulating factor to increase WBC count recovery. Severe neutropenia is reversible up to cumulative dose of 6.5 mg/kg in a single course.
• Therapeutic effects are frequently accompanied by toxicity.
• To prevent bleeding, avoid all I.M. injections when platelet count is below 50,000/mm³.
• Anticipate blood transfusions during treatment because of cumulative anemia. Patient may receive injections of RBC colony-stimulating factor to promote RBC production and decrease need for blood transfusions.

PATIENT TEACHING

• Advise patient to watch for signs of infection (fever, sore throat, fatigue) and bleeding (easy bruising, nosebleeds, bleeding gums, tarry stools). Tell patient to take temperature daily.
• Instruct patient to avoid OTC products containing aspirin and NSAIDs.
• Advise women to stop breast-feeding during therapy because of risk of toxicity to infant.
• Advise women of childbearing age to avoid becoming pregnant during therapy and to notify prescriber immediately if pregnancy is suspected.

chlorpheniramine maleate
klor-fen-IR-a-meen

Aller-Chlor ◊*, Allergy ◊,
Chlo-Amine ◊,
Chlor-Trimeton Allergy
4 Hour ◊, Chlor-Trimeton Allergy
8 Hour ◊, Chlor-Trimeton Allergy
12 Hour ◊, Efidac ◊

Pharmacologic class: alkylamine
Pregnancy risk category B

AVAILABLE FORMS
Capsules (sustained-release) ◊: 8 mg,
12 mg
Syrup ◊: 2 mg/5 ml*
Tablets ◊: 4 mg
Tablets (chewable) ◊: 2 mg
Tablets (extended-release) ◊: 8 mg,
12 mg, 16 mg

INDICATIONS & DOSAGES
➤ **Allergic rhinitis**
Adults and children age 12 and older:
4 mg P.O. every 4 to 6 hours, not to exceed
24 mg daily. Or, 8 to 12 mg timed-release
P.O. every 8 to 12 hours, not to exceed
24 mg daily. Or, 16 mg timed-release P.O.
once daily.
Children ages 6 to 12 years: Give 2 mg
P.O. every 4 to 6 hours, not to exceed
12 mg daily. Or, 8 mg timed-release P.O. at
bedtime.
Children ages 2 to 5 years: Give 1 mg P.O.
every 4 to 6 hours, not to exceed 6 mg daily.

ADMINISTRATION
P.O.
● Give extended-release tablets whole and
not crushed or divided.

ACTION
Competes with histamine for H_1-receptor
sites on effector cells. Drug prevents,
but doesn't reverse, histamine-mediated
responses.

Route	Onset	Peak	Duration
P.O.	15–60 min	2–6 hr	24 hr

Half-life: Adults with normal renal and hepatic function, 12 to 43 hours; children with
normal renal and hepatic function, 9½ to 13
hours; chronic renal failure on hemodialysis,
11½ to 13¾ days.

ADVERSE REACTIONS
CNS: *drowsiness, stimulation,* sedation,
excitability in children.
CV: hypotension, palpitations, weak pulse.
GI: *dry mouth,* epigastric distress.
GU: urine retention.
Respiratory: thick bronchial secretions.
Skin: rash, urticaria, pallor.

INTERACTIONS
Drug-drug. *CNS depressants:* May in-
crease sedation. Use together cautiously.
MAO inhibitors: May increase anticholin-
ergic effects. Avoid using together.
Drug-lifestyle. *Alcohol use:* May increase
CNS depression. Discourage use together.

EFFECTS ON LAB TEST RESULTS
● May prevent, reduce, or mask positive
result in diagnostic skin test.

CONTRAINDICATIONS & CAUTIONS
● Contraindicated in patients having acute
asthmatic attacks and in those with angle-
closure glaucoma, symptomatic prostatic
hyperplasia, pyloroduodenal obstruction,
or bladder neck obstruction.
● Contraindicated in breast-feeding women
and in patients taking MAO inhibitors.
● Use cautiously in elderly patients and in
those with increased intraocular pressure,
hyperthyroidism, CV or renal disease, hypertension, bronchial asthma, urine retention, prostatic hyperplasia, and stenosing
peptic ulcerations.

NURSING CONSIDERATIONS
● Stop drug 4 days before diagnostic skin
testing because antihistamines can prevent,
reduce, or mask positive skin test response.

PATIENT TEACHING
● Warn patient to avoid alcohol and hazardous activities that require alertness until
CNS effects of drug are known.
● Inform patient that sugarless gum,
hard candy, or ice chips may relieve dry
mouth.
● Instruct patient to notify prescriber if
tolerance develops because a different
antihistamine may need to be prescribed.
● Advise patient that extended-release
tablets should be swallowed whole and not
crushed, chewed, or divided.

---

ciclesonide
si-CLEH-son-ide

Alvesco†, Omnaris

Pharmacologic class: nonhalo-genated glucocorticoid
Pregnancy risk category C

AVAILABLE FORMS
Nasal spray: 50 mcg/metered spray

INDICATIONS & DOSAGES
➤ **Symptoms of seasonal or peren-nial allergic rhinitis**
Adults and children age 12 and older:
2 sprays in each nostril once daily
(200 mcg/day).

ADMINISTRATION
Intranasal
• Before first use, gently shake container, then prime by spraying eight times. If not used for 4 consecutive days, gently shake and reprime with 1 spray or until a fine mist appears.

ACTION
Hydrolyzed by the nasal mucosa to a biologically active metabolite with anti-inflammatory properties.

Route	Onset	Peak	Duration
Nasal	1–2 days	1–5 wk	Unknown

Half-life: Unknown.

ADVERSE REACTIONS
CNS: headache.
EENT: epistaxis, nasopharyngitis, ear pain, nasal discomfort.
Metabolic: growth retardation.

INTERACTIONS
None significant.

EFFECTS ON LAB TEST RESULTS
None reported.

CONTRAINDICATIONS & CAUTIONS
• Contraindicated in patients hypersensi-tive to the drug or its components.
• Contraindicated in patients who have had recent nasal septal ulcers, nasal surgery, or nasal trauma until healing has occurred.

• Use cautiously in patients who have changed from systemic to inhaled cor-ticosteroids; renal insufficiency, steroid withdrawal (pain, lassitude, depression) or acute worsening of symptoms may occur.
• Use cautiously in immunosuppressed patients or in those with wounds; cortico-steroids suppress the immune system.
• Use cautiously in children; may cause a decline in growth rate.
• Use cautiously in breast-feeding women.

NURSING CONSIDERATIONS
• Monitor infants born to mothers using drug during pregnancy for hypoadrenal-ism.
• Monitor patients who are switched from systemic to inhaled corticosteroids for worsening of symptoms and other side effects of withdrawal.
• Monitor children for decline in growth rate; potential to regain growth after drug is stopped hasn't been studied.
• Monitor patient for nasal side effects.

PATIENT TEACHING
• Teach patient how to use the spray prop-erly. Refer patient to package insert.
• Instruct patient to contact his prescriber if he has no relief from symptoms after 1 week.
• Advise patient to use drug every day, as directed.
• Warn patient to avoid exposure to people with infections, such as chickenpox or measles; corticosteroids have immunosup-pressant effects.

cidofovir
sye-DOE-fo-veer

Vistide

Pharmacologic class: nucleotide analogue
Pregnancy risk category C

AVAILABLE FORMS
Injection: 75 mg/ml in 5-ml vial

INDICATIONS & DOSAGES
➤ **CMV retinitis in patients with AIDS**
Adults: Initially, 5 mg/kg I.V. infused over 1 hour once weekly for 2 consecutive

weeks; then maintenance dose of
5 mg/kg I.V. infused over 1 hour once
every 2 weeks. Give probenecid and prehydration with normal saline solution I.V.
simultaneously to reduce risk of nephrotoxicity.

Adjust-a-dose: For patients with creatinine
level of 0.3 to 0.4 mg/dl above baseline,
reduce dosage to 3 mg/kg at same rate and
frequency. If creatinine level reaches
0.5 mg/dl or more above baseline, or
patient develops 3+ or higher proteinuria,
stop drug.

ADMINISTRATION
I.V.
• Drug has mutagenic effects; prepare it
in a class II laminar flow biological safety
cabinet and wear surgical gloves and a
closed-front surgical gown with knit cuffs.
• If drug contacts skin, wash and flush
thoroughly with water.
• Place excess drug and all materials used
to prepare and give it in a leak-proof,
puncture-proof container.
• Let drug reach room temperature before
use.
• Using a syringe, withdraw prescribed
dose and add to an I.V. bag containing
100 ml of normal saline solution.
• Infuse over 1 hour using an infusion
pump.
• Because of the risk of nephrotoxicity,
don't exceed recommended dosages or
frequency or rate of infusion.
• Discard any partially used vials.
• Give within 24 hours of preparing.
Admixture may be refrigerated at 36° to
46° F (2° to 8° C) for up to 24 hours.
• *Alert:* Give 1 L normal saline solution
I.V. over 1- to 2-hour period, immediately
before giving drug.
• *Alert:* Give probenecid with cidofovir.
• Compatibility of admixture with
Ringer's, lactated Ringer's, and bacte-
riostatic solutions hasn't been evaluated.
• **Incompatibilities:** Other drugs or sup-
plements.

ACTION
Suppresses CMV replication by selective
inhibition of viral DNA synthesis.

Route	Onset	Peak	Duration
I.V.	Unknown	Unknown	Unknown

Half-life: Unknown.

ADVERSE REACTIONS
CNS: *asthenia, fever, headache,* **seizures,**
abnormal gait, amnesia, anxiety, confusion, depression, dizziness, hallucinations,
insomnia, neuropathy, paresthesia, somnolence, malaise.
CV: hypotension, orthostatic hypotension,
pallor, syncope, tachycardia, vasodilation.
EENT: *ocular hypotony,* abnormal vision,
amblyopia, conjunctivitis, eye disorders,
iritis, pharyngitis, retinal detachment,
rhinitis, sinusitis, uveitis.
GI: *abdominal pain, anorexia, diarrhea,
nausea, vomiting,* aphthous stomatitis,
colitis, constipation, dry mouth, dyspepsia,
dysphagia, flatulence, gastritis, melena,
mouth ulcers, oral candidiasis, rectal
disorders, stomatitis, taste perversion,
tongue discoloration.
GU: *proteinuria,* **nephrotoxicity,** glycosuria, hematuria, urinary incontinence,
UTI.
Hematologic: anemia, **neutropenia,
thrombocytopenia.**
Hepatic: hepatomegaly.
Metabolic: fluid imbalance, hyperglycemia, hyperlipemia, hypocalcemia,
hypokalemia, weight loss.
Musculoskeletal: arthralgia, myalgia,
myasthenia, pain in back, chest, or neck.
Respiratory: *dyspnea,* asthma, bronchitis,
coughing, hiccups, increased sputum, lung
disorders, pneumonia.
Skin: *alopecia, rash,* acne, dry skin,
pruritus, skin discoloration, sweating,
urticaria.
Other: *chills, infections,* **sarcoma, sepsis,**
allergic reactions, facial edema, herpes
simplex.

INTERACTIONS
Drug-drug. *Nephrotoxic drugs (such
as aminoglycosides, amphotericin B,
foscarnet, I.V. pentamidine):* May increase
nephrotoxicity. Avoid using together.

EFFECTS ON LAB TEST RESULTS
• May increase alkaline phosphatase, ALT,
AST, BUN, creatinine, LDH, and urine

protein levels. May decrease bicarbonate and hemoglobin levels.
• May decrease neutrophil and platelet counts.

CONTRAINDICATIONS & CAUTIONS

• Contraindicated in patients hypersensitive to drug, probenecid, and other sulfa drugs.
• Contraindicated in patients receiving other drugs with nephrotoxic potential (stop such drugs at least 7 days before starting cidofovir therapy) and in those with creatinine level exceeding 1.5 mg/dl, creatinine clearance of 55 ml/minute or less, or urine protein level of 100 mg/dl or more (equivalent to 2+ proteinuria or more).
• Use within 1 month of placement of a ganciclovir ocular implant may cause profound hypotony.
• Safety and effectiveness in children haven't been established.
• Use cautiously in patients with renal impairment. Monitor renal function tests and patient's fluid balance.

NURSING CONSIDERATIONS

• Safety and effectiveness of drug haven't been established for treating other CMV infections, congenital or neonatal CMV disease, or CMV disease in patients not infected with HIV.
• Monitor creatinine and urine protein levels and WBC counts with differential before each dose.
• Drug may cause Fanconi syndrome and decreased bicarbonate level with renal tubular damage. Monitor patient closely.
• Drug may cause granulocytopenia.
• Stop zidovudine therapy or reduce dosage by 50% on the days when cidofovir is given; probenecid reduces metabolic clearance of zidovudine.

PATIENT TEACHING

• Inform patient that drug doesn't cure CMV retinitis and that regular ophthalmologic examinations are needed.
• Alert patient taking zidovudine that he'll need to obtain dosage guidelines on days cidofovir is given.
• Tell patient that close monitoring of kidney function will be needed and that abnormalities may require a change in therapy.
• Stress importance of completing a full course of probenecid with each cidofovir dose. Tell patient to take probenecid after a meal to decrease nausea.
• Patients with AIDS should use effective contraception, especially during and for 1 month after treatment.
• Advise men to practice barrier contraception during and for 3 months after treatment.

---

ciprofloxacin
si-proe-FLOX-a-sin

Cipro, Cipro I.V., Cipro XR, Proquin XR

Pharmacologic class:
fluoroquinolone
Pregnancy risk category C

AVAILABLE FORMS

Infusion (premixed): 200 mg in 100 ml D_5W, 400 mg in 200 ml D_5W
Injection: 200 mg, 400 mg
Suspension (oral): 5 g/100 ml (5%), 10 g/100 ml (10%)
Tablets (extended-release, film-coated): 500 mg, 1,000 mg
Tablets (film-coated): 100 mg, 250 mg, 500 mg, 750 mg

INDICATIONS & DOSAGES

➤ **Complicated intra-abdominal infection**
Adults: 500 mg P.O. or 400 mg I.V. every 12 hours for 7 to 14 days. Give with metronidazole.
➤ **Severe or complicated bone or joint infection, severe respiratory tract infection, severe skin or skin-structure infection**
Adults: 750 mg P.O. every 12 hours or 400 mg I.V. every 8 hours.
➤ **Severe or complicated UTI; mild to moderate bone or joint infection; mild to moderate respiratory infection; mild to moderate skin or skin-structure infection; infectious diarrhea; typhoid fever**

Adults: 500 mg P.O. or 400 mg I.V. every 12 hours. Or, 1,000 mg extended-release tablets P.O. every 24 hours.

➤ **Complicated UTI or pyelonephritis**

Children age 1 to 17: 6 to 10 mg/kg I.V. every 8 hours for 10 to 21 days. Maximum I.V. dose, 400 mg. Or, 10 to 20 mg/kg P.O. every 12 hours. Maximum P.O. dose, 750 mg. Don't exceed maximum dose, even in patients who weigh more than 51 kg (112 lb).

➤ **Nosocomial pneumonia**

Adults: 400 mg I.V. every 8 hours for 10 to 14 days.

➤ **Mild to moderate UTI**

Adults: 250 mg P.O. or 200 mg I.V. every 12 hours for 7 to 14 days.

➤ **Uncomplicated UTI**

Adults: 500 mg extended-release tablet P.O. once daily for 3 days.

➤ **Chronic bacterial prostatitis**

Adults: 500 mg P.O. every 12 hours or 400 mg I.V. every 12 hours for 28 days.

➤ **Acute uncomplicated cystitis**

Adults: 100 mg or 250 mg P.O. every 12 hours for 3 days.

➤ **Mild to moderate acute sinusitis**

Adults: 500 mg P.O. or 400 mg I.V. every 12 hours for 10 days.

➤ **Empirical therapy in febrile neutropenic patients**

Adults: 400 mg I.V. every 8 hours used with piperacillin 50 mg/kg I.V. every 4 hours (not to exceed 24 g/day).

➤ **Inhalation anthrax (postexposure)**

Adults: 400 mg I.V. every 12 hours initially until susceptibility test results are known; then 500 mg P.O. b.i.d. Give drug with one or two additional antimicrobials. Switch to oral therapy when appropriate. Treat for 60 days (I.V. and P.O. combined).
Children: 10 mg/kg I.V. every 12 hours; then 15 mg/kg P.O. every 12 hours. Don't exceed 800 mg/day I.V. or 1,000 mg/day P.O. Give drug with one or two additional antimicrobials. Switch to oral therapy when appropriate. Treat for 60 days (I.V. and P.O. combined).

➤ **Cutaneous anthrax ♦**

Adults: 500 mg P.O. b.i.d. for 60 days.
Children: 10 to 15 mg/kg every 12 hours. Don't exceed 1,000 mg/day. Treat for 60 days.

Adjust-a-dose: For patients with a creatinine clearance of 30 to 50 ml/minute, give 250 to 500 mg P.O. every 12 hours or the usual I.V. dose; if clearance is 5 to 29 ml/minute, give 250 to 500 mg P.O. every 18 hours or 200 to 400 mg I.V. every 18 to 24 hours. If patient is receiving hemodialysis, give 250 to 500 mg P.O. every 24 hours after dialysis.

ADMINISTRATION
P.O.
• Obtain specimen for culture and sensitivity tests before giving first dose. Begin therapy while awaiting results.
• To avoid decreasing the effects of ciprofloxacin, separate dosage of certain drugs by up to 6 hours. Food doesn't affect absorption but may delay peak levels.
• Caffeine should be avoided during therapy with this drug because of potential for increased caffeine effects.
• Give drug with plenty of fluids to reduce risk of urine crystals.
• Don't crush or split the extended-release tablets.
I.V.
• Obtain specimen for culture and sensitivity tests before giving first dose. Begin therapy while awaiting results.
• Dilute drug to 1 to 2 mg/ml using D_5W or normal saline solution for injection.
• If giving drug through a Y-type set, stop the other I.V. solution while infusing.
• Infuse over 1 hour into a large vein to minimize discomfort and vein irritation.
• **Incompatibilities:** Aminophylline, ampicillin-sulbactam, azithromycin, cefepime, clindamycin phosphate, dexamethasone sodium phosphate, furosemide, heparin sodium, methylprednisolone sodium succinate, phenytoin sodium.

ACTION
Inhibits bacterial DNA synthesis, mainly by blocking DNA gyrase; bactericidal.

Route	Onset	Peak	Duration
P.O.	Unknown	30–120 min	Unknown
P.O. (extended-release)	Unknown	1–4 hr	Unknown
I.V.	Unknown	Immediate	Unknown

Half-life: 4 hours; Cipro XR, 6 hours in adults with normal renal function.

ADVERSE REACTIONS

CNS: *seizures,* confusion, depression, dizziness, drowsiness, fatigue, hallucinations, headache, insomnia, lightheadedness, paresthesia, restlessness, tremor.
CV: chest pain, edema, thrombophlebitis.
GI: *pseudomembranous colitis, diarrhea, nausea,* abdominal pain or discomfort, constipation, dyspepsia, flatulence, oral candidiasis, vomiting.
GU: crystalluria, interstitial nephritis.
Hematologic: *leukopenia, neutropenia, thrombocytopenia,* eosinophilia.
Musculoskeletal: aching, arthralgia, arthropathy, joint inflammation, joint or back pain, joint stiffness, neck pain, tendon rupture.
Skin: *rash, Stevens-Johnson syndrome, toxic epidermal necrolysis,* burning, erythema, exfoliative dermatitis, photosensitivity, pruritus.
Other: hypersensitivity reactions.

INTERACTIONS

Drug-drug. *Aluminum hydroxide, aluminum-magnesium hydroxide, calcium carbonate, didanosine (chewable tablets, buffered tablets, or pediatric powder for oral solution), magnesium hydroxide, products containing zinc:* May decrease ciprofloxacin absorption and effects. Give ciprofloxacin 2 hours before or 6 hours after these drugs.
Cyclosporine: May increase risk for cyclosporine toxicity. Monitor cyclosporine level.
Iron salts: May decrease absorption of ciprofloxacin, reducing anti-infective response. Give at least 2 hours apart.
NSAIDs: May increase risk of CNS stimulation. Monitor patient closely.

Probenecid: May elevate level of ciprofloxacin. Monitor patient for toxicity.
Sucralfate: May decrease ciprofloxacin absorption, reducing anti-infective response. If use together can't be avoided, give at least 6 hours apart.
Theophylline: May increase theophylline level and prolong theophylline half-life. Monitor level of theophylline and watch for adverse effects.
Tizanidine: Increases tizanidine levels, causing low blood pressure, somnolence, dizziness, and slowed psychomotor skills. Avoid using together.
Warfarin: May increase anticoagulant effects. Monitor PT and INR closely.
Drug-herb. *Dong quai, St. John's wort:* May cause photosensitivity. Advise patient to avoid excessive sunlight exposure.
Yerba maté: May decrease clearance of herb's methylxanthines and cause toxicity. Discourage use together.
Drug-food. *Caffeine:* May increase effect of caffeine. Monitor patient closely.
Dairy products, other foods: May delay peak drug levels. Advise patient to take drug on an empty stomach.
Orange juice fortified with calcium: May decrease GI absorption of drug, reducing its effects. Discourage use together.
Drug-lifestyle. *Sun exposure:* May cause photosensitivity reactions. Advise patient to avoid excessive sunlight exposure.

EFFECTS ON LAB TEST RESULTS

● May increase alkaline phosphatase, ALT, AST, bilirubin, BUN, creatinine, LDH, and GGT levels.
● May increase eosinophil count. May decrease WBC, neutrophil, and platelet counts.

CONTRAINDICATIONS & CAUTIONS

● Contraindicated in patients sensitive to fluoroquinolones.
● Use cautiously in patients with CNS disorders, such as severe cerebral arteriosclerosis or seizure disorders, and in those at risk for seizures. Drug may cause CNS stimulation.
● Drug is associated with increased risk of adverse reactions involving joints, tendons, and surrounding tissues in children younger than age 18.

NURSING CONSIDERATIONS

- Monitor patient's intake and output and observe patient for signs of crystalluria.
- Tendon rupture may occur in patients receiving quinolones. If pain or inflammation occurs or if patient ruptures a tendon, stop drug.
- Long-term therapy may result in overgrowth of organisms resistant to drug.
- Cutaneous anthrax patients with signs of systemic involvement, extensive edema, or lesions on the head or neck need I.V. therapy and a multidrug approach.
- Additional antimicrobials for anthrax multidrug regimens can include rifampin, vancomycin, penicillin, ampicillin, chloramphenicol, imipenem, clindamycin, and clarithromycin.
- Steroids may be used as adjunctive therapy for anthrax patients with severe edema and for meningitis.
- Follow current Centers for Disease Control and Prevention (CDC) recommendations for anthrax.
- Pregnant women and immunocompromised patients should receive the usual doses and regimens for anthrax.

PATIENT TEACHING

- Tell patient to take drug as prescribed, even after he feels better.
- Advise patient to drink plenty of fluids to reduce risk of urine crystals.
- Advise patient not to crush, split, or chew the extended-release tablets.
- Warn patient to avoid hazardous tasks that require alertness, such as driving, until effects of drug are known.
- Instruct patient to avoid caffeine while taking drug because of potential for increased caffeine effects.
- Advise patient that hypersensitivity reactions may occur even after first dose. If a rash or other allergic reaction occurs, tell him to stop drug immediately and notify prescriber.
- Tell patient that tendon rupture can occur with drug and to notify prescriber if he experiences pain or inflammation.
- Tell patient to avoid excessive sunlight or artificial ultraviolet light during therapy.
- Because drug appears in breast milk, advise woman to stop breast-feeding during treatment or to consider treatment with another drug.

SAFETY ALERT!

cisplatin (CDDP)
SIS-pla-tin

Platinol, Platinol AQ

Pharmacologic class: platinum coordination complex
Pregnancy risk category D

AVAILABLE FORMS
Injection: 0.5 mg/ml†, 1 mg/ml

INDICATIONS & DOSAGES
➤ **Adjunctive therapy in metastatic testicular cancer**
Adults: 20 mg/m² I.V. daily for 5 days. Repeat every 3 weeks for three or four cycles.
➤ **Adjunctive therapy in metastatic ovarian cancer**
Adults: 100 mg/m² I.V.; repeat every 4 weeks. Or, 75 to 100 mg/m² I.V. once every 4 weeks with cyclophosphamide.
➤ **Advanced bladder cancer**
Adults: 50 to 70 mg/m² I.V. every 3 to 4 weeks. Give 50 mg/m² every 4 weeks in patients who have received other antineoplastics or radiation therapy.
➤ **Cervical cancer** ♦
Adults: 40 to 75 mg/m² I.V. weekly or daily as monotherapy, in combination therapy, or with radiation therapy.
➤ **Non small-cell lung cancer** ♦
Adults: 75 to 100 mg/m² I.V. every 3 to 4 weeks in combination therapy.
➤ **Osteogenic sarcoma or neuroblastoma** ♦
Children ♦: 90 mg/m² I.V. every 3 weeks, or 30 mg/m² I.V. once weekly.
➤ **Recurrent brain tumor** ♦
Children: 60 mg/m² I.V. daily for 2 consecutive days every 3 to 4 weeks.
➤ **Head and neck cancer** ♦
Adults: 80 to 120 mg/m² I.V. every 3 weeks or 50 mg/m² I.V. on days 1 and 8 every 4 weeks. Doses of 50 to 120 mg/m² I.V. may be used in combination therapy.

ADMINISTRATION
I.V.
- Preparing and giving parenteral form of drug may be mutagenic, teratogenic,

or carcinogenic. Follow facility policy to reduce risks.
• Hydrate patient with normal saline solution before giving drug. Maintain urine output of at least 100 ml/hour for 4 consecutive hours before therapy and for 24 hours after therapy.
• Reconstitute powder using sterile water for injection. Add 10 ml to 10-mg vial or 50 ml to 50-mg vial to make a solution containing 1 mg/ml.
• Infusions are most stable in solutions containing chloride (such as normal or half-normal saline solution and 0.22% sodium chloride). Don't use D_5W alone.
• Further dilute with dextrose 5% in 0.3% sodium chloride injection or dextrose 5% in half-normal saline solution for injection.
• Give mannitol or furosemide boluses or infusions before and during cisplatin infusion to maintain diuresis of 100 to 400 ml/hour during and for 24 hours after therapy.
• Add potassium chloride (10 to 20 mEq/L) to I.V. fluids before and after cisplatin therapy to prevent hypokalemia. Add magnesium sulfate to I.V. fluids before and after therapy to prevent hypomagnesemia.
• Give drug as an I.V. infusion in 2 L of dextrose 5% in half-normal saline solution or dextrose 5% in 0.33% sodium chloride solution with 37.5 g of mannitol over 6 to 8 hours.
• Solutions are stable for 20 hours at room temperature. Don't refrigerate.
• **Incompatibilities:** Aluminum administration sets, amifostine, amphotericin B cholesteryl sulfate complex, cefepime, D_5W, etoposide with mannitol and potassium chloride, fluorouracil, mesna, 0.1% sodium chloride solution, paclitaxel, piperacillin sodium with tazobactam sodium, sodium bicarbonate, sodium bisulfate, sodium thiosulfate, solutions with a chloride content less than 2%, thiotepa.

ACTION
May cross-link strands of cellular DNA and interfere with RNA transcription, causing an imbalance of growth that leads to cell death. Not specific to cell cycle.

Route	Onset	Peak	Duration
I.V.	Unknown	Unknown	Several days

Half-life: Initial phase, 25 to 79 minutes; terminal phase, 58 to 78 hours.

ADVERSE REACTIONS
CNS: *peripheral neuritis,* **seizures.**
EENT: *tinnitus, hearing loss, ototoxicity,* vestibular toxicity, optic neuritis, papilledema, cerebral blindness, blurred vision.
GI: loss of taste, *nausea, vomiting.*
GU: PROLONGED RENAL TOXICITY WITH REPEATED COURSES OF THERAPY.
Hematologic: MYELOSUPPRESSION, *leukopenia, thrombocytopenia,* anemia.
Metabolic: *hypomagnesemia,* hypokalemia, hypocalcemia, hyponatremia, hypophosphatemia, hyperuricemia.
Other: **anaphylactoid reaction.**

INTERACTIONS
Drug-drug. *Aminoglycosides:* May increase nephrotoxicity. Carefully monitor renal function study results.
Aminoglycosides, bumetanide, ethacrynic acid, furosemide, torsemide: May increase ototoxicity. Avoid using together, if possible.
Aspirin, NSAIDs: May increase risk of bleeding. Avoid using together.
Fosphenytoin, phenytoin: May decrease phenytoin and fosphenytoin levels. Monitor levels.
Myelosuppressives: May increase myelosuppression. Monitor patient.

EFFECTS ON LAB TEST RESULTS
• May increase uric acid level. May decrease calcium, hemoglobin, magnesium, phosphate, potassium, and sodium levels.
• May decrease platelet and WBC counts.

CONTRAINDICATIONS & CAUTIONS
• Contraindicated in patients hypersensitive to drug or other platinum-containing compounds and in those with severe renal disease, hearing impairment, or myelosuppression.
• Use cautiously in patients previously treated with radiation or cytotoxic drugs and in those with peripheral neuropathies;

also use cautiously with other ototoxic and nephrotoxic drugs.

NURSING CONSIDERATIONS
● Monitor CBC, electrolyte levels (especially potassium and magnesium), platelet count, and renal function studies before initial and subsequent doses.
● To detect hearing loss, obtain audiometry tests before initial and subsequent doses.
● Prehydration and mannitol diuresis may significantly reduce renal toxicity and ototoxicity.
● Therapeutic effects are frequently accompanied by toxicity.
● Some prescribers use I.V. sodium thiosulfate or amifostine to minimize toxicity. Check current protocol.
● Patients may experience vomiting 3 to 5 days after treatment, requiring prolonged antiemetic treatment. Some prescribers combine metoclopramide with dexamethasone and antihistamines, or ondansetron or granisetron with dexamethasone to control vomiting. Monitor intake and output. Continue I.V. hydration until patient can tolerate adequate oral intake.
● Renal toxicity is cumulative; don't give next dose until renal function returns to normal.
● Don't repeat dose unless platelet count exceeds $100,000/mm^3$, WBC count exceeds $4,000/mm^3$, creatinine level is below 1.5 mg/dl, creatinine clearance is 50 ml/minute or more, and BUN level is below 25 mg/dl.
● To prevent bleeding, avoid all I.M. injections when platelet count is less than $50,000/mm^3$.
● Anticipate need for blood transfusions during treatment because of cumulative anemia.
● *Alert:* Immediately give epinephrine, corticosteroids, or antihistamines for anaphylactoid reactions.
● Safety of drug in children hasn't been established.
● *Look alike–sound alike:* Don't confuse cisplatin with carboplatin; they aren't interchangeable.

PATIENT TEACHING
● Advise patient to watch for signs and symptoms of infection (fever, sore throat, fatigue) and bleeding (easy bruising,

nosebleeds, bleeding gums, tarry stools). Tell patient to take temperature daily.
● Tell patient to immediately report ringing in the ears or numbness in hands or feet.
● Instruct patient to avoid OTC products containing aspirin.
● Advise women to stop breast-feeding during therapy because of risk of toxicity to infant.
● Advise women of childbearing age to consult prescriber before becoming pregnant.

clemastine fumarate
KLEM-as-teen

Dayhist-1 ◊, Tavist Allergy ◊

Pharmacologic class: ethanolamine
Pregnancy risk category B

AVAILABLE FORMS
Syrup: 0.67 mg (equivalent to 0.5 mg clemastine)/5 ml*
Tablets: 1.34 mg (equivalent to 1 mg clemastine) ◊, 2.68 mg (equivalent to 2 mg clemastine)

INDICATIONS & DOSAGES
➤ **Rhinitis, allergy symptoms**
Adults and children age 12 and older: 1.34 mg P.O. b.i.d.; not to exceed 8.04 mg/day for syrup and 2.68 mg/day for tablets.
Children ages 6 to 11: Give 0.67 mg syrup P.O. b.i.d.; not to exceed 4.02 mg/day.
➤ **Allergic skin manifestation of urticaria and angioedema**
Adults and children age 12 and older: 2.68 mg P.O. b.i.d.; not to exceed 8.04 mg daily.
Children ages 6 to 11: Give 1.34 mg syrup P.O. b.i.d.; not to exceed 4.02 mg/day.

ADMINISTRATION
P.O.
● Give drug without regard for food.

ACTION
Competes with histamine for H_1-receptor sites effector cells. Drug prevents, but doesn't reverse, histamine-mediated responses.

Route	Onset	Peak	Duration
P.O.	15–60 min	5–7 hr	12 hr

Half-life: Unknown.

ADVERSE REACTIONS
CNS: *incoordination, dizziness, sleepiness, sedation, drowsiness,* **seizures,** nervousness, tremor, confusion, restlessness, vertigo, headache, fatigue.
CV: hypotension, palpitations, tachycardia.
GI: *dry mouth, epigastric distress,* anorexia, diarrhea, nausea, vomiting, constipation.
GU: urine retention, urinary frequency.
Hematologic: hemolytic anemia, ***thrombocytopenia, agranulocytosis.***
Respiratory: *thick bronchial secretions.*
Skin: rash, urticaria, photosensitivity, diaphoresis.
Other: *anaphylactic shock.*

INTERACTIONS
Drug-drug. *CNS depressants:* May increase sedation. Use together cautiously.
MAO inhibitors: May increase anticholinergic effects. Avoid using together.
Drug-lifestyle. *Alcohol use:* May increase CNS depression. Discourage use together.
Sun exposure: May cause photosensitivity reactions. Advise patient to avoid extensive sunlight exposure.

EFFECTS ON LAB TEST RESULTS
• May decrease hemoglobin level and hematocrit.
• May decrease granulocyte and platelet counts.
• May prevent, reduce, or mask positive result in diagnostic skin test.

CONTRAINDICATIONS & CAUTIONS
• Contraindicated in patients hypersensitive to drug or other antihistamines of similar chemical structure, in those taking MAO inhibitors, and in those with acute asthma, angle-closure glaucoma, stenosing peptic ulcer, symptomatic prostatic hyperplasia, bladder neck obstruction, or pyloroduodenal obstruction.
• Contraindicated in neonates, premature infants, and breast-feeding women.
• Use cautiously in elderly patients and in those with increased intraocular pressure, hyperthyroidism, CV disease, hypertension, bronchial asthma, and prostatic hyperplasia.
• Use in children younger than age 12 only as directed by prescriber.

NURSING CONSIDERATIONS
• Stop drug 4 days before diagnostic skin testing because antihistamines can prevent, reduce, or mask positive skin test result.
• Monitor blood counts during long-term therapy; observe for signs of blood dyscrasias.

PATIENT TEACHING
• Warn patient to avoid alcohol and hazardous activities that require alertness until CNS effects of drug are known.
• Inform patient that sugarless gum, hard candy, or ice chips may relieve dry mouth.
• Warn patient of possible photosensitivity reactions. Advise use of a sunblock.
• Tell patient to notify prescriber if tolerance develops because a different antihistamine may need to be prescribed.

clomipramine hydrochloride
kloe-MI-pra-meen

Anafranil

Pharmacologic class: tricyclic antidepressant (TCA)
Pregnancy risk category C

AVAILABLE FORMS
Capsules: 25 mg, 50 mg, 75 mg

INDICATIONS & DOSAGES
➤ **Obsessive-compulsive disorder**
Adults: Initially, 25 mg P.O. daily with meals, gradually increased to 100 mg daily in divided doses during first 2 weeks. Thereafter, increase to maximum dose of 250 mg daily in divided doses with meals, as needed. After adjustment, give total daily dose at bedtime.
Children and adolescents: Initially, 25 mg P.O. daily with meals, gradually increased over first 2 weeks to daily maximum of 3 mg/kg or 100 mg P.O. in divided doses, whichever is smaller. Maximum daily dose is 3 mg/kg or 200 mg, whichever is smaller; give at bedtime after adjustment. Reassess and adjust dosage periodically.

➤ **To manage panic disorder with or without agoraphobia**
Adults: 12.5 to 150 mg P.O. daily (maximum 200 mg).
➤ **Depression, chronic pain ♦**
Adults: 100 to 250 mg P.O. daily.
➤ **Cataplexy and related narcolepsy ♦**
Adults: 25 to 200 mg P.O. daily.

ADMINISTRATION
P.O.
● Give drug without regard for food.

ACTION
Unknown. Inhibits reuptake of serotonin and norepinephrine at the presynaptic neuron.

Route	Onset	Peak	Duration
P.O.	Unknown	2–6 hr	Unknown

Half-life: Parent compound, 32 hours; active metabolite, 69 hours.

ADVERSE REACTIONS
CNS: *somnolence, tremor, dizziness, headache, insomnia, nervousness, myoclonus, fatigue, **seizures,** EEG changes.*
CV: orthostatic hypotension, palpitations, tachycardia.
EENT: *pharyngitis, rhinitis, visual changes.*
GI: *dry mouth, constipation, nausea, dyspepsia, increased appetite, anorexia, abdominal pain,* diarrhea.
GU: *urinary hesitancy,* UTI, *dysmenorrhea, ejaculation failure, impotence.*
Hematologic: purpura.
Metabolic: *weight gain.*
Musculoskeletal: *myalgia.*
Skin: *diaphoresis,* rash, pruritus, dry skin.
Other: *altered libido.*

INTERACTIONS
Drug-drug. *Barbiturates:* May decrease TCA level. Watch for decreased antidepressant effect.
*Cimetidine, **fluoxetine, fluvoxamine, paroxetine, sertraline:** May increase TCA level.
Monitor drug level and patient for signs of toxicity.
Clonidine: May cause life-threatening hypertension. Avoid using together.
CNS depressants: May enhance CNS depression. Avoid using together.

Epinephrine, norepinephrine: May increase hypertensive effect. Use together cautiously.
MAO inhibitors: May cause hyperpyretic crisis, seizures, coma, or death. Avoid using within 14 days of MAO inhibitor therapy.
Quinolones: May increase the risk of life-threatening arrhythmias. Avoid using together.
Drug-herb. *Evening primrose oil:* May cause additive or synergistic effect, resulting in lower seizure threshold and increasing the risk of seizure. Discourage use together.
St. John's wort, SAM-e, yohimbe: May cause serotonin syndrome. Discourage use together.
Drug-lifestyle. *Alcohol use:* May enhance CNS depression. Discourage use together.
Sun exposure: May increase risk of photosensitivity reactions. Advise patient to avoid excessive sunlight exposure.

EFFECTS ON LAB TEST RESULTS
None reported.

CONTRAINDICATIONS & CAUTIONS
● Contraindicated in patients hypersensitive to drug or other tricyclic antidepressants, in those who have taken MAO inhibitors within previous 14 days, and in patients in acute recovery period after MI.
● Use cautiously in patients with history of seizure disorders or with brain damage of varying cause; in patients receiving other seizure threshold–lowering drugs; in patients at risk for suicide; in patients with history of urine retention or angle-closure glaucoma, increased intraocular pressure, CV disease, impaired hepatic or renal function, or hyperthyroidism; in patients with tumors of the adrenal medulla; in patients receiving thyroid drug or electroconvulsive therapy; and in those undergoing elective surgery.

NURSING CONSIDERATIONS
● Monitor mood and watch for suicidal tendencies. Allow patient to have only the minimum amount of drug.
● *Alert:* Drug may increase risk of suicidal thinking and behavior in children, adolescents, and young adults ages 18 to 24 during the first 2 months of treatment,

---

Reactions may be *common,* uncommon, *life-threatening,* or COMMON AND LIFE-THREATENING.
Interaction may have a *rapid onset* or ***delayed onset.***

especially in those with major depressive disorder or other psychiatric disorder.
• Don't withdraw drug abruptly.
• Because patients may suffer hypertensive episodes during surgery, stop drug gradually several days before surgery.
• Relieve dry mouth with sugarless candy or gum. Saliva substitutes may be needed.
• *Look alike–sound alike:* Don't confuse clomipramine with chlorpromazine or clomiphene, or Anafranil with enalapril, nafarelin, or alfentanil.

PATIENT TEACHING
• Warn patient to avoid hazardous activities requiring alertness and good coordination, especially during adjustment. Daytime sedation and dizziness may occur.
• Tell patient to avoid alcohol during drug therapy.
• Warn patient not to stop drug suddenly.
• Advise patient to use sunblock, wear protective clothing, and avoid prolonged exposure to strong sunlight to prevent oversensitivity to the sun.

SAFETY ALERT!

codeine phosphate
koe-DEEN

codeine sulfate

Pharmacologic class: opioid
Pregnancy risk category C
Controlled substance schedule II

AVAILABLE FORMS
codeine phosphate
Injection: 15 mg/ml, 30 mg/ml, 60 mg/ml†
Oral solution: 15 mg/5 ml, 10 mg/ml†
codeine sulfate
Tablets: 15 mg, 30 mg, 60 mg

INDICATIONS & DOSAGES
➤ **Mild to moderate pain**
Adults: 15 to 60 mg P.O. or 15 to 60 mg (phosphate) subcutaneously, I.M., or I.V. every 4 to 6 hours p.r.n. Maximum daily dose is 360 mg.
Children older than age 1: Give 0.5 mg/kg P.O., subcutaneously, or I.M. every 4 to 6 hours p.r.n. Don't give I.V. in children.

➤ **Nonproductive cough**
Adults: 10 to 20 mg P.O. every 4 to 6 hours. Maximum daily dose is 120 mg.
Children ages 6 to 12: 5 to 10 mg P.O. every 4 to 6 hours. Maximum daily dose is 60 mg.
Children ages 2 to 5: Give 2.5 to 5 mg P.O. every 4 to 6 hours. Maximum daily dose is 30 mg.

ADMINISTRATION
P.O.
• Give drug with milk or meals to avoid GI upset.
I.V.
• Don't give discolored solution.
• Give drug by direct injection into a large vein. Give very slowly.
• **Incompatibilities:** Aminophylline, ammonium chloride, amobarbital, bromides, chlorothiazide, heparin, iodides, pentobarbital, phenobarbital, phenytoin, salts of heavy metals, sodium bicarbonate, sodium iodide, thiopental.
I.M.
• Document injection site.
Subcutaneous
• Assess injection site for local irritation, pain, and induration.

ACTION
May bind with opioid receptors in the CNS, altering perception of and emotional response to pain. Also suppresses the cough reflex by direct action on the cough center in the medulla.

Route	Onset	Peak	Duration
P.O.	30–45 min	1–2 hr	4–6 hr
I.V.	Immediate	Immediate	4–6 hr
I.M.	10–30 min	30–60 min	4–6 hr
Subcut	10–30 min	Unknown	4–6 hr

Half-life: 2½ to 4 hours.

ADVERSE REACTIONS
CNS: *clouded sensorium, sedation,* dizziness, euphoria, light-headedness, physical dependence.
CV: *bradycardia,* flushing, hypotension.
GI: *constipation,* dry mouth, ileus, nausea, vomiting.
GU: urine retention.
Respiratory: *respiratory depression.*
Skin: *diaphoresis,* pruritus.

INTERACTIONS
Drug-drug. *CNS depressants, general anesthetics, hypnotics, MAO inhibitors, other opioid analgesics, sedatives, tranquilizers, tricyclic antidepressants:* May cause additive effects. Use together cautiously; monitor patient response.
Drug-lifestyle. *Alcohol use:* May cause additive effects. Discourage use together.

EFFECTS ON LAB TEST RESULTS
● May increase amylase and lipase levels.

CONTRAINDICATIONS & CAUTIONS
● Contraindicated in patients hypersensitive to drug.
● I.V. use contraindicated in children.
● Use cautiously in elderly or debilitated patients and in those with head injury, increased intracranial pressure, increased CSF pressure, hepatic or renal disease, hypothyroidism, Addison disease, acute alcoholism, seizures, severe CNS depression, bronchial asthma, COPD, respiratory depression, and shock.
● *Alert:* Breast-feeding mothers may put their infants at increased risk of morphine overdose if the mother is an ultra-rapid codeine metabolizer.

NURSING CONSIDERATIONS
● Reassess patient's level of pain at least 15 and 30 minutes after use.
● Codeine and aspirin or acetaminophen are commonly prescribed together to provide enhanced pain relief.
● For full analgesic effect, give drug before patient has intense pain.
● Drug is an antitussive and shouldn't be used when cough is a valuable diagnostic sign or is beneficial (as after thoracic surgery).
● Monitor cough type and frequency.
● Monitor respiratory and circulatory status.
● Opioids may cause constipation. Assess bowel function and need for stool softeners and stimulant laxatives.
● Codeine may delay gastric emptying, increase biliary tract pressure from contraction of the sphincter of Oddi, and interfere with hepatobiliary imaging studies.
● *Look alike–sound alike:* Don't confuse codeine with Cardene, Lodine, or Cordran.

PATIENT TEACHING
● Advise patient that GI distress caused by taking drug P.O. can be eased by taking drug with milk or meals.
● Instruct patient to ask for or to take drug before pain is intense.
● Caution ambulatory patient about getting out of bed or walking. Warn outpatient to avoid driving and other hazardous activities that require mental alertness until drug's effects on the CNS are known.
● Advise patient to avoid alcohol during therapy.
● Warn breast-feeding woman to watch for increased sleepiness, difficulty breast-feeding, or breathing, or limpness of infant. Tell her to immediately seek medical attention if this occurs.

SAFETY ALERT!

cyclophosphamide
sye-kloe-FOSS-fa-mide

Cytoxan, Cytoxan Lyophilized, Neosar, Procytox†

Pharmacologic class: nitrogen mustard
Pregnancy risk category D

AVAILABLE FORMS
Injection: 100-mg, 200-mg, 500-mg, 1-g, 2-g vials
Tablets: 25 mg, 50 mg

INDICATIONS & DOSAGES
➤ **Breast or ovarian cancer, Hodgkin lymphoma, chronic lymphocytic leukemia, chronic myelocytic leukemia, acute lymphoblastic leukemia, acute myelocytic leukemia, acute monocytic leukemia, neuroblastoma, retinoblastoma, malignant lymphoma, multiple myeloma, mycosis fungoides, sarcoma**
Adults: Initially for induction, 40 to 50 mg/kg I.V. in divided doses over 2 to 5 days. Or, 10 to 15 mg/kg I.V. every 7 to 10 days, 3 to 5 mg/kg I.V. twice weekly, or 1 to 5 mg/kg P.O. daily, based on patient tolerance.
Children: Initially for induction, 2 to 8 mg/kg or 60 to 250 mg/m^2 P.O. or I.V.

daily. Maintenance dose is 2 to 5 mg/kg P.O. or 50 to 150 mg/m² P.O. twice weekly.

Adjust subsequent doses according to evidence of antitumor activity or leukopenia.

➤ **Minimal-change nephrotic syndrome**
Children: 2 to 3 mg/kg P.O. daily for 60 to 90 days.

ADMINISTRATION
P.O.
● Don't give drug at bedtime; infrequent urination during the night may increase possibility of cystitis.
I.V.
● Preparing and giving parenteral form of drug may be mutagenic, teratogenic, or carcinogenic. Follow facility policy to reduce risks.
● Reconstitute powder using sterile water for injection or bacteriostatic water for injection containing only parabens.
● For the nonlyophilized product, add 5 ml to 100-mg vial, 10 ml to 200-mg vial, 25 ml to 500-mg vial, 50 ml to 1-g vial, or 100 ml to 2-g vial to produce a solution containing 20 mg/ml. Shake vigorously to dissolve. If powder doesn't dissolve completely, let vial stand for a few minutes.
● Lyophilized product is much easier to reconstitute; check package insert for amount of diluent needed.
● Check reconstituted solution for small particles. Filter solution, if needed.
● Give by direct I.V. injection or infusion.
● For infusion, further dilute with D₅W, dextrose 5% in normal saline solution for injection, dextrose 5% in Ringer's injection, lactated Ringer's injection, sodium lactate injection, or half-normal saline solution for injection.
● Reconstituted solution is stable 6 days if refrigerated or 24 hours at room temperature. Use stored solutions cautiously because drug contains no preservatives.
● **Incompatibilities:** Amphotericin B cholesteryl sulfate complex.

ACTION
Cross-links strands of cellular DNA and interferes with RNA transcription, causing an imbalance of growth that leads to cell death. Not specific to cell cycle.

Route	Onset	Peak	Duration
P.O.	Unknown	Unknown	Unknown
I.V.	Unknown	2–3 hr	Unknown

Half-life: 3 to 12 hours.

ADVERSE REACTIONS
CV: *cardiotoxicity with very high doses and with doxorubicin,* flushing.
GI: *nausea and vomiting,* anorexia, abdominal pain, stomatitis, mucositis.
GU: HEMORRHAGIC CYSTITIS, impaired fertility.
Hematologic: *leukopenia, thrombocytopenia,* anemia.
Hepatic: *hepatotoxicity.*
Metabolic: hyperuricemia, SIADH.
Respiratory: *pulmonary fibrosis with high doses.*
Skin: *reversible alopecia,* rash, pigmentation, nail changes, itching.
Other: *secondary malignant disease, anaphylaxis,* hypersensitivity reactions.

INTERACTIONS
Drug-drug. *Allopurinol, myelosuppressives:* May increase myelosuppression. Monitor patient for toxicity.
Anticoagulants: May increase anticoagulant effect. Monitor patient for bleeding.
Aspirin, NSAIDs: May increase risk of bleeding. Avoid using together.
Barbiturates: May enhance cyclophosphamide toxicity. Monitor patient closely.
Cardiotoxic drugs: May increase adverse cardiac effects. Monitor patient for toxicity.
Chloramphenicol, corticosteroids: May reduce activity of cyclophosphamide. Use together cautiously.
Ciprofloxacin: May decrease antimicrobial effect. Monitor patient for effect.
Digoxin: May decrease digoxin level. Monitor level closely.
Succinylcholine: May prolong neuromuscular blockade. Avoid using together.
Thiazide diuretics: May prolong antineoplastic-induced leukopenia. Monitor patient closely.

EFFECTS ON LAB TEST RESULTS
● May increase uric acid level. May decrease hemoglobin and pseudocholinesterase levels.

• May decrease platelet, RBC, and WBC counts.

• May suppress positive reaction to *Candida*, mumps, *Trichophyton*, and tuberculin skin test results. May cause a false-positive Papanicolaou test result.

CONTRAINDICATIONS & CAUTIONS

• Contraindicated in patients hypersensitive to drug and in those with severe bone marrow suppression.

• Use cautiously in patients with leukopenia, thrombocytopenia, malignant cell infiltration of bone marrow, or hepatic or renal disease and in those who have recently undergone radiation therapy or chemotherapy.

NURSING CONSIDERATIONS

• If cystitis occurs, stop drug and notify prescriber. Cystitis can occur months after therapy ends. Mesna may be given to reduce frequency and severity of bladder toxicity. Test urine for blood.

• Adequately hydrate patients before and after dose to decrease risk of cystitis.

• Use caution to ensure correct dose to decrease risk of cardiac toxicity.

• Monitor CBC and renal and liver function test results.

• Monitor patient closely for leukopenia (nadir between days 8 and 15, recovery in 17 to 28 days).

• Monitor uric acid level. To prevent hyperuricemia with resulting uric acid nephropathy, allopurinol may be used with adequate hydration.

• To prevent bleeding, avoid all I.M. injections when platelet count is less than 50,000/mm^3.

• Anticipate blood transfusions because of cumulative anemia. Patients may receive injections of RBC colony-stimulating factor to promote RBC production and decrease need for blood transfusions.

• Therapeutic effects are often accompanied by toxicity.

• In boys, using drug for nephrotic syndrome for more than 60 days increases the incidence of oligospermia and azoospermia. Use for more than 90 days increases the risk of sterility.

• Drug may be used to treat nononcologic disorders, such as lupus, nephritis, and rheumatoid arthritis.

PATIENT TEACHING

• Warn patient that hair loss is likely to occur but is reversible.

• Advise patient to watch for signs and symptoms of infection (fever, sore throat, fatigue) and bleeding (easy bruising, nosebleeds, bleeding gums, tarry stools). Tell patient to take temperature daily.

• Instruct patient to avoid OTC products that contain aspirin.

• To minimize risk of hemorrhagic cystitis, encourage patient to urinate every 1 to 2 hours while awake and to drink at least 3 L of fluid daily.

• If patient is taking tablets, tell him not to take it at bedtime because infrequent urination increases risk of cystitis.

• Advise both men and women to practice contraception during therapy and for 4 months afterward; drug may cause birth defects.

• Advise women to stop breast-feeding during therapy because of risk of toxicity to infant.

• Drug can cause irreversible sterility in both men and women. Before therapy, counsel patients who are considering parenthood. Also recommend that women consult prescriber before becoming pregnant.

---

cycloserine
sye-kloe-SER-een

Seromycin

Pharmacologic class: isoxazolidine derivative, d-alanine analogue
Pregnancy risk category C

AVAILABLE FORMS
Capsules: 250 mg

INDICATIONS & DOSAGES

➤ **Adjunctive treatment for pulmonary or extrapulmonary tuberculosis (TB)**

Adults: Initially, 250 mg P.O. every 12 hours for 2 weeks; then, if levels are below 25 to 30 mcg/ml and no toxicity has developed, increase dosage to 250 mg every 8 hours for 2 weeks. If optimum levels still aren't achieved and no toxicity has developed, then increase dosage to

---

250 mg every 6 hours. Maximum dosage is 1 g daily. If CNS toxicity occurs, stop drug for 1 week, then resume at 250 mg daily for 2 weeks. If no serious toxic effects occur, increase dosage by 250-mg increments every 10 days until level of 25 to 30 mcg/ml is obtained.
Children ♦: 10 to 20 mg/kg/day P.O. in two divided doses. Maximum dosage is 1 g daily.
➤ **Acute UTIs**
Adults: 250 mg P.O. every 12 hours for 2 weeks.

ADMINISTRATION
P.O.
● Drug is considered a second-line drug in TB treatment and should always be given with other antituberculotics to prevent the development of resistant organisms.

ACTION
Inhibits cell-wall biosynthesis by interfering with the bacterial use of amino acids; may be bacteriostatic or bactericidal, depending on the drug level attained at the site of infection and the organism's susceptibility.

Route	Onset	Peak	Duration
P.O.	Unknown	4–8 hr	Unknown

Half-life: 10 hours.

ADVERSE REACTIONS
CNS: *coma, seizures, suicidal behavior,* drowsiness, somnolence, headache, tremor, dysarthria, vertigo, confusion, loss of memory, psychosis, hyperirritability, paresthesia, paresis, hyperreflexia.
CV: *sudden heart failure.*
Other: hypersensitivity reactions (rash, photosensitivity).

INTERACTIONS
Drug-drug. *Ethionamide:* May increase neurotoxic adverse reactions. Monitor patient closely.
Isoniazid: May increase risk of CNS toxicity, causing dizziness or drowsiness. Monitor patient closely.

Drug-lifestyle. *Alcohol use:* May increase risk of CNS toxicity, causing seizures. Discourage use together.

EFFECTS ON LAB TEST RESULTS
● May increase transaminase levels.

CONTRAINDICATIONS & CAUTIONS
● Contraindicated in patients hypersensitive to drug, in those who use alcohol excessively, and in those with seizure disorders, depression, severe anxiety, psychosis, or severe renal insufficiency.
● Use cautiously in patients with impaired renal function; reduce dosage in these patients.

NURSING CONSIDERATIONS
● Obtain specimen for culture and sensitivity tests before therapy begins and then periodically to detect possible resistance.
● Use to treat UTIs only when better alternatives are contraindicated and susceptibility to cycloserine is confirmed.
● Monitor level periodically, especially in patients receiving high dosages (more than 500 mg daily), because toxic reactions may occur with levels above 30 mcg/ml.
● Watch patient receiving dosages of more than 500 mg daily for signs and symptoms of CNS toxicity, such as seizures, anxiety, and tremor. Giving 200 to 300 mg pyridoxine daily may help prevent neurotoxic effects.
● Monitor results of hematologic tests and renal and liver function tests.
● Observe patient for psychotic symptoms, hallucinations, and suicidal behavior.
● Monitor patient for hypersensitivity reactions, such as allergic dermatitis.
● Give anticonvulsant, tranquilizer, or sedative to relieve adverse reactions.

PATIENT TEACHING
● Warn patient to avoid alcohol, which may cause serious neurologic reactions.
● Advise patient not to perform hazardous activities if drowsiness occurs.
● Tell patient to report adverse reactions promptly; dosage may need to be adjusted or other drugs prescribed to relieve adverse reactions.

cyclosporine
SYE-kloe-spor-een

Sandimmune

cyclosporine, modified
Gengraf, Neoral

Pharmacologic class: immunosuppressive
Pregnancy risk category C

AVAILABLE FORMS
Capsules for microemulsion (modified):
25 mg, 50 mg, 100 mg
Capsules (nonmodified): 25 mg, 50 mg,
100 mg
Injection: 50 mg/ml
Oral solution (modified and nonmodified):
100 mg/ml

INDICATIONS & DOSAGES
➤ **To prevent organ rejection in
renal, hepatic, or cardiac transplantation**
Adults and children: 15 mg/kg P.O. 4 to
12 hours before transplantation and
continue daily for 1 to 2 weeks postoperatively. Then reduce dosage by 5%
each week to maintenance level of 5 to
10 mg/kg daily. Or, 5 to 6 mg/kg I.V.
concentrate 4 to 12 hours before transplantation as a continuous infusion. Postoperatively, repeat dose daily until patient can
tolerate P.O. forms.

For conversion from Sandimmune
to Gengraf or Neoral, use same daily
dose as previously used for Sandimmune.
Monitor blood levels every 4 to 7 days after conversion, and monitor blood pressure
and creatinine level every 2 weeks during
the first 2 months.
➤ **Severe, active rheumatoid arthritis (RA) that hasn't adequately
responded to methotrexate**
Adults: 2.5 mg/kg Gengraf or Neoral daily
P.O., taken b.i.d. as divided doses. Dosage
may be increased by 0.5 to 0.75 mg/kg
daily after 8 weeks and again after
12 weeks to a maximum of 4 mg/kg daily.
If no response is seen after 16 weeks, stop
therapy.

➤ **Psoriasis**
Adults: 1.25 mg/kg Gengraf or Neoral
daily P.O. b.i.d. for at least 4 weeks. Increase dosage by 0.5 mg/kg daily once
every 2 weeks as needed to a maximum of
4 mg/kg daily.
Adjust-a-dose: For patients with adverse
effects such as hypertension, creatinine
level 30% above pretreatment level, or
abnormal CBC count or liver function test
results, decrease dosage by 25% to 50%.

ADMINISTRATION
P.O.
● Give Neoral or Gengraf on an empty
stomach.
● Measure oral solution doses carefully in
an oral syringe. Don't rinse dosing syringe
with water. If syringe is cleaned, it must be
completely dry before reuse.
● To improve the taste of Sandimmune
oral solution, mix it with milk, chocolate
milk, or orange juice. Gengraf or Neoral
oral solution may be mixed with orange or
apple juice (not grapefruit juice); it's less
palatable when mixed with milk.
● Use a glass container to mix, and have
patient drink at once.
I.V.
● This form is usually reserved for patients
who can't tolerate oral drugs.
● Immediately before use, dilute each
milliliter of concentrate in 20 to 100 ml
of D_5W or normal saline solution for
injection. Give at one-third the oral dose.
● Infuse over 2 to 6 hours.
● Protect diluted drug from light.
● **Incompatibilities:** Amphotericin B
cholesteryl sulfate complex, magnesium
sulfate.

ACTION
May inhibit proliferation and function of
T lymphocytes and inhibit production and
release of lymphokines.

Route	Onset	Peak	Duration
P.O.	Unknown	90 min–3 hr	Unknown
I.V.	Unknown	Unknown	Unknown

Half-life: Initial phase, about 1 hour;
terminal phase, 8½ to 27 hours.

ADVERSE REACTIONS
CNS: *tremor, headache,* confusion, paresthesia.

CV: *hypertension,* flushing.
EENT: *gum hyperplasia,* sinusitis.
GI: *nausea, vomiting,* diarrhea, oral thrush, abdominal discomfort.
GU: NEPHROTOXICITY.
Hematologic: anemia, *leukopenia, thrombocytopenia.*
Hepatic: *hepatotoxicity.*
Metabolic: hyperglycemia.
Skin: *hirsutism,* acne.
Other: infections, *anaphylaxis,* gynecomastia.

INTERACTIONS
Drug-drug. *Acyclovir, aminoglycosides, amphotericin B, cimetidine, cotrimoxazole, diclofenac, gentamicin, ketoconazole, melphalan, NSAIDs, ranitidine, sulfamethoxazole and trimethoprim, tacrolimus, tobramycin, vancomycin:* May increase risk of nephrotoxicity. Avoid using together.
Allopurinol, **azole antifungals,** *bromocriptine,* **caspofungin,** *cimetidine, clarithromycin, danazol, diltiazem, erythromycin, imipenem and cilastatin, methylprednisolone, metoclopramide,* **micafungin,** *nicardipine, prednisolone, verapamil:* May increase cyclosporine level. Monitor patient for increased toxicity.
Azathioprine, corticosteroids, cyclophosphamide, verapamil: May increase immunosuppression. Monitor patient closely.
Carbamazepine, isoniazid, nafcillin, octreotide, **orlistat,** *phenobarbital,* **phenytoin, rifabutin, rifampin,** *ticlopidine:* May decrease immunosuppressant effect from low cyclosporine level. Cyclosporine dosage may need to be increased.
Digoxin, lovastatin, prednisolone: May decrease clearance of these drugs. Use together cautiously.
Mycophenolate mofetil: May decrease mycophenolate level. Monitor patient closely when cyclosporine is added to or removed from therapy.
Potassium-sparing diuretics: May induce hyperkalemia. Monitor patient closely.
Sirolimus: May increase sirolimus level. Take sirolimus at least 4 hours after cyclosporine dose. If separating doses isn't possible, monitor patient for increased adverse effects.
Vaccines: May decrease immune response. Delay routine immunization.

Drug-herb. *Astragalus, echinacea, licorice:* May interfere with drug's effect. Discourage use together.
St. John's wort: May reduce drug level, resulting in transplant failure. Discourage use together.
Drug-food. *Alfalfa sprouts:* May interfere with drug's effect. Discourage use together.
Grapefruit and grapefruit juices: May increase drug level and cause toxicity. Advise patient to avoid use together.
Drug-lifestyle. *Sunlight:* May increase risk of sensitivity to sunlight. Advise patient to avoid excessive sunlight exposure.

EFFECTS ON LAB TEST RESULTS
● May increase ALT, AST, bilirubin, BUN, creatinine, glucose, and LDL levels. May decrease hemoglobin and magnesium levels.
● May decrease platelet and WBC counts.

CONTRAINDICATIONS & CAUTIONS
● Contraindicated in patients hypersensitive to drug or polyoxyethylated castor oil (found in injectable form).
● Contraindicated in patients with RA or psoriasis with abnormal renal function, uncontrolled hypertension, or malignancies (Neoral or Gengraf).

NURSING CONSIDERATIONS
● Psoriasis patients previously treated with psoralen and ultraviolet light A, methotrexate or other immunosuppressive agents, UVB, coal tar, or radiation therapy are at an increased risk for skin malignancies when taking Neoral or Gengraf.
● Drug can cause nephrotoxicity and hepatotoxicity.
● Monitor elderly patient for renal impairment and hypertension.
● Monitor drug level at regular intervals. Absorption of oral solution can be erratic.
● Neoral and Gengraf have greater bioavailability than Sandimmune. A lower dose of Neoral or Gengraf may be needed to provide blood level similar to that achieved with Sandimmune. Monitor blood level when switching patients between these two brands.
● Gengraf is bioequivalent to and interchangeable with Neoral capsules.

• Always give with corticosteroids; however, don't give Sandimmune with other immunosuppressants.
• Use Neoral or Gengraf to treat RA or psoriasis.
• *Look alike–sound alike:* Don't confuse cyclosporine with cyclophosphamide or cycloserine. Don't confuse Sandimmune with Sandoglobulin or Sandostatin.

RA
• Before starting treatment, measure blood pressure at least twice and obtain two creatinine levels to estimate baseline.
• Evaluate blood pressure and creatinine level every 2 weeks during first 3 months and then monthly if patient is stable.
• Monitor blood pressure and creatinine level after an increase in NSAID dosage or introduction of a new NSAID. Monitor CBC and liver function tests monthly if patient also receives methotrexate.
• If hypertension occurs, decrease dosage of Gengraf or Neoral by 25% to 50%. If hypertension persists, decrease dosage further or control blood pressure with antihypertensives.

Psoriasis
• Measure blood pressure at least twice to determine a baseline.
• Evaluate patient for occult infection and tumors initially and throughout treatment.
• Obtain baseline creatinine level (on two occasions), CBC, and BUN, magnesium, uric acid, potassium, and lipid levels.
• Evaluate creatinine and BUN levels every 2 weeks during first 3 months and then monthly thereafter if patient is stable.
• If creatinine level is 25% above pretreatment levels, repeat creatinine level measurement within 2 weeks. If creatinine level stays 25% to 50% above baseline, reduce dosage by 25% to 50%. If creatinine level is ever 50% above baseline, reduce dosage by 25% to 50%. Stop therapy if creatinine level isn't reversed after two dosage modifications.
• Monitor creatinine level after increasing NSAID dose or starting a new NSAID.
• Evaluate blood pressure, CBC, and uric acid, potassium, lipid, and magnesium levels every 2 weeks for the first 3 months and then monthly if patient is stable, or more frequently if a dosage is adjusted.
• If an adverse reaction occurs, reduce dosage by 25% to 50%.

• Improvement in psoriasis takes 12 to 16 weeks of therapy.

PATIENT TEACHING
• Encourage patient to take drug at same time each day and to be consistent with relation to meals.
• Teach patient how to measure dosage and mask taste of oral solution. Tell him not to take drug with grapefruit juice.
• Instruct patient to fill glass with water after dose and drink it to make sure he consumes all of drug.
• Advise patient to take drug with meals if nausea occurs.
• Advise patient to take Neoral or Gengraf on an empty stomach.
• Tell patient being treated for psoriasis that improvement may not occur until after 12 to 16 weeks of therapy.
• Stress that drug shouldn't be stopped without prescriber's approval.
• Explain to patient the importance of frequent laboratory monitoring while receiving therapy.
• Tell patient to avoid people with infections because drug lowers resistance to infection.
• Advise patient to perform careful oral care and to see a dentist regularly because drug can cause gum disease.
• Advise woman to use barrier contraception, not hormonal contraceptives, during therapy. Advise her of the potential risk during pregnancy and the increased risk of tumors, high blood pressure, and renal problems.
• Warn patient to wear protection in the sun and to avoid excessive sun exposure.

SAFETY ALERT!

dalteparin sodium
DAHL-tep-ah-rin

Fragmin

Pharmacologic class:
low–molecular-weight heparin
Pregnancy risk category B

AVAILABLE FORMS
Injection: 2,500 antifactor Xa international units/0.2 ml syringe, 5,000 antifactor Xa international units/0.2 ml syringe,

7,500 antifactor Xa international units/0.3 ml syringe, 10,000 antifactor Xa international units/ml syringe, 10,000 antifactor Xa international units/ml in 9.5-ml multidose vial, 25,000 antifactor Xa international units/ml in 3.8-ml multidose vial. Each multidose vial contains 14 mg/ml of benzyl alcohol.

INDICATIONS & DOSAGES
➤ **To prevent deep vein thrombosis (DVT) in patients undergoing abdominal surgery who are at moderate to high risk for thromboembolic complications**
Adults: 2,500 international units subcutaneously daily, starting 1 to 2 hours before surgery and repeated once daily for 5 to 10 days postoperatively. Or, for patients at high risk, give 5,000 international units subcutaneously the evening before surgery, then once daily postoperatively for 5 to 10 days.
➤ **To prevent DVT in patients undergoing hip replacement surgery**
Adults: 2,500 international units subcutaneously within 2 hours before surgery and second dose 2,500 international units subcutaneously in the evening after surgery (at least 6 hours after first dose). If surgery is performed in the evening, omit second dose on day of surgery. Starting on first postoperative day, give 5,000 international units subcutaneously once daily for 5 to 10 days. Or, give 5,000 international units subcutaneously on the evening before surgery; then 5,000 international units subcutaneously once daily starting in the evening of surgery for 5 to 10 days postoperatively.
➤ **Unstable angina non–Q-wave MI**
Adults: 120 international units/kg subcutaneously every 12 hours with aspirin (75 to 165 mg daily) P.O., unless contraindicated. Maximum dose, 10,000 international units. Treatment usually lasts 5 to 8 days.
➤ **To prevent DVT in patients at risk for thromboembolic complications because of severely restricted mobility during acute illness**
Adults: 5,000 international units subcutaneously once daily for 12 to 14 days.
✱*NEW INDICATION:* Symptomatic venous thromboembolism in cancer patients

Adults: Initially, 200 international units/kg (maximum, 18,000 international units) subcutaneously daily for 30 days; then 150 international units/kg (maximum, 18,000 international units) subcutaneously daily months 2 through 6.
Adjust-a-dose: In patients with platelet count 50,000 to 100,000/mm³, reduce dose by 2,500 international units until platelet count exceeds 100,000/mm³. In patients with platelet count less than 50,000/mm³, stop drug until platelet count exceeds 50,000/mm³. For patients with creatinine clearance of 30 ml/minute or less, monitor anti-Xa levels to determine appropriate dose. Target anti-Xa range is 0.5 to 1.5 international units/ml. Draw anti-Xa 4 to 6 hours after dose and only after the patient has received three to four doses.

ADMINISTRATION
Subcutaneous
● Before giving injection, obtain complete list of all prescribed and OTC medications, and supplements, including herbs.
● Have patient sit or lie supine when giving drug.
● Injection sites include a U-shaped area around the navel, upper outer side of thigh, and upper outer quadrangle of buttock. Rotate sites daily.
● When area around the navel or thigh is used, use thumb and forefinger to lift up a fold of skin while giving injection.
● Give subcutaneous injection deeply, inserting the entire length of needle at a 45- to 90-degree angle.

ACTION
Enhances inhibition of factor Xa and thrombin by antithrombin.

Route	Onset	Peak	Duration
Subcut	Unknown	4 hr	Unknown

Half-life: 3 to 5 hours.

ADVERSE REACTIONS
CNS: fever.
GU: hematuria.
Hematologic: *thrombocytopenia, hemorrhage,* ecchymoses, bleeding complications.
Skin: pruritus, rash, *hematoma at injection site,* injection site pain.
Other: *anaphylaxis.*

INTERACTIONS

Drug-drug. *Antiplatelet drugs (aspirin, NSAIDs, clopidogrel, dipyridamole, ticlodipine), oral anticoagulants, thrombolytics:* May increase risk of bleeding. Use together cautiously.

Drug-herb. *Angelica (dong quai), boldo, bromelains, capsicum, chamomile, dandelion, danshen, devil's claw, fenugreek, feverfew, garlic, ginger, ginkgo, ginseng, horse chestnut, licorice, meadowsweet, onion, passion flower, red clover, willow:* May increase risk of bleeding. Discourage use together.

EFFECTS ON LAB TEST RESULTS

- May increase ALT and AST levels.
- May decrease platelet count.

CONTRAINDICATIONS & CAUTIONS

- Contraindicated in patients hypersensitive to drug, heparin, or pork products; in those with active major bleeding; and in those with thrombocytopenia and antiplatelet antibodies in presence of drug.
- Contraindicated in patients with unstable angina or non-Q-wave MI who are undergoing regional anesthesia because of an increased risk of bleeding associated with the dose of dalteparin recommended for these indications.
- Use with caution in patients with history of heparin-induced thrombocytopenia and in patients at increased risk for hemorrhage, such as those with severe uncontrolled hypertension, bacterial endocarditis, congenital or acquired bleeding disorders, active ulceration, angiodysplastic GI disease, or hemorrhagic stroke; also use with caution shortly after brain, spinal, or ophthalmic surgery. Monitor vital signs.
- Use with caution in patients with bleeding diathesis, thrombocytopenia, platelet defects, severe hepatic or renal insufficiency, hypertensive or diabetic retinopathy, or recent GI bleeding.

NURSING CONSIDERATIONS

- *Alert:* Patients who have received epidural or spinal anesthesia are at increased risk for developing an epidural or spinal hematoma, which may result in long-term or permanent paralysis. Monitor these patients closely for neurologic impairment.
- DVT is a risk factor in patients who are candidates for therapy, including those older than age 40, those who are obese, those undergoing surgery under general anesthesia lasting longer than 30 minutes, and those who have additional risk factors (such as malignancy or history of DVT or pulmonary embolism).
- Never give drug I.M.
- Don't mix with other injections or infusions unless specific compatibility data support such mixing.
- Multidose vial shouldn't be used in pregnant women because of benzyl alcohol content. Benzyl alcohol has been associated with fatal "gasping syndrome" in premature neonates.
- *Alert:* Drug isn't interchangeable (unit for unit) with unfractionated heparin or other low–molecular-weight heparin.
- Periodic, routine CBC and fecal occult blood tests are recommended during therapy. Patients don't need regular monitoring of PT or activated PTT.
- Monitor patient closely for thrombocytopenia.
- Stop drug if a thromboembolic event occurs despite dalteparin prophylaxis. May use alternative therapy, or may have been inadequate dose.
- Obtain a complete list of patient's prescription and OTC drugs and supplements, including herbs.

PATIENT TEACHING

- Instruct patient and family to watch for and report signs of bleeding (bruising and blood in stools).
- Tell patient to avoid OTC drugs containing aspirin or other salicylates unless ordered by prescriber.
- Advise patient to consult with prescriber prior to initiating any herbal therapy; many herbs have anticoagulant, antiplatelet, and fibrinolytic properties.
- Tell patient to use a soft toothbrush and electric razor during treatment.

---

desloratadine
dess-lor-AT-a-deen

Clarinex, Clarinex RediTabs

Pharmacologic class: piperidine
Pregnancy risk category C

AVAILABLE FORMS
Syrup: 2.5 mg/5 ml
Tablets: 5 mg
Tablets (orally disintegrating): 2.5 mg,
5 mg

INDICATIONS & DOSAGES
➤ **Seasonal allergic rhinitis (patients age 2 and older); perennial allergic rhinitis; chronic idiopathic urticaria**
Adults and children age 12 and older:
5 mg P.O. tablets or syrup once daily.
Children ages 6 to 11: 2.5 mg orally disintegrating tablet (ODT) or syrup P.O. once daily.
Children ages 12 months to 5 years:
1.25 mg P.O. once daily.
Infants ages 6 to 11 months: 1 mg P.O. once daily.
Adjust-a-dose: In adults with hepatic or renal impairment, start dosage at 5 mg P.O. every other day.

ADMINISTRATION
P.O.
● Give drug without regard for meals.
● Give ODTs with or without water.
● Store tablets at 36° to 86° F (2° to 30° C); store ODTs at 59° to 86° F (15° to 30° C).

ACTION
Long-acting tricyclic antihistamine with selective H_1-receptor histamine antagonist activity. It inhibits histamine release from human mast cells in vitro. Drug doesn't cross the blood-brain barrier.

Route	Onset	Peak	Duration
P.O.	< 1 hr	3 hr	Up to 24 hr
P.O. (orally disintegrating)	< 1 hr	2½–4 hr	Up to 24 hr

Half-life: 27 hours.

ADVERSE REACTIONS
CNS: *headache,* somnolence, fatigue, dizziness.
EENT: pharyngitis, dry throat.
GI: nausea, dry mouth.
Musculoskeletal: myalgia.
Other: flulike symptoms.

INTERACTIONS
None reported.

EFFECTS ON LAB TEST RESULTS
● May prevent, reduce, or mask positive result in diagnostic skin test.

CONTRAINDICATIONS & CAUTIONS
● Contraindicated in breast-feeding women and in patients hypersensitive to drug, to any of its components, or to loratadine.
● Use cautiously in elderly patients because of the greater likelihood of decreased hepatic, renal, or cardiac function, and concomitant disease or other drug therapy.

NURSING CONSIDERATIONS
● Stop drug 4 days before diagnostic skin testing because antihistamines can prevent, reduce, or mask positive skin test response.

PATIENT TEACHING
● Advise patient not to exceed recommended dosage. Higher doses don't increase effectiveness and may cause somnolence.
● Tell patient that drug can be taken without regard to meals.
● Instruct patient to remove ODTs from blister pack and place on tongue immediately to dissolve.
● ODTs may be taken with or without water.
● Tell patient to report adverse effects.

dextromethorphan hydrobromide
dex-troe-meth-OR-fan

Belminil DM † ◊, Benylin Adult ◊, Benylin Pediatric ◊, Creomulsion ◊, Creo-Terpin ◊*, Delsym ◊, DexAlone ◊, Hold DM ◊, Koffex DM† ◊, Pertussin DM ◊*, Robitussin ◊, Robitussin Pediatric ◊, Scot-Tussin ◊, Simply Cough ◊, Sucrets Cough ◊, Theraflu Thin Strips ◊*, Triaminic ◊*, Trocal ◊, Vicks Formula 44 ◊

Pharmacologic class: levorphanol derivative
Pregnancy risk category C

AVAILABLE FORMS
Gelcaps: 15 mg ◊, 30 mg ◊
Liquid (extended-release): 30 mg/5 ml ◊
Lozenges: 5 mg ◊, 7.5 mg ◊, 10 mg ◊
Solution: 3.5 mg/5 ml, 5 mg/5 ml ◊*, 7.5 mg/5 ml ◊, 10 mg/5 ml ◊*, 15 mg/ 5 ml ◊*, 15 mg/5 ml ◊*
Strips (orally disintegrating): 7.5 mg ◊*, 15 mg ◊*

INDICATIONS & DOSAGES
➤ **Nonproductive cough**
Adults and children age 12 and older: 10 to 20 mg P.O. every 4 hours, or 30 mg every 6 to 8 hours. Or, 60 mg extended-release liquid b.i.d. Maximum, 120 mg daily. Or, give lozenges, 5 to 15 mg, every 1 to 4 hours, up to 120 mg/day.
Children ages 6 to 11: Give 5 to 10 mg P.O. every 4 hours, or 15 mg every 6 to 8 hours. Or, 30 mg extended-release liquid b.i.d. Maximum, 60 mg daily. Or, give lozenges, 5 to 10 mg, every 1 to 4 hours, up to 60 mg/day.
Children ages 2 to 5: Give 2.5 to 5 mg P.O. every 4 hours, or 7.5 mg every 6 to 8 hours. Or, 15 mg extended-release liquid b.i.d. Maximum, 30 mg daily.

ADMINISTRATION
P.O.
• Store at controlled room temperature (59° to 86° F [15° to 30° C]).

ACTION
Suppresses the cough reflex by direct action on the cough center in the medulla.

Route	Onset	Peak	Duration
P.O.	< 30 min	Unknown	3–6 hr

Half-life: About 11 hours.

ADVERSE REACTIONS
CNS: drowsiness, dizziness.
GI: nausea, vomiting, stomach pain.

INTERACTIONS
Drug-drug. *MAO inhibitors:* May cause risk of hypotension, coma, hyperpyrexia, and death. Avoid using together.
Quinidine: May increase the risk of dextromethorphan adverse effects. Consider decreasing dextromethorphan dose if needed.
Sibutramine: Serotonin syndrome may occur. Avoid using together.
Drug-herb. *Parsley:* May promote or produce serotonin syndrome. Discourage use together.

EFFECTS ON LAB TEST RESULTS
None reported.

CONTRAINDICATIONS & CAUTIONS
• Contraindicated in patients currently taking MAO inhibitors or within 2 weeks of stopping MAO inhibitors.
• Use cautiously in atopic children, sedated or debilitated patients, and patients confined to the supine position.
• Use cautiously in patients sensitive to aspirin or tartrazine dyes.
• *Alert:* Use of OTC cough products is not recommended for neonates and children under 2 years.

NURSING CONSIDERATIONS
• Don't use dextromethorphan when cough is a valuable diagnostic sign or is beneficial (such as after thoracic surgery).
• Dextromethorphan 15 to 30 mg is equivalent to codeine 8 to 15 mg as an antitussive.
• Drug produces no analgesia or addiction and little or no CNS depression.
• Use drug with chest percussion and vibration.
• Monitor cough type and frequency.

PATIENT TEACHING
• Instruct patient to take drug exactly as prescribed.
• Tell patient to report adverse reactions.
• Tell patient to contact his health care provider if cough lasts longer than 1 week, recurs frequently, or is accompanied by high fever, rash, or severe headache.

SAFETY ALERT!

digoxin
di-JOX-in

Digitek, Digoxin, Lanoxicaps, Lanoxin*

Pharmacologic class: cardiac glycoside
Pregnancy risk category C

AVAILABLE FORMS
Capsules: 0.05 mg, 0.1 mg, 0.2 mg
Elixir: 0.05 mg/ml (pediatric)
Injection: 0.05 mg/ml†, 0.1 mg/ml (pediatric), 0.25 mg/ml
Tablets: 0.125 mg, 0.25 mg

INDICATIONS & DOSAGES
➤ **Heart failure, paroxysmal supraventricular tachycardia, atrial fibrillation and flutter**
Capsules
Adults: For rapid digitalization, give 0.4 to 0.6 mg P.O. initially, followed by 0.1 to 0.3 mg every 6 to 8 hours, as needed and tolerated, for 24 hours. For slow digitalization, give 0.05 to 0.35 mg daily in two divided doses. Therapeutic levels are reached in 7 to 22 days. Maintenance dose is 0.05 to 0.35 mg daily in one or two divided doses.
Children: Digitalizing dose is based on child's age and is given in three or more divided doses over the first 24 hours. First dose is 50% of the total dose; subsequent doses are given as 25% of total dose for two doses every 6 to 8 hours as needed and tolerated.
Children age 10 and older: For rapid digitalization, give 8 to 12 mcg/kg P.O. over 24 hours, divided as described previously. Maintenance dose is 25% to 35% of total digitalizing dose, given daily as a single dose.

Children ages 5 to 10: For rapid digitalization, give 15 to 30 mcg/kg P.O. over 24 hours, divided as described previously. Maintenance dose is 25% to 35% of total digitalizing dose, divided and given in two or three equal portions daily.
Children ages 2 to 5: For rapid digitalization, give 25 to 35 mcg/kg P.O. over 24 hours, divided as described previously. Maintenance dose is 25% to 35% of total digitalizing dose, divided and given in two or three equal portions daily.
Elixir, tablets
Adults: For rapid digitalization, give 0.75 to 1.25 mg P.O. over 24 hours in two or more divided doses every 6 to 8 hours. For slow digitalization, give 0.0625 to 0.5 mg daily. Titrate every 2 weeks as needed. Maintenance dose is 0.0625 to 0.5 mg daily.
Children age 10 and older: 10 to 15 mcg/kg P.O. over 24 hours in two or more divided doses every 6 to 8 hours. Maintenance dose is 25% to 35% of total digitalizing dose.
Children ages 5 to 10: 20 to 35 mcg/kg P.O. over 24 hours in two or more divided doses every 6 to 8 hours. Maintenance dose is 25% to 35% of total digitalizing dose.
Children ages 2 to 5: 30 to 40 mcg/kg P.O. over 24 hours in two or more divided doses every 6 to 8 hours. Maintenance dose is 25% to 35% of total digitalizing dose.
Infants ages 1 month to 2 years: 35 to 60 mcg/kg P.O. over 24 hours in two or more divided doses every 6 to 8 hours. Maintenance dose is 25% to 35% of total digitalizing dose.
Neonates: 25 to 35 mcg/kg P.O. over 24 hours in two or more divided doses every 6 to 8 hours. Maintenance dose is 25% to 35% of total digitalizing dose.
Premature infants: 20 to 30 mcg/kg P.O. over 24 hours in two or more divided doses every 6 to 8 hours. Maintenance dose is 20% to 30% of total digitalizing dose.
Injection
Adults: For rapid digitalization, give 0.4 to 0.6 mg I.V. initially, followed by 0.1 to 0.3 mg I.V. every 6 to 8 hours, as needed and tolerated, for 24 hours. For slow digitalization, give appropriate daily maintenance dose for 7 to 22 days until therapeutic levels are reached. Maintenance dose

is 0.075 to 0.35 mg I.V. daily in one or two divided doses.

Children: Digitalizing dose is based on child's age; give in three or more divided doses over the first 24 hours. First dose is 50% of total dose; subsequent doses are given every 6 to 8 hours as needed and tolerated.

Children age 10 and older: For rapid digitalization, give 8 to 12 mcg/kg I.V. over 24 hours, divided as described previously. Maintenance dose is 25% to 35% of total digitalizing dose, given daily as a single dose.

Children ages 5 to 10: For rapid digital-ization, give 15 to 30 mcg/kg I.V. over 24 hours, divided as described previously. Maintenance dose is 25% to 35% of total digitalizing dose, divided and given in two or three equal portions daily.

Children ages 2 to 5: For rapid digital-ization, give 25 to 35 mcg/kg I.V. over 24 hours, divided as described previously. Maintenance dose is 25% to 35% of total digitalizing dose, divided and given in two or three equal portions daily.

Infants ages 1 month to 2 years: For rapid digitalization, give 30 to 50 mcg/kg I.V. over 24 hours, divided as described previ-ously. Maintenance dose is 25% to 35% of total digitalizing dose, divided and given in two or three equal portions daily.

Neonates: For rapid digitalization, give 20 to 30 mcg/kg I.V. over 24 hours, divided as described previously. Maintenance dose is 25% to 35% of the total digitalizing dose, divided and given in two or three equal portions daily.

Premature infants: For rapid digitalization, give 15 to 25 mcg/kg I.V. over 24 hours, divided as described previously. Main-tenance dose is 20% to 30% of the total digitalizing dose, divided and given in two or three equal portions daily.

Adjust-a-dose: For patients with impaired renal function, give smaller loading and maintenance doses; extended dosing intervals may be needed.

ADMINISTRATION
P.O.
● Before giving loading dose, obtain baseline data (heart rate and rhythm, blood pressure, and electrolytes) and ask patient

about use of cardiac glycosides within the previous 2 to 3 weeks.
● Before giving drug, take apical-radial pulse for 1 minute. Record and notify prescriber of significant changes (sudden increase or decrease in pulse rate, pulse deficit, irregular beats and, particularly, regularization of a previously irregular rhythm). If these occur, check blood pres-sure and obtain a 12-lead ECG.
I.V.
● Before giving loading dose, obtain baseline data (heart rate and rhythm, blood pressure, and electrolytes) and ask patient about use of cardiac glycosides within the previous 2 to 3 weeks.
● Before giving drug, take apical-radial pulse for 1 minute. Record and notify prescriber of significant changes (sudden increase or decrease in pulse rate, pulse deficit, irregular beats and, particularly, regularization of a previously irregular rhythm). If these occur, check blood pres-sure and obtain a 12-lead ECG.
● Dilute fourfold with D_5W, normal saline solution, or sterile water for injection to reduce the chance of precipitation.
● Infuse drug slowly over at least 5 min-utes.
● Protect solution from light.
● **Incompatibilities:** Amiodarone, am-photericin B cholesteryl sulfate complex, dobutamine, doxapram, fluconazole, fos-carnet, propofol, remifentanil. Mixing with other drugs isn't recommended.

ACTION
Inhibits sodium-potassium–activated adenosine triphosphatase, promoting movement of calcium from extracellular to intracellular cytoplasm and strengthening myocardial contraction. Also acts on CNS to enhance vagal tone, slowing conduction through the SA and AV nodes.

Route	Onset	Peak	Duration
P.O.	30–120 min	2–6 hr	3–4 days
I.V.	5–30 min	1–4 hr	3–4 days

Half-life: 30 to 40 hours.

ADVERSE REACTIONS
CNS: *agitation, fatigue, generalized mus-cle weakness, hallucinations,* dizziness, headache, malaise, paresthesia, stupor, vertigo.

CV: *arrhythmias, heart block.*
EENT: blurred vision, diplopia, light flashes, photophobia, yellow-green halos around visual images.
GI: *anorexia, nausea,* diarrhea, vomiting.

INTERACTIONS

Drug-drug. *Amiloride:* May decrease digoxin effect and increase renal clearance of digoxin. Monitor patient for altered digoxin effect.

Amiodarone, *diltiazem, indomethacin,* **nifedipine,** *quinidine,* **verapamil:** May increase digoxin level. Monitor patient for toxicity.

Amphotericin B, carbenicillin, corticosteroids, **diuretics (such as chlorthalidone, loop diuretics, metolazone, thiazides),** *ticarcillin:* May cause hypokalemia, predisposing patient to digitalis toxicity. Monitor potassium level.

Antacids, kaolin-pectin: May decrease absorption of oral digoxin. Separate doses as much as possible.

Antibiotics (azole antifungals, macrolides, telithromycin, tetracyclines), *propafenone,* **ritonavir:** May increase risk of toxicity. Monitor patient for toxicity.

Anticholinergics: May increase digoxin absorption of oral digoxin tablets. Monitor drug level and observe for toxicity.

Beta-blockers, calcium channel blockers: May have additive effects on AV node conduction causing advanced or complete heart block. Use cautiously.

Cholestyramine, colestipol, metoclopramide: May decrease absorption of oral digoxin. Monitor patient for decreased digoxin level and effect. Give digoxin $1\frac{1}{2}$ hours before or 2 hours after other drugs.

Parenteral calcium, thiazides: May cause hypercalcemia and hypomagnesemia, predisposing patient to digitalis toxicity. Monitor calcium and magnesium levels.

Drug-herb. *Betel palm, foxglove, fumitory, goldenseal, hawthorn, lily of the valley, motherwort, rue, shepherd's purse:* May increase cardiac effects. Discourage use together.

Gossypol, horsetail, licorice, oleander, Siberian ginseng, squill: May increase toxicity. Monitor patient closely.

Plantain, St. John's wort: May decrease effectiveness of drug. Discourage use together.

EFFECTS ON LAB TEST RESULTS

● May prolong PR interval or depress ST segment.

CONTRAINDICATIONS & CAUTIONS

● Contraindicated in patients hypersensitive to drug and in those with digitalis-induced toxicity, ventricular fibrillation, or ventricular tachycardia unless caused by heart failure.

● Don't use in patients with Wolff-Parkinson-White syndrome unless the conduction accessory pathway has been pharmacologically or surgically disabled.

● Use with extreme caution in elderly patients and in those with acute MI, incomplete AV block, sinus bradycardia, PVCs, chronic constrictive pericarditis, hypertrophic cardiomyopathy, renal insufficiency, severe pulmonary disease, or hypothyroidism.

NURSING CONSIDERATIONS

● Drug-induced arrhythmias may increase the severity of heart failure and hypotension.

● In children, cardiac arrhythmias, including sinus bradycardia, are usually early signs of toxicity.

● Patients with hypothyroidism are extremely sensitive to cardiac glycosides and may need lower doses.

● Loading dose is usually divided over the first 24 hours with about half the loading dose given in the first dose.

● Toxic effects on the heart may be life-threatening and require immediate attention.

● Absorption of digoxin from liquid-filled capsules is superior to absorption from tablets or elixir. Expect dosage reduction of 20% to 25% when changing from tablets or elixir to liquid-filled capsules or parenteral therapy.

● Monitor digoxin level. Therapeutic level ranges from 0.8 to 2 nanogram/ml. Obtain blood for digoxin level at least 6 to 8 hours after last oral dose, preferably just before next scheduled dose.

● **Alert:** Excessively slow pulse rate (60 beats/minute or less) may be a sign of digitalis toxicity. Withhold drug and notify prescriber.

● Monitor potassium level carefully. Take corrective action before hypokalemia

occurs. Hyperkalemia may result from digoxin toxicity.
• Reduce drug dose for 1 or 2 days before elective cardioversion. Adjust dosage after cardioversion.
• *Look alike–sound alike:* Don't confuse digoxin with doxepin.

PATIENT TEACHING
• Teach patient and a responsible family member about drug action, dosage regimen, how to take pulse, reportable signs, and follow-up care.
• Tell patient to report pulse less than 60 beats/minute or more than 110 beats/minute, or skipped beats or other rhythm changes.
• Instruct patient to report adverse reactions promptly. Nausea, vomiting, diarrhea, appetite loss, and visual disturbances may be indicators of toxicity.
• Encourage patient to eat a consistent amount of potassium-rich foods.
• Tell patient not to substitute one brand for another.
• Advise patient to avoid the use of herbal drugs or to consult his prescriber before taking one.

---

diltiazem hydrochloride
dil-TYE-a-zem

Apo-Diltiaz†, Cardizem, Cardizem CD, Cardizem LA, Cartia XT, Dilacor XR, Diltia XT, Dilt-XR, Nu-Diltiaz†, Nu-Diltiaz CD†, Taztia XT, Tiazac, Tiazac XC†

Pharmacologic class: calcium channel blocker
Pregnancy risk category C

AVAILABLE FORMS
Capsules (extended-release): 120 mg, 180 mg, 240 mg, 300 mg, 360 mg, 420 mg
Injection: 5 mg/ml in 5-, 10-, 25-ml vials
Powder for injection: 25 mg
Tablets: 30 mg, 60 mg, 90 mg, 120 mg
Tablets (extended-release): 120 mg, 180 mg, 240 mg, 300 mg, 360 mg, 420 mg

INDICATIONS & DOSAGES
➤ **To manage Prinzmetal's or variant angina or chronic stable angina pectoris**
Adults: 30 mg P.O. q.i.d. before meals and at bedtime. Increase dose gradually to maximum of 360 mg/day divided into three or four doses, as indicated. Or, give 120- or 180-mg extended-release capsule or 180-mg extended-release tablet P.O. once daily. Adjust over a 7- to 14-day period as needed and tolerated up to a maximum dose of 360 mg/day (Cardizem LA), 480 mg/day (Cardizem CD, Cartia XT, Dilacor XR, Dilacor XT), or 540 mg/day (Tiazac).
➤ **Hypertension**
Adults: 180- to 240-mg extended-release capsule P.O. once daily. Adjust dosage based on patient response to a maximum dose of 480 mg/day. Or, 120 to 240 mg P.O. (Cardizem LA) once daily. Dosage can be adjusted about every 2 weeks to a maximum of 540 mg daily.
➤ **Atrial fibrillation or flutter; paroxysmal supraventricular tachycardia**
Adults: 0.25 mg/kg I.V. as a bolus injection over 2 minutes. Repeat after 15 minutes if response isn't adequate with a dose of 0.35 mg/kg I.V. over 2 minutes. Follow bolus with continuous I.V. infusion at 5 to 15 mg/hour (for up to 24 hours).

ADMINISTRATION
P.O.
• Don't crush or allow patient to chew extended-release tablets; they should be swallowed whole.
• Tiazac extended-release capsules can be opened and the contents sprinkled onto a spoonful of applesauce. The applesauce must be eaten immediately and without chewing, followed by a glass of cool water.
I.V.
• For 100-mg Cardizem Monovials, reconstitute according to manufacturer's directions.
• For direct injection, you need not dilute the 5 mg/ml injection.
• For continuous infusion, add 25 ml of drug to 100 ml solution, 50 ml of drug to 250 ml solution, or 50 ml of drug to 500 ml solution of 5 mg/ml injection to yield 1 mg/ml, 0.83 mg/ml, or

0.45 mg/ml, respectively. Compatible solutions include normal saline solution, D₅W, or 5% dextrose and half-normal saline solution.

• For direct injection or continuous infusion; give slowly while monitoring ECG and blood pressure continuously.

• Don't infuse for longer than 24 hours.

• **Incompatibilities:** Acetazolamide, acyclovir, aminophylline, ampicillin, ampicillin sodium and sulbactam sodium, cefoperazone, diazepam, furosemide, heparin, hydrocortisone, insulin, methylprednisolone, nafcillin, phenytoin, rifampin, sodium bicarbonate, thiopental.

ACTION

A calcium channel blocker that inhibits calcium ion influx across cardiac and smooth-muscle cells, decreasing myocardial contractility and oxygen demand. Drug also dilates coronary arteries and arterioles.

Route	Onset	Peak	Duration
P.O.	30–60 min	2–3 hr	6–8 hr
P.O. (extended-release capsule)	2–3 hr	10–14 hr	12–24 hr
P.O. (Cardizem LA)	3–4 hr	11–18 hr	6–9 hr
I.V.	< 3 min	2–7 min	1–10 hr

Half-life: 3 to 9 hours.

ADVERSE REACTIONS

CNS: *headache,* dizziness, asthenia, somnolence.

CV: *edema, arrhythmias, AV block, bradycardia, heart failure,* flushing, hypotension, conduction abnormalities, abnormal ECG.

GI: nausea, constipation, abdominal discomfort.

Hepatic: *acute hepatic injury.*

Skin: rash.

INTERACTIONS

Drug-drug. *Anesthetics:* May increase effects of anesthetics. Monitor patient.

Carbamazepine: May increase level of carbamazepine. Monitor carbamazepine level, and watch for signs and symptoms of toxicity.

Cimetidine: May inhibit diltiazem metabolism, increasing additive AV node conduction slowing. Monitor patient for toxicity.

Cyclosporine: May increase cyclosporine level, possibly by decreasing its metabolism, leading to increased risk of cyclosporine toxicity. Monitor cyclosporine level with each dosage change.

Diazepam, midazolam, triazolam: May increase CNS depression and prolonged effects of these drugs. Use lower dose of these benzodiazepines.

Digoxin: May increase digoxin level. Monitor patient for digoxin toxicity.

Furosemide: May form a precipitate when mixed with diltiazem injection. Give through separate I.V. lines.

Lithium: May reduce lithium levels, causing loss of mania control, and neurotoxic and psychotic symptoms. Monitor patient for signs of neurotoxicity.

Propranolol, other beta blockers: May precipitate heart failure or prolong conduction time. Use together cautiously.

Sirolimus, tacrolimus: May increase level of these drugs. Monitor drug level and patient for toxicity.

Theophylline: May enhance action of theophylline, causing intoxication. Monitor theophylline levels.

EFFECTS ON LAB TEST RESULTS
None reported.

CONTRAINDICATIONS & CAUTIONS

• Contraindicated in patients hypersensitive to drug and in those with sick sinus syndrome or second- or third-degree AV block in the absence of an artificial pacemaker, cardiogenic shock, ventricular tachycardia, systolic blood pressure below 90 mm Hg, acute MI, or pulmonary congestion (documented by X-ray).

• Contraindicated in I.V. form for patients who have atrial fibrillation or flutter with an accessory bypass tract, as in Wolff-Parkinson-White syndrome or short PR interval syndrome.

• Use cautiously in elderly patients and in those with heart failure or impaired hepatic or renal function.

NURSING CONSIDERATIONS

● Patients controlled on drug alone or with other drugs may be switched to Cardizem LA tablets once a day at the nearest equivalent total daily dose.
● Monitor blood pressure and heart rate when starting therapy and during dosage adjustments.
● Maximal antihypertensive effect may not be seen for 14 days.
● If systolic blood pressure is below 90 mm Hg or heart rate is below 60 beats/minute, withhold dose and notify prescriber.

PATIENT TEACHING

● Instruct patient to take drug as prescribed, even when he feels better.
● Advise patient to avoid hazardous activities during start of therapy.
● If nitrate therapy is prescribed during dosage adjustment, stress patient compliance. Tell patient that S.L. nitroglycerin may be taken with drug, as needed, when angina symptoms are acute.
● *Alert:* Tell patient to swallow extended-release tablets whole, and not to crush or chew them.
● If patient is taking Tiazac extended-release capsules, inform him that these capsules can be opened and the contents sprinkled onto a spoonful of applesauce. He must eat the applesauce immediately and without chewing, and then drink a glass of cool water.

---

diphenhydramine hydrochloride
dye-fen-HYE-drah-meen

Allerdryl † ◊, AllerMax ◊*, Aller-Max Caplets ◊, Allernix† ◊, Altaryl Children's Allergy† ◊, Banophen ◊, Benadryl ◊, Benadryl Allergy ◊, Children's Pedia Care Nightime Cough† ◊, Compoz ◊, Diphen Cough ◊, Diphenhist ◊, Diphenhist Captabs ◊, Dytan ◊, Genahist ◊, Hydramine Cough ◊*, Siladryl ◊*, Silphen ◊*, Sominex ◊, Triaminic MultiSymptom ◊*, Tusstat ◊*, Twilite Caplets ◊

Pharmacologic class: ethanolamine
Pregnancy risk category B

AVAILABLE FORMS

Capsules: 25 mg ◊, 50 mg ◊
Elixir: 12.5 mg/5 ml ◊*
Injection: 50 mg/ml
Strips (orally disintegrating): 12.5 mg ◊*, 25 mg ◊*
Syrup: 12.5 mg/5 ml ◊*
Tablets: 25 mg ◊, 50 mg ◊
Tablets (chewable): 12.5 mg ◊

INDICATIONS & DOSAGES

➤ **Rhinitis, allergy symptoms, motion sickness, Parkinson's disease**
Adults and children age 12 and older: 25 to 50 mg P.O. every 4 to 6 hours. Maximum, 300 mg P.O. daily. Or, 10 to 50 mg I.V. or deep I.M. Maximum I.V. or I.M. dosage, 400 mg daily.
Children ages 6 to 11: 12.5 to 25 mg P.O. every 4 to 6 hours. Maximum dose is 150 mg daily. Or, 5 mg/kg day divided into four doses P.O., deep I.M., or I.V. Maximum dose is 300 mg daily.
Children ages 2 to 5: 6.25 mg every 4 to 6 hours. Maximum dose is 37.5 mg daily. Or, 5 mg/kg day divided into four doses P.O., deep I.M., or I.V. Maximum dose is 300 mg daily.
Children weighing less than 9.1 kg (20 lb): 5 mg/kg day divided into four doses P.O., deep I.M., or I.V. Maximum dose is 300 mg daily.
➤ **Sedation**
Adults: 25 to 50 mg P.O. or deep I.M. as needed.
➤ **Nighttime sleep aid**
Adults: 25 to 50 mg P.O. at bedtime.
➤ **Nonproductive cough**
Adults and children age 12 and older: 25 mg (syrup) P.O. every 4 hours. Don't exceed 150 mg daily. Or, 25 to 50 mg (liquid) every 4 hours. Don't exceed 300 mg daily.
Children ages 6 to 11: 12.5 mg (syrup) P.O. every 4 hours. Don't exceed 75 mg daily. Or, 12.5 to 25 mg (liquid) every 4 hours. Don't exceed 150 mg daily.
Children ages 2 to 5: 6.25 mg (syrup) P.O. every 4 hours. Don't exceed 25 mg daily.
➤ **Antipsychotic-induced dystonia** ◆
Adults: 50 mg I.M. or I.V.

ADMINISTRATION
P.O.
• Give drug with food or milk to reduce GI distress.
I.V.
• Don't exceed 25 mg/minute.
• **Incompatibilities:** Allopurinol, amobarbital, amphotericin B, cefepime, dexamethasone, foscarnet, haloperidol lactate, pentobarbital, phenobarbital, phenytoin, thiopental.
I.M.
• Give I.M. injection deep into large muscle.
• Alternate injection sites to prevent irritation.

ACTION
Competes with histamine for H_1-receptor sites. Prevents, but doesn't reverse, histamine-mediated responses, particularly those of the bronchial tubes, GI tract, uterus, and blood vessels. Structurally related to local anesthetics, drug provides local anesthesia and suppresses cough reflex.

Route	Onset	Peak	Duration
P.O.	15 min	1–4 hr	6–8 hr
I.V.	Immediate	1–4 hr	6–8 hr
I.M.	Unknown	1–4 hr	6–8 hr

Half-life: 2.4 to 9.3 hours.

ADVERSE REACTIONS
CNS: *drowsiness, sedation, sleepiness, dizziness, incoordination, seizures,* confusion, insomnia, headache, vertigo, fatigue, restlessness, tremor, nervousness.
CV: palpitations, hypotension, tachycardia.
EENT: diplopia, blurred vision, nasal congestion, tinnitus.
GI: *dry mouth, nausea, epigastric distress,* vomiting, diarrhea, constipation, anorexia.
GU: dysuria, urine retention, urinary frequency.
Hematologic: *thrombocytopenia, agranulocytosis,* hemolytic anemia.
Respiratory: *thickening of bronchial secretions.*
Skin: urticaria, photosensitivity, rash.
Other: *anaphylactic shock.*

INTERACTIONS
Drug-drug. *CNS depressants:* May increase sedation. Use together cautiously.
MAO inhibitors: May increase anticholinergic effects. Avoid using together.
Other products that contain diphenhydramine (including topical therapy): May increase risk of adverse reactions. Avoid using together.
Drug-lifestyle. *Alcohol use:* May increase CNS depression. Discourage use together.
Sun exposure: May cause photosensitivity reactions. Advise patient to avoid extensive sunlight exposure.

EFFECTS ON LAB TEST RESULTS
• May decrease hemoglobin level and hematocrit.
• May decrease granulocyte and platelet counts.
• May prevent, reduce, or mask positive result in diagnostic skin test.

CONTRAINDICATIONS & CAUTIONS
• Contraindicated in patients hypersensitive to drug; newborns; premature neonates; breast-feeding women; patients with angle-closure glaucoma, stenosing peptic ulcer, symptomatic prostatic hyperplasia, bladder neck obstruction, or pyloroduodenal obstruction; and those having an acute asthmatic attack.
• Avoid use in patients taking MAO inhibitors.
• Use with caution in patients with prostatic hyperplasia, asthma, COPD, increased intraocular pressure, hyperthyroidism, CV disease, and hypertension.
• Children younger than age 12 should use drug only as directed by prescriber.

NURSING CONSIDERATIONS
• Stop drug 4 days before diagnostic skin testing.
• Dizziness, excessive sedation, syncope, toxicity, paradoxical stimulation, and hypotension are more likely to occur in elderly patients.
• *Look alike–sound alike:* Don't confuse diphenhydramine with dimenhydrinate; don't confuse Benadryl with Bentyl or benazepril.

PATIENT TEACHING
• Warn patient not to take this drug with any other products that contain diphenhydramine (including topical therapy) because of increased adverse reactions.

• Instruct patient to take drug 30 minutes before travel to prevent motion sickness.
• Tell patient to take diphenhydramine with food or milk to reduce GI distress.
• Warn patient to avoid alcohol and hazardous activities that require alertness until CNS effects of drug are known.
• Inform patient that sugarless gum, hard candy, or ice chips may relieve dry mouth.
• Tell patient to notify prescriber if tolerance develops because a different antihistamine may need to be prescribed.
• Drug is in many OTC sleep and cold products. Advise patient to consult prescriber before using these products.
• Warn patient of possible photosensitivity reactions. Advise use of a sunblock.

SAFETY ALERT!

dobutamine hydrochloride
DOE-byoo-ta-meen

Pharmacologic class: adrenergic, beta$_1$ agonist
Pregnancy risk category B

AVAILABLE FORMS
Injection: 12.5 mg/ml in 20-ml vials (parenteral)
Dobutamine in 5% dextrose: 0.5 mg/ml (125 or 250 mg); 1 mg/ml (250 or 500 mg); 2 mg/ml (500 mg); 4 mg/ml (1,000 mg)

INDICATIONS & DOSAGES
➤ **Increased cardiac output in short-term treatment of cardiac decompensation caused by depressed contractility, such as during refractory heart failure; adjunctive therapy in cardiac surgery**
Adults: 0.5 to 1 mcg/kg/minute I.V. infusion, titrating to optimum dosage of 2 to 20 mcg/kg/minute. Usual effective range to increase cardiac output is 2.5 to 10 mcg/kg/minute. Rarely, rates up to 40 mcg/kg/minute may be needed.

ADMINISTRATION
I.V.
• Before starting therapy, give a plasma volume expander to correct hypovolemia and a cardiac glycoside.

• Dilute concentrate before injecting. Compatible solutions include D$_5$W, D$_{10}$W, half-normal or normal saline solution for injection, lactated Ringer's injection, Isolyte-M with D$_5$W, Normosol-M in D$_5$W, and 20% Osmitrol.
• Diluting one vial (250 mg) with 1,000 ml of solution yields 250 mcg/ml. Diluting with 500 ml yields 500 mcg/ml. Diluting with 250 ml yields 1,000 mcg/ml.
• Oxidation may slightly discolor admixture. This doesn't indicate a significant loss of potency, provided drug is used within 24 hours of reconstitution.
• Give through a central venous catheter or large peripheral vein using an infusion pump.
• Titrate rate according to patient's condition. Don't exceed 5 mg/ml.
• Infusions lasting up to 72 hours produce no more adverse effects than shorter infusions.
• Watch for irritation and infiltration; extravasation can cause tissue damage and necrosis. Change I.V. sites regularly to avoid phlebitis.
• Solution remains stable for 24 hours. Don't freeze.
• **Incompatibilities:** Acyclovir, alkaline solutions, alteplase, aminophylline, bretylium, bumetanide, calcium chloride, calcium gluconate, cefamandole, cefazolin, cefepime, diazepam, digoxin, ethacrynate, furosemide, heparin, hydrocortisone sodium succinate, indomethacin, insulin, magnesium sulfate, midazolam, penicillin, phenytoin, phytonadione, piperacillin with tazobactam, potassium chloride, sodium bicarbonate, thiopental, verapamil, warfarin. Don't give through same line with other drugs.

ACTION
Stimulates heart's beta$_1$ receptors to increase myocardial contractility and stroke volume. At therapeutic dosages, drug increases cardiac output by decreasing peripheral vascular resistance, reducing ventricular filling pressure, and facilitating AV node conduction.

Route	Onset	Peak	Duration
I.V.	1–2 min	10 min	< 5 min after infusion

Half-life: 2 minutes.

ADVERSE REACTIONS
CNS: headache.
CV: *hypertension, increased heart rate,* angina, PVCs, phlebitis, nonspecific chest pain, palpitations, ventricular ectopy, hypotension.
GI: nausea, vomiting.
Respiratory: *asthma attack,* shortness of breath.
Other: *anaphylaxis,* hypersensitivity reactions.

INTERACTIONS
Drug-drug. *Beta blockers:* May antagonize dobutamine effects. Avoid using together.
Bretylium: May increase risk of arrhythmias. Monitor ECG.
General anesthetics: May have greater risk of ventricular arrhythmias. Monitor ECG closely.
Guanethidine, oxytocic drugs: May increase pressor response, causing severe hypertension. Monitor blood pressure closely.
Tricyclic antidepressants: May potentiate pressor response and cause arrhythmias. Use together cautiously.
Drug-herb. *Rue:* May increase inotropic potential. Discourage use together.

EFFECTS ON LAB TEST RESULTS
● May decrease potassium level.
● May decrease platelet count.

CONTRAINDICATIONS & CAUTIONS
● Contraindicated in patients hypersensitive to drug or its components and in those with idiopathic hypertrophic subaortic stenosis.
● Use cautiously in patients with history of hypertension because drug may increase pressor response.
● Use cautiously after acute MI.
● Use cautiously in patients with history of sulfite sensitivity.

NURSING CONSIDERATIONS
● Because drug increases AV node conduction, patients with atrial fibrillation may develop a rapid ventricular rate.
● Continuously monitor ECG, blood pressure, pulmonary artery wedge pressure, cardiac output, and urine output.

● Monitor electrolyte levels. Drug may lower potassium level.
● *Look alike–sound alike:* Don't confuse dobutamine with dopamine.

PATIENT TEACHING
● Tell patient to report adverse reactions promptly, especially labored breathing and drug-induced headache.
● Instruct patient to report discomfort at I.V. insertion site.

SAFETY ALERT!

dopamine hydrochloride
DOE-pa-meen

Pharmacologic class: adrenergic
Pregnancy risk category C

AVAILABLE FORMS
Injection: 40 mg/ml, 80 mg/ml, 160 mg/ml parenteral concentrate for injection for I.V. infusion; 0.8 mg/ml (200 or 400 mg) in D_5W; 1.6 mg/ml (400 or 800 mg) in D_5W; 3.2 mg/ml (800 mg) in D_5W parenteral injection for I.V. infusion

INDICATIONS & DOSAGES
➤ **To treat shock and correct hemodynamic imbalances; to improve perfusion to vital organs; to increase cardiac output; to correct hypotension**
Adults: Initially, 2 to 5 mcg/kg/minute by I.V. infusion. Titrate dosage to desired hemodynamic or renal response. Increase by 1 to 4 mcg/kg/minute at 10- to 30-minute intervals. In seriously ill patients, start with 5 mcg/kg/minute and increase gradually in increments of 5 to 10 mcg/kg/minute to a rate of 20 to 50 mcg/kg/minute, as needed.
Adjust-a-dose: In patients with occlusive vascular disease, initial dose is 1 mcg/kg/minute or less.

ADMINISTRATION
I.V.
● Dilute with D_5W, normal saline solution, D_5W in normal saline or 0.45% saline, lactated Ringer's, or D_5W in lactated Ringer's. Mix just before use.

- Use a central line or large vein, as in the antecubital fossa, to minimize risk of extravasation.
- Use a continuous infusion pump to regulate flow rate.
- Watch infusion site carefully for extravasation; if it occurs, stop infusion immediately and call prescriber. You may need to infiltrate area with 5 to 10 mg phentolamine in 10 to 15 ml normal saline solution.
- Because solution will deteriorate rapidly, discard after 24 hours or earlier if it's discolored.
- **Incompatibilities:** Acyclovir sodium, additives with a dopamine and dextrose solution, alteplase, amphotericin B, cefepime, furosemide, gentamicin, indomethacin sodium trihydrate, iron salts, insulin, oxidizing agents, penicillin G potassium, sodium bicarbonate or other alkaline solutions, thiopental. Don't mix other drugs in I.V. container with dopamine.

ACTION
Stimulates dopaminergic and alpha and beta receptors of the sympathetic nervous system resulting in a positive inotropic effect and increased cardiac output. Action is dose-related; large doses cause mainly alpha stimulation.

Route	Onset	Peak	Duration
I.V.	5 min	Unknown	< 10 min after infusion

Half-life: 2 minutes.

ADVERSE REACTIONS
CNS: headache, anxiety.
CV: *hypotension, ventricular arrhythmias (high doses),* ectopic beats, tachycardia, angina, palpitations, vasoconstriction.
GI: nausea, vomiting.
Metabolic: azotemia, hyperglycemia.
Respiratory: *asthmatic episodes,* dyspnea.
Skin: necrosis and tissue sloughing with extravasation, piloerection.
Other: *anaphylactic reactions.*

INTERACTIONS
Drug-drug. *Alpha and beta blockers:* May antagonize dopamine effects. Monitor patient closely.
Ergot alkaloids: May cause extremely high blood pressure. Avoid using together.
Inhaled anesthetics: May increase risk of arrhythmias or hypertension. Monitor patient closely.
MAO inhibitors (phenelzine, tranylcypromine): May cause fever, hypertensive crisis, or severe headache. Avoid using together; if patient received an MAO inhibitor in the past 2 to 3 weeks, initial dopamine dose is less than or equal to 10% of the usual dose.
Oxytocics: May cause severe, persistent hypertension. Use together cautiously.
Phenytoin: May cause severe hypotension, bradycardia, and cardiac arrest. Monitor patient carefully.
Tricyclic antidepressants: May decrease pressor response. Monitor patient closely.

EFFECTS ON LAB TEST RESULTS
- May increase catecholamine, glucose, and urine urea levels.

CONTRAINDICATIONS & CAUTIONS
- Contraindicated in patients with uncorrected tachyarrhythmias, pheochromocytoma, or ventricular fibrillation.
- Use cautiously in patients with occlusive vascular disease, cold injuries, diabetic endarteritis, and arterial embolism; in pregnant or breast-feeding women; in those with a history of sulfite sensitivity; and in those taking MAO inhibitors.

NURSING CONSIDERATIONS
- Most patients receive less than 20 mcg/kg/minute. Doses of 0.5 to 2 mcg/kg/minute mainly stimulate dopamine receptors and dilate the renal vasculature. Doses of 2 to 10 mcg/kg/minute stimulate beta receptors for a positive inotropic effect. Higher doses also stimulate alpha receptors, constricting blood vessels and increasing blood pressure.
- Drug isn't a substitute for blood or fluid volume deficit. If deficit exists, replace fluid before giving vasopressors.
- During infusion, frequently monitor ECG, blood pressure, cardiac output,

central venous pressure, pulmonary artery wedge pressure, pulse rate, urine output, and color and temperature of limbs.
• If diastolic pressure rises disproportionately with a significant decrease in pulse pressure, decrease infusion rate, and watch carefully for further evidence of predominant vasoconstrictor activity, unless such an effect is desired.
• Observe patient closely for adverse reactions; dosage may need to be adjusted or drug stopped.
• Check urine output often. If urine flow decreases without hypotension, notify prescriber because dosage may need to be reduced.
• *Alert:* After drug is stopped, watch closely for sudden drop in blood pressure. Taper dosage slowly to evaluate stability of blood pressure.
• Acidosis decreases effectiveness of drug.
• *Look alike–sound alike:* Don't confuse dopamine with dobutamine.

PATIENT TEACHING
• Tell patient to report adverse reactions promptly.
• Instruct patient to report discomfort at I.V. insertion site.

doxepin hydrochloride
DOKS-eh-pin

Sinequan

Pharmacologic class: tricyclic antidepressant (TCA)
Pregnancy risk category C

AVAILABLE FORMS
Capsules: 10 mg, 25 mg, 50 mg, 75 mg, 100 mg, 150 mg
Oral concentrate: 10 mg/ml

INDICATIONS & DOSAGES
➤ **Depression; anxiety**
Adults: Initially, 75 mg P.O. daily. Usual dosage range is 75 to 150 mg daily to maximum of 300 mg daily in divided doses. Or, entire maintenance dose may be given once daily with maximum dose of 150 mg.

ADMINISTRATION
P.O.
• Dilute oral concentrate with 4 ounces (120 ml) of water, milk, or juice (orange, grapefruit, tomato, prune, or pineapple, but not grape); don't mix preparation with carbonated beverages.
• Give at bedtime, if possible, because it may cause drowsiness and dizziness.

ACTION
Unknown. Increases amount of norepinephrine, serotonin, or both in the CNS by blocking their reuptake by the presynaptic neurons.

Route	Onset	Peak	Duration
P.O.	Unknown	2 hr	Unknown

Half-life: 6 to 8 hours.

ADVERSE REACTIONS
CNS: *drowsiness, dizziness, seizures,* confusion, numbness, hallucinations, paresthesia, ataxia, weakness, headache, extrapyramidal reactions.
CV: *orthostatic hypotension, tachycardia,* ECG changes.
EENT: *blurred vision,* tinnitus.
GI: *dry mouth, constipation,* nausea, vomiting, anorexia.
GU: urine retention.
Metabolic: *hypoglycemia,* hyperglycemia.
Skin: *diaphoresis,* rash, urticaria, photosensitivity reactions.
Other: hypersensitivity reactions.

INTERACTIONS
Drug-drug. *Barbiturates, CNS depressants:* May enhance CNS depression. Avoid using together.
Cimetidine, fluoxetine, fluvoxamine, paroxetine, sertraline: May increase doxepin level. Monitor drug levels and patient for signs of toxicity.
Clonidine: May cause life-threatening hypertension. Avoid using together.
Epinephrine, norepinephrine: May increase hypertensive effect. Use together cautiously.
MAO inhibitors: May cause severe excitation, hyperpyrexia, or seizures, usually with high dosage. Avoid using within 14 days of MAO inhibitor therapy.

Quinolones: May increase the risk of life-threatening arrhythmias. Avoid using together.

Drug-herb. *Evening primrose oil:* May cause additive or synergistic effect, resulting in lower seizure threshold and increasing the risk of seizure. Discourage use together.

St. John's wort, SAM-e, yohimbe: May cause serotonin syndrome. Discourage use together.

Drug-lifestyle. *Alcohol use:* May enhance CNS depression. Discourage use together. *Sun exposure:* May increase risk of photosensitivity reactions. Advise patient to avoid excessive sunlight exposure.

EFFECTS ON LAB TEST RESULTS
• May increase or decrease glucose level.
• May increase liver function test values.

CONTRAINDICATIONS & CAUTIONS
• Contraindicated in patients hypersensitive to drug and in those with glaucoma or tendency toward urine retention; also contraindicated in those who have received an MAO inhibitor within past 14 days and during acute recovery phase of an MI.

NURSING CONSIDERATIONS
• Don't withdraw drug abruptly.
• Monitor patient for nausea, headache, and malaise after abrupt withdrawal of long-term therapy; these symptoms don't indicate addiction.
• *Alert:* Because hypertensive episodes may occur during surgery in patients receiving drug, stop it gradually several days before surgery.
• If signs or symptoms of psychosis occur or increase, expect prescriber to reduce dosage. Record mood changes. Monitor patient for suicidal tendencies and allow only a minimum supply of drug.
• *Alert:* Drug may increase risk of suicidal thinking and behavior in children, adolescents, and young adults ages 18 to 24 during the first 2 months of treatment, especially in those with major depressive disorder or other psychiatric disorder.
• Drug has strong anticholinergic effects and is one of the most sedating TCAs. Adverse anticholinergic effects can occur rapidly.

• Recommend use of sugarless hard candy or gum to relieve dry mouth.
• *Look alike–sound alike:* Don't confuse doxepin with doxazosin, digoxin, doxapram, or Doxidan; don't confuse Sinequan with saquinavir.

PATIENT TEACHING
• Tell patient to dilute oral concentrate with 4 ounces (120 ml) of water, milk, or juice (orange, grapefruit, tomato, prune, or pineapple, but not grape); preparation shouldn't be mixed with carbonated beverages.
• Tell patient to take full dose at bedtime whenever he can, but warn him of possible morning dizziness on standing up quickly.
• Advise patient to consult prescriber before taking other prescription or OTC drugs.
• Warn patient to avoid hazardous activities that require alertness and good psychomotor coordination until effects of drug are known. Drowsiness and dizziness usually subside after a few weeks.
• Tell patient to avoid alcohol during drug therapy.
• Tell patient that maximal effect may not be evident for 2 to 3 weeks.
• Warn patient not to stop drug suddenly.
• To prevent sensitivity to the sun, advise patient to use sunblock, wear protective clothing, and avoid prolonged exposure to strong sunlight.

SAFETY ALERT!

doxorubicin hydrochloride
dox-oh-ROO-bi-sin

Adriamycin PFS, Adriamycin RDF

Pharmacologic class: anthracycline glycoside antibiotic
Pregnancy risk category D

AVAILABLE FORMS
Injection (preservative-free): 2 mg/ml
Powder for injection: 10-mg, 20-mg, 50-mg, 100-mg, 150-mg vials

INDICATIONS & DOSAGES
➤ **Bladder, breast, lung, ovarian, stomach, and thyroid cancers;**

Reactions may be *common,* uncommon, *life-threatening,* or COMMON AND LIFE-THREATENING.
Interaction may have a *rapid onset* or **delayed onset**.

non-Hodgkin lymphoma; Hodgkin lymphoma; acute lymphoblastic and myeloblastic leukemia; Wilms tumor; neuroblastoma; lymphoma; soft tissue and bone sarcomas
Adults: 60 to 75 mg/m^2 I.V. as single dose every 3 weeks; or when used in combination with other chemotherapy drugs, 40 to 60 mg/m^2 I.V. every 21 to 28 days.
Elderly patients: May need reduced dosages.
Adjust-a-dose: Reduce dosage for patients with myelosuppression or impaired cardiac or liver function. Be prepared to decrease dosage if bilirubin level rises: Give 50% of dose when bilirubin level is 1.2 to 3 mg/100 ml; 25% when it's 3.1 to 5 mg/100 ml.

ADMINISTRATION
I.V.
• Preparing and giving parenteral drug may be mutagenic, teratogenic, or carcinogenic. Follow facility policy to reduce risks.
• If drug leaks or spills, inactivate with 5% sodium hypochlorite solution (household bleach).
• Reconstitute with preservative-free normal saline solution for injection to yield 2 mg/ml; add 5 ml to 10-mg vial, 10 ml to 20-mg vial, or 25 ml to 50-mg vial. Shake vial to dissolve drug.
• Don't place I.V. line over joints or in limbs with poor venous or lymphatic drainage.
• Give by direct injection over at least 3 minutes into the tubing of a free-flowing I.V. solution containing D$_5$W or normal saline solution for injection.
• If vein streaking occurs, slow administration rate. If welts appear, stop drug and notify prescriber.
• Some protocols give doxorubicin as a prolonged infusion, which requires central venous access.
• If extravasation occurs, stop infusion immediately, apply ice to area for 24 to 48 hours, and notify prescriber. Monitor area closely because extravasation may be progressive. Drug is a strong vesicant and may cause tissue necrosis. Early consultation with a plastic surgeon may be advisable.

• Refrigerated, reconstituted solution is stable 48 hours; at room temperature, it's stable 24 hours.
• **Incompatibilities:** Allopurinol, aluminum, aminophylline, bacteriostatic diluents, cefepime, dexamethasone sodium phosphate, diazepam, fluorouracil, furosemide, ganciclovir, heparin sodium, hydrocortisone sodium succinate, piperacillin with tazobactam.

ACTION
May interfere with DNA-dependent RNA synthesis by intercalation.

Route	Onset	Peak	Duration
I.V.	Unknown	Unknown	Unknown

Half-life: Initial, 30 minutes; terminal, 16½ hours.

ADVERSE REACTIONS
CV: cardiac depression, *arrhythmias, acute left ventricular failure, irreversible cardiomyopathy.*
EENT: conjunctivitis.
GI: *nausea, vomiting,* diarrhea, *stomatitis,* esophagitis, anorexia.
GU: transient red urine.
Hematologic: *leukopenia, thrombocytopenia,* MYELOSUPPRESSION.
Metabolic: hyperuricemia.
Skin: *severe cellulitis and tissue sloughing with drug extravasation,* urticaria, facial flushing, *complete alopecia within 3 to 4 weeks,* hyperpigmentation of nail beds and dermal creases, radiation recall effect.
Other: chills, *anaphylaxis.*

INTERACTIONS
Drug-drug. *Aminophylline, cephalothin, dexamethasone, fluorouracil, heparin, hydrocortisone:* May form a precipitate. Don't mix together.
Calcium channel blockers: May increase cardiotoxic effects. Monitor patient's ECG closely.
Cyclosporine: May increase doxorubicin concentration. Monitor patient for toxicity.
Digoxin: May decrease digoxin level. Monitor digoxin level closely.
Fosphenytoin, phenytoin: May decrease level of phenytoin or fosphenytoin. Monitor drug level.

Paclitaxel: May decrease doxorubicin clearance. Monitor patient for toxicity.
Phenobarbital: May increase doxorubicin clearance. Monitor patient closely.
Progesterone: May enhance neutropenia and thrombocytopenia. Monitor patient and laboratory values closely.
Streptozocin: May increase and prolong doxorubicin level. Doxorubicin dosage may have to be adjusted.

EFFECTS ON LAB TEST RESULTS
• May increase uric acid level.
• May decrease platelet and WBC counts.

CONTRAINDICATIONS & CAUTIONS
• Contraindicated in patients with a history of sensitivity reactions to drug or its components.
• Contraindicated in patients with marked myelosuppression induced by previous treatment with other antitumor drugs or radiotherapy and in those who have received a lifetime cumulative dose of 550 mg/m^2 of doxorubicin or daunorubicin.

NURSING CONSIDERATIONS
• Perform cardiac function studies, including ECG and ejection fraction, before treatment and then periodically throughout therapy. Dexrazoxane may be given within 30 minutes of doxorubicin if the accumulated dose of doxorubicin has reached 300 mg/m^2.
• Take preventive measures, including adequate hydration of the patient, before starting treatment. Rapid lysis of leukemic cells may cause hyperuricemia. Allopurinol may be ordered.
• Premedicate with antiemetic to reduce nausea.
• If skin or mucosal contact occurs, immediately wash with soap and water.
• Never give drug I.M. or subcutaneously.
• Dosage modification may be needed in patients with myelosuppression or impaired cardiac or hepatic function, and in elderly patients.

• Monitor CBC with differential and hepatic function tests; monitor ECG monthly during therapy. If WBC count falls below 2,000/mm^3 or granulocyte count falls below 1,000/mm^3, follow institutional policy for infection control in immunocompromised patients.
• Monitor ECG for changes, such as sinus tachycardia, T-wave flattening, ST-segment depression, and voltage reduction.
• Leukopenia may occur during days 10 to 15, with recovery by day 21.
• If tachycardia develops, stop drug or slow rate of infusion, and notify prescriber.
• *Alert:* If signs of heart failure develop, stop drug and notify prescriber. Heart failure can often be prevented by limiting cumulative dose to 550 mg/m^2 (400 mg/m^2 when patient is also receiving or has received cyclophosphamide or radiation therapy to cardiac area).
• *Look alike–sound alike:* Reddish color of drug is similar to that of daunorubicin; don't confuse the two drugs.
• Esophagitis is common in patients who also have received radiation therapy.
• *Alert:* If patient has previously received radiation therapy, he's susceptible to radiation recall effect.
• *Look alike–sound alike:* Don't confuse doxorubicin with doxorubicin liposomal.

PATIENT TEACHING
• Advise patient to report any pain or burning at site of injection during or after administration.
• Advise patient to watch for signs and symptoms of infection (fever, sore throat, fatigue) and bleeding (easy bruising, nosebleeds, bleeding gums, tarry stools) and to take temperature daily.
• Advise patient that orange to red urine for 1 to 2 days is normal and doesn't indicate presence of blood.
• Inform patient that hair loss may occur but that it's usually reversible. Hair may regrow 2 to 5 months after drug is stopped.

Reactions may be *common*, uncommon, *life-threatening*, or COMMON AND LIFE-THREATENING.
Interaction may have a *rapid onset* or *delayed onset*.

enalaprilat
eh-NAH-leh-prel-at

enalapril maleate
Vasotec

Pharmacologic class: ACE inhibitor
*Pregnancy risk category C; D in 2nd
and 3rd trimesters*

AVAILABLE FORMS
enalaprilat
Injection: 1.25 mg/ml
enalapril maleate
Tablets: 2.5 mg, 5 mg, 10 mg, 20 mg

INDICATIONS & DOSAGES
➤ **Hypertension**
Adults: In patients not taking diuretics, initially, 5 mg P.O. once daily; then adjusted based on response. Usual dosage range is 10 to 40 mg daily as a single dose or two divided doses. Or, 1.25 mg I.V. infusion over 5 minutes every 6 hours.
Children ages 1 month to 16 years:
0.08 mg/kg (up to 5 mg) P.O. once daily; dosage should be adjusted as needed up to 0.58 mg/kg (maximum 40 mg). Don't use if creatinine clearance is less than 30 ml/minute.
Adjust-a-dose: If patient is taking diuretics or creatinine clearance is 30 ml/minute or less, initially, 2.5 mg P.O. once daily. Or, 0.625 mg I.V. over 5 minutes, and repeat in 1 hour, if needed; then 1.25 mg I.V. every 6 hours.
➤ **To convert from I.V. therapy to oral therapy**
Adults: Initially, 2.5 mg P.O. once daily; if patient was receiving 0.625 mg I.V. every 6 hours, then 2.5 mg P.O. once daily. Adjust dosage based on response.
➤ **To convert from oral therapy to I.V. therapy**
Adults: 1.25 mg I.V. over 5 minutes every 6 hours. Higher dosages aren't more effective.
Adjust-a-dose: If creatinine level is more than 1.6 mg/dl or sodium level below 130 mEq/L, initially, 2.5 mg P.O. daily and adjust slowly.

➤ **To manage symptomatic heart failure**
Adults: Initially, 2.5 mg P.O. daily or b.i.d., increased gradually over several weeks. Maintenance is 5 to 20 mg daily in two divided doses. Maximum daily dose is 40 mg in two divided doses.
➤ **Asymptomatic left ventricular dysfunction**
Adults: Initially, 2.5 mg P.O. b.i.d. Increase as tolerated to target daily dose of 20 mg P.O. in divided doses.

ADMINISTRATION
P.O.
● Give drug without regard for food.
● Request oral suspension for patient who has difficulty swallowing.
I.V.
● Compatible solutions include D_5W, normal saline solution for injection, dextrose 5% in lactated Ringer injection, dextrose 5% in normal saline solution for injection, and Isolyte E.
● Inject drug slowly over at least 5 minutes, or dilute in 50 ml of a compatible solution and infuse over 15 minutes.
● **Incompatibilities:** Amphotericin B, cefepime hydrochloride, phenytoin sodium.

ACTION
May inhibit ACE, preventing conversion of angiotensin I to angiotensin II, a potent vasoconstrictor. Less angiotensin II decreases peripheral arterial resistance, decreasing aldosterone secretion, reducing sodium and water retention, and lowering blood pressure.

Route	Onset	Peak	Duration
P.O.	1 hr	4–6 hr	24 hr
I.V.	15 min	1–4 hr	6 hr

Half-life: 12 hours.

ADVERSE REACTIONS
CNS: *asthenia,* headache, dizziness, fatigue, vertigo, syncope.
CV: hypotension, chest pain, angina pectoris.
GI: diarrhea, nausea, abdominal pain, vomiting.

GU: decreased renal function (in patients with bilateral renal artery stenosis or heart failure).
Hematologic: bone marrow depression.
Respiratory: *dry, persistent, tickling, nonproductive cough,* dyspnea.
Skin: rash.
Other: *angioedema.*

INTERACTIONS

Drug-drug. *Azathioprine:* May increase risk of anemia or leukopenia. Monitor hematologic study results if used together.
Diuretics: May excessively reduce blood pressure. Use together cautiously.
Insulin, oral antidiabetics: May cause hypoglycemia, especially at start of enalapril therapy. Monitor patient closely.
Lithium: May cause lithium toxicity. Monitor lithium level.
NSAIDs: May reduce antihypertensive effect. Monitor blood pressure.
Potassium-sparing diuretics, potassium supplements: May cause hyperkalemia. Avoid using together unless hypokalemia is confirmed.
Drug-herb. *Capsaicin:* May cause cough. Discourage use together.
Ma huang: May decrease antihypertensive effects. Discourage use together.
Drug-food. *Salt substitutes containing potassium:* May cause hyperkalemia. Monitor patient closely.

EFFECTS ON LAB TEST RESULTS

● May increase bilirubin, BUN, creatinine, and potassium levels. May decrease sodium and hemoglobin levels and hematocrit.
● May increase liver function test values.

CONTRAINDICATIONS & CAUTIONS

● Contraindicated in patients hypersensitive to drug and in those with a history of angioedema related to previous treatment with an ACE inhibitor.
● Use cautiously in renally impaired patients or those with aortic stenosis or hypertrophic cardiomyopathy.

NURSING CONSIDERATIONS

● Closely monitor blood pressure response to drug.
● *Look alike–sound alike:* Similar packaging and labeling of enalaprilat injection and pancuronium, a neuromuscular-blocking drug, could result in a fatal medication error. Check all labels carefully.
● Monitor CBC with differential counts before and during therapy.
● Diabetic patients, those with impaired renal function or heart failure, and those receiving drugs that can increase potassium level may develop hyperkalemia. Monitor potassium intake and potassium level.
● *Look alike–sound alike:* Don't confuse enalapril with Anafranil or Eldepryl.

PATIENT TEACHING

● Instruct patient to report breathing difficulty or swelling of face, eyes, lips, or tongue. Swelling of the face and throat (including swelling of the larynx) may occur, especially after first dose.
● Advise patient to report signs of infection, such as fever and sore throat.
● Inform patient that light-headedness can occur, especially during first few days of therapy. Tell him to rise slowly to minimize this effect and to notify prescriber if symptoms develop. If he faints, he should stop taking drug and call prescriber immediately.
● Tell patient to use caution in hot weather and during exercise. Inadequate fluid intake, vomiting, diarrhea, and excessive perspiration can lead to light-headedness and fainting.
● Advise patient to avoid salt substitutes; these products may contain potassium, which can cause high potassium levels in patients taking this drug.
● Tell woman of childbearing age to notify prescriber if pregnancy occurs. Drug will need to be stopped.

enoxaparin sodium
en-OCKS-a-par-in

Lovenox

Pharmacologic class:
low–molecular-weight heparin
Pregnancy risk category B

AVAILABLE FORMS
Syringes (graduated prefilled): 60 mg/
0.6 ml, 80 mg/0.8 ml, 100 mg/ml, 120 mg/
0.8 ml, 150 mg/ml
Syringes (prefilled): 30 mg/0.3 ml,
40 mg/0.4 ml
Vial (multidose): 300 mg/3 ml (contains
15 mg/ml of benzyl alcohol)

INDICATIONS & DOSAGES
➤ **To prevent pulmonary embolism
and deep vein thrombosis (DVT)
after hip or knee replacement
surgery**
Adults: 30 mg subcutaneously every
12 hours for 7 to 10 days. Give initial dose
between 12 and 24 hours postoperatively,
as long as hemostasis has been established.
Continue treatment during postoperative
period until risk of DVT has diminished.
Hip replacement patients may receive
40 mg subcutaneously given 12 hours pre-
operatively. After initial phase of therapy,
hip replacement patients should continue
with 40 mg subcutaneously daily for
3 weeks.
➤ **To prevent pulmonary embolism
and DVT after abdominal surgery**
Adults: 40 mg subcutaneously daily with
initial dose 2 hours before surgery. Give
subsequent dose, as long as hemostasis
has been established, 24 hours after initial
preoperative dose and continue once daily
for 7 to 10 days. Continue treatment during
postoperative period until risk of DVT has
diminished.
➤ **To prevent pulmonary embolism
and DVT in patients with acute
illness who are at increased risk
because of decreased mobility**
Adults: 40 mg once daily subcutaneously
for 6 to 11 days. Treatment for up to
14 days has been well tolerated.

Adjust-a-dose: In patients with creatinine clearance less than 30 ml/minute
receiving drug as prophylaxis after abdominal surgery or hip or knee replacement
surgery, and in medical patients for prophylaxis during acute illness, give 30 mg
subcutaneously once daily.
➤ **To prevent ischemic complications of unstable angina and non–Q-
wave MI with oral aspirin therapy**
Adults: 1 mg/kg subcutaneously every
12 hours until clinical stabilization (minimum 2 days) with aspirin 100 to 325 mg
P.O. once daily.
✳*NEW INDICATION:* **Acute ST-segment
elevation MI**
Adults younger than age 75: 30 mg single
I.V. bolus plus 1 mg/kg subcutaneously
followed by 1 mg/kg subcutaneously every
12 hours (maximum of 100 mg for the first
two doses only) with aspirin. When given
with a thrombolytic, give enoxaparin from
15 minutes before to 30 minutes after the
start of fibrinolytic therapy. For patients
with percutaneous coronary intervention
(PCI), if the last subcutaneous dose was
given less than 8 hours before balloon
inflation, no additional dose is needed. If
the last dose was given more than 8 hours
before balloon inflation, give 0.3 mg/kg
I.V. bolus.
Adults age 75 and older: 0.75 mg/kg
subcutaneously every 12 hours (maximum
75 mg for the first two doses only).
Adjust-a-dose: In adults younger than
age 75 with severe renal impairment,
30 mg single I.V. bolus plus 1 mg/kg
subcutaneously followed by 1 mg/kg
subcutaneously once daily. In adults age
75 and older with severe renal impairment,
1 mg/kg subcutaneously once daily with no
initial bolus.
➤ **Inpatient treatment of acute
DVT with and without pulmonary
embolism when given with warfarin
sodium**
Adults: 1 mg/kg subcutaneously every
12 hours. Or, 1.5 mg/kg subcutaneously
once daily (at same time daily) for 5 to
7 days until therapeutic oral anticoagulant
effect (INR 2 to 3) is achieved. Warfarin
sodium therapy is usually started within
72 hours of enoxaparin injection.

> ➤ **Outpatient treatment of acute DVT without pulmonary embolism when given with warfarin sodium**
Adults: 1 mg/kg subcutaneously every 12 hours for 5 to 7 days until therapeutic oral anticoagulant effect (INR 2 to 3) is achieved. Warfarin sodium therapy usually is started within 72 hours of enoxaparin injection.
Adjust-a-dose: In patients with creatinine clearance less than 30 ml/minute receiving drug for acute DVT or prophylaxis of ischemic complications of unstable angina and non–Q-wave MI, give 1 mg/kg subcutaneously once daily.

ADMINISTRATION
Subcutaneous
• With patient lying down, give by deep subcutaneous injection, alternating doses between left and right anterolateral and posterolateral abdominal walls.
• Don't massage after subcutaneous injection. Watch for signs of bleeding at site. Rotate sites and keep record.

ACTION
Accelerates formation of antithrombin III–thrombin complex and deactivates thrombin, preventing conversion of fibrinogen to fibrin. Drug has a higher antifactor-Xa-to-antifactor-IIa activity ratio than heparin.

Route	Onset	Peak	Duration
Subcut	Unknown	4 hr	Unknown

Half-life: 4½ hours.

ADVERSE REACTIONS
CNS: confusion, fever, pain.
CV: edema, peripheral edema.
GI: nausea, diarrhea.
Hematologic: *thrombocytopenia, hemorrhage,* ecchymoses, bleeding complications, hypochromic anemia.
Skin: irritation, pain, hematoma, and erythema at injection site, *rash, urticaria.*
Other: *angioedema, anaphylaxis.*

INTERACTIONS
Drug-drug. *Anticoagulants, antiplatelet drugs, NSAIDs:* May increase risk of bleeding. Use together cautiously. Monitor PT and INR.

Drug-herb. *Angelica (dong quai), boldo, bromelains, capsicum, chamomile, dandelion, danshen, devil's claw, fenugreek, feverfew, garlic, ginger, ginkgo, ginseng, horse chestnut, licorice, meadowsweet, onion, passion flower, red clover, willow:* May increase risk of bleeding. Discourage use together.

EFFECTS ON LAB TEST RESULTS
• May increase ALT and AST levels. May decrease hemoglobin level.
• May decrease platelet count.

CONTRAINDICATIONS & CAUTIONS
• Contraindicated in patients hypersensitive to drug, heparin, or pork products; in those with active major bleeding; and in those with thrombocytopenia and antiplatelet antibodies in presence of drug.
• Use cautiously in patients with history of heparin-induced thrombocytopenia, aneurysms, cerebrovascular hemorrhage, spinal or epidural punctures (as with anesthesia), uncontrolled hypertension, or threatened abortion.
• Use cautiously in elderly patients and in those with conditions that place them at increased risk for hemorrhage, such as bacterial endocarditis, congenital or acquired bleeding disorders, ulcer disease, angiodysplastic GI disease, hemorrhagic stroke, or recent spinal, eye, or brain surgery.
• Use cautiously in patients with prosthetic heart valves, with regional or lumbar block anesthesia, blood dyscrasias, recent childbirth, pericarditis or pericardial effusion, renal insufficiency, or severe CNS trauma.

NURSING CONSIDERATIONS
• It's important to achieve hemostasis at the puncture site after PCI. The vascular access sheath for instrumentation should remain in place for 6 hours after a dose if manual compression method is used; give next dose no sooner than 6 to 8 hours after sheath removal. Monitor vital signs and site for hematoma and bleeding.
• Monitor pregnant women closely. Warn pregnant women and women of childbearing age about the potential risk of therapy to her and the fetus.

• Multidose vial shouldn't be used in pregnant women because of benzyl alcohol content.
• Monitor anti-Xa levels in pregnant women with mechanical heart valves.
• *Alert:* Patients who receive epidural or spinal anesthesia during therapy are at increased risk for developing an epidural or spinal hematoma, which may result in long-term or permanent paralysis. Monitor these patients closely for neurologic impairment.
• Draw blood to establish baseline coagulation parameters before therapy.
• Never give drug I.M.
• *Alert:* Don't try to expel the air bubble from the 30- or 40-mg prefilled syringes. This may lead to loss of drug and an incorrect dose.
• Avoid I.M. injections of other drugs to prevent or minimize hematoma.
• Monitor platelet counts regularly. Patients with normal coagulation won't need close monitoring of PT or PTT.
• Regularly inspect patient for bleeding gums, bruises on arms or legs, petechiae, nosebleeds, melena, tarry stools, hematuria, hematemesis.
• To treat severe overdose, give protamine sulfate (a heparin antagonist) by slow I.V. infusion at concentration of 1% to equal dose of drug injected.
• *Alert:* Drug isn't interchangeable with heparin or other low–molecular-weight heparins.

PATIENT TEACHING
• Instruct patient and family to watch for signs of bleeding or abnormal bruising and to notify prescriber immediately if any occur.
• Tell patient to avoid OTC drugs containing aspirin or other salicylates unless ordered by prescriber.
• Advise patient to consult with prescriber before initiating any herbal therapy; many herbs have anticoagulant, antiplatelet, or fibrinolytic properties.

ephedrine sulfate
e-FED-rin

Pharmacologic class: adrenergic
Pregnancy risk category C

AVAILABLE FORMS
Capsules: 25 mg, 50 mg
Injection: 25 mg/ml, 50 mg/ml

INDICATIONS & DOSAGES
➤ **Hypotension**
Adults: 25 mg P.O. once daily to q.i.d. Or, 5 to 25 mg I.V., p.r.n., to maximum of 150 mg/24 hours. Or, 25 to 50 mg I.M. or subcutaneously.
Children: 3 mg/kg P.O. or 0.5 mg/kg or 16.7 mg/m^2 subcutaneously or I.M. every 4 to 6 hours.
➤ **Bronchodilation**
Adults and children older than age 12: 12.5 to 25 mg P.O. every 4 hours, as needed, not to exceed 150 mg in 24 hours.
Children age 2 to 12: 2 to 3 mg/kg or 100 mg/m^2 P.O. daily in four to six divided doses. Or, for children ages 6 to 12, 6.25 to 12.5 mg P.O. every 4 hours, not to exceed 75 mg in 24 hours.

ADMINISTRATION
P.O.
• Give last dose of the day at least 2 hours before bedtime, to prevent insomnia.
I.V.
• Drug is compatible with most common solutions.
• Give slowly by direct injection.
• If needed, repeat in 5 to 10 minutes.
• **Incompatibilities:** Fructose 10% in normal saline solution; hydrocortisone sodium succinate; Ionosol B, D-CM, and D solutions; pentobarbital sodium; phenobarbital sodium; thiopental.
I.M.
• Don't use solution with particulate matter or discoloration.
• Document injection site.
Subcutaneous
• Don't use solution with particulate matter or discoloration.
• Document injection site.

ACTION

Relaxes bronchial smooth muscle by stimulating $beta_2$ receptors; also stimulates alpha and beta receptors and is a direct- and indirect-acting sympathomimetic.

Route	Onset	Peak	Duration
P.O.	15–60 min	Unknown	3–5 hr
I.V.	5 min	Unknown	60 min
I.M., Subcut	10–20 min	Unknown	30–60 min

Half-life: 3 to 6 hours.

ADVERSE REACTIONS

CNS: *insomnia, nervousness, cerebral hemorrhage,* dizziness, headache, muscle weakness, euphoria, confusion, delirium, tremor.
CV: *palpitations, arrhythmias,* tachycardia, hypertension, precordial pain.
EENT: dry nose and throat.
GI: nausea, vomiting, anorexia.
GU: urine retention, painful urination from visceral sphincter spasm.
Skin: diaphoresis.

INTERACTIONS

Drug-drug. *Acetazolamide:* May increase ephedrine level. Monitor patient for toxicity.
Alpha blockers: May reduce vasopressor response. Monitor patient closely.
Antihypertensives: May decrease effects. Monitor blood pressure.
Beta blockers: May block the effects of ephedrine. Monitor patient closely.
Cardiac glycosides, general anesthetics (halogenated hydrocarbons): May increase risk of ventricular arrhythmias. Monitor ECG closely.
Guanethidine: May decrease pressor effects of ephedrine. Monitor patient closely.
MAO inhibitors (phenelzine, tranyl-cypromine): May cause severe headache, hypertension, fever, and hypertensive crisis. Avoid using together.

Methyldopa, reserpine: May inhibit ephedrine effects. Use together cautiously.
Oxytocics: May cause severe hypertension. Avoid using together.
Tricyclic antidepressants: May decrease pressor response. Monitor patient closely.

EFFECTS ON LAB TEST RESULTS

None reported.

CONTRAINDICATIONS & CAUTIONS

• Contraindicated in patients hypersensitive to ephedrine and other sympathomimetics and in those with porphyria, severe coronary artery disease, arrhythmias, angle-closure glaucoma, psychoneurosis, angina pectoris, substantial organic heart disease, or CV disease.
• Contraindicated in those receiving MAO inhibitors or general anesthesia with cyclopropane or halothane.
• Use with caution in elderly patients and in those with hypertension, hyperthyroidism, nervous or excitable states, diabetes, or prostatic hyperplasia.

NURSING CONSIDERATIONS

• *Alert:* Hypoxia, hypercapnia, and acidosis must be identified and corrected before or during therapy because they may reduce effectiveness or increase adverse reactions.
• Drug isn't a substitute for blood or fluid volume replenishment. Volume deficit must be corrected before giving vasopressors.
• Effectiveness decreases after 2 to 3 weeks as tolerance develops. Prescriber may increase dosage. Drug isn't addictive.
• *Look alike–sound alike:* Don't confuse ephedrine with epinephrine.

PATIENT TEACHING

• Tell patient taking oral form of drug at home to take last dose of day at least 2 hours before bedtime to prevent insomnia.
• Warn patient not to take OTC drugs or herbs that contain ephedrine without consulting prescriber.

epinephrine (adrenaline)
ep-i-NEF-rin

Primatene Mist ◊

epinephrine hydrochloride
Adrenalin Chloride, EpiPen,
EpiPen Jr, microNefrin ◊,
Nephron ◊

Pharmacologic class: adrenergic
Pregnancy risk category C

AVAILABLE FORMS
Aerosol inhaler: 220 mcg ◊
Injection: 0.1 mg/ml (1:10,000),
0.5 mg/ml (1:2,000), 1 mg/ml (1:1,000)
parenteral
Nebulizer inhaler: 1% (1:100) ◊,
1.125% ◊

INDICATIONS & DOSAGES
➤ **Bronchospasm, hypersensitivity
reactions, anaphylaxis**
Adults: 0.1 to 0.5 ml of 1:1,000 solution
I.M. or subcutaneously. Repeat every
10 to 15 minutes as needed. Or, 0.1 to
0.25 ml of 1:1,000 solution I.V. slowly over
5 to 10 minutes (1 to 2.5 ml of a commercially available 1:10,000 injection or of
a 1:10,000 dilution prepared by diluting
1 ml of a commercially available 1:1,000
injection with 10 ml of water for injection
or normal saline solution for injection).
May repeat every 5 to 15 minutes as
needed, or follow with a continuous I.V.
infusion, starting at 1 mcg/minute and
increasing to 4 mcg/minute, as needed.
Children: 0.01 ml/kg (10 mcg) of
1:1,000 solution subcutaneously; repeat
every 20 minutes to 4 hours, as needed.
Maximum single dose shouldn't exceed
0.5 mg.
➤ **Hemostasis**
Adults: 1:50,000 to 1:1,000, sprayed or
applied topically.
➤ **Acute asthma attacks**
Adults and children age 4 and older:
One inhalation, repeated once if needed
after at least 1 minute; don't give subsequent doses for at least 3 hours. Or, 1
to 3 deep inhalations using a hand-bulb
nebulizer containing 1% (1:100) solution

of epinephrine repeated every 3 hours, as
needed.
➤ **To prolong local anesthetic effect**
Adults and children: With local anesthetics, may be used in concentrations of
1:500,000 to 1:50,000; most commonly,
1:200,000.
➤ **To restore cardiac rhythm in
cardiac arrest**
Adults: 0.5 to 1 mg I.V., repeated every
3 to 5 minutes, if needed. A higher dose
may be used if 1 mg fails: 3 to 5 mg (about
0.1 mg/kg); repeat every 3 to 5 minutes.
Children: 0.01 mg/kg (0.1 ml/kg of
1:10,000 injection) I.V. First endotracheal dose is 0.1 mg/kg (0.1 ml/kg of a
1:1,000 injection) diluted in 1 to 2 ml of
half-normal or normal saline solution.
Give subsequent I.V. or intratracheal doses
from 0.1 to 0.2 mg/kg (0.1 to 0.2 ml/kg of
a 1:1,000 injection), repeated every 3 to
5 minutes, if needed.

ADMINISTRATION
I.V.
● Keep solution in light-resistant container,
and don't remove before use.
● Just before use, mix with D_5W, normal
saline solution for injection, lactated
Ringer's injection, or combinations of
dextrose in saline solution.
● Monitor blood pressure, heart rate, and
ECG when therapy starts and frequently
thereafter.
● Discard solution if it's discolored or
contains precipitate or after 24 hours.
● **Incompatibilities:** Aminophylline;
ampicillin sodium; furosemide;
hyaluronidase; Ionosol D-CM, PSL, and
T solutions with D_5W; mephentermine;
thiopental sodium. Compatible with most
other I.V. solutions. Rapidly destroyed
by alkalies or oxidizing drugs, including
halogens, nitrates, nitrites, permanganates,
sodium bicarbonate, and salts of easily
reducible metals, such as iron, copper, and
zinc. Don't mix with alkaline solutions.
I.M.
● Avoid I.M. use of parenteral suspension
into buttocks. Gas gangrene may occur
because drug reduces oxygen tension
of the tissues, encouraging growth of
contaminating organisms.
● Massage site after I.M. injection to counteract vasoconstriction. Repeated local

injection can cause necrosis at injection site.

Subcutaneous
● Don't refrigerate; protect from light.
● Preferred route. Don't inject too deeply and enter muscle.

Inhalational
● Teach patient to perform oral inhalation correctly. See "Patient teaching" for complete instructions.
● Epinephrine 1:100 will turn from pink to brown if exposed to air, light, heat, alkalies, and some metals. Don't use solution that's discolored or has a precipitate.

ACTION
Relaxes bronchial smooth muscle by stimulating $beta_2$ receptors and alpha and beta receptors in the sympathetic nervous system.

Route	Onset	Peak	Duration
I.V.	Immediate	5 min	Short
I.M.	Variable	Unknown	1–4 hr
Subcut	5–15 min	30 min	1–4 hr
Inhalation	1–5 min	Unknown	1–3 hr

Half-life: Unknown.

ADVERSE REACTIONS
CNS: *drowsiness, headache, nervousness, tremor,* **cerebral hemorrhage, stroke,** vertigo, pain, disorientation, agitation, fear, dizziness, weakness.
CV: *palpitations,* **ventricular fibrillation, shock,** widened pulse pressure, hypertension, tachycardia, anginal pain, altered ECG (including a decreased T-wave amplitude).
GI: *nausea, vomiting.*
Respiratory: dyspnea.
Skin: urticaria, hemorrhage at injection site, pallor.
Other: tissue necrosis.

INTERACTIONS
Drug-drug. *Alpha blockers:* May cause hypotension from unopposed beta-adrenergic effects. Avoid using together.
Antihistamines, thyroid hormones: When given with sympathomimetics, may cause severe adverse cardiac effects. Avoid using together.
Cardiac glycosides, general anesthetics (halogenated hydrocarbons): May increase

risk of ventricular arrhythmias. Monitor ECG closely.
Carteolol, nadolol, penbutolol, pindolol, propranolol, timolol: May cause hypertension followed by bradycardia. Stop beta blocker 3 days before starting epinephrine.
Doxapram, methylphenidate: May enhance CNS stimulation or pressor effects. Monitor patient closely.
Ergot alkaloids: May decrease vasoconstrictor activity. Monitor patient closely.
Guanadrel, guanethidine: May enhance pressor effects of epinephrine. Monitor patient closely.
Levodopa: May enhance risk of arrhythmias. Monitor ECG closely.
MAO inhibitors: May increase risk of hypertensive crisis. Monitor blood pressure closely.
Tricyclic antidepressants: May potentiate the pressor response and cause arrhythmias. Use together cautiously.

EFFECTS ON LAB TEST RESULTS
● May increase BUN, glucose, and lactic acid levels.

CONTRAINDICATIONS & CAUTIONS
● Contraindicated in patients with angle-closure glaucoma, shock (other than anaphylactic shock), organic brain damage, cardiac dilation, arrhythmias, coronary insufficiency, or cerebral arteriosclerosis.
● Contraindicated in patients receiving general anesthesia with halogenated hydrocarbons or cyclopropane and in patients in labor (may delay second stage).
● Commercial products containing sulfites contraindicated in patients with sulfite allergies, except when epinephrine is being used to treat serious allergic reactions or other emergency situations.
● Contraindicated for use in fingers, toes, ears, nose, or genitalia when used with local anesthetic.
● Use cautiously in patients with longstanding bronchial asthma or emphysema who have developed degenerative heart disease.
● Use cautiously in elderly patients and in those with hyperthyroidism, CV disease, hypertension, psychoneurosis, and diabetes.

NURSING CONSIDERATIONS
● In patients with Parkinson disease, drug increases rigidity and tremor.
● Drug interferes with tests for urinary catecholamines.
● One mg equals 1 ml of 1:1,000 solution or 10 ml of 1:10,000 solution.
● Epinephrine is drug of choice in emergency treatment of acute anaphylactic reactions.
● Observe patient closely for adverse reactions. Notify prescriber if adverse reactions develop; adjusting dosage or stopping drug may be necessary.
● If blood pressure increases sharply, give rapid-acting vasodilators, such as nitrates and alpha blockers, to counteract the marked pressor effect of large doses.
● Drug is rapidly destroyed by oxidizing products, such as iodine, chromates, nitrites, oxygen, and salts of easily reducible metals (such as iron).
● When treating patient with reactions caused by other drugs given I.M. or subcutaneously, inject this drug into the site where the other drug was given to minimize further absorption.
● *Look alike–sound alike:* Don't confuse epinephrine with ephedrine or norepinephrine.

PATIENT TEACHING
● Teach patient to perform oral inhalation correctly. Give the following instructions for using a metered-dose inhaler:
– Shake canister.
– Clear nasal passages and throat.
– Breathe out, expelling as much air from lungs as possible.
– Place mouthpiece well into mouth, and inhale deeply as you release dose from inhaler. Or, hold inhaler about 1 inch (two fingerwidths) from open mouth, and inhale while releasing dose.
– Hold breath for several seconds, remove mouthpiece, and exhale slowly.
● If more than one inhalation is prescribed, advise patient to wait at least 2 minutes before repeating procedure.
● Tell patient that use of a spacer device may improve drug delivery to lungs.
● If patient is also using a corticosteroid inhaler, instruct him to use the bronchodilator first and then to wait about 5 minutes before using the corticosteroid.

This lets the bronchodilator open the air passages for maximal effectiveness.
● Instruct patient to remove canister and wash inhaler with warm, soapy water at least once weekly.
● If patient has acute hypersensitivity reactions (such as to bee stings), you may need to teach him to self-inject drug.

SAFETY ALERT!

erlotinib
ur-LOE-tih-nib

Tarceva

Pharmacologic class: epidermal growth factor receptor inhibitor
Pregnancy risk category D

AVAILABLE FORMS
Tablets: 25 mg, 100 mg, 150 mg

INDICATIONS & DOSAGES
➤ **With gemcitabine, first-line treatment of locally advanced, unresectable, or metastatic pancreatic cancer**
Adults: 100 mg P.O. once daily taken at least 1 hour before or 2 hours after meals. Continue until disease progresses or intolerable toxicity occurs.
➤ **Locally advanced or metastatic non–small cell lung cancer after failure of at least one chemotherapy regimen**
Adults: 150 mg P.O. once daily taken at least 1 hour before or 2 hours after meals. Continue until disease progresses or intolerable toxicity occurs.
Adjust-a-dose: In patients with severe skin reactions or severe diarrhea refractory to loperamide, reduce dose in 50-mg decrements or stop therapy.

ADMINISTRATION
P.O.
● Give drug 1 hour before or 2 hours after a meal.

ACTION
Probably inhibits tyrosine kinase activity in epidermal growth factor receptors, which are expressed on the surface of

normal and cancer cells. Is particularly selective for human epidermal growth factor receptor 1.

Route	Onset	Peak	Duration
P.O.	Unknown	4 hr	Unknown

Half-life: About 36 hours.

ADVERSE REACTIONS
CNS: *fatigue.*
EENT: *conjunctivitis, keratoconjuctivitis sicca.*
GI: *abdominal pain, anorexia, diarrhea, nausea, stomatitis, vomiting.*
Respiratory: *cough, dyspnea, **pulmonary toxicity.***
Skin: *dry skin, pruritus, rash.*
Other: *infection.*

INTERACTIONS
Drug-drug. *Anticoagulants, such as warfarin:* May increase risk of bleeding. Monitor PT and INR.
CYP3A4 inducers, such as carbamazepine, phenobarbital, phenytoin, rifabutin, rifampin: May increase erlotinib metabolism. Increase erlotinib dosage, as needed.
Strong CYP3A4 inhibitors, such as atazanavir, clarithromycin, indinavir, itraconazole, ketoconazole, nefazodone, nelfinavir, ritonavir, saquinavir, telithromycin, troleandomycin, voriconazole: May decrease erlotinib metabolism. Use together cautiously, and consider reducing erlotinib dosage.
Drug-herb. *St. John's wort:* May increase drug metabolism. Drug dosage may need to be increased. Discourage use together.

EFFECTS ON LAB TEST RESULTS
• May increase ALT, AST, and bilirubin levels.
• May increase INR and PT.

CONTRAINDICATIONS & CAUTIONS
• Use cautiously in patients with pulmonary disease or liver impairment. Also use cautiously in patients who have received or are receiving chemotherapy because it may worsen adverse pulmonary effects.

NURSING CONSIDERATIONS
• Monitor liver function tests periodically during therapy. Notify prescriber of abnormal findings.
• *Alert:* Rarely, serious interstitial lung disease may occur. If patient develops dyspnea, cough, and fever, notify prescriber. Therapy may need to be interrupted or stopped.
• Monitor patient for severe diarrhea, and give loperamide if needed.
• Women shouldn't breast-feed while taking this drug.
• Drug has been used to treat squamous cell head and neck cancer.

PATIENT TEACHING
• *Alert:* Tell patient to immediately report new or worsened cough, shortness of breath, eye irritation, or severe or persistent diarrhea, nausea, anorexia, or vomiting.
• Instruct patient to take drug 1 hour before or 2 hours after food.
• Advise women to avoid pregnancy while taking this drug and for 2 weeks after treatment ends. Drug can harm fetus.
• Explain the likelihood of serious interactions with other drugs and herbal supplements and the need to tell prescriber about any change in drugs and supplements taken.

ethambutol hydrochloride
e-THAM-byoo-tole

Etibi†, Myambutol

Pharmacologic class: synthetic antituberculotic
Pregnancy risk category B

AVAILABLE FORMS
Tablets: 100 mg, 400 mg

INDICATIONS & DOSAGES
➤ **Adjunctive treatment for pulmonary tuberculosis**
Adults and children older than age 13: In patients who haven't received prior antitubercular therapy, 15 mg/kg P.O. daily as a single dose, combined with other antituberculotics. For retreatment, 25 mg/kg P.O. daily as a single dose for

60 days (or until bacteriologic smears and cultures become negative) with at least one other antituberculotic; then decrease to 15 mg/kg/day as a single dose.

ADMINISTRATION
P.O.
• Obtain baseline visual acuity and color discrimination tests and AST and ALT levels before starting therapy.
• Always give drug with other antituberculotics to prevent development of resistant organisms.

ACTION
May inhibit synthesis of one or more metabolites of susceptible bacteria, changing cell metabolism during cell division; bacteriostatic.

Route	Onset	Peak	Duration
P.O.	Unknown	2–4 hr	Unknown

Half-life: About 3½ hours.

ADVERSE REACTIONS
CNS: dizziness, fever, hallucinations, headache, malaise, mental confusion, peripheral neuritis.
EENT: optic neuritis.
GI: abdominal pain, anorexia, GI upset, nausea, vomiting.
Hematologic: *thrombocytopenia.*
Metabolic: hyperuricemia.
Musculoskeletal: joint pain.
Respiratory: bloody sputum.
Skin: *toxic epidermal necrolysis,* dermatitis, pruritus.
Other: *anaphylactoid reactions,* precipitation of acute gout.

INTERACTIONS
Drug-drug. *Aluminum salts:* May delay and reduce absorption of ethambutol. Separate doses by several hours.

EFFECTS ON LAB TEST RESULTS
• May increase ALT, AST, bilirubin, and uric acid levels. May decrease glucose level.
• May decrease platelet count.

CONTRAINDICATIONS & CAUTIONS
• Contraindicated in children younger than age 13, patients hypersensitive to drug, and patients with optic neuritis.

• Use cautiously in patients with impaired renal function, cataracts, recurrent eye inflammation, gout, or diabetic retinopathy.

NURSING CONSIDERATIONS
• Perform visual acuity and color discrimination tests before and during therapy.
• Ensure that any changes in vision don't result from an underlying condition.
• Obtain AST and ALT levels before therapy, and monitor these levels every 3 to 4 weeks.
• In patients with impaired renal function, base dosage on drug level.
• Monitor uric acid level; observe patient for signs and symptoms of gout.

PATIENT TEACHING
• Reassure patient that visual disturbances usually disappear several weeks to months after drug is stopped. Inflammation of the optic nerve is related to dosage and duration of treatment.
• Inform patient that drug is given with other antituberculotics.
• Stress importance of compliance with drug therapy.
• Advise patient to report adverse reactions to prescriber.

SAFETY ALERT!

etoposide (VP-16-213)
e-toe-POE-side

Toposar, VePesid

etoposide phosphate
Etopophos

Pharmacologic class: podophyllotoxin derivative
Pregnancy risk category D

AVAILABLE FORMS
etoposide
Capsules: 50 mg
Injection: 20 mg/ml in 5-, 12.5-, and 25-ml vials
etoposide phosphate
Injection: 119.3-mg vials equivalent to 100 mg etoposide

INDICATIONS & DOSAGES
➤ **Testicular cancer**
Adults: 50 to 100 mg/m^2 daily I.V. on 5 consecutive days every 3 to 4 weeks. Or, 100 mg/m^2 daily I.V. on days 1, 3, and 5 every 3 to 4 weeks for three or four courses of therapy.
➤ **Small cell carcinoma of the lung**
Adults: 35 mg/m^2 daily I.V. for 4 days. Or, 50 mg/m^2 daily I.V. for 5 days. P.O. dose is two times I.V. dose, rounded to nearest 50 mg.
Adjust-a-dose: For patients with creatinine clearance of 15 to 50 ml/minute, reduce dose by 25%.
➤ **Kaposi sarcoma ♦**
Adults: 150 mg/m^2 I.V. daily for 3 days every 4 weeks. Repeat as needed, based on response.

ADMINISTRATION
P.O.
• Give drug without regard for food.
• Don't give drug with grapefruit juice.
I.V.
• Preparing and giving parenteral drug may be mutagenic, teratogenic, or carcinogenic. Follow facility policy to reduce risks.
• For etoposide infusion, dilute to 0.2 or 0.4 mg/ml in either D$_5$W or normal saline solution. Higher concentrations may crystallize.
• Give etoposide by slow infusion over at least 30 minutes to prevent severe hypotension.
• For etoposide phosphate, give without further dilution or dilute to as low as 0.1 mg/ml in either D$_5$W or normal saline solution.
• Give etoposide phosphate over 5 to 210 minutes.
• Check blood pressure every 15 minutes during infusion. Hypotension may occur if infusion is too rapid. If systolic pressure falls below 90 mm Hg, stop infusion and notify prescriber.
• Etoposide diluted to 0.2 mg/ml is stable 96 hours at room temperature in plastic or glass, unprotected from light; at 0.4 mg/ml, it's stable 24 hours under same conditions. Diluted etoposide phosphate solution is stable for same times at room temperature or 24 hours refrigerated.

• **Incompatibilities:** Cefepime hydrochloride, filgrastim, gallium nitrate, idarubicin.

ACTION
Inhibits topoisomerase II enzyme, causing inability to repair DNA strand breaks, which leads to cell death. Cell cycle specific to G$_2$ portion of cell cycle.

Route	Onset	Peak	Duration
P.O., I.V.	Unknown	Unknown	Unknown

Half-life: Initial phase, ½ to 2 hours; terminal phase, 5¼ hours.

ADVERSE REACTIONS
CNS: peripheral neuropathy.
CV: hypotension.
GI: *anorexia, diarrhea, nausea, vomiting,* abdominal pain, stomatitis.
Hematologic: LEUKOPENIA, NEUTROPENIA, THROMBOCYTOPENIA, *anemia, myelosuppression.*
Hepatic: *hepatotoxicity.*
Skin: *reversible alopecia,* rash.
Other: *anaphylaxis,* hypersensitivity reactions.

INTERACTIONS
Drug-drug. *Cyclosporine:* May increase etoposide level and toxicity. Monitor CBC and adjust etoposide dose.
Phosphatase inhibitors such as levamisole hydrochloride: May decrease etoposide effectiveness. Monitor drug effects.
Warfarin: May further prolong PT. Monitor PT and INR closely.
Drug-food. *Grapefruit juice:* May reduce etoposide concentrations. Avoid using together.

EFFECTS ON LAB TEST RESULTS
• May decrease hemoglobin level.
• May decrease neutrophil, platelet, RBC, and WBC counts.

CONTRAINDICATIONS & CAUTIONS
• Contraindicated in patients hypersensitive to drug.
• Use cautiously in patients who have had cytotoxic or radiation therapy and in those with hepatic impairment.

NURSING CONSIDERATIONS
- Obtain baseline blood pressure before starting therapy.
- Anticipate need for antiemetics.
- Have diphenhydramine, hydrocortisone, epinephrine, and emergency equipment available to establish an airway in case anaphylaxis occurs.
- Store capsules in refrigerator.
- Monitor CBC. Watch for evidence of bone marrow suppression.
- Observe patient's mouth for signs of ulceration.
- To prevent bleeding, avoid all I.M. injections when platelet count is below 50,000/mm^3.
- Anticipate need for RBC colony-stimulating factors or blood transfusions.
- Etoposide phosphate dose is expressed as etoposide equivalents; 119.3 mg of etoposide phosphate is equivalent to 100 mg of etoposide.

PATIENT TEACHING
- Tell patient to watch for signs and symptoms of infection (fever, sore throat, fatigue) and bleeding (easy bruising, nosebleeds, bleeding gums, tarry stools). Tell patient to take temperature daily.
- Inform patient of need for frequent blood pressure readings during I.V. administration.
- Caution woman of childbearing age to avoid pregnancy and breast-feeding during therapy.

---

fexofenadine hydrochloride
fecks-oh-FEN-a-deen

Allegra

Pharmacologic class: piperidine
Pregnancy risk category C

AVAILABLE FORMS
Capsules: 60 mg
Oral suspension: 30 mg/5 ml
Tablets: 30 mg, 60 mg, 180 mg
Tablets (orally disintegrating): 30 mg

INDICATIONS & DOSAGES
➤ **Seasonal allergic rhinitis**
Adults and children age 12 and older:
60 mg P.O. b.i.d. or 180 mg P.O. once daily.
Children ages 2 to 11: Give 30 mg P.O. b.i.d. either as a tablet or 5 ml oral suspension.
➤ **Chronic idiopathic urticaria**
Adults and children age 12 and older:
60 mg P.O. b.i.d. or 180 mg P.O. once daily.
Children ages 2 to 11: Give 30 mg P.O. b.i.d. either as a tablet or 5 ml oral suspension.
Children ages 6 months to 2 years: 15 mg (2.5 ml) P.O. b.i.d.
Adjust-a-dose: For patients with impaired renal function or a need for dialysis, give adults 60 mg daily, children ages 2 to 11, 30 mg daily, and children ages 6 months to 2 years, 15 mg daily.

ADMINISTRATION
P.O.
- Don't give antacid within 2 hours of this drug.
- Give orally disintegrating tablets (ODTs) to patient with an empty stomach. Allow ODT to disintegrate on the patient's tongue; and it may be swallowed with or without water.
- Don't remove ODT from blister package until time of administration.

ACTION
A long-acting nonsedating antihistamine that selectively inhibits peripheral H$_1$ receptors.

Route	Onset	Peak	Duration
P.O.	Rapid	3 hr	14 hr

Half-life: 14½ hours.

ADVERSE REACTIONS
CNS: fatigue, drowsiness, headache.
GI: nausea, dyspepsia.
GU: dysmenorrhea.
Other: viral infection.

INTERACTIONS
Drug-drug. *Aluminum or magnesium antacids:* May decrease fexofenadine level. Separate dosage times.
Erythromycin, ketoconazole: May increase fexofenadine level. Monitor patient for side effects.
Drug-food. *Apple juice, grapefruit juice, orange juice:* May decrease drug effects. Patients should take drug with liquid other than these juices.
Drug-lifestyle. *Alcohol use:* May increase CNS depression. Discourage use together.

EFFECTS ON LAB TEST RESULTS
● May prevent, reduce, or mask positive result in diagnostic skin test.

CONTRAINDICATIONS & CAUTIONS
● Contraindicated in patients hypersensitive to drug or its components.
● Use cautiously in patients with impaired renal function.

NURSING CONSIDERATIONS
● Stop drug 4 days before patient undergoes diagnostic skin tests because drug can prevent, reduce, or mask positive skin test response.
● It's unknown if drug appears in breast milk; use caution when using drug in breast-feeding woman.

PATIENT TEACHING
● Instruct patient or parent not to exceed prescribed dosage and to use drug only when needed.
● Warn patient to avoid alcohol and hazardous activities that require alertness until CNS effects of drug are known. Explain that drug may cause drowsiness.
● Tell patient not to take antacids within 2 hours of this drug.
● Advise patient with dry mouth to try sugarless gum, hard candy, or ice chips.
● Tell parents to keep the oral suspension in a cool, dry place, tightly closed, and to shake well before using.
● Instruct patient to let ODT disintegrate on the tongue then swallow with or without water.
● Tell patient ODT should be taken on an empty stomach.
● Tell patient to keep ODT in original blister package until time of use.

flunisolide
floo-NISS-oh-lide

AeroBid, AeroBid-M, Nasarel, Rhinalar†

flunisolide hemihydrate
AeroSpan HFA

Pharmacologic class: glucocorticoid
Pregnancy risk category C

AVAILABLE FORMS
flunisolide
Nasal solution: 25 mcg/metered spray
Oral inhalant: 250 mcg/metered spray (at least 100 metered inhalations/container)
flunisolide hemihydrate
Oral inhalant in a hydrofluoroalkane (HFA) inhaler: 80 mcg/metered dose

INDICATIONS & DOSAGES
➤ **Chronic asthma**
Adults and adolescents older than age 15: Give 2 inhalations (500 mcg) with chlorofluorocarbon (CFC) inhaler b.i.d. Maximum, 8 inhalations (2,000 mcg) daily.
Children ages 6 to 15: Give 2 inhalations (500 mcg) with CFC inhaler b.i.d. Maximum, 1,000 mcg daily.
➤ **Chronic asthma**
Adults and children age 12 and older: Give 2 inhalations (160 mcg) with HFA inhaler b.i.d. Don't exceed 320 mcg twice daily.
Children ages 6 to 11: Give 1 inhalation (80 mcg) with HFA inhaler b.i.d. Don't exceed 160 mcg twice daily.
➤ **Seasonal or perennial rhinitis**
Adults and adolescents older than age 14: Give 2 sprays (50 mcg) in each nostril b.i.d. May be increased to t.i.d., as needed. Maximum dose is 8 sprays in each nostril daily (400 mcg).
Children ages 6 to 14: Give 1 spray (25 mcg) in each nostril t.i.d. or 2 sprays (50 mcg) in each nostril b.i.d. Maximum dose is 4 sprays in each nostril daily (200 mcg).

ADMINISTRATION
Inhalational
● Warm the canister to room temperature before using.

• Allow 1 minute between doses.
Intranasal
• Before the first use, prime the nasal spray by pushing down on the pump 5 or 6 times until a fine mist appears.

ACTION
A corticosteroid that may decrease inflammation of asthma by inhibiting macrophages, T-cells, eosinophils, and mediators such as leukotrienes, while reducing the number of mast cells within the airway.

Route	Onset	Peak	Duration
Inhalation (nasal)	< 3 wk	Unknown	Unknown
Inhalation (oral)	1–4 wk	Unknown	Unknown

Half-life: 1.8 hours.

ADVERSE REACTIONS
CNS: *headache,* dizziness, fever, irritability, nervousness.
CV: chest pain, edema, palpitations.
EENT: *nasal congestion, sore throat,* altered taste, hoarseness, nasal burning or stinging, nasal irritation, nasopharyngeal fungal infections, throat irritation.
GI: *diarrhea, nausea, unpleasant taste, upset stomach, vomiting,* abdominal pain, decreased appetite, dry mouth.
Respiratory: *cold symptoms, upper respiratory tract infection.*
Skin: pruritus, rash.
Other: *influenza.*

INTERACTIONS
None significant.

EFFECTS ON LAB TEST RESULTS
None reported.

CONTRAINDICATIONS & CAUTIONS
• Contraindicated in patients hypersensitive to drug and in those with status asthmaticus or respiratory tract infections.
• Drug isn't recommended in patients with nonasthmatic bronchial diseases or with asthma controlled by bronchodilator or other noncorticosteroid alone.

NURSING CONSIDERATIONS
• All patients with asthma should have routine tests of adrenal cortical function, including measurement of early morning resting cortisol levels to establish a baseline in the event of an emergency.
• *Alert:* Withdraw drug slowly in patients who have received long-term oral corticosteroid therapy.
• After withdrawing systemic corticosteroids, patient may need supplemental systemic corticosteroids if stress (trauma, surgery, or infection) causes adrenal insufficiency.
• Store drug at room temperature.
• *Look alike–sound alike:* Don't confuse flunisolide with fluocinonide.
• Stop nasal spray after 3 weeks if symptoms don't improve.

PATIENT TEACHING
Oral inhalant
• Warn patient that drug doesn't relieve acute asthma attacks.
• *Alert:* Instruct patient to immediately contact prescriber if asthma episodes unresponsive to bronchodilators occur during treatment.
• Advise patient to ensure delivery of proper dose by gently warming the canister to room temperature before using. Some patients carry the canister in a pocket to keep it warm.
• Tell patient who also uses a bronchodilator to use it several minutes before beginning flunisolide treatment.
• Instruct patient to begin inhaling immediately before activating the canister to get the full dose.
• Instruct patient to allow 1 minute to elapse before repeating inhalations and to hold his breath for a few seconds to enhance drug action.
• Teach patient to keep inhaler clean and unobstructed. If he's using a CFC inhaler, tell him to wash it with warm water and dry it thoroughly after use. The HFA inhaler doesn't need cleaning during normal use.
• Teach patient to check mucous membranes frequently for signs and symptoms of fungal infection.
• Advise patient to prevent oral fungal infections by gargling or rinsing mouth with water after each inhaler use. Caution him not to swallow the water.

• Warn patient to avoid exposure to chickenpox or measles. If exposed, contact prescriber immediately.
• Advise parents of a child receiving long-term therapy that the child should have periodic growth measurements and be checked for evidence of hypothalamic-pituitary-adrenal axis suppression.

Nasal spray

• Tell patient to prime the nasal inhaler (5 to 6 sprays) before first use and after long periods of no use.
• Advise patient to clear nasal passageways before use.
• Patient should follow manufacturer's instructions for use and cleaning. Tell him to discard open containers after 3 months.
• Advise patient that therapeutic results may take several weeks.

---

fluticasone furoate
FLOO-tih-ka-sone

Veramyst

fluticasone propionate
Flonase, Flovent Diskus†, Flovent HFA

Pharmacologic class: corticosteroid
Pregnancy risk category C

AVAILABLE FORMS
Nasal spray (furoate): 27.5 mcg/spray
Nasal spray (propionate): 50 mcg/metered spray
Oral inhalation aerosol: 44 mcg, 110 mcg, 220 mcg
Oral inhalation powder†: 50 mcg, 100 mcg, 250 mcg

INDICATIONS & DOSAGES
➤ **As preventative in maintenance of chronic asthma in patients requiring oral corticosteroid**
Flovent Diskus †
Adults and children ages 12 and older: In patients previously taking bronchodilators alone, initially, inhaled dose of 100 mcg b.i.d. to maximum of 500 mcg b.i.d.
Adults and children age 12 and older previously taking inhaled corticosteroids: Initially, inhaled dose of 100 to 250 mcg b.i.d. to maximum of 500 mcg b.i.d.

Adults and children ages 12 and older previously taking oral corticosteroids: Inhaled dose of 500 to 1,000 mcg b.i.d. Maximum dose, 1,000 mcg b.i.d.
Children ages 4 to 11: For patients previously on bronchodilators alone or on inhaled corticosteroids, initially, inhaled dose of 50 mcg b.i.d. to maximum of 100 mcg b.i.d.
Flovent HFA
Adults and children age 12 and older: In those previously taking bronchodilators alone, initially, inhaled dose of 88 mcg b.i.d. to maximum of 440 mcg b.i.d.
Adults and children age 12 and older previously taking inhaled corticosteroids: Initially, inhaled dose of 88 to 220 mcg b.i.d. to maximum of 440 mcg b.i.d.
Adults and children age 12 and older previously taking oral corticosteroids: Initially, inhaled dose of 440 mcg b.i.d. to maximum of 880 mcg b.i.d.
Children ages 4 to 11: 88 mcg inhaled b.i.d. regardless of prior therapy.
➤ **Nasal symptoms of seasonal and perennial allergic and nonallergic rhinitis**
Flonase
Adults: Initially, 2 sprays (100 mcg) in each nostril daily or 1 spray b.i.d. Once symptoms are controlled, decrease to 1 spray in each nostril daily. Or, for seasonal allergic rhinitis, 2 sprays in each nostril once daily, as needed, for symptom control.
Adolescents and children age 4 and older: Initially, 1 spray (50 mcg) in each nostril daily. If not responding, increase to 2 sprays in each nostril daily. Once symptoms are controlled, decrease to 1 spray in each nostril daily. Maximum dose is 2 sprays in each nostril daily.
Veramyst
Adults and children age 12 and older: 110 mcg once daily administered as 2 sprays (27.5 mcg/spray) in each nostril.
Children ages 2 to 11: 55 mcg once daily administered as 1 spray (27.5 mcg/spray) in each nostril.

ADMINISTRATION
Inhalational
• Prime and shake well before each use.

Intranasal
● Prime and shake well before use.

ACTION
Anti-inflammatory and vasoconstrictor that may decrease inflammation by inhibiting mast cells, macrophages, and mediators such as leukotrienes.

Route	Onset	Peak	Duration
Inhalation (nasal)	12 hr	Several days	1–2 wk
Inhalation (oral)	24 hr	Several days	1–2 wk

Half-life: 3 hours.

ADVERSE REACTIONS
CNS: *headache,* dizziness, fever, migraine, nervousness.
EENT: *pharyngitis,* blood in nasal mucus, cataracts, conjunctivitis, dry eye, dysphonia, epistaxis, eye irritation, hoarseness, laryngitis, nasal burning or irritation, nasal discharge, rhinitis, sinusitis.
GI: *oral candidiasis,* abdominal discomfort, abdominal pain, diarrhea, mouth irritation, nausea, viral gastroenteritis, vomiting.
GU: UTI.
Hematologic: eosinophilia.
Metabolic: cushingoid features, growth retardation in children, hyperglycemia, weight gain.
Musculoskeletal: aches and pains, disorder or symptoms of neck sprain or strain, joint pain, muscular soreness, osteoporosis.
Respiratory: *upper respiratory tract infection, bronchospasm,* asthma symptoms, bronchitis, chest congestion, cough, dyspnea.
Skin: dermatitis, urticaria.
Other: *angioedema,* influenza, viral infections.

INTERACTIONS
Drug-drug. *Ketoconazole and other cytochrome P-450 3A4 inhibitors:* May increase mean fluticasone level. Use together cautiously.
Ritonavir: May cause systemic corticosteroid effects, such as Cushing syndrome and adrenal suppression. Avoid using together.

EFFECTS ON LAB TEST RESULTS
● May cause an abnormal response to the 6-hour cosyntropin stimulation test in patients taking high doses of fluticasone.

CONTRAINDICATIONS & CAUTIONS
● Contraindicated in patients hypersensitive to ingredients in these preparations.
● Contraindicated as primary treatment of patients with status asthmaticus or other acute, intense episodes of asthma.
● Use cautiously in breast-feeding women.

NURSING CONSIDERATIONS
● Because of risk of systemic absorption of inhaled corticosteroids, observe patient carefully for evidence of systemic corticosteroid effects.
● Monitor patient, especially postoperatively or during periods of stress, for evidence of inadequate adrenal response.
● During withdrawal from oral corticosteroids, some patients may experience signs and symptoms of systemically active corticosteroid withdrawal, such as joint or muscle pain, lassitude, and depression, despite maintenance or even improvement of respiratory function.
● For patients starting therapy who are currently receiving oral corticosteroid therapy, reduce dose of prednisone to no more than 2.5 mg/day on a weekly basis, beginning after at least 1 week of therapy with fluticasone.
● *Alert:* As with other inhaled asthma drugs, bronchospasm may occur with an immediate increase in wheezing after a dose. If bronchospasm occurs after a dose of inhalation aerosol, treat immediately with a fast-acting inhaled bronchodilator.

PATIENT TEACHING
● Tell patient that drug isn't indicated for the relief of acute bronchospasm.
● For proper use of drug and to attain maximal improvement, tell patient to carefully follow the accompanying patient instructions.
● Advise patient to use drug at regular intervals, as directe.

• Instruct patient to contact prescriber if nasal spray doesn't improve condition after 4 days of treatment.

• Instruct patient to immediately contact prescriber if asthma episodes unresponsive to bronchodilators occur during treatment with fluticasone. During such episodes, patient may need therapy with oral corticosteroids.

• Warn patient to avoid exposure to chickenpox or measles and, if exposed, to consult prescriber immediately.

• Tell patient to carry or wear medical identification indicating that he may need supplementary corticosteroids during stress or a severe asthma attack.

• During periods of stress or a severe asthma attack, instruct patient who has been withdrawn from systemic corticosteroids to resume prescribed oral corticosteroids immediately and to contact prescriber for further instruction.

• Tell patient to prime inhaler with 4 test sprays (away from his face) before first use, shaking well before each spray. Also, prime with 1 spray if inhaler has been dropped or not used for 1 week or longer.

• Advise patient to avoid spraying inhalation aerosol into eyes.

• Instruct patient to shake canister well before using inhalation aerosol.

• Instruct patient to rinse his mouth and spit water out after inhalation.

• Advise patient to store fluticasone powder in a dry place.

Flonase nasal spray

• Tell patient to prime the nasal inhaler before first use or after 1 week or longer of nonuse.

• Have patient clear nasal passages before use.

• Advise patient to follow manufacturer's recommendations for use and cleaning.

• Advise patient to use at regular intervals for full benefit.

• Tell patient to contact provider if signs or symptoms don't improve within 4 days or if signs or symptoms worsen.

• Tell patient that the correct amount of spray can't be guaranteed after 120 sprays, even though the bottle may not be completely empty.

fluticasone propionate and salmeterol inhalation powder
FLOO-tih-ka-sone and sal-MEE-ter-ol

Advair Diskus 100/50, Advair Diskus 250/50, Advair Diskus 500/50, Advair HFA 45/21, Advair HFA 115/21, Advair HFA 230/21

Pharmacologic class: corticosteroid, long-acting beta$_2$ adrenergic agonist
Pregnancy risk category C

AVAILABLE FORMS
Inhalation powder: 100 mcg fluticasone and 50 mcg salmeterol, 250 mcg fluticasone and 50 mcg salmeterol, 500 mcg fluticasone and 50 mcg salmeterol
Aerosol spray: 45 mcg fluticasone propionate and 21 mcg salmeterol, 115 mcg fluticasone propionate and 21 mcg salmeterol, 230 mcg fluticasone propionate and 21 mcg salmeterol

INDICATIONS & DOSAGES
➤ **Long-term maintenance of asthma**
Adults and children age 12 and older:
1 inhalation b.i.d., at least 12 hours apart of Advair Diskus; or 2 inhalations twice daily of Advair HFA. Starting doses are dependent on the patient's current asthma therapy.
Adults and children age 12 and older not currently taking an inhaled corticosteroid:
1 inhalation of fluticasone 100 mcg/salmeterol 50 mcg Diskus or fluticasone 250 mcg/salmeterol 50 mcg Diskus twice daily; or 2 inhalations of fluticasone 45 mcg/salmeterol 21 mcg HFA or fluticasone 115 mcg/salmeterol 21 mcg HFA twice daily.
Adults and children age 12 and older currently on and not adequately controlled by an inhaled corticosteroid: Consult the table on the following page.
For patients already using an inhaled corticosteroid: Maximum inhalation of Advair Diskus is 500/50 b.i.d. and maximum dose of Advair HFA is 2 inhalations of fluticasone 230 mcg/salmeterol 21 mcg b.i.d.

Name of current corticosteroid	Dose of current corticosteroid	Recommended strength of Advair Diskus (1 inhalation b.i.d.)	Recommended strength of Advair HFA (2 inhalations b.i.d.)
Beclomethasone dipropionate HFA inhalation aerosol	≤ 160 mcg 320 mcg 640 mcg	100 mcg/50 mcg 250 mcg/50 mcg 500 mcg/50 mcg	45 mcg/21 mcg 115 mcg/21 mcg 230 mcg/21 mcg
Budesonide inhalation aerosol/powder	≤ 400 mcg 800 to 1,200 mcg 1,600 mcg	100 mcg/50 mcg 250 mcg/50 mcg 500 mcg/50 mcg	45 mcg/21 mcg 115 mcg/21 mcg 230 mcg/21 mcg
Flunisolide CFC inhalation aerosol	≤ 1,000 mcg 1,250 to 2,000 mcg	100 mcg/50 mcg 250 mcg/50 mcg	45 mcg/21 mcg 115 mcg/21 mcg
Flunisolide HFA inhalation aerosol	≤ 320 mcg 640 mcg	100 mcg/50 mcg 250 mcg/50 mcg	45 mcg/21 mcg 115 mcg/21 mcg
Fluticasone propionate HFA inhalation aerosol	≤ 176 mcg 440 mcg 660 to 880 mcg	100 mcg/50 mcg 250 mcg/50 mcg 500 mcg/50 mcg	45 mcg/21 mcg 115 mcg/21 mcg 230 mcg/21 mcg
Fluticasone propionate inhalation powder	≤ 200 mcg 500 mcg 1,000 mcg	100 mcg/50 mcg 250 mcg/50 mcg 500 mcg/50 mcg	45 mcg/21 mcg 115 mcg/21 mcg 230 mcg/21 mcg
Mometasone furoate inhalation powder	220 mcg 440 mcg 880 mcg	100 mcg/50 mcg 250 mcg/50 mcg 500 mcg/50 mcg	45 mcg/21 mcg 115 mcg/21 mcg 230 mcg/21 mcg
Triamcinolone acetonide inhalation aerosol	≤ 1,000 mcg 1,100 to 1,600 mcg	100 mcg/50 mcg 250 mcg/50 mcg	45 mcg/21 mcg 115 mcg/21 mcg

➤ **Asthma in children who remain symptomatic while taking an inhaled corticosteroid**

Children ages 4 to 11: Give 1 inhalation (100 mg fluticasone and 50 mg salmeterol) b.i.d., morning and evening, about 12 hours apart.

➤ **Maintenance therapy for airflow obstruction in patients with COPD from chronic bronchitis**

Adults: 1 inhalation of Advair Diskus 250/50 only, b.i.d., about 12 hours apart.

ADMINISTRATION

Inhalational

• Prime Advair HFA before first use.
• After administration, have the patient rinse his mouth without swallowing.

ACTION

Fluticasone is a synthetic corticosteroid with potent anti-inflammatory activity. Salmeterol xinafoate, a long-acting beta agonist, relaxes bronchial smooth muscle and inhibits release of mediators.

Route	Onset	Peak	Duration
Inhalation (fluticasone)	Unknown	1–2 hr	Unknown
Inhalation (salmeterol)	Unknown	5 min	Unknown

Half-life: Fluticasone: 8 hours; salmeterol: 5½ hours.

ADVERSE REACTIONS

CNS: *headache,* compressed nerve syndromes, hypnagogic effects, sleep disorders, tremors, pain.
CV: palpitations.
EENT: *pharyngitis,* blood in nasal mucosa, congestion, conjunctivitis, dental discomfort and pain, eye redness, hoarseness or dysphonia, keratitis, nasal irritation, rhinorrhea, rhinitis, sinusitis, sneezing, viral eye infections.
GI: abdominal pain and discomfort, appendicitis, constipation, diarrhea, gastroenteritis, nausea, oral candidiasis, oral discomfort and pain, oral erythema and

rashes, oral ulcerations, unusual taste, vomiting.

Musculoskeletal: arthralgia, articular rheumatism, bone and cartilage disorders, muscle pain, muscle stiffness, rigidity, tightness.

Respiratory: *upper respiratory tract infection,* bronchitis, cough, lower respiratory tract infections, pneumonia.

Skin: disorders of sweat and sebum, infection, skin flakiness, sweating, urticaria.

Other: allergic reactions, chest symptoms, fluid retention, viral or bacterial infections.

INTERACTIONS

Drug-drug. *Beta blockers:* Blocked pulmonary effect of salmeterol may produce severe bronchospasm in patients with asthma. Avoid using together. If necessary, use a cardioselective beta blocker cautiously.

Ketoconazole, other inhibitors of cytochrome P-450: May increase fluticasone level and adverse effects. Use together cautiously.

Loop diuretics, thiazide diuretics: Potassium-wasting diuretics may cause or worsen ECG changes or hypokalemia. Use together cautiously.

MAO inhibitors, tricyclic antidepressants: May potentiate the action of salmeterol on the vascular system. Separate doses by 2 weeks.

EFFECTS ON LAB TEST RESULTS

• May increase liver enzyme levels.

CONTRAINDICATIONS & CAUTIONS

• Contraindicated in patients hypersensitive to drug or its components.

• Contraindicated as primary treatment of status asthmaticus or other acute asthmatic episodes.

• Use cautiously, if at all, in patients with active or quiescent respiratory tuberculosis infection; untreated systemic fungal, bacterial, viral, or parasitic infection; or ocular herpes simplex.

• Use cautiously in patients with CV disorders, seizure disorders or thyrotoxicosis; in patients unusually responsive to sympathomimetic amines; and in patients with hepatic impairment.

NURSING CONSIDERATIONS

• *Alert:* Patient shouldn't be switched from systemic corticosteroids to Advair Diskus or Advair HFA because of hypothalamic-pituitary-adrenal axis suppression. Death from adrenal insufficiency can occur. Several months are required for recovery of hypothalamic-pituitary-adrenal function after withdrawal of systemic corticosteroids.

• Don't start therapy during rapidly deteriorating or potentially life-threatening episodes of asthma. Serious acute respiratory events, including fatality, can occur.

• The benefit of Advair 250/50 in treating patients with COPD for more than 6 months is unknown. If drug is used for longer than 6 months, periodically reevaluate patient to assess for benefits or risks of therapy.

• Monitor patient for urticaria, angioedema, rash, bronchospasm, or other signs of hypersensitivity.

• Don't use this drug to stop an asthma attack. Patients should carry an inhaled, short-acting beta$_2$ agonist (such as albuterol) for acute symptoms.

• If drug causes paradoxical bronchospasm, treat immediately with a short-acting inhaled bronchodilator (such as albuterol), and notify prescriber.

• *Alert:* Rare, serious asthma episodes or asthma-related deaths have occurred in patients taking salmeterol; black patients may be at a greater risk.

• Monitor patient for increased use of inhaled short-acting beta$_2$ agonist. The dose of Advair may need to be increased.

• Closely monitor children for growth suppression.

PATIENT TEACHING

• Instruct patient on proper use of the prescribed inhaler to provide effective treatment.

• Tell patient to avoid exhaling into the dry-powder multidose inhaler, to activate and use the dry-powder multidose inhaler in a level, horizontal position and not to use Advair Diskus with a spacer device.

• Instruct patient to keep the dry-powder multidose inhaler in a dry place, away from direct heat or sunlight, and to avoid washing the mouthpiece or other parts of the device. Patient should discard device 1 month after removal from the moisture-protective overwrap pouch or after every blister has been used, whichever comes first. He shouldn't attempt to take device apart.

• Instruct patient to rinse mouth after inhalation to prevent oral candidiasis.

• Inform patient that improvement may occur within 30 minutes after dose, but the full benefit may not occur for 1 week or more.

• Advise patient not to exceed recommended prescribing dose.

• Instruct patient not to relieve acute symptoms with Advair. Treat acute symptoms with an inhaled short-acting beta$_2$ agonist.

• Instruct patient to report decreasing effects or use of increasing doses of their short-acting inhaled beta$_2$ agonist.

• Tell patient to report palpitations, chest pain, rapid heart rate, tremor, or nervousness.

• Instruct patient to call immediately if exposed to chickenpox or measles.

SAFETY ALERT!

fondaparinux sodium
fon-dah-PEAR-ah-nucks

Arixtra

Pharmacologic class: activated factor X inhibitor
Pregnancy risk category B

AVAILABLE FORMS
Injection: 2.5 mg/0.5 ml, 5 mg/0.4 ml, 7.5 mg/0.6 ml, 10 mg/0.8 ml single-dose prefilled syringe

INDICATIONS & DOSAGES
➤ **To prevent deep vein thrombosis (DVT), which may lead to pulmonary embolism, in patients undergoing surgery for hip fracture, hip replacement, knee replacement, or abdominal surgery**
Adults who weigh 50 kg (110 lb) or more: 2.5 mg subcutaneously once daily for 5 to 9 days. Give first dose after hemostasis is established, 6 to 8 hours after surgery.

Giving the dose earlier than 6 hours after surgery increases the risk of major bleeding. Patients undergoing hip fracture surgery should receive an extended prophylaxis course of up to 24 additional days; a total of 32 days (perioperative and extended prophylaxis) has been tolerated.
➤ **Acute DVT (with warfarin); acute pulmonary embolism (with warfarin) when treatment is started in the hospital**
Adults who weigh more than 100 kg (220 lb): Give 10 mg subcutaneously daily for 5 to 9 days, and until INR level is 2 to 3. Begin warfarin therapy as soon as possible, usually within 72 hours.
Adults who weigh 50 to 100 kg: Give 7.5 mg subcutaneously daily for 5 to 9 days, and until INR level is 2 to 3. Begin warfarin therapy as soon as possible, usually within 72 hours.
Adults who weigh less than 50 kg: Give 5 mg subcutaneously daily for 5 to 9 days, and until INR level is 2 to 3. Begin warfarin therapy as soon as possible, usually within 72 hours.

ADMINISTRATION
Subcutaneous
• Give subcutaneously only, never I.M. Inspect the single-dose, prefilled syringe for particulate matter and discoloration before giving.
• Give the drug in fatty tissue, rotating injection sites. If the drug has been properly injected, the needle will pull back into the syringe security sleeve and the white safety indicator will appear above the blue upper body. A soft click may be heard or felt when the syringe plunger is fully released. After injection of the syringe contents, the plunger automatically rises while the needle withdraws from the skin and retracts into the security sleeve. Don't recap the needle.
• **Incompatibilities:** Other injections or infusions.

ACTION
Binds to antithrombin III (AT-III) and potentiates the neutralization of factor Xa by AT-III, which interrupts coagulation and inhibits formation of thrombin and blood clots.

Route	Onset	Peak	Duration
Subcut	Unknown	2–3 hr	Unknown

Half-life: 17 to 21 hours.

ADVERSE REACTIONS

CNS: *fever,* insomnia, dizziness, confusion, headache, pain.
CV: hypotension, edema.
GI: *nausea,* constipation, vomiting, diarrhea, dyspepsia.
GU: UTI, urine retention.
Hematologic: *hemorrhage, anemia,* hematoma, *postoperative hemorrhage, thrombocytopenia.*
Metabolic: hypokalemia.
Skin: mild local irritation (injection site bleeding, rash, pruritus), bullous eruption, purpura, rash, increased wound drainage.

INTERACTIONS

Drug-drug. *Drugs that increase risk of bleeding (NSAIDs, platelet inhibitors, anticoagulants):* May increase risk of hemorrhage. Stop these drugs before starting fondaparinux. If use together is unavoidable, monitor patient closely.
Drug-herb. *Angelica (dong quai), boldo, bromelains, capsicum, chamomile, dandelion, danshen, devil's claw, fenugreek, feverfew, garlic, ginger, ginkgo, ginseng, horse chestnut, licorice, meadowsweet, onion, passion flower, red clover, willow:* May increase risk of bleeding. Discourage use together.

EFFECTS ON LAB TEST RESULTS

• May increase AST, ALT, and bilirubin levels. May decrease potassium and hemoglobin levels and hematocrit.
• May decrease platelet count.

CONTRAINDICATIONS & CAUTIONS

• Contraindicated in patients with creatinine clearance less than 30 ml/minute and in those who are hypersensitive to the drug.
• Contraindicated for prophylaxis in patients who weigh less than 50 kg who are undergoing hip fracture, hip replacement, knee replacement, or abdominal surgery.
• Contraindicated in patients with active major bleeding, bacterial endocarditis, or thrombocytopenia with a positive test result for antiplatelet antibody after taking fondaparinux.
• Use cautiously in patients being treated with platelet inhibitors; in those at increased risk for bleeding, such as congenital or acquired bleeding disorders; in those with active ulcerative and angiodysplastic GI disease; in those with hemorrhagic stroke; and in patients shortly after brain, spinal, or ophthalmologic surgery.
• Use cautiously in patients who have had epidural or spinal anesthesia or spinal puncture; they are at increased risk for developing an epidural or spinal hematoma (which may cause paralysis).
• Use cautiously in elderly patients, in patients with creatinine clearance of 30 to 50 ml/minute, and in those with a history of heparin-induced thrombocytopenia, a bleeding diathesis, uncontrolled arterial hypertension, or a history of recent GI ulceration, diabetic retinopathy, or hemorrhage.

NURSING CONSIDERATIONS

• Don't use interchangeably with heparin, low–molecular-weight heparins, or heparinoids.
• *Alert:* To avoid loss of drug, don't expel air bubble from the syringe.
• *Alert:* Patients who receive epidural or spinal anesthesia are at increased risk for developing an epidural or spinal hematoma, which may result in long-term or permanent paralysis. Monitor these patients closely for neurologic impairment.
• Monitor renal function periodically and stop drug in patients who develop unstable renal function or severe renal impairment while receiving therapy.
• Routinely assess patient for signs and symptoms of bleeding, and regularly monitor CBC, platelet count, creatinine level, and stool occult blood test results. Stop use if platelet count is less than 100,000/mm^3.
• Anticoagulant effects may last for 2 to 4 days after stopping drug in patients with normal renal function.
• PT and activated PTT aren't suitable monitoring tests to measure drug activity. If coagulation parameters change unexpectedly or patient develops major bleeding, stop drug.

Reactions may be *common,* uncommon, *life-threatening,* or COMMON AND LIFE-THREATENING.
Interaction may have a *rapid onset* or *delayed onset.*

PATIENT TEACHING
- Tell patient to report signs and symptoms of bleeding.
- Instruct patient to avoid OTC products that contain aspirin or other salicylates.
- Advise patient to consult with prescriber before starting herbal therapy; many herbs have anticoagulant, antiplatelet, or fibrinolytic properties.
- Teach patient the correct technique for subcutaneous use, if needed.

---

formoterol fumarate
for-MOH-te-rol

Foradil Aerolizer, Performist

Pharmacologic class: selective beta$_2$-adrenergic agonist
Pregnancy risk category C

AVAILABLE FORMS
Capsules for inhalation: 12 mcg
Inhalation solution: 20 mcg/2-ml vial

INDICATIONS & DOSAGES
➤ **Maintenance treatment and prevention of bronchospasm in patients with reversible obstructive airway disease or nocturnal asthma, who usually require treatment with short-acting inhaled beta$_2$ agonists**
Adults and children age 5 and older: One 12-mcg capsule by inhalation via Aerolizer inhaler every 12 hours. Total daily dosage shouldn't exceed 1 capsule b.i.d. (24 mcg/day). If symptoms occur between doses, use a short-acting beta$_2$ agonist for immediate relief.
➤ **To prevent exercise-induced bronchospasm**
Adults and children age 5 and older: One 12-mcg capsule by inhalation via Aerolizer inhaler at least 15 minutes before exercise p.r.n. Don't give additional doses within 12 hours of first dose.
➤ **Maintenance treatment of bronchoconstriction in patients with COPD (chronic bronchitis, emphysema)**
Adults: One 20-mcg/2 ml vial (Performist) by oral inhalation through a jet nebulizer every 12 hours. Maximum dose, 40 mcg/day. Or, one 12-mcg capsule

(Foradil) by inhalation via Aerolizer inhaler every 12 hours; total daily dosage shouldn't exceed 24 mcg/day.

ADMINISTRATION
Inhalational
Foradil
- Give Foradil capsules only by oral inhalation and only with the Aerolizer inhaler. They aren't for oral ingestion. Patient shouldn't exhale into the device. Capsules should remain in the unopened blister until administration time and be removed immediately before use.
- Pierce Foradil capsules only once. In rare instances, the gelatin capsule may break into small pieces and get delivered to the mouth or throat upon inhalation. The Aerolizer contains a screen that should catch any broken pieces before they leave the device. To minimize the possibility of shattering the capsule, strictly follow storage and use instructions.
Performist
- Give Performist inhalational solution through a standard jet nebulizer connected to an air compressor.

ACTION
Long-acting selective beta$_2$ agonist that causes bronchodilation. It ultimately increases cAMP, leading to relaxation of bronchial smooth muscle and inhibition of mediator release from mast cells.

Route	Onset	Peak	Duration
Inhalation	15 min	1–3 hr	12 hr

Half-life: 7 hours for Performist.

ADVERSE REACTIONS
CNS: tremor, dizziness, insomnia, nervousness, headache, fatigue, malaise.
CV: *arrhythmias,* chest pain, angina, hypertension, hypotension, tachycardia, palpitations.
EENT: dry mouth, tonsillitis, dysphonia, nasopharyngitis.
GI: nausea, vomiting, diarrhea.
Metabolic: *metabolic acidosis,* hypokalemia, hyperglycemia.
Musculoskeletal: muscle cramps.
Respiratory: bronchitis, chest infection, dyspnea.
Skin: rash.
Other: viral infection.

INTERACTIONS
Drug-drug. *Adrenergics:* May potentiate sympathetic effects of formoterol. Use together cautiously.

Beta blockers: May antagonize effects of beta agonists, causing bronchospasm in asthmatic patients. Avoid use except when benefit outweighs risks. Use cardioselective beta blockers with caution to minimize risk of bronchospasm.

Diuretics, steroids, xanthine derivatives: May increase hypokalemic effect of formoterol. Use together cautiously.

MAO inhibitors, tricyclic antidepressants, other drugs that prolong QT interval: May increase risk of ventricular arrhythmias. Use together cautiously.

Non–potassium-sparing diuretics, such as loop or thiazide diuretics: May worsen ECG changes or hypokalemia. Use together cautiously, and monitor patient for toxicity.

EFFECTS ON LAB TEST RESULTS
● May increase glucose level. May decrease potassium level.

CONTRAINDICATIONS & CAUTIONS
● Contraindicated in patients hypersensitive to drug or its components.
● Use cautiously in patients with CV disease, especially coronary insufficiency, cardiac arrhythmias, and hypertension, and in those who are unusually responsive to sympathomimetic amines.
● Use cautiously in patients with diabetes mellitus because hyperglycemia and ketoacidosis have occurred rarely with the use of beta agonists.
● Use cautiously in patients with seizure disorders or thyrotoxicosis and in breast-feeding women.

NURSING CONSIDERATIONS
● Drug isn't indicated for patients who can control asthma symptoms with just occasional use of inhaled, short-acting beta$_2$ agonists or for treatment of acute bronchospasm requiring immediate reversal with short-acting beta$_2$ agonists or in patients with rapidly deteriorating or significantly worsening asthma.
● Drug may be used along with short-acting beta agonists, inhaled corticosteroids, and theophylline therapy for asthma management.
● *Alert:* Drug isn't a substitute for short-acting beta$_2$ agonists for immediate relief of bronchospasm or as substitute for inhaled or oral corticosteroids.
● Patients using drug twice daily shouldn't take additional doses to prevent exercise-induced bronchospasm.
● For patients formerly using regularly scheduled short-acting beta$_2$ agonists, decrease use of the short-acting drug to an as-needed basis when starting long-acting formoterol.
● *Alert:* As with all beta$_2$ agonists, drug may produce life-threatening paradoxical bronchospasm. If bronchospasm occurs, notify prescriber immediately.
● *Alert:* If patient develops tachycardia, hypertension, or other CV adverse effects, drug may need to be stopped.
● Watch for immediate hypersensitivity reactions, such as anaphylaxis, urticaria, angioedema, rash, and bronchospasm.
● *Look alike–sound alike:* Don't confuse Foradil with Toradol.

PATIENT TEACHING
● Tell patient not to increase the dosage or frequency of use without medical advice.
● Warn patient not to stop or reduce other medication taken for asthma.
● Advise patient that drug isn't to be used for acute asthmatic episodes. Prescriber should give a short-acting beta$_2$ agonist for this use.
● Advise patient to report worsening symptoms, treatment that becomes less effective, or increased use of short-acting beta agonists.
● Tell patient to report nausea, vomiting, shakiness, headache, fast or irregular heart beat, or sleeplessness.
● Tell patient using drug for exercise-induced bronchospasm to take it at least 15 minutes before exercise and to wait 12 hours before taking additional doses.
● Tell patient not to use the Foradil Aerolizer with a spacer device or to exhale or blow into the Aerolizer.
● Advise patient to avoid washing the Aerolizer and to always keep it dry. Each refill contains a new device to replace the old one.

Reactions may be *common*, uncommon, ***life-threatening***, or COMMON AND LIFE-THREATENING.
Interaction may have a *rapid onset* or ***delayed onset***.

- Tell patient to avoid exposing capsules to moisture and to handle them only with dry hands.
- Advise woman to notify prescriber if she becomes pregnant or is breast-feeding.

---

furosemide
fur-OH-se-mide

Furosemide Special†, Lasix*, Novo-semide†

Pharmacologic class: loop diuretic
Pregnancy risk category C

AVAILABLE FORMS
Injection: 10 mg/ml
Oral solution: 10 mg/ml, 40 mg/5 ml
Tablets: 20 mg, 40 mg, 80 mg, 500 mg†

INDICATIONS & DOSAGES
➤ **Acute pulmonary edema**
Adults: 40 mg I.V. injected slowly over 1 to 2 minutes; then 80 mg I.V. in 60 to 90 minutes if needed.
➤ **Edema**
Adults: 20 to 80 mg P.O. daily in the morning. If response is inadequate, give a second dose, and each succeeding dose, every 6 to 8 hours. Carefully increase dose in 20- to 40-mg increments up to 600 mg daily. Once effective dose is attained, may give once or twice daily. Or, 20 to 40 mg I.V. or I.M., increased by 20 mg every 2 hours until desired effect achieved.
Infants and children: 2 mg/kg P.O. daily, increased by 1 to 2 mg/kg in 6 to 8 hours if needed; carefully adjusted up to 6 mg/kg daily if needed.
➤ **Hypertension**
Adults: 40 mg P.O. b.i.d. Dosage adjusted based on response. May be used as adjunct to other antihypertensives if needed.
Children ♦: 0.5 to 2 mg/kg P.O. once or twice daily. Increase dose as needed up to 6 mg/kg daily.

ADMINISTRATION
P.O.
- To prevent nocturia, give in the morning. Give second dose if ordered in early afternoon, 6 to 8 hours after morning dose.
- Give drug with food to prevent GI upset.
- Store tablets in light-resistant container to prevent discoloration (doesn't affect potency). Refrigerate oral solution to ensure drug stability.
I.V.
- If discolored yellow, don't use.
- For direct injection, give over 1 to 2 minutes.
- For infusion, dilute with D_5W, normal saline solution, or lactated Ringer solution.
- To avoid ototoxicity, infuse no more than 4 mg/minute.
- Use prepared infusion solution within 24 hours.
- **Incompatibilities:** Acidic solutions, aminoglycosides, amiodarone, ascorbic acid, azithromycin, bleomycin, buprenorphine, chlorpromazine, ciprofloxacin, diazepam, diltiazem, dobutamine, doxapram, doxorubicin, droperidol, epinephrine, erythromycin, esmolol, filgrastim, fluconazole, fructose 10% in water, gentamicin, hydralazine, idarubicin, invert sugar 10% in electrolyte #2, isoproterenol, levofloxacin, mannitol, meperidine, methocarbamol, metoclopramide, midazolam, milrinone, morphine, netilmicin, norepinephrine, ondansetron, oxytetracycline, prochlorperazine, promethazine, protamine, quinidine, tetracycline, thiamine, vinblastine, vincristine, vitamins B and C.
I.M.
- To prevent nocturia, give in the morning. Give second dose if ordered in early afternoon, 6 to 8 hours after morning dose.
- Record administration site.

ACTION
Inhibits sodium and chloride reabsorption at the proximal and distal tubules and the ascending loop of Henle.

Route	Onset	Peak	Duration
P.O.	20–60 min	1–2 hr	6–8 hr
I.V.	Within 5 min	30 min	2 hr
I.M.	Unknown	30 min	2 hr

Half-life: 30 minutes.

ADVERSE REACTIONS
CNS: vertigo, headache, dizziness, paresthesia, weakness, restlessness, fever.
CV: orthostatic hypotension, thrombophlebitis with I.V. administration.

EENT: transient deafness, blurred or yellowed vision, tinnitus.
GI: abdominal discomfort and pain, diarrhea, anorexia, nausea, vomiting, constipation, *pancreatitis.*
GU: azotemia, nocturia, polyuria, frequent urination, oliguria.
Hematologic: *agranulocytosis, aplastic anemia, leukopenia, thrombocytopenia,* anemia.
Hepatic: hepatic dysfunction, jaundice.
Metabolic: volume depletion and dehydration, asymptomatic hyperuricemia, impaired glucose tolerance, hypokalemia, hypochloremic alkalosis, hyperglycemia, dilutional hyponatremia, hypocalcemia, hypomagnesemia.
Musculoskeletal: muscle spasm.
Skin: dermatitis, purpura, photosensitivity reactions, transient pain at I.M. injection site.
Other: gout.

INTERACTIONS
Drug-drug. *Aminoglycoside antibiotics, cisplatin:* May increase ototoxicity. Use together cautiously.
Amphotericin B, corticosteroids, corticotropin, metolazone: May increase risk of hypokalemia. Monitor potassium level closely.
Antidiabetics: May decrease hypoglycemic effects. Monitor glucose level.
Antihypertensives: May increase risk of hypotension. Use together cautiously. Decrease antihypertensive dose if needed.
Cardiac glycosides, neuromuscular blockers: May increase toxicity of these drugs from furosemide-induced hypokalemia. Monitor potassium level.
Chlorothiazide, chlorthalidone, hydrochlorothiazide, indapamide, metolazone: May cause excessive diuretic response, causing serious electrolyte abnormalities or dehydration. Adjust doses carefully, and monitor patient closely for signs and symptoms of excessive diuretic response.
Ethacrynic acid: May increase risk of ototoxicity. Avoid using together.
Lithium: May decrease lithium excretion, resulting in lithium toxicity. Monitor lithium level.

NSAIDs: May inhibit diuretic response. Use together cautiously.
Phenytoin: May decrease diuretic effects of furosemide. Use together cautiously.
Propranolol: May increase propranolol level. Monitor patient closely.
Salicylates: May cause salicylate toxicity. Use together cautiously.
Sucralfate: May reduce diuretic and antihypertensive effect. Separate doses by 2 hours.
Drug-herb. *Aloe:* May increase drug effect. Discourage use together.
Dandelion: May interfere with drug activity. Discourage use together.
Ginseng: May decrease drug effect. Discourage use together.
Licorice: May cause unexpected rapid potassium loss. Discourage use together.
Drug-lifestyle. *Sun exposure:* May increase risk for photosensitivity reactions. Advise patient to avoid excessive sunlight exposure.

EFFECTS ON LAB TEST RESULTS
● May increase cholesterol, glucose, BUN, creatinine, and uric acid levels. May decrease calcium, hemoglobin, magnesium, potassium, and sodium levels.
● May decrease granulocyte, platelet, and WBC counts.

CONTRAINDICATIONS & CAUTIONS
● Contraindicated in patients hypersensitive to drug and in those with anuria.
● Use cautiously in patients with hepatic cirrhosis and in those allergic to sulfonamides. Use during pregnancy only if potential benefits to mother clearly outweigh risks to fetus.

NURSING CONSIDERATIONS
● *Alert:* Monitor weight, blood pressure, and pulse rate routinely with long-term use and during rapid diuresis. Use can lead to profound water and electrolyte depletion.
● If oliguria or azotemia develops or increases, drug may need to be stopped.
● Monitor fluid intake and output and electrolyte, BUN, and carbon dioxide levels frequently.
● Watch for signs of hypokalemia, such as muscle weakness and cramps.

• Consult prescriber and dietitian about a high-potassium diet or potassium supplements. Foods rich in potassium include citrus fruits, tomatoes, bananas, dates, and apricots.

• Monitor glucose level in diabetic patients.

• Drug may not be well absorbed orally in patient with severe heart failure. Drug may need to be given I.V. even if patient is taking other oral drugs.

• Monitor uric acid level, especially in patients with a history of gout.

• Monitor elderly patients, who are especially susceptible to excessive diuresis, because circulatory collapse and thromboembolic complications are possible.

• *Look alike–sound alike:* Don't confuse furosemide with torsemide or Lasix with Lonox, Lidex, or Luvox.

PATIENT TEACHING

• Advise patient to take drug with food to prevent GI upset, and to take drug in morning to prevent need to urinate at night. If patient needs second dose, tell him to take it in early afternoon, 6 to 8 hours after morning dose.

• Inform patient of possible need for potassium or magnesium supplements.

• Instruct patient to stand slowly to prevent dizziness and to limit alcohol intake and strenuous exercise in hot weather to avoid worsening dizziness upon standing quickly.

• Advise patient to immediately report ringing in ears, severe abdominal pain, or sore throat and fever; these symptoms may indicate toxicity.

• *Alert:* Discourage patient from storing different types of drugs in the same container, increasing the risk of drug errors. The most popular strengths of this drug and digoxin are white tablets about equal in size.

• Tell patient to check with prescriber or pharmacist before taking OTC drugs.

• Teach patient to avoid direct sunlight and to use protective clothing and a sunblock because of risk of photosensitivity reactions.

---

gemifloxacin mesylate
jem-ah-FLOX-a-sin

Factive

Pharmacologic class: fluoroquinolone
Pregnancy risk category C

AVAILABLE FORMS
Tablets: 320 mg

INDICATIONS & DOSAGES
➤ **Acute bacterial worsening of chronic bronchitis caused by** *Streptococcus pneumoniae, Haemophilus influenzae, H. parainfluenzae,* **or** *Moraxella catarrhalis*
Adults: 320 mg P.O. once daily for 5 days.
➤ **Mild to moderate community-acquired pneumonia caused by** *S. pneumoniae* **(including multidrug-resistant strains),** *H. influenzae, M. catarrhalis, Mycoplasma pneumoniae, Chlamydia pneumoniae,* **or** *Klebsiella pneumoniae*
Adults: 320 mg P.O. once daily for 7 days.
Adjust-a-dose: If creatinine clearance is 40 ml/minute or less, or if patient receives routine hemodialysis or continuous ambulatory peritoneal dialysis, reduce dosage to 160 mg P.O. once daily.

ADMINISTRATION
P.O.
• Give drug with or without food; however it must be given 2 hours before or 3 hours after an antacid.
• Give plenty of fluids during treatment.

ACTION
Prevents cell growth by inhibiting DNA gyrase and topoisomerase IV, which interferes with DNA synthesis.

Route	Onset	Peak	Duration
P.O.	Unknown	½–2 hr	Unknown

Half-life: 4 to 12 hours.

ADVERSE REACTIONS
CNS: headache.
GI: diarrhea, nausea.
Musculoskeletal: ruptured tendons.

Skin: rash.
Other: hypersensitivity reactions.

INTERACTIONS
Drug-drug. *Antacids (magnesium or aluminum), didanosine (chewable tablets, buffered tablets, or pediatric powder for oral solution), ferrous sulfate, multivitamins containing metal cations (such as zinc):* May decrease gemifloxacin level. Give these drugs at least 3 hours before or 2 hours after gemifloxacin.
Antiarrhythmics of class IA (procainamide, quinidine) or class III (amiodarone, sotalol): May increase risk of prolonged QTc interval. Avoid using together.
Antipsychotics, erythromycin, tricyclic antidepressants: May increase risk of prolonged QTc interval. Use together cautiously.
Probenecid: May increase gemifloxacin level. May use with probenecid for this reason.
Sucralfate: May decrease gemifloxacin level. Use together cautiously.
Warfarin: May increase anticoagulation effect. Monitor PT and INR.
Drug-lifestyle. *Sun exposure:* May increase risk of photosensitivity. Advise patient to avoid excessive sunlight exposure.

EFFECTS ON LAB TEST RESULTS
• May increase alkaline phosphatase, ALT, AST, bilirubin, BUN, CK, creatinine, GGT, and potassium levels. May decrease albumin, protein, and sodium levels. May increase or decrease calcium and hemoglobin levels and hematocrit.
• May increase or decrease neutrophil, platelet, and RBC counts.

CONTRAINDICATIONS & CAUTIONS
• Contraindicated in patients hypersensitive to fluoroquinolones, gemifloxacin, or their components.
• Contraindicated in patients with a history of prolonged QTc interval, those with uncorrected electrolyte disorders (such as hypokalemia or hypomagnesemia), and those taking a drug that could prolong the QTc interval.
• Use cautiously in patients with a proarrhythmic condition (such as bradycardia or

acute myocardial ischemia), epilepsy, or a predisposition to seizures.
• Safety and efficacy haven't been established for children younger than age 18.

NURSING CONSIDERATIONS
• Use drug only for infections caused by susceptible bacteria.
• *Alert:* Don't exceed recommended dosage because this increases the risk of prolonging the QTc interval.
• Mild to moderate maculopapular rash may appear, usually 8 to 10 days after therapy starts. It's more likely in women younger than age 40, especially those taking hormone therapy. Stop drug if rash appears.
• *Alert:* Serious, occasionally fatal, hypersensitivity reactions may occur. Stop drug immediately if hypersensitivity reaction occurs.
• Fluoroquinolones may cause tendon rupture, arthropathy, or osteochondrosis; stop drug if patient reports pain or inflammation or ruptures a tendon.
• Stop drug if patient has a photosensitivity reaction.
• Fluoroquinolones may cause CNS effects, such as tremors and anxiety. Monitor patient carefully.
• Serious diarrhea may reflect pseudomembranous colitis; drug may need to be stopped.
• Keep patient adequately hydrated to avoid concentration of urine.

PATIENT TEACHING
• Urge patient to finish full course of treatment, even if symptoms improve.
• Tell patient that drug may be taken with or without food, but that it shouldn't be taken within 3 hours after or 2 hours before an antacid.
• Tell patient to stop drug and seek medical care if evidence of hypersensitivity reaction develops.
• Instruct patient to drink fluids liberally during treatment.
• Warn patient against taking OTC drugs or dietary supplements without consulting his prescriber.
• Tell patient to avoid excessive exposure to sunlight or ultraviolet light.

- Urge patient to report pain, inflammation, or rupture of tendons.
- Warn patient to avoid driving or other hazardous activities until effects of drug are known.

gentamicin sulfate
jen-ta-MYE-sin

Pharmacologic class: aminoglycoside
Pregnancy risk category D

AVAILABLE FORMS
Injection: 40 mg/ml (adults), 10 mg/ml (children)
I.V. infusion (premixed): 60 mg, 70 mg, 80 mg, 90 mg, 100 mg, in normal saline solution

INDICATIONS & DOSAGES
➤ **Serious infections caused by sensitive strains of** *Pseudomonas aeruginosa, Escherichia coli, Proteus, Klebsiella, Serratia,* **or** *Staphylococcus*
Adults: 3 mg/kg daily in three divided doses I.M. or I.V. infusion every 8 hours. For life-threatening infections, may give up to 5 mg/kg daily in three or four divided doses; reduce dosage to 3 mg/kg daily as soon as patient improves.
Children: 2 to 2.5 mg/kg every 8 hours I.M. or by I.V. infusion.
Neonates older than 1 week and infants: 2.5 mg/kg every 8 hours I.M. or by I.V. infusion.
Neonates younger than 1 week and preterm infants: 2.5 mg/kg every 12 hours I.M. or by I.V. infusion.
➤ **To prevent endocarditis before GI or GU procedure or surgery**
Adults: 1.5 mg/kg I.M. or I.V. 30 minutes before procedure or surgery. Maximum dose is 80 mg. Give with ampicillin (vancomycin in penicillin-allergic patients).
Children: 2 mg/kg I.M. or I.V. 30 minutes before procedure or surgery. Maximum dose is 80 mg. Give with ampicillin (vancomycin in penicillin-allergic patients).
Adjust-a-dose: For adults with impaired renal function, doses and frequency are determined by drug level and renal function. To maintain therapeutic levels, adults should receive 1 to 1.7 mg/kg I.M. or by

I.V. infusion after each dialysis session, and children should receive 2 to 2.5 mg/kg I.M. or by I.V. infusion after each dialysis session.

ADMINISTRATION
I.V.
- Obtain specimen for culture and sensitivity tests before giving. Begin therapy while awaiting results.
- For intermittent infusion, dilute with 50 to 200 ml of D_5W or normal saline solution for injection.
- Infuse over 30 minutes to 2 hours.
- After completing infusion, flush the line with normal saline solution or D_5W.
- **Incompatibilities:** Allopurinol, amphotericin B, ampicillin, azithromycin, cefazolin, cefepime, cefotaxime, ceftazidime, ceftriaxone sodium, cefuroxime, certain parenteral nutrition formulations, cytarabine, dopamine, fat emulsions, furosemide, heparin, hetastarch, idarubicin, indomethacin sodium trihydrate, nafcillin, propofol, ticarcillin, warfarin.
I.M.
- Obtain specimen for culture and sensitivity tests before giving. Begin therapy while awaiting results.
- Obtain blood for peak level 1 hour after I.M. injection or 30 minutes after I.V. infusion finishes; for trough levels, draw blood just before next dose. Don't collect blood in a heparinized tube; heparin is incompatible with aminoglycosides.

ACTION
Inhibits protein synthesis by binding directly to the 30S ribosomal subunit; bactericidal.

Route	Onset	Peak	Duration
I.V.	Immediate	30–90 min	Unknown
I.M.	Unknown	30–90 min	Unknown

Half-life: 2 to 3 hours.

ADVERSE REACTIONS
CNS: *encephalopathy, seizures,* fever, headache, lethargy, confusion, dizziness, numbness, peripheral neuropathy, vertigo, ataxia, tingling.
CV: hypotension.
EENT: *ototoxicity,* blurred vision, tinnitus.

GI: vomiting, nausea.
GU: *nephrotoxicity,* possible increase in urinary excretion of casts.
Hematologic: *agranulocytosis, leukopenia, thrombocytopenia,* anemia, eosinophilia.
Musculoskeletal: muscle twitching, myasthenia gravis–like syndrome.
Respiratory: *apnea.*
Skin: rash, urticaria, pruritus, injection site pain.
Other: *anaphylaxis.*

INTERACTIONS

Drug-drug. *Acyclovir, amphotericin B, cephalosporins, cidofovir, cisplatin, methoxyflurane, vancomycin, other aminoglycosides:* May increase ototoxicity and nephrotoxicity. Monitor hearing and renal function test results.
Atracurium, pancuronium, rocuronium, vecuronium: May increase effects of nondepolarizing muscle relaxants, including prolonged respiratory depression. Use together only when necessary, and expect to reduce dosage of nondepolarizing muscle relaxant.
Dimenhydrinate: May mask ototoxicity symptoms. Monitor patient's hearing.
General anesthetics: May increase neuromuscular blockade. Monitor patient closely.
Indomethacin: May increase peak and trough levels of gentamicin. Monitor gentamicin level.
I.V. loop diuretics (such as furosemide): May increase risk of ototoxicity. Monitor patient's hearing.
Parenteral penicillins (such as ampicillin and ticarcillin): May inactivate gentamicin in vitro. Don't mix together.

EFFECTS ON LAB TEST RESULTS

• May increase ALT, AST, bilirubin, BUN, creatinine, LDH, and nonprotein nitrogen levels. May decrease hemoglobin level.
• May increase eosinophil count. May decrease granulocyte, platelet, and WBC counts.

CONTRAINDICATIONS & CAUTIONS

• Contraindicated in patients hypersensitive to drug or other aminoglycosides.

• Use cautiously in neonates, infants, elderly patients, and patients with impaired renal function or neuromuscular disorders.

NURSING CONSIDERATIONS

• *Alert:* Evaluate patient's hearing before and during therapy. Notify prescriber if patient complains of tinnitus, vertigo, or hearing loss.
• Weigh patient and review renal function studies before therapy begins.
• *Alert:* Use preservative-free form when intrathecal route is used adjunctively for serious CNS infections, such as meningitis and ventriculitis.
• Maintain peak levels at 4 to 12 mcg/ml and trough levels at 1 to 2 mcg/ml. The maximum peak level is usually 8 mcg/ml, except in patients with cystic fibrosis, who need increased lung penetration. Prolonged peak levels of 10 to 12 mcg/ml or prolonged trough levels greater than 2 mcg/ml may increase risk of toxicity.
• *Alert:* Monitor renal function: urine output, specific gravity, urinalysis, BUN and creatinine levels, and creatinine clearance. Report to prescriber evidence of declining renal function.
• Hemodialysis for 8 hours may remove up to 50% of drug from blood.
• Watch for signs and symptoms of superinfection (especially of upper respiratory tract), such as continued fever, chills, and increased pulse rate.
• Therapy usually continues for 7 to 10 days. If no response occurs in 3 to 5 days, stop therapy and obtain new specimens for culture and sensitivity testing.

PATIENT TEACHING

• Instruct patient to promptly report adverse reactions, such as dizziness, vertigo, unsteady gait, ringing in the ears, hearing loss, numbness, tingling, or muscle twitching.
• Encourage patient to drink plenty of fluids.
• Warn patient to avoid hazardous activities if adverse CNS reactions occur.

Reactions may be *common,* uncommon, *life-threatening,* or COMMON AND LIFE-THREATENING.
Interaction may have a *rapid onset* or **delayed onset.**

guaifenesin (glyceryl guaiacolate)
gwye-FEN-e-sin

Allfen Jr, Altarussin ◊, Balminil† ◊, Benylin E† ◊, Diabetic Tussin ◊, Ganidin NR, Guiatuss ◊, Humibid ◊, Hytuss ◊, Hytuss 2X ◊, Liquibid ◊, Mucinex ◊, Mucinex Mini-Melts ◊, Naldecon Senior EX ◊, Organidin NR, Robitussin ◊, Scot-Tussin Expectorant ◊, Siltussin ◊

Pharmacologic class: propanediol derivative
Pregnancy risk category C

AVAILABLE FORMS
Capsules: 200 mg ◊
Granules: 50 mg ◊, 100 mg ◊
Liquid: 100 mg/5 ml* ◊, 200 mg/5 ml ◊
Syrup: 100 mg/5 ml ◊
Tablets: 100 mg ◊, 200 mg ◊, 400 mg
Tablets (extended-release): 600 mg ◊, 1,200 mg ◊

INDICATIONS & DOSAGES
➤ **Expectorant**
Adults and children age 12 and older: 200 to 400 mg P.O. every 4 hours, or 600 to 1,200 mg extended-release capsules or tablets every 12 hours. Maximum, 2,400 mg daily.
Children ages 6 to 11: Give 100 to 200 mg P.O. every 4 hours. Maximum, 1,200 mg daily.
Children ages 2 to 5: Give 50 to 100 mg P.O. every 4 hours. Maximum, 600 mg daily.

ADMINISTRATION
P.O.
• Don't break or crush extended-release products.
• Empty entire contents of granule packet on the patient's tongue. Tell patient to swallow without chewing for best taste.

ACTION
Increases production of respiratory tract fluids to help liquefy and reduce the viscosity of tenacious secretions.

Route	Onset	Peak	Duration
P.O.	Unknown	Unknown	Unknown

Half-life: Unknown.

ADVERSE REACTIONS
CNS: dizziness, headache.
GI: vomiting, nausea.
Skin: rash.

INTERACTIONS
None significant.

EFFECTS ON LAB TEST RESULTS
• May interfere with uric acid level determination and with 5-hydroxyindoleacetic acid and vanillylmandelic tests.

CONTRAINDICATIONS & CAUTIONS
• Contraindicated in patients hypersensitive to drug.

NURSING CONSIDERATIONS
• Some liquid formulations contain alcohol.
• Drug is used to liquefy thick, tenacious sputum. Evidence suggests that guaifenesin is effective as an expectorant, but no evidence exists to support its role as an antitussive.
• Monitor cough type and frequency.
• Stop use 48 hours before 5-hydroxyindoleacetic acid and vanillylmandelic tests.
• *Look alike–sound alike:* Don't confuse guaifenesin with guanfacine.

PATIENT TEACHING
• Tell patient to contact his health care provider if cough lasts longer than 1 week, recurs frequently, or is accompanied by high fever, rash, or severe headache.
• Inform patient that drug shouldn't be used for chronic or persistent cough, such as with smoking, asthma, chronic bronchitis, or emphysema.
• Advise patient to take each dose with one glass of water; increasing fluid intake may prove beneficial.
• Tell patient to empty entire contents of granule packet onto the tongue and to swallow without chewing for best taste.
• Encourage deep-breathing exercises.

heparin sodium
HEP-ah-rin

Hepalean†, Heparin Lock Flush Solution (with Tubex), Heparin Sodium Injection, Hep-Lock, Hep-Pak

Pharmacologic class: anticoagulant
Pregnancy risk category C

AVAILABLE FORMS
Products are derived from beef lung or pork intestinal mucosa.
heparin sodium
Carpuject: 5,000 units/ml
Premixed I.V. solutions: 1,000 units in 500 ml of normal saline solution; 2,000 units in 1,000 ml of normal saline solution; 12,500 units in 250 ml of half-normal saline solution; 25,000 units in 250 ml of half-normal saline solution; 25,000 units in 500 ml of half-normal saline solution; 10,000 units in 100 ml of D_5W; 12,500 units in 250 ml of D_5W; 20,000 units in 500 ml of D_5W; 25,000 units in 250 ml D_5W; 25,000 units in 500 ml D_5W
Single-dose ampules and vials: 1,000 units/ml, 5,000 units/ml, 10,000 units/ml, 20,000 units/ml, 40,000 units/ml
Syringes: 1,000 units/ml, 2,500 units/ml, 5,000 units/ml, 7,500 units/ml, 10,000 units/ml, 20,000 units/ml
Unit-dose vials: 1,000 units/ml, 2,500 units/ml, 5,000 units/ml, 7,500 units/ml, 10,000 units/ml, 20,000 units/ml
Vials (multidose): 1,000 units/ml, 2,000 units/ml, 2,500 units/ml, 5,000 units/ml, 10,000 units/ml, 20,000 units/ml, 40,000 units/ml
heparin sodium flush
Syringes: 10 units/ml, 100 units/ml
Vials: 10 units/ml, 100 units/ml

INDICATIONS & DOSAGES
➤ **Full-dose continuous I.V. infusion therapy for deep vein thrombosis (DVT), MI, pulmonary embolism**
Adults: Initially, 5,000 units by I.V. bolus; then 750 to 1,500 units/hour by I.V. infusion with pump. Titrate hourly rate based on PTT results (every 4 to 6 hours in the early stages of treatment).
Children: Initially, 50 units/kg I.V.; then 25 units/kg/hour or 20,000 units/m^2 daily by I.V. infusion pump. Titrate dosage based on PTT.
➤ **Full-dose subcutaneous therapy for DVT, MI, pulmonary embolism**
Adults: Initially, 5,000 units I.V. bolus and 10,000 to 20,000 units in a concentrated solution subcutaneously; then 8,000 to 10,000 units subcutaneously every 8 hours or 15,000 to 20,000 units in a concentrated solution every 12 hours.
➤ **Full-dose intermittent I.V. therapy for DVT, MI, pulmonary embolism**
Adults: Initially, 10,000 units by I.V. bolus; then titrated according to PTT, and 5,000 to 10,000 units I.V. every 4 to 6 hours.
Children: Initially, 100 units/kg by I.V. bolus; then 50 to 100 units/kg every 4 hours.
➤ **Fixed low-dose therapy for prevention of venous thrombosis, pulmonary embolism, embolism associated with atrial fibrillation, and postoperative DVT**
Adults: 5,000 units subcutaneously every 12 hours. In surgical patients, give first dose 1 to 2 hours before procedure; then 5,000 units subcutaneously every 8 to 12 hours for 5 to 7 days or until patient can walk.
➤ **Consumptive coagulopathy (such as disseminated intravascular coagulation)**
Adults: 50 to 100 units/kg by I.V. bolus or continuous I.V. infusion every 4 hours.
Children: 25 to 50 units/kg by I.V. bolus or continuous I.V. infusion every 4 hours. If no improvement within 4 to 8 hours, stop heparin.
➤ **Open-heart surgery**
Adults: For total body perfusion, 150 to 400 units/kg continuous I.V. infusion.
➤ **Patency maintenance of I.V. indwelling catheters**
Adults: 10 to 100 units I.V. flush. Use sufficient volume to fill device. Not intended for therapeutic use.

ADMINISTRATION
I.V.
• Draw blood to establish baseline coagulation parameters before therapy.
• Use an infusion pump to provide maximum safety. Check constant infusions regularly, even when pumps are in good working order, to ensure correct dosing. Place notice above patient's bed to caution I.V. team or laboratory personnel to apply pressure dressings after taking blood.
• During intermittent infusion, always draw blood 30 minutes before next scheduled dose to avoid falsely elevated PTT. Blood for PTT may be drawn 4 hours after continuous I.V. heparin therapy starts. Never draw blood for PTT from the tubing of the heparin infusion or from the infused vein, because falsely elevated PTT will result. Always draw blood from the opposite arm.
• Don't skip a dose or try to "catch up" with a solution containing heparin. If solution runs out, restart it as soon as possible, and reschedule bolus dose immediately. Monitor PTT.
• Concentrated heparin solutions (more than 100 units/ml) can irritate blood vessels.
• Never piggyback other drugs into an infusion line while heparin infusion is running. Never mix another drug and heparin in same syringe when giving a bolus.
• **Incompatibilities:** Alteplase; amikacin; amiodarone; amphotericin B cholesteryl; ampicillin sodium; atracurium; caspofungin; chlorpromazine; ciprofloxacin; codeine phosphate; cytarabine; dacarbazine; dantrolene; daunorubicin; dextrose 4.3% in sodium chloride solution 0.18%; diazepam; diltiazem; dobutamine; doxorubicin; doxycycline hyclate; droperidol; ergotamine; erythromycin glucceptate or lactobionate; filgrastim; gentamicin; haloperidol lactate; hydrocortisone sodium succinate; hydroxyzine hydrochloride; idarubicin; kanamycin; labetalol; levofloxacin; levorphanol; meperidine; methadone; methylprednisolone sodium succinate; morphine sulfate; nesiritide; netilmicin; nicardipine; penicillin G potassium; penicillin G sodium; pentazocine lactate; phenytoin sodium; polymyxin B sulfate; prochlorperazine edisylate; promethazine hydrochloride; quinidine gluconate; reteplase; 1/6 M sodium lactate; solutions containing a phosphate buffer, sodium carbonate, or sodium oxalate; streptomycin; sulfamethoxazole and trimethoprim; tobramycin sulfate; trifluoperazine; triflupromazine; vancomycin; vinblastine; warfarin.
Subcutaneous
• Give low-dose injections sequentially between iliac crests in lower abdomen deep into subcutaneous fat. Inject drug subcutaneously slowly into fat pad.
• Don't massage injection site; watch for signs of bleeding there.
• Alternate sites every 12 hours—right for morning, left for evening. Record location.

ACTION
Accelerates formation of antithrombin III-thrombin complex and deactivates thrombin, preventing conversion of fibrinogen to fibrin.

Route	Onset	Peak	Duration
I.V.	Immediate	Unknown	Variable
Subcut	20–60 min	2–4 hr	Variable

Half-life: 1 to 2 hours. Half-life is dose-dependent and nonlinear and may be disproportionately prolonged at higher doses.

ADVERSE REACTIONS
CNS: fever.
EENT: rhinitis.
Hematologic: *hemorrhage, overly prolonged clotting time, thrombocytopenia, white clot syndrome.*
Metabolic: *hyperkalemia,* hypoaldosteronism.
Skin: irritation, mild pain, hematoma, ulceration, cutaneous or subcutaneous necrosis, pruritus, urticaria.
Other: hypersensitivity reactions, including chills, *anaphylactoid reactions.*

INTERACTIONS
Drug-drug. *Antihistamines, digoxin, quinine, tetracycline:* May interfere with anticoagulant effect of heparin. Monitor patient for therapeutic effect.
Antiplatelet drugs, salicylates: May increase anticoagulant effect. Use together cautiously. Monitor coagulation studies and patient closely.

Cephalosporins, penicillins: May increase risk of bleeding. Monitor patient closely.
Nitroglycerin: May decrease effects of heparin. Monitor patient closely.
Oral anticoagulants: May increase additive anticoagulation. Monitor PT, INR, and PTT.
Thrombolytics: May increase risk of hemorrhage. Monitor patient closely.
Drug-herb. *Angelica (dong quai), boldo, bromelains, capsicum, chamomile, dandelion, danshen, devil's claw, fenugreek, feverfew, garlic, ginger, ginkgo, ginseng, horse chestnut, licorice, meadowsweet, motherwort, onion, passion flower, red clover, white willow:* May increase risk of bleeding. Discourage herb use.
Drug-lifestyle. *Smoking:* May interfere with anticoagulant effect of heparin. Discourage smoking.

EFFECTS ON LAB TEST RESULTS
● May increase ALT, AST, and potassium levels.
● May increase INR, PT, and PTT. May decrease platelet count.
● Drug may cause false elevations in some tests for thyroxine level.

CONTRAINDICATIONS & CAUTIONS
● Contraindicated in patients hypersensitive to drug. Conditionally contraindicated in patients with active bleeding, blood dyscrasia, or bleeding tendencies, such as hemophilia, thrombocytopenia, or hepatic disease with hypoprothrombinemia; suspected intracranial hemorrhage; suppurative thrombophlebitis; inaccessible ulcerative lesions (especially of GI tract) and open ulcerative wounds; extensive denudation of skin; ascorbic acid deficiency and other conditions that cause increased capillary permeability.
● Conditionally contraindicated during or after brain, eye, or spinal cord surgery; during spinal tap or spinal anesthesia; during continuous tube drainage of stomach or small intestine; and in subacute bacterial endocarditis, shock, advanced renal disease, threatened abortion, or severe hypertension.

● Use cautiously in women during menses or after childbirth and in patients with mild hepatic or renal disease, alcoholism, occupations with high risk of physical injury, or history of allergies, asthma, or GI ulcerations.

NURSING CONSIDERATIONS
● Although heparin use is clearly hazardous in certain conditions, its risks and benefits must be evaluated.
● If a woman needs anticoagulation during pregnancy, most prescribers use heparin.
● Some commercially available heparin injections contain benzyl alcohol. Avoid using these products in neonates and pregnant women if possible.
● Drug requirements are higher in early phases of thrombogenic diseases and febrile states; they are lower when patient's condition stabilizes.
● Elderly patients should usually start at lower dosage.
● Check order and vial carefully; heparin comes in various concentrations.
● *Alert:* USP and international units aren't equivalent for heparin.
● *Alert:* Heparin, low–molecular-weight heparins, and danaparoid aren't interchangeable.
● *Alert:* Don't change concentrations of infusions unless absolutely necessary. This is a common source of dosage errors.
● *Alert:* There is the potential for delayed onset of heparin-induced thrombocytopenia (HIT), a serious antibody-mediated reaction resulting from irreversible aggregation of platelets. HIT may progress to the development of venous and arterial thromboses, a condition referred to as heparin-induced thrombocytopenia and thrombosis (HITT). Thrombotic events may be the initial presentation for HITT, which can occur up to several weeks after stopping heparin therapy. Evaluate patients presenting with thrombocytopenia or thrombosis after stopping heparin for HIT and HITT.
● Draw blood for PTT 4 to 6 hours after dose given subcutaneously.
● Avoid I.M. injections of other drugs to prevent or minimize hematoma.

- Measure PTT carefully and regularly. Anticoagulation is present when PTT values are $1\frac{1}{2}$ to 2 times the control values.
- Monitor platelet count regularly. When new thrombosis accompanies thrombocytopenia (white clot syndrome), stop heparin.
- Regularly inspect patient for bleeding gums, bruises on arms or legs, petechiae, nosebleeds, melena, tarry stools, hematuria, and hematemesis.
- Monitor vital signs.
- **Alert:** To treat severe overdose, use protamine sulfate, a heparin antagonist. Dosage is based on the dose of heparin, its route of administration, and the time since it was given. Generally, 1 to 1.5 mg of protamine per 100 units of heparin is given if only a few minutes have elapsed; 0.5 to 0.75 mg protamine per 100 units heparin, if 30 to 60 minutes have elapsed; and 0.25 to 0.375 mg protamine per 100 units heparin, if 2 hours or more have elapsed. Don't give more than 50 mg protamine in a 10-minute period.
- Abrupt withdrawal may cause increased coagulability; warfarin therapy usually overlaps heparin therapy for continuation of prophylaxis or treatment.
- **Look alike–sound alike:** Don't confuse heparin with Hespan.
- **Look alike–sound alike:** Don't confuse heparin sodium injection 10,000 units/ml and Hep-Lock 10 units/ml.

PATIENT TEACHING
- Instruct patient and family to watch for signs of bleeding or bruising and to notify prescriber immediately if any occur.
- Tell patient to avoid OTC drugs containing aspirin, other salicylates, or drugs that may interact with heparin unless ordered by prescriber.
- Advise patient to consult with prescriber before starting herbal therapy; many herbs have anticoagulant, antiplatelet, or fibrinolytic properties.

hydromorphone hydrochloride (dihydromorphinone hydrochloride)
hye-droe-MOR-fone

Dilaudid, Dilaudid-5, Dilaudid-HP

Pharmacologic class: opioid
Pregnancy risk category C
Controlled substance schedule II

AVAILABLE FORMS
Cough syrup: 1 mg/5 ml
Injection: 1 mg/ml, 2 mg/ml, 3 mg/ml, 4 mg/ml, 10 mg/ml
Liquid: 5 mg/5 ml
Lyophilized powder for injection: 10 mg/ml
Suppositories: 3 mg
Tablets: 1 mg, 2 mg, 3 mg, 4 mg, 8 mg

INDICATIONS & DOSAGES
➤ **Moderate to severe pain**
Adults: 2 to 4 mg P.O. every 4 to 6 hours p.r.n. Or, 1 to 4 mg I.M., subcutaneously, or I.V. (slowly over at least 2 to 5 minutes) every 4 to 6 hours p.r.n. Or, 3 mg P.R. suppository every 6 to 8 hours p.r.n.
➤ **Cough**
Adults and children older than age 12: Give 1 mg cough syrup P.O. every 3 to 4 hours p.r.n.
Children ages 6 to 12: Give 0.5 mg cough syrup P.O. every 3 to 4 hours p.r.n.

ADMINISTRATION
P.O.
- Give drug with food if GI upset occurs.
I.V.
- For infusion, drug may be mixed in D_5W, normal saline solution, dextrose 5% in normal saline solution, dextrose 5% in half-normal saline solution, or Ringer or lactated Ringer solutions.
- Give by direct injection over no less than 2 minutes.
- Respiratory depression and hypotension can occur. Give slowly, and monitor patient constantly. Keep resuscitation equipment available.
- **Incompatibilities:** Alkalies, amphotericin B cholesterol complex, ampicillin sodium, bromides, cefazolin, dexamethasone, diazepam, gallium

nitrate, haloperidol, heparin sodium, io-
dides, minocycline, phenobarbital sodium,
phenytoin sodium, prochlorperazine edi-
sylate, sargramostim, sodium bicarbonate,
sodium phosphate, thiopental.
I.M.
• Document administration site.
Subcutaneous
• Rotate injection sites to avoid induration
with subcutaneous injection.
Rectal
• Refrigerate suppositories.

ACTION

Unknown. Binds with opioid receptors in
the CNS, altering perception of and emotional response to pain. Also suppresses
the cough reflex by direct action on the
cough center in the medulla.

Route	Onset	Peak	Duration
P.O.	15–30 min	30–60 min	4–5 hr
I.V.	10–15 min	15–30 min	2–3 hr
I.M.	15 min	30–60 min	4–5 hr
Subcut	15 min	30–90 min	4 hr
P.R.	Unknown	Unknown	4 hr

Half-life: 2½ to 4 hours.

ADVERSE REACTIONS

CNS: sedation, somnolence, clouded
sensorium, dizziness, euphoria, light-
headedness.
CV: hypotension, flushing, *bradycardia.*
EENT: blurred vision, diplopia, nystag-
mus.
GI: nausea, vomiting, *constipation,* ileus,
dry mouth.
GU: urine retention.
Respiratory: *respiratory depression,*
bronchospasm.
Skin: diaphoresis, pruritus.
Other: induration with repeated subcuta-
neous injections, physical dependence.

INTERACTIONS

Drug-drug. *CNS depressants, general*
anesthetics, hypnotics, MAO inhibitors,
other opioid analgesics, sedatives, tran-
quilizers, tricyclic antidepressants: May
cause additive effects. Use together with
caution; reduce hydromorphone dose and
monitor patient response.
Drug-lifestyle. *Alcohol use:* May cause
additive effects. Discourage use together.

EFFECTS ON LAB TEST RESULTS

• May increase amylase and lipase levels.
• May interfere with hepatobiliary imaging studies because delayed gastric emptying and contraction of sphincter of Oddi
may increase biliary tract pressure.

CONTRAINDICATIONS & CAUTIONS

• Contraindicated in patients hypersensitive to drug; in those with intracranial
lesions that cause increased intracranial
pressure; and in those with depressed
ventilation, such as in status asthmaticus,
COPD, cor pulmonale, emphysema, and
kyphoscoliosis.
• Use with caution in elderly or debilitated
patients and in those with hepatic or
renal disease, hypothyroidism, Addison's
disease, prostatic hyperplasia, or urethral
stricture.

NURSING CONSIDERATIONS

• Reassess patient's level of pain at least 15
and 30 minutes after administration.
• For better analgesic effect, give drug on a
regular schedule, before patient has intense
pain.
• Dilaudid-HP, a highly concentrated
form (10 mg/ml), may be given in smaller
volumes to prevent the discomfort of large-
volume I.M. or subcutaneous injections.
Check dosage carefully.
• Monitor respiratory and circulatory
status and bowel function.
• Keep opioid antagonist (naloxone)
available.
• Drug may worsen or mask gallbladder
pain.
• Drug is a commonly abused opioid.
• Drug may cause constipation. Assess
bowel function and need for stool softeners
and stimulant laxatives.
• *Alert:* Cough syrup may contain tartrazine.
• *Look alike–sound alike:* Don't confuse
hydromorphone with morphine or oxymor-
phone or Dilaudid with Dilantin.

PATIENT TEACHING

• Instruct patient to request or take drug
before pain becomes intense.
• Tell patient to store suppositories in
refrigerator.
• Advise patient to take drug with food if
GI upset occurs.

Reactions may be *common,* uncommon, *life-threatening,* or COMMON AND LIFE-THREATENING.
Interaction may have a *rapid onset* or *delayed onset.*

• When drug is used after surgery, encourage patient to turn, cough, and breathe deeply to avoid lung problems.
• Caution patient about getting out of bed or walking. Warn outpatient to avoid hazardous activities that require mental alertness until drug's CNS effects are known.
• Advise patient to avoid alcohol during therapy.

SAFETY ALERT!

ifosfamide
eye-FOSS-fa-mide

Ifex

Pharmacologic class: nitrogen mustard
Pregnancy risk category D

AVAILABLE FORMS
Powder for injection: 1 g, 3 g

INDICATIONS & DOSAGES
➤ **Testicular cancer**
Adults: 1.2 g/m² daily I.V. for 5 consecutive days. Repeat treatment every 3 weeks or after patient recovers from hematologic toxicity. Don't repeat doses until WBC count exceeds 4,000/mm³ and platelet count exceeds 100,000/mm³.
➤ **Sarcomas; small-cell lung, cervical, ovarian, and uterine cancer ♦**
Adults: 1.2 to 2.5 g/m² I.V. daily for 3 to 5 days. Repeat cycle, as needed, based on patient response.

ADMINISTRATION
I.V.
• Preparing and giving drug may be mutagenic, teratogenic, or carcinogenic. Follow facility policy to reduce risks.
• Give a protective drug such as mesna to prevent hemorrhagic cystitis. Ifosfamide and mesna are physically compatible and may be mixed in the same I.V. solution.
• Obtain urinalysis before each dose. If microscopic hematuria occurs, notify prescriber. Adjust dosage of mesna, if needed. Adequate fluid intake (2 L daily, either P.O. or I.V.) is essential before, and 72 hours after, therapy.

• Reconstitute each gram of drug with 20 ml of diluent to yield a solution of 50 mg/ml. Use sterile water for injection or bacteriostatic water for injection. Solutions may then be further diluted with sterile water, dextrose 2.5% or 5% in water, half-normal or normal saline solution for injection, dextrose 5% and normal saline solution for injection, or lactated Ringer's injection.
• Infuse each dose over at least 30 minutes.
• Reconstituted solution is stable for 1 week at room temperature or 6 weeks if refrigerated. However, use solution within 6 hours if drug was reconstituted with sterile water without a preservative (such as benzyl alcohol or parabens).
• **Incompatibilities:** Cefepime, mesna with epirubicin, methotrexate sodium.

ACTION
Cross-links strands of cellular DNA and interferes with RNA transcription, causing an imbalance of growth that leads to cell death. Not specific to cell cycle.

Route	Onset	Peak	Duration
I.V.	Unknown	Unknown	Unknown

Half-life: About 14 hours.

ADVERSE REACTIONS
CNS: *somnolence, confusion, coma, seizures,* ataxia, hallucinations, depressive psychosis, dizziness, disorientation, cranial nerve dysfunction.
GI: *nausea, vomiting,* diarrhea.
GU: *hemorrhagic cystitis, hematuria, nephrotoxicity,* Fanconi syndrome.
Hematologic: *leukopenia, thrombocytopenia, myelosuppression.*
Hepatic: *hepatotoxicity.*
Metabolic: *metabolic acidosis.*
Skin: *alopecia.*
Other: infection, phlebitis.

INTERACTIONS
Drug-drug. *Anticoagulants, aspirin, NSAIDs:* May increase risk of bleeding. Avoid using together.
Barbiturates, chloral hydrate, fosphenytoin, phenytoin: May increase ifosfamide toxicity. Monitor patient closely.
Corticosteroids: May inhibit hepatic enzymes, reducing ifosfamide's effect. Monitor patient for increased ifosfamide

toxicity if corticosteroid dosage is suddenly reduced or stopped.
Cyclophosphamide: May increase risk of cardiac tamponade in patients with thalassemia. Monitor patient closely.
Myelosuppressives: May enhance hematologic toxicity. Dosage adjustment may be needed.

EFFECTS ON LAB TEST RESULTS
● May increase liver enzyme levels.
● May decrease WBC and platelet counts.

CONTRAINDICATIONS & CAUTIONS
● Contraindicated in patients hypersensitive to drug and in those with severe bone marrow suppression.
● Use cautiously in patients with renal impairment or compromised bone marrow reserve as indicated by leukopenia, granulocytopenia, extensive bone marrow metastases, previous radiation therapy, or previous therapy with cytotoxic drugs.

NURSING CONSIDERATIONS
● Give antiemetic before drug, to reduce nausea.
● Ensure that patient is adequately hydrated during therapy.
● Don't give drug at bedtime; infrequent urination during the night may increase possibility of cystitis. If cystitis develops, stop drug and notify prescriber.
● Bladder irrigation with normal saline solution may be done to treat cystitis.
● Monitor CBC and renal and liver function tests.
● To prevent bleeding, avoid all I.M. injections when platelet count is less than 50,000/mm³.
● Anticipate blood transfusions because of cumulative anemia. Patients may receive injections of RBC colony-stimulating factor to promote RBC production and decrease need for blood transfusions.
● Assess patient for mental status changes; dosage may have to be decreased.
● *Look alike–sound alike:* Don't confuse ifosfamide with cyclophosphamide.

PATIENT TEACHING
● Remind patient to urinate frequently to minimize contact of drug and its metabolites with the lining of the bladder.

● Advise patient to watch for signs and symptoms of infection (fever, sore throat, fatigue) and bleeding (easy bruising, nosebleeds, bleeding gums, tarry stools). Tell patient to take temperature daily.
● Instruct patient to avoid OTC products that contain aspirin.
● Advise women to stop breast-feeding during therapy because of possible risk of toxicity to infant.
● Caution woman of childbearing age to avoid becoming pregnant during therapy. Recommend that she consult prescriber before becoming pregnant.

---

iloprost
EYE-loe-prost

Ventavis

Pharmacologic class: prostacyclin analog
Pregnancy risk category C

AVAILABLE FORMS
Inhalation solution: 10 mcg/ml in 1- and 2-ml single-dose ampules

INDICATIONS & DOSAGES
➤ **Pulmonary arterial hypertension in patients with New York Heart Association (NYHA) Class III or IV symptoms**
Adults: Initially, 2.5 mcg inhaled using the I-neb or the Prodose Adaptive Aerosol Delivery (AAD) systems. As tolerated, increase to 5 mcg inhaled six to nine times daily while patient is awake, as needed, but to no more than every 2 hours. Maximum, 5 mcg nine times daily.

ADMINISTRATION
Inhalational
● Use only I-neb AAD or Prodose AAD delivery devices, per manufacturer's instructions.

ACTION
Lowers pulmonary arterial pressure by dilating systemic and pulmonary arterial beds. Drug also affects platelet aggregation, although effect in pulmonary hypertension treatment isn't known.

Route	Onset	Peak	Duration
Inhalation	Unknown	Unknown	30-60 min

Half-life: 20 to 30 minutes.

ADVERSE REACTIONS
CNS: *headache,* insomnia, syncope.
CV: *hypotension, vasodilation, chest pain, heart failure, supraventricular tachycardia,* palpitations, peripheral edema.
GI: *nausea,* tongue pain, vomiting.
GU: *renal failure.*
Musculoskeletal: *trismus,* back pain, muscle cramps.
Respiratory: *cough,* dyspnea, hemoptysis, pneumonia.
Other: *flulike syndrome.*

INTERACTIONS
Drug-drug. *Anticoagulants:* May increase risk of bleeding. Monitor patient closely.
Antihypertensives, vasodilators: May increase effects of these drugs. Monitor patient's blood pressure.

EFFECTS ON LAB TEST RESULTS
• May increase alkaline phosphatase and GGT levels.

CONTRAINDICATIONS & CAUTIONS
• No contraindications known. Avoid using in patients whose systolic blood pressure is less than 85 mm Hg.
• Use cautiously in elderly patients, patients with hepatic or renal impairment, and patients with COPD, severe asthma, or acute pulmonary infection.

NURSING CONSIDERATIONS
• Keep drug away from skin and eyes.
• The 2-ml ampule must be used with the Prodose AAD System and may be used with the I-neb AAD System. The 1-ml ampule must be used only with the I-neb AAD System.
• Take care not to inhale drug while providing treatment.
• Monitor patient's vital signs carefully at start of treatment.
• Watch for syncope.
• If patient develops evidence of pulmonary edema, stop treatment immediately.

PATIENT TEACHING
• Advise patient to take drug exactly as prescribed and using Prodose AAD or I-neb AAD.
• Urge patient to follow manufacturer's instructions for preparing and inhaling drug.
• Advise patient to keep a backup Prodose AAD or I-neb AAD in case the original malfunctions.
• Tell patient to keep drug away from skin and eyes and to rinse the area immediately if contact occurs.
• Caution patient not to ingest drug solution.
• Inform patient that drug may cause dizziness and fainting. Urge him to stand up slowly from a sitting or lying position and to report to prescriber worsening of symptoms.
• Tell patient to take drug before physical exertion but no more than every 2 hours.
• Tell patient not to expose others, especially pregnant women and infants, to drug.
• Teach patient how to clean equipment and safely dispose of used ampules after each treatment. Caution patient not to save or use leftover solution.

infliximab
in-FLICKS-ih-mab

Remicade

Pharmacologic class: monoclonal antibody immunoglobulin G1k
Pregnancy risk category B

AVAILABLE FORMS
Lyophilized powder for injection: 100-mg vial

INDICATIONS & DOSAGES
➤ **Moderately to severely active Crohn's disease; reduction in the number of draining enterocutaneous and rectovaginal fistulas and maintenance of fistula closure in patients with fistulizing Crohn's disease**
Adults: 5 mg/kg I.V. infusion over at least 2 hours. Repeat at 2 and 6 weeks, then every 8 weeks thereafter. For patients

who respond and then lose their response, consider 10 mg/kg. Patients who don't respond by week 14 are unlikely to respond with continued therapy. In those patients, consider stopping drug.

Children age 6 to 17: For Crohn's disease, 5 mg/kg I.V. infusion over at least 2 hours. Repeat at 2 and 6 weeks, then every 8 weeks thereafter.

➤ **Moderately to severely active rheumatoid arthritis**

Adults: 3 mg/kg I.V. infusion over at least 2 hours. Repeat at 2 and 6 weeks after first infusion and every 8 weeks thereafter. Dose may be increased up to 10 mg/kg, or doses may be given every 4 weeks if response is inadequate. Use with methotrexate.

➤ **Moderate to severe ulcerative colitis**

Adults: Induction dose, 5 mg/kg I.V. over at least 2 hours. Repeat at 2 and 6 weeks, then every 8 weeks thereafter.

➤ **Ankylosing spondylitis**

Adults: 5 mg/kg I.V. infusion over at least 2 hours. Repeat at 2 and 6 weeks, then every 6 weeks thereafter.

➤ **Psoriatic arthritis, with or without methotrexate**

Adults: 5 mg/kg I.V. infusion over at least 2 hours. Repeat at 2 and 6 weeks after first infusion, then every 8 weeks thereafter.

➤ **Chronic severe plaque psoriasis**

Adults: 5 mg/kg I.V. infusion over at least 2 hours. Repeat dose in 2 and 6 weeks, then give 5 mg/kg every 8 weeks thereafter.

ADMINISTRATION

I.V.

● Reconstitute with 10 ml sterile water for injection, using syringe with 21G or smaller needle. Don't shake; gently swirl to dissolve powder. Solution should be colorless to light yellow and opalescent. It may also develop a few translucent particles; don't use if other types of particles develop or discoloration occurs.

● Dilute total volume of reconstituted drug to 250 ml with normal saline solution for injection. Infusion concentration range is 0.4 to 4 mg/ml.

● Use an in-line, sterile, nonpyrogenic, low–protein-binding filter with a pore size less than 1.2 micrometer.

● Begin infusion within 3 hours of preparation and give over at least 2 hours.

● **Incompatibilities:** Other I.V. drugs.

ACTION

Binds to human tumor necrosis factor (TNF)-alpha to neutralize its activity and inhibit its binding with receptors, thereby reducing the infiltration of inflammatory cells and TNF-alpha production in inflamed areas of the intestine.

Route	Onset	Peak	Duration
I.V.	Unknown	Unknown	Unknown

Half-life: 9½ days.

ADVERSE REACTIONS

CNS: *fatigue, fever, headache,* dizziness, depression, insomnia, malaise, pain, systemic and cutaneous vasculitis.

CV: *hypertension,* chest pain, flushing, hypotension, pericardial effusion, tachycardia.

EENT: *pharyngitis, rhinitis, sinusitis,* conjunctivitis.

GI: *abdominal pain, diarrhea, dyspepsia, nausea,* **intestinal obstruction,** constipation, flatulence, oral pain, ulcerative stomatitis, vomiting.

GU: *UTI,* dysuria, increased urinary frequency.

Hematologic: **leukopenia, neutropenia, pancytopenia, thrombocytopenia,** anemia, hematoma.

Musculoskeletal: *arthralgia, back pain,* arthritis, myalgia.

Respiratory: *coughing, upper respiratory tract infections,* bronchitis, dyspnea, respiratory tract allergic reaction.

Skin: *rash,* acne, alopecia, candidiasis, dry skin, eczema, erythema, erythematous rash, increased sweating, maculopapular rash, papular rash, urticaria.

Other: abscess, chills, ecchymosis, flulike syndrome, hot flashes, peripheral edema, toothache.

INTERACTIONS
Drug-drug. *Abatacept, anakinra:* May increase the risk of serious infections and neutropenia. Avoid using together.
Vaccines: May affect normal immune response. Postpone live-virus vaccine until therapy stops.

EFFECTS ON LAB TEST RESULTS
• May increase liver enzyme level. May decrease hemoglobin level and hematocrit.
• May decrease WBC and platelet counts.
• May cause false-positive antinuclear antibody test result.

CONTRAINDICATIONS & CAUTIONS
• Contraindicated in patients hypersensitive to murine proteins or other components of drug. Doses greater than 5 mg/kg are contraindicated in patients with moderate to severe heart failure.
• Use cautiously in elderly patients and in patients with active infection, history of chronic or recurrent infections, a history of hematologic abnormalities, or preexisting or recent onset of CNS demyelinating or seizure disorders; or in those who have lived in regions where histoplasmosis is endemic.

NURSING CONSIDERATIONS
• *Alert:* Watch for infusion-related reactions, including fever, chills, pruritus, urticaria, dyspnea, hypotension, hypertension, and chest pain during administration and for 2 hours afterward. If an infusion-related reaction occurs, stop drug, notify prescriber, and give acetaminophen, antihistamines, corticosteroids, and epinephrine.
• Give for Crohn's disease and ulcerative colitis only after patient has an inadequate response to conventional therapy.
• Consider stopping treatment in patient who develops significant hematologic abnormalities or CNS adverse reactions.
• Notify prescriber for symptoms of new or worsening heart failure.
• Watch for development of lymphoma and infection. A patient with chronic Crohn's disease and long-term exposure to immunosuppressants is more likely to develop lymphoma and infection.

• Drug may affect normal immune responses. Patient may develop autoimmune antibodies and lupus-like syndrome; stop drug if this happens. Symptoms should resolve.
• *Alert:* Drug may cause disseminated or extrapulmonary tuberculosis and fatal opportunistic infections.
• Evaluate patient for latent tuberculosis infection with a tuberculin skin test. Treat latent tuberculosis infection before therapy.
• *Look alike–sound alike:* Don't confuse Remicade with Renacidin.

PATIENT TEACHING
• Tell patient about infusion-reaction symptoms and adverse effects and the need to report them promptly.
• Advise patient to seek immediate medical attention for signs and symptoms of infection or unusual bleeding or bruising.
• Tell woman to stop breast-feeding during therapy.
• Tell patient that before he receives vaccines, he should alert prescriber to therapy.
• Advise parent to get child up-to-date for all vaccines before therapy.

ipratropium bromide
ih-pra-TROE-pee-um

Atrovent, Atrovent HFA

Pharmacologic class: anticholinergic
Pregnancy risk category B

AVAILABLE FORMS
Inhaler: 18 mcg/metered dose (Atrovent), 17 mcg/metered dose (Atrovent HFA)
Nasal spray: 0.03% (21 mcg/metered dose), 0.06% (42 mcg/metered dose)
Solution (for inhalation): 0.02% (500 mcg/vial)

INDICATIONS & DOSAGES
➤ **Bronchospasm in chronic bronchitis and emphysema**
Adults: Usually, 2 inhalations q.i.d.; patient may take additional inhalations as needed but shouldn't exceed 12 inhalations in 24 hours. Or, 250 to 500 mcg every 6 to 8 hours via oral nebulizer.

➤ **Rhinorrhea caused by allergic and nonallergic perennial rhinitis**
Adults and children age 6 and older: Two 0.03% nasal sprays (42 mcg) per nostril b.i.d. or t.i.d.
➤ **Rhinorrhea caused by the common cold**
Adults and children age 12 and older: Two 0.06% nasal sprays (84 mcg) per nostril t.i.d. or q.i.d.
Children ages 5 to 11: Two 0.06% nasal sprays (84 mcg) per nostril t.i.d.
➤ **Rhinorrhea caused by seasonal allergic rhinitis**
Adults and children age 5 and older: Two 0.06% nasal sprays (84 mcg) per nostril q.i.d.

ADMINISTRATION
Inhalational
● Shake canister before use, except for Atrovent HFA.
● If more than 1 inhalation is ordered, wait at least 2 minutes between inhalations.
● Use spacer device to improve drug delivery, if appropriate.
Intranasal
● Prime nasal spray before first use and after unused for more than 24 hours.
● Tilt patient's head backward after dose to allow drug to spread to back of nose.

ACTION
Inhibits vagally mediated reflexes by antagonizing acetylcholine at muscarinic receptors on bronchial smooth muscle.

Route	Onset	Peak	Duration
Inhalation	5–15 min	1–2 hr	3–6 hr

Half-life: About 2 hours.

ADVERSE REACTIONS
CNS: dizziness, pain, headache, nervousness.
CV: palpitations, hypertension, chest pain.
EENT: blurred vision, rhinitis, pharyngitis, sinusitis, epistaxis.
GI: nausea, GI distress, dry mouth.
Musculoskeletal: back pain.
Respiratory: *upper respiratory tract infection, bronchitis, **bronchospasm,*** cough, dyspnea, increased sputum.
Skin: rash.

Other: flulike symptoms, hypersensitivity reactions.

INTERACTIONS
Drug-drug. *Anticholinergics:* May increase anticholinergic effects. Avoid using together.
Drug-herb. *Jaborandi tree:* May decrease effect of drug. Advise patient to use cautiously.
Pill-bearing spurge: May decrease effect of drug. Advise patient to use cautiously.

EFFECTS ON LAB TEST RESULTS
None reported.

CONTRAINDICATIONS & CAUTIONS
● Contraindicated in patients hypersensitive to drug, atropine, or its derivatives.
● Use cautiously in patients with angle-closure glaucoma, prostatic hyperplasia, or bladder-neck obstruction.
● Safety and effectiveness of nebulization or inhaler in children younger than age 12 haven't been established.

NURSING CONSIDERATIONS
● If patient uses a face mask for a nebulizer, take care to prevent leakage around the mask because eye pain or temporary blurring of vision may occur.
● Safety and effectiveness of use beyond 4 days in patients with a common cold haven't been established.
● *Look alike–sound alike:* Don't confuse Atrovent with Alupent.

PATIENT TEACHING
● Warn patient that drug isn't effective for treating acute episodes of bronchospasm when rapid response is needed.
● Teach patient to perform oral inhalation correctly. Give the following instructions for using an MDI:
–Shake canister. The HFA form doesn't need to be shaken.
–Clear nasal passages and throat.
–Breathe out, expelling as much air from lungs as possible.
–Place mouthpiece well into mouth, and inhale deeply as you release dose from inhaler. (Patient should close his eyes.)
–Hold breath for several seconds, remove mouthpiece, and exhale slowly.

• Inform patient that use of a spacer device with MDI may improve drug delivery to lungs.

• Warn patient to avoid accidentally spraying drug into eyes. Temporary blurring of vision may result.

• If more than 1 inhalation is prescribed, tell patient to wait at least 2 minutes before repeating procedure.

• Instruct patient to remove canister and wash inhaler in warm, soapy water at least once weekly.

• If patient is also using a corticosteroid inhaler, instruct him to use ipratropium first and then to wait about 5 minutes before using the corticosteroid. This lets the bronchodilator open air passages for maximal effectiveness of the corticosteroid.

• Instruct patient to prime nasal spray by pumping seven times before first use and after unused for 1 week. Prime with two pumps after unused for 1 day.

• Instruct patient to sniff deeply after each spray and to breathe out through mouth. Tell him to tilt head backward to allow drug to spread to back of nose.

---

isoniazid (INH, isonicotinic acid hydrazide)
Isotamine†, Nydrazid

Pharmacologic class: isonicotinic acid hydrazine
Pregnancy risk category C

AVAILABLE FORMS
Injection: 100 mg/ml
Oral solution: 50 mg/5 ml
Tablets: 100 mg, 300 mg

INDICATIONS & DOSAGES
➤ **Actively growing tubercle bacilli**
Adults and children age 15 and older: 5 mg/kg daily P.O. or I.M. in a single dose, up to 300 mg/day, with other drugs, continued for 6 months to 2 years. For intermittent multiple-drug regimen, 15 mg/kg (up to 900 mg) P.O. or I.M. up to three times a week.
Infants and children: 10 to 15 mg/kg daily P.O. or I.M. in a single dose, up to 300 mg/day, continued long enough to prevent relapse. Give with at least one other antituberculotic. For intermittent

multidrug regimen, 20 to 40 mg/kg (up to 900 mg) P.O. or I.M. two or three times weekly.
➤ **To prevent tubercle bacilli in those exposed to tuberculosis (TB) or those with positive skin test results whose chest X-rays and bacteriologic study results indicate nonprogressive TB**
Adults: 300 mg daily P.O. in a single dose, continued for 6 months to 1 year.
Infants and children: 10 mg/kg daily P.O. in a single dose, up to 300 mg/day, continued for up to 1 year.

ADMINISTRATION
P.O.
• Always give drug with other antituberculotics to prevent development of resistant organisms.
• Give drug 1 hour before or 2 hours after meals.
I.M.
• Solution may crystallize at a low temperature. Warm vial to room temperature before use to redissolve crystals.

ACTION
May inhibit cell-wall biosynthesis by interfering with lipid and DNA synthesis; bactericidal.

Route	Onset	Peak	Duration
P.O., I.M.	Unknown	1–2 hr	Unknown

Half-life: 1 to 4 hours.

ADVERSE REACTIONS
CNS: *peripheral neuropathy, seizures, toxic encephalopathy,* memory impairment, toxic psychosis.
EENT: optic neuritis and atrophy.
GI: epigastric distress, nausea, vomiting.
Hematologic: *agranulocytosis, aplastic anemia, thrombocytopenia,* eosinophilia, hemolytic anemia, sideroblastic anemia.
Hepatic: *hepatitis,* bilirubinemia, jaundice.
Metabolic: hyperglycemia, hypocalcemia, hypophosphatemia, *metabolic acidosis.*
Skin: irritation at injection site.
Other: gynecomastia, hypersensitivity reactions, pyridoxine deficiency, rheumatic and lupuslike syndromes.

INTERACTIONS

Drug-drug. *Antacids and laxatives containing aluminum:* May decrease isoniazid absorption. Give isoniazid at least 1 hour before antacid or laxative.

Benzodiazepines, such as diazepam, triazolam: May inhibit metabolic clearance of benzodiazepines that undergo oxidative metabolism, possibly increasing benzodiazepine activity. Monitor patient for adverse reactions.

Carbamazepine, phenytoin: May increase levels of these drugs. Monitor drug levels closely.

Cycloserine: May increase CNS adverse reactions. Use safety precautions.

Disulfiram: May cause neurologic symptoms, including changes in behavior and coordination. Avoid using together.

Enflurane: In rapid acetylators of isoniazid, may cause high-output renal failure because of nephrotoxic inorganic fluoride level. Monitor renal function.

Ketoconazole: May decrease ketoconazole level. Monitor patient for lack of efficacy.

Meperidine: May increase CNS adverse reactions and hypotension. Use safety precautions.

Oral anticoagulants: May enhance anticoagulant activity. Monitor PT and INR.

Phenytoin: May inhibit phenytoin metabolism and increase phenytoin level. Monitor patient for phenytoin toxicity.

Rifampin: May increase the risk of hepatotoxicity. Monitor liver function tests closely.

Drug-food. *Foods containing tyramine (such as aged cheese, beer, and chocolate):* May cause hypertensive crisis. Tell patient to avoid such foods or eat in small quantities.

Drug-lifestyle. *Alcohol use:* May increase risk of drug-related hepatitis. Discourage use of alcohol.

EFFECTS ON LAB TEST RESULTS

• May increase transaminase, glucose, and bilirubin levels. May decrease calcium, phosphate, and hemoglobin levels.

• May increase eosinophil count. May decrease granulocyte and platelet counts.

• May alter result of urine glucose tests that use cupric sulfate method, such as Benedict's reagent and Diastix.

CONTRAINDICATIONS & CAUTIONS

• Contraindicated in patients with acute hepatic disease or isoniazid-related liver damage.

• Use cautiously in elderly patients, in those with chronic non–isoniazid-related liver disease or chronic alcoholism, in those with seizure disorders (especially if taking phenytoin), and in those with severe renal impairment.

NURSING CONSIDERATIONS

• Drug's pharmacokinetics vary among patients because drug is metabolized in the liver by genetically controlled acetylation. Fast acetylators metabolize drug up to five times faster than slow acetylators. About 50% of blacks and whites are fast acetylators; more than 80% of Chinese, Japanese, and Inuits are fast acetylators.

• Peripheral neuropathy is more common in patients who are slow acetylators, malnourished, alcoholic, or diabetic.

• Monitor hepatic function closely for changes. Elevated liver function study results occur in about 15% of patients; most abnormalities are mild and transient, but some may persist throughout treatment.

• *Alert:* Severe and sometimes fatal hepatitis may develop, even after many months of treatment. Risk increases with age. Monitor liver study results closely.

• Give pyridoxine to prevent peripheral neuropathy, especially in malnourished patients.

PATIENT TEACHING

• Instruct patient to take drug exactly as prescribed; warn against stopping drug without prescriber's consent.

• Advise patient to take drug 1 hour before or 2 hours after meals.

• Tell patient to notify prescriber immediately if signs and symptoms of liver impairment occur, such as appetite loss, fatigue, malaise, yellow skin or eye discoloration, and dark urine.

• Advise patient to avoid alcoholic beverages while taking drug. Also tell him to avoid certain foods: fish, such as skipjack and tuna, and products containing tyramine, such as aged cheese, beer, and chocolate, because drug has some MAO inhibitor activity.

Reactions may be *common*, uncommon, *life-threatening*, or COMMON AND LIFE-THREATENING.
Interaction may have a *rapid onset* or **delayed onset**.

• Encourage patient to comply fully with treatment, which may take months or years.

---

isoproterenol hydrochloride
eye-soe-proe-TER-e-nole

Isuprel

Pharmacologic class: nonselective beta-adrenergic agonist
Pregnancy risk category C

AVAILABLE FORMS
Injection: 20 mcg/ml in 10-ml prefilled syringes, 200 mcg/ml in 1- and 5-ml ampules and 5- and 10-ml vials

INDICATIONS & DOSAGES
➤ **Bronchospasm during anesthesia**
Adults: Dilute 1 ml of a 1:5,000 solution with 10 ml of normal saline or D_5W. Give 0.01 to 0.02 mg I.V. and repeat as necessary. Or, give 1:50,000 solution undiluted using same dose.
➤ **Heart block, ventricular arrhythmias**
Adults: Initially, 0.02 to 0.06 mg I.V.; then 0.01 to 0.2 mg I.V. or 5 mcg/minute I.V. Or, initially, 0.2 mg I.M.; then 0.02 to 1 mg I.M., as needed.
Children: Initial I.V. infusion of 0.1 mcg/kg/minute. Adjust dosage based on patient's response. Usual dosage range is 0.1 to 1 mcg/kg/minute.
➤ **Shock**
Adults and children: 0.5 to 5 mcg/minute isoproterenol hydrochloride by continuous I.V. infusion. Usual concentration is 1 mg or 5 ml in 500 ml D_5W. Titrate infusion rate according to heart rate, central venous pressure, blood pressure, and urine flow.
➤ **Postoperative cardiac patients with bradycardia ♦**
Children: I.V. infusion of 0.029 mcg/kg/minute.
➤ **As an aid in diagnosing the cause of mitral regurgitation ♦**
Adults: 4 mcg/minute I.V. infusion.
➤ **As an aid in diagnosing coronary artery disease or lesions ♦**
Adults: 1 to 3 mcg/minute I.V. infusion.

ADMINISTRATION
I.V.
• For infusion, dilute with most common I.V. solutions, but don't use with sodium bicarbonate injection; drug decomposes rapidly in alkaline solutions.
• Don't use solution if it's discolored or contains precipitate.
• Give by direct injection or I.V. infusion.
• For shock, closely monitor blood pressure, central venous pressure, ECG, arterial blood gas measurements, and urine output. Carefully titrate infusion rate according to these measurements. Use a continuous infusion pump to regulate flow rate.
• Store at room temperature. Protect from light.
• **Incompatibilities:** Alkalies, aminophylline, furosemide, metals, sodium bicarbonate.

ACTION
Relaxes bronchial smooth muscle by stimulating $beta_2$ receptors. As a cardiac stimulant, acts on $beta_1$ receptors in the heart.

Route	Onset	Peak	Duration
I.V.	Immediate	Unknown	< 60 min

Half-life: Unknown.

ADVERSE REACTIONS
CNS: headache, mild tremor, weakness, dizziness, nervousness, insomnia, anxiety.
CV: *palpitations, rapid rise and fall in blood pressure, tachycardia, angina, arrhythmias, cardiac arrest.*
GI: nausea, vomiting.
Metabolic: hyperglycemia.
Skin: diaphoresis.
Other: swelling of parotid glands with prolonged use.

INTERACTIONS
Drug-drug. *Epinephrine, other sympathomimetics:* May increase risk of arrhythmias. Use together cautiously. If used together, give at least 4 hours apart.
Halogenated general anesthetics or cyclopropane: May increase risk of arrhythmias. Avoid using together.
Propranolol, other beta blockers: May block bronchodilating effect of isoproterenol. Monitor patient carefully.

EFFECTS ON LAB TEST RESULTS
• May increase glucose level.

CONTRAINDICATIONS & CAUTIONS
• Contraindicated in patients with tachycardia or AV block caused by digoxin intoxication, arrhythmias other than those that may respond to drug, angina pectoris, or angle-closure glaucoma.
• Contraindicated when used with general anesthetics, with halogenated drugs, or with cyclopropane.
• Use cautiously in elderly patients and in those with renal or CV disease, coronary insufficiency, diabetes, hyperthyroidism, or history of sensitivity to sympathomimetic amines.

NURSING CONSIDERATIONS
• Correct volume deficit before giving vasopressors.
• *Alert:* If heart rate exceeds 110 beats/minute during I.V. infusion, notify prescriber. Doses that increase the heart rate to more than 130 beats/minute may induce ventricular arrhythmias.
• Drug may cause a slight increase in systolic blood pressure and a slight to marked decrease in diastolic blood pressure.
• Monitor patient for adverse reactions.
• *Look alike–sound alike:* Don't confuse Isuprel with Isordil.

PATIENT TEACHING
• Tell patient to report chest pain, fluttering in chest, or other adverse reactions.
• Remind patient to report pain at the I.V. injection site.

---

levalbuterol hydrochloride
lev-al-BYOO-ter-ol

Xopenex, Xopenex HFA

Pharmacologic class: beta$_2$ agonist
Pregnancy risk category C

AVAILABLE FORMS
Inhalation aerosol: 15 g containing 200 actuations
Solution for inhalation: 0.31 mg, 0.63 mg, or 1.25 mg in 3-ml vials; 1.25 mg/0.5-ml vials (concentrate)

INDICATIONS & DOSAGES
➤ **To prevent or treat bronchospasm in patients with reversible obstructive airway disease**
Adults and adolescents age 12 and older: 0.63 mg given t.i.d. every 6 to 8 hours, by oral inhalation via a nebulizer. Patients with more severe asthma who don't respond adequately to 0.63 mg t.i.d. may benefit from 1.25 mg t.i.d.
Children ages 6 to 11: Give 0.31 mg inhaled t.i.d. by nebulizer. Routine dosage shouldn't exceed 0.63 mg t.i.d.
Adults and children age 4 and older: 2 inhalations Xopenex HFA (90 mcg) every 4 to 6 hours. In some patients, 1 inhalation every 4 hours is sufficient.

ADMINISTRATION
Inhalational
• Keep unopened vial in foil pouch. After opened, vial must be used within 2 weeks and protected from light.
• Release four test sprays before first use of inhaler or after unused for more than 3 days.
• Shake canister well before use.
• Use a spacer device to improve inhalation, as appropriate.

ACTION
Relaxes bronchial smooth muscle by stimulating beta$_2$ receptors; also, inhibits release of mediators from mast cells in the airway.

Route	Onset	Peak	Duration
Inhalation	5–15 min	1 hr	3–4 hr

Half-life: 3$\frac{1}{4}$ to 4 hours.

ADVERSE REACTIONS
CNS: dizziness, migraine, nervousness, pain, tremor, anxiety.
CV: tachycardia.
EENT: *rhinitis,* sinusitis, turbinate edema.
GI: dyspepsia.
Musculoskeletal: leg cramps.
Respiratory: increased cough.
Other: *viral infection,* flulike syndrome, accidental injury.

INTERACTIONS
Drug-drug. *Beta blockers:* May block pulmonary effect of the drug and cause severe bronchospasm. Avoid using together, if

---

possible. If use together is unavoidable, consider a cardioselective beta blocker, but use cautiously.

Digoxin: May decrease digoxin level up to 22%. Monitor digoxin level.

Loop or thiazide diuretics: May cause ECG changes and hypokalemia. Use together cautiously.

MAO inhibitors, tricyclic antidepressants: May potentiate action of levalbuterol on the vascular system. Avoid using within 2 weeks of MAO inhibitor or tricyclic antidepressant therapy.

Other short-acting sympathomimetic aerosol bronchodilators, epinephrine: May increase adrenergic adverse effects. Use together cautiously.

EFFECTS ON LAB TEST RESULTS
None reported.

CONTRAINDICATIONS & CAUTIONS
• Contraindicated in patients hypersensitive to drug or to racemic albuterol.
• Use cautiously in patients with CV disorders (especially coronary insufficiency, hypertension, and arrhythmias), seizure disorders, hyperthyroidism, or diabetes mellitus, and in those who are unusually responsive to sympathomimetic amines.

NURSING CONSIDERATIONS
• *Alert:* As with other inhaled beta agonists, drug can produce paradoxical bronchospasm or life-threatening CV effects. If this occurs, stop drug immediately and notify prescriber.
• Drug may worsen diabetes mellitus and ketoacidosis.
• Drug may temporarily decrease potassium level, but potassium supplementation is usually unnecessary.
• The compatibility of levalbuterol mixed with other drugs in a nebulizer hasn't been established.

PATIENT TEACHING
• Warn patient that he may experience worsened breathing. Tell him to stop drug and contact prescriber immediately if this occurs.
• Tell patient not to increase dosage without consulting prescriber.
• Urge patient to seek medical attention immediately if levalbuterol becomes

less effective, if signs and symptoms become worse, or if he's using drug more frequently than usual.
• Tell patient that the effects of levalbuterol may last up to 8 hours.
• Tell patient not to double the next dose if he misses one. Tell him to take doses at least 6 hours apart.
• Advise patient to use other inhalations and antiasthmatics only as directed while taking levalbuterol.
• Inform patient that common adverse reactions include palpitations, rapid heart rate, headache, dizziness, tremor, and nervousness.
• Encourage woman to contact prescriber if she becomes pregnant or is breastfeeding.
• Tell patient to keep unopened vials in foil pouch. After the foil pouch is opened, vials must be used within 2 weeks. Inform patient that vials removed from the pouch, if not used immediately, should be protected from light and excessive heat and used within 1 week.
• Teach patient to use drug correctly when inhaling by nebulizer.
• Instruct patient to breathe as calmly, deeply, and evenly as possible until no more mist is formed in the nebulizer reservoir (5 to 15 minutes).
• Tell patient using the inhaler to release four test sprays into the air away from the face before the first use or if it hasn't been used for more than 3 days.

✳ NEW DRUG
levocetirizine dihydrochloride
LEE-voe-se-TIR-a-zeen

Xyzal

Pharmacologic class: H$_1$-receptor antagonist
Pregnancy risk category B

AVAILABLE FORMS
Tablets: 5 mg

INDICATIONS & DOSAGES
➤ **Seasonal and perennial allergic rhinitis**
Adults and children ages 12 and older: 5 mg P.O. once daily in the evening.

Children ages 6 to 11: Give 2.5 mg P.O. once daily in the evening.

➤ **Uncomplicated skin manifestations of chronic idiopathic urticaria**
Adults and children ages 12 and older: Give 5 mg P.O. once daily in the evening.
Children ages 6 to 11: Give 2.5 mg P.O. once daily in the evening.

Adjust-a-dose: For patients ages 12 and older with creatinine clearance of 50 to 80 ml/minute, give 2.5 mg P.O. once daily; with creatinine clearance of 30 to 50 ml/minute, give 2.5 mg P.O. every other day; and with creatinine clearance 10 to 30 ml/minute, give 2.5 mg P.O. twice weekly (once every 3 to 4 days). Avoid use in patients with end-stage renal disease or those undergoing hemodialysis. Avoid use in children ages 6 to 11 with impaired renal function.

ADMINISTRATION
P.O.
• Give drug without regard for food.

ACTION
H_1-receptor inhibition creates antihistamine effect, relieving allergy symptoms.

Route	Onset	Peak	Duration
P.O.	Unknown	1 hr	24 hr

Half-life: 8 hours.

ADVERSE REACTIONS
CNS: fatigue, pyrexia, somnolence.
EENT: dry mouth, epistaxis, nasopharyngitis, pharyngitis.
Respiratory: cough.

INTERACTIONS
Drug-drug. *CNS depressants:* May have additive effects when taken together. Avoid using together.
Ritonavir: May increase serum concentration and increase half-life of levocetirizine. Use cautiously together.
Theophylline: May decrease the clearance of levocetirizine. Use cautiously together.
Drug-lifestyle. *Alcohol use:* May have additive effect when taken with levocetirizine. Discourage use together.

EFFECTS ON LAB TEST RESULTS
• None significant.

CONTRAINDICATIONS & CAUTIONS
• Contraindicated in patients hypersensitive to drug or to cetirizine.
• Contraindicated in patients with creatinine clearance less than 10 ml/minute or those undergoing hemodialysis.
• Contraindicated in patients age 6 to 11 with impaired renal function.

NURSING CONSIDERATIONS
• Monitor patient's renal function.
• Patient should avoid engaging in hazardous occupations requiring mental alertness and motor coordination, such as operating machinery or driving a motor vehicle.
• Drug is excreted in breast milk; avoid use in nursing mothers.
• Safety and effectiveness in patients younger than age 6 haven't been established.
• Use drug during pregnancy only if benefits to mother clearly outweigh risk to fetus.

PATIENT TEACHING
• Warn patient not to perform hazardous tasks or those requiring alertness and coordination until CNS effects are known.
• Advise patient to avoid use of alcohol and other CNS depressants while taking this drug.
• Advise patient not to take more than the recommended dose because of increased risk of somnolence at higher doses.

---

levofloxacin
lee-voe-FLOX-a-sin

Levaquin

Pharmacologic class: fluoroquinolone
Pregnancy risk category C

AVAILABLE FORMS
Infusion (premixed): 250 mg in 50 ml D_5W, 500 mg in 100 ml D_5W, 750 mg in 150 ml D_5W
Oral solution: 25 mg/ml
Single-use vials: 500 mg, 750 mg
Tablets: 250 mg, 500 mg, 750 mg

INDICATIONS & DOSAGES

➤ **Acute bacterial sinusitis caused by susceptible strains of** *Streptococcus pneumoniae, Moraxella catarrhalis,* **or** *Haemophilus influenzae*
Adults: 500 mg P.O. or I.V. infusion over 60 minutes every 24 hours for 10 to 14 days or 750 mg P.O. every 24 hours for 5 days.

➤ **Mild to moderate skin and skin-structure infections caused by** *Staphylococcus aureus* **or** *S. pyogenes*
Adults: 500 mg P.O. or I.V. infusion over 60 minutes every 24 hours for 7 to 10 days.

➤ **Acute bacterial worsening of chronic bronchitis caused by** *S. aureus, S. pneumoniae, M. catarrhalis, H. influenzae,* **or** *H. parainfluenzae*
Adults: 500 mg P.O. or I.V. infusion over 60 minutes every 24 hours for 7 days.

➤ **Community-acquired pneumonia from** *S. pneumoniae* **(resistant to two or more of the following antibiotics: penicillin, second-generation cephalosporins, macrolides, trimethoprim-sulfamethoxazole, tetracyclines),** *S. aureus, M. catarrhalis, H. influenzae, H. parainfluenzae, Klebsiella pneumoniae, Chlamydia pneumoniae, Legionella pneumophila,* **or** *Mycoplasma pneumoniae*
Adults: 500 mg P.O. or I.V. infusion over 60 minutes every 24 hours for 7 to 14 days.

➤ **To prevent inhalation anthrax after confirmed or suspected exposure to** *Bacillus anthracis*
Adults: 500 mg I.V. infusion or P.O. every 24 hours for 60 days.

➤ **Chronic bacterial prostatitis caused by** *Escherichia coli, Enterococcus faecalis,* **or** *Staphylococcus epidermidis*
Adults: 500 mg P.O. or I.V. over 60 minutes every 24 hours for 28 days.
Adjust-a-dose: In patients with a creatinine clearance of 20 to 49 ml/minute, give first dose of 500 mg and then 250 mg daily. If clearance is 10 to 19 ml/minute, give first dose of 500 mg and then 250 mg every 48 hours. For patients receiving dialysis or chronic ambulatory peritoneal dialysis, give first dose of 500 mg and then 250 mg every 48 hours. For patients

using the 5-day regimen for acute bacterial sinusitis, use the Adjust-a-dose schedule for nosocomial pneumonia.

➤ **Community-acquired pneumonia from** *S. pneumoniae* **(excluding multidrug-resistant strains),** *H. influenzae, H. parainfluenzae, M. pneumoniae,* **and** *C. pneumoniae*
Adults: 750 mg P.O. or I.V. over 90 minutes every 24 hours for 5 days.

➤ **Complicated skin and skin-structure infections caused by methicillin-sensitive** *S. aureus, E. faecalis, S. pyogenes,* **or** *Proteus mirabilis*
Adults: 750 mg P.O. or I.V. infusion over 90 minutes every 24 hours for 7 to 14 days.

➤ **Nosocomial pneumonia caused by methicillin-susceptible** *S. aureus, Pseudomonas aeruginosa, Serratia marcescens, E. coli, K. pneumoniae, H. influenzae,* **or** *S. pneumoniae*
Adults: 750 mg P.O. or I.V. infusion over 90 minutes every 24 hours for 7 to 14 days.
Adjust-a-dose: If creatinine clearance is 20 to 49 ml/minute, give 750 mg initially and then 750 mg every 48 hours; if clearance is 10 to 19 ml/minute, or patient is receiving hemodialysis or chronic ambulatory peritoneal dialysis, give 750 mg initially and then 500 mg every 48 hours.

➤ **Complicated UTI caused by** *E. faecalis, Enterobacter cloacae, E. coli, K. pneumoniae, P. mirabilis,* **or** *P. aeruginosa;* **acute pyelonephritis caused by** *E. coli*
Adults: 250 mg P.O. or I.V. over 60 minutes every 24 hours for 10 days.
Adjust-a-dose: If creatinine clearance is 10 to 19 ml/minute, increase dosage interval to every 48 hours.

➤ **Complicated UTI caused by** *E. coli, K. pneumoniae,* **or** *P. mirabilis;* **acute pyelonephritis caused by** *E. coli*
Adults: 750 mg P.O. or I.V. over 90 minutes daily for 5 days.
Adjust-a-dose: If creatinine clearance is 20 to 49 ml/minute, increase dosage interval to every 48 hours. If creatinine clearance is 10 to 19 ml/minute or patient is receiving dialysis, give 750 mg P.O. or I.V. initial dose, then 500 mg every 48 hours.

➤ **Mild to moderate uncomplicated UTI caused by** *E. coli, K. pneumoniae,* **or** *S. saprophyticus*
Adults: 250 mg P.O. daily for 3 days.
➤ **Traveler's diarrhea** ♦
Adults: 500 mg P.O. daily for up to 3 days.
➤ **To prevent traveler's diarrhea** ♦
Adults: 500 mg P.O. once daily during period of risk, for up to 3 weeks.
➤ **Uncomplicated cervical, urethral, or rectal gonorrhea** ♦
Adults: 250 mg P.O. as a single dose. Or, if chlamydia isn't ruled out, combine with 1 g azithromycin as single dose or 100 mg doxycycline P.O. b.i.d. for 7 days.
➤ **Disseminated gonococcal infection** ♦
Adults: 250 mg I.V. once daily and continued for 24 to 48 hours after patient starts to improve. Therapy may be switched to 500 mg P.O. daily to complete at least 1 week of therapy.
➤ **Nongonococcal urethritis; chlamydia** ♦
Adults: 500 mg P.O. once daily for 7 days.
➤ **Acute pelvic inflammatory disease** ♦
Adults: 500 mg I.V. once daily with or without metronidazole 500 mg every 8 hours. Stop parenteral therapy 24 hours after patient improves; then begin doxycycline 100 mg P.O. b.i.d. to complete 14 days of treatment. Or, 500 mg P.O. once daily for 14 days with or without metronidazole 500 mg b.i.d. for 14 days.

ADMINISTRATION
P.O.
• Obtain specimen for culture and sensitivity tests before therapy and as needed to determine if bacterial resistance has occurred.
• Give drug with plenty of fluids.
• Give 2 hours before or 6 hours after antacids, sucralfate, and products containing iron or zinc.
• Give oral solution 1 hour before or 2 hours after a meal.
I.V.
• Obtain specimen for culture and sensitivity tests before therapy and as needed to determine if bacterial resistance has occurred.
• Give this form only by infusion.

• Dilute drug in single-use vials, according to manufacturer's instructions, with D_5W or normal saline solution for injection to a final concentration of 5 mg/ml.
• Infuse doses of 500 mg or less over 60 minutes and doses of 750 mg over 90 minutes.
• Reconstituted solution should be clear, slightly yellow, and free of particulate matter.
• Reconstituted drug is stable for 72 hours at room temperature, for 14 days when refrigerated in plastic containers, and for 6 months when frozen.
• Thaw at room temperature or in refrigerator.
• **Incompatibilities:** Acyclovir sodium, alprostadil, azithromycin, furosemide, heparin sodium, indomethacin sodium trihydrate, insulin, mannitol 20%, nitroglycerin, propofol, sodium bicarbonate, sodium nitroprusside. The manufacturer recommends not mixing or infusing other drugs with levofloxacin.

ACTION
Inhibits bacterial DNA gyrase and prevents DNA replication, transcription, repair, and recombination in susceptible bacteria.

Route	Onset	Peak	Duration
P.O., I.V.	Unknown	1–2 hr	Unknown

Half-life: About 6 to 8 hours.

ADVERSE REACTIONS
CNS: *encephalopathy, seizures,* dizziness, headache, insomnia, pain, paresthesia.
CV: chest pain, palpitations, vasodilation.
GI: *pseudomembranous colitis,* abdominal pain, constipation, diarrhea, dyspepsia, flatulence, nausea, vomiting.
GU: vaginitis.
Hematologic: *lymphopenia,* eosinophilia, hemolytic anemia.
Metabolic: *hypoglycemia.*
Musculoskeletal: back pain, tendon rupture.
Respiratory: allergic pneumonitis.
Skin: *erythema multiforme, Stevens-Johnson syndrome,* photosensitivity, pruritus, rash.
Other: *anaphylaxis, multisystem organ failure,* hypersensitivity reactions.

Reactions may be *common,* uncommon, *life-threatening,* or COMMON AND LIFE-THREATENING.
Interaction may have a *rapid onset* or *delayed onset.*

INTERACTIONS

Drug-drug. *Aluminum hydroxide, aluminum–magnesium hydroxide, calcium carbonate, didanosine, magnesium hydroxide, products containing zinc, sucralfate:* May interfere with GI absorption of levofloxacin. Give levofloxacin 2 hours before or 6 hours after these products.
Antidiabetics: May alter glucose level. Monitor glucose level closely.
Iron salts: May decrease absorption of levofloxacin, reducing anti-infective response. Separate doses by at least 2 hours.
NSAIDs: May increase CNS stimulation. Monitor patient for seizure activity.
Theophylline: May decrease clearance of theophylline. Monitor theophylline level.
Warfarin and derivatives: May increase effect of oral anticoagulant. Monitor PT and INR.
Drug-herb. *Dong quai, St. John's wort:* May cause photosensitivity reactions. Advise patient to avoid excessive sunlight exposure.
Drug-lifestyle. *Sun exposure:* May cause photosensitivity reactions. Advise patient to avoid excessive sunlight exposure.

EFFECTS ON LAB TEST RESULTS

- May decrease glucose and hemoglobin levels.
- May increase eosinophil count. May decrease WBC count.
- May produce false-positive opioid assay results.

CONTRAINDICATIONS & CAUTIONS

- Contraindicated in patients hypersensitive to drug, its components, or other fluoroquinolones.
- Use cautiously in patients with history of seizure disorders or other CNS diseases, such as cerebral arteriosclerosis.
- Use cautiously and with dosage adjustment in patients with renal impairment.
- Safety and efficacy of drug in children younger than age 18 and in pregnant and breast-feeding women haven't been established.

NURSING CONSIDERATIONS

- If patient experiences symptoms of excessive CNS stimulation (restlessness, tremor, confusion, hallucinations), stop drug and notify prescriber. Begin seizure precautions.
- Patients with acute hypersensitivity reactions may need treatment with epinephrine, oxygen, I.V. fluids, antihistamines, corticosteroids, pressor amines, and airway management.
- Most antibacterials can cause pseudomembranous colitis. If diarrhea occurs, notify prescriber; drug may be stopped.
- Drug may cause an abnormal ECG.
- **Alert:** If *P. aeruginosa* is a confirmed or suspected pathogen, use with a beta-lactam.
- Monitor glucose level and results of renal, hepatic, and hematopoietic blood studies.

PATIENT TEACHING

- Tell patient to take drug as prescribed, even if signs and symptoms disappear.
- Advise patient to take drug with plenty of fluids and to space antacids, sucralfate, and products containing iron or zinc.
- Tell patient to take oral solution 1 hour before or 2 hours after eating.
- Warn patient to avoid hazardous tasks until adverse effects of drug are known.
- Advise patient to avoid excessive sunlight, use sunscreen, and wear protective clothing when outdoors.
- Instruct patient to stop drug and notify prescriber if rash or other signs or symptoms of hypersensitivity develop.
- Tell patient that tendon rupture may occur with drug and to notify prescriber if he experiences pain or inflammation.
- Instruct diabetic patient to monitor glucose level and notify prescriber about low-glucose reaction.
- Instruct patient to notify prescriber of loose stools or diarrhea.

loratadine
lor-AT-a-deen

Alavert ◊, Alavert Children's ◊, Claritin ◊, Claritin Hives Relief ◊, Claritin 24-Hour Allergy ◊, Claritin RediTabs ◊, Claritin Syrup ◊, Dimetapp Children's Non-Drowsy Allergy ◊, Tavist ND ◊, Triaminic Allerchews ◊

Pharmacologic class: piperidine
Pregnancy risk category B

AVAILABLE FORMS
Syrup: 1 mg/ml ◊
Tablets: 10 mg ◊
Tablets (chewable): 5 mg ◊
Tablets (orally disintegrating): 5 mg ◊, 10 mg ◊

INDICATIONS & DOSAGES
➤ **Seasonal allergic rhinitis; chronic idiopathic urticaria**
Adults and children age 6 and older: 10 mg P.O. daily.
Children ages 2 to 5 years: 5 mg P.O. daily.
Adjust-a-dose: In adults and children age 6 and older with hepatic impairment or GFR less than 30 ml/minute, give 10 mg every other day. In children ages 2 to 5 years with hepatic or renal impairment, give 5 mg every other day.

ADMINISTRATION
P.O.
• Give Claritin Reditabs on the tongue, where it disintegrates within a few seconds.
• Give drug with or without water.

ACTION
Blocks effects of histamine at H_1-receptor sites. Drug is a nonsedating antihistamine; its chemical structure prevents entry into the CNS.

Route	Onset	Peak	Duration
P.O.	Rapid	1.3–2.5 hr	24 hr

Half-life: 8½ hours.

ADVERSE REACTIONS
CNS: *headache,* drowsiness, fatigue, insomnia, nervousness.
GI: dry mouth.

INTERACTIONS
Drug-drug. *Cimetidine, ketoconazole, macrolide antibiotics (clarithromycin, erythromycin, troleandomycin):* May increase loratadine level. Monitor patient closely.
Drug-lifestyle. *Alcohol use:* May increase CNS depression. Discourage use together.

EFFECTS ON LAB TEST RESULTS
• May prevent, reduce, or mask positive result in diagnostic skin test.

CONTRAINDICATIONS & CAUTIONS
• Contraindicated in patients hypersensitive to drug.
• Use cautiously in patients with hepatic or renal impairment and in breast-feeding women.

NURSING CONSIDERATIONS
• Stop drug 4 days before patient undergoes diagnostic skin tests because drug can prevent, reduce, or mask positive skin test response.

PATIENT TEACHING
• Make sure patient understands to take drug once daily. If symptoms persist or worsen, tell him to contact prescriber.
• Tell patient taking Claritin Reditabs to use tablet immediately after opening individual blister.
• Advise patient taking Claritin Reditabs to place tablet on the tongue, where it disintegrates within a few seconds. It can be swallowed with or without water.
• Warn patient to avoid alcohol and hazardous activities that require alertness until CNS effects of drug are known.
• Tell patient that dry mouth can be relieved with sugarless gum, hard candy, or ice chips.

lorazepam
lor-AZ-e-pam

Ativan, Lorazepam Intensol,
Novo-Lorazem†

Pharmacologic class: benzodi-
azepine
Pregnancy risk category D
Controlled substance schedule IV

AVAILABLE FORMS
Injection: 2 mg/ml, 4 mg/ml
Oral solution (concentrated): 2 mg/ml
Tablets: 0.5 mg, 1 mg, 2 mg

INDICATIONS & DOSAGES
➤ **Anxiety**
Adults: 2 to 6 mg P.O. daily in divided
doses. Maximum, 10 mg daily.
Elderly patients: 1 to 2 mg P.O. daily in
divided doses. Maximum, 10 mg daily.
➤ **Insomnia from anxiety**
Adults: 2 to 4 mg P.O. at bedtime.
➤ **Preoperative sedation**
Adults: 2 mg I.V. total or 0.044 mg/kg
I.V., whichever is smaller. Larger doses up
to 0.05 mg/kg I.V., to total of 4 mg, may
be needed. Or, 0.05 mg/kg I.M. 2 hours
before procedure. Total dose shouldn't
exceed 4 mg.
➤ **Status epilepticus**
Adults: 4 mg I.V. If seizures continue
or recur after 10 to 15 minutes; then,
an additional 4-mg dose may be given.
Drug may be given I.M. if I.V. access isn't
available.
Children ♦: 0.05 to 0.1 mg/kg I.V.
➤ **Nausea and vomiting caused by
emetogenic cancer chemotherapy ♦**
Adults: 2.5 mg P.O. the evening before
and just after starting chemotherapy. Or,
1.5 mg/m^2 (usually up to a maximum dose
of 3 mg) I.V. (over 5 minutes) 45 minutes
before starting chemotherapy.

ADMINISTRATION
P.O.
● Mix oral solution with liquid or
semisolid food, such as water, juices,
carbonated beverages, applesauce, or
pudding.

I.V.
● Keep emergency resuscitation equipment
and oxygen available.
● Dilute with an equal volume of sterile
water for injection, normal saline solution
for injection, or D$_5$W. Give slowly at no
more than 2 mg/minute.
● Monitor respirations every 5 to
15 minutes and before each I.V. dose.
● Contains benzyl alcohol. Avoid use in
neonates.
● Refrigerate intact vials and protect from
light.
● **Incompatibilities:** Aldesleukin, aztreonam, buprenorphine, caffeine citrate,
floxacillin, foscarnet, idarubicin,
imipenem-cilastatin sodium, omeprazole,
ondansetron hydrochloride, sargramostim,
sufentanil citrate, thiopental.
I.M.
● For status epilepticus, drug may be given
I.M. if I.V. access isn't available.
● For I.M. use, inject deeply into a muscle.
Don't dilute.
● Refrigerate parenteral form to prolong
shelf life.

ACTION
May potentiate the effects of GABA,
depress the CNS, and suppress the spread
of seizure activity.

Route	Onset	Peak	Duration
P.O.	1 hr	2 hr	12–24 hr
I.V.	5 min	60–90 min	6–8 hr
I.M.	15–30 min	60–90 min	6–8 hr

Half-life: 10 to 20 hours.

ADVERSE REACTIONS
CNS: *drowsiness, sedation,* amnesia,
insomnia, agitation, dizziness, weakness,
unsteadiness, disorientation, depression,
headache.
CV: hypotension.
EENT: visual disturbances, nasal congestion.
GI: abdominal discomfort, nausea, change
in appetite.

INTERACTIONS
Drug-drug. *CNS depressants:* May increase CNS depression. Use together
cautiously.

Digoxin: May increase digoxin level and risk of toxicity. Monitor patient and digoxin level closely.
Drug-herb. *Kava:* May increase sedation. Discourage use together.
Drug-lifestyle. *Alcohol use:* May cause additive CNS effects. Discourage use together.
Smoking: May decrease drug's effectiveness. Monitor patient closely.

EFFECTS ON LAB TEST RESULTS
● May increase liver function test values.

CONTRAINDICATIONS & CAUTIONS
● Contraindicated in patients hypersensitive to drug, other benzodiazepines, or the vehicle used in parenteral dosage form; in patients with acute angle-closure glaucoma; and in pregnant women, especially in the first trimester.
● Use cautiously in patients with pulmonary, renal, or hepatic impairment.
● Use cautiously in elderly, acutely ill, or debilitated patients.

NURSING CONSIDERATIONS
● Monitor hepatic, renal, and hematopoietic function periodically in patients receiving repeated or prolonged therapy.
● *Alert:* Use of this drug may lead to abuse and addiction. Don't stop drug abruptly after long-term use because withdrawal symptoms may occur.
● *Look alike–sound alike:* Don't confuse lorazepam with alprazolam.

PATIENT TEACHING
● When used before surgery, drug causes substantial preoperative amnesia. Patient teaching requires extra care to ensure adequate recall. Provide written materials or inform a family member, if possible.
● Warn patient to avoid hazardous activities that require alertness or good coordination until effects of drug are known.
● Tell patient to avoid use of alcohol while taking drug.
● Notify patient that smoking may decrease drug's effectiveness.
● Warn patient not to stop drug abruptly because withdrawal symptoms may occur.
● Advise woman to avoid becoming pregnant while taking drug.

medroxyprogesterone acetate
me-DROX-ee-proe-JESS-te-rone

Depo-Provera, Depo-subQ
Provera 104, Provera

Pharmacologic class: progestin
Pregnancy risk category X

AVAILABLE FORMS
Injection (suspension): 104 mg/0.65 ml, 150 mg/ml, 400 mg/ml
Tablets: 2.5 mg, 5 mg, 10 mg

INDICATIONS & DOSAGES
➤ **Abnormal uterine bleeding caused by hormonal imbalance**
Women: 5 to 10 mg P.O. daily for 5 to 10 days beginning on day 16 of menstrual cycle. If patient also has received estrogen, give 10 mg P.O. daily for 10 days beginning on day 16 or 21 of cycle.
➤ **Secondary amenorrhea**
Women: 5 to 10 mg P.O. daily for 5 to 10 days. Start at any time during menstrual cycle (usually during latter half of cycle).
➤ **Endometrial or renal cancer**
Adults: 400 to 1,000 mg I.M. weekly. Dosage may be decreased to 400 mg/month when disease has stabilized.
➤ **Contraception**
Women: 150 mg (Depo-Provera) I.M. once every 3 months. Or, 104 mg Depo-subQ Provera subcutaneously once every 3 months.
➤ **Endometriosis**
Adults: 104 mg Depo-subQ Provera subcutaneously once every 3 months. Therapy for longer than 2 years isn't recommended.

ADMINISTRATION
P.O.
● Give drug with food if GI upset occurs.
I.M.
● Shake vigorously before use.
● Give by deep I.M. injection in the gluteal or deltoid muscle.
● I.M. injection may be painful. Monitor sites for evidence of sterile abscess. Rotate injection sites to prevent muscle atrophy.
Subcutaneous
● Shake vigorously before use.
● Give subcutaneous injection into the anterior thigh or abdomen.

ACTION
Suppresses ovulation, possibly by inhibiting pituitary gonadotropin secretion,
thus preventing follicular maturation and
causing endometrial thinning.

Route	Onset	Peak	Duration
P.O.	Rapid	2 to 4 hr	3 to 5 days
I.M.	Slow	24 hr	3 to 4 mo
Subcut	Unknown	Unknown	Unknown

Half-life: 2¼ to 9 hours P.O., 50 days I.M.,
40 days subcutaneous.

ADVERSE REACTIONS
CNS: depression, *stroke,* pain, dizziness.
CV: thrombophlebitis, *pulmonary em-
bolism,* edema, *thromboembolism,* syn-
cope.
EENT: exophthalmos, diplopia.
GI: *bloating, abdominal pain.*
GU: *breakthrough bleeding,* dysmen-
orrhea, *amenorrhea,* cervical erosion,
abnormal secretions.
Hepatic: cholestatic jaundice.
Metabolic: weight changes.
Skin: rash, induration, sterile abscesses,
acne, pruritus, melasma, alopecia, hir-
sutism.
Other: breast tenderness, enlargement, or
secretion, hot flashes.

INTERACTIONS
Drug-drug. *Aminoglutethimide, carbamazepine, fosphenytoin, phenobarbital,
phenytoin, rifampin:* May decrease progestin effects. Monitor patient for diminished therapeutic response. Tell patient to
use a nonhormonal contraceptive during
therapy with these drugs.
Drug-food. *Caffeine:* May increase caffeine level. Advise caution.
Drug-lifestyle. *Smoking:* May increase
risk of adverse CV effects. If smoking
continues, may need alternative therapy.

EFFECTS ON LAB TEST RESULTS
● May increase liver function test values,
coagulation tests, and prothrombin factors
VII, VIII, IX, and X.
● May reduce metyrapone test results.
May cause abnormal thyroid function test
results.

CONTRAINDICATIONS & CAUTIONS
● Contraindicated in patients hypersensitive to drug and in those with active
thromboembolic disorders or history of
thromboembolic disorders, cerebrovascular disease, apoplexy, breast cancer,
undiagnosed abnormal vaginal bleeding,
missed abortion, or hepatic dysfunction;
also contraindicated during pregnancy.
Tablets are contraindicated in patients with
liver dysfunction or known or suspected
malignant disease of genital organs.
● Use cautiously in patients with diabetes, seizures, migraine, cardiac or renal
disease, asthma, or depression.

NURSING CONSIDERATIONS
● Drug shouldn't be used as test for pregnancy; it may cause birth defects and
masculinization of female fetus.
● Depo-Provera and Depo-subQ Provera
may cause a significant loss of bone mineral density.
● Monitor patient for pain, swelling,
warmth, or redness in calves; sudden,
severe headaches; visual disturbances;
numbness in extremities; signs of depression; signs of liver dysfunction (abdominal
pain, dark urine, jaundice).

PATIENT TEACHING
● According to FDA regulations, patient
must read package insert explaining possible adverse effects of progestins before
receiving first dose. Also, give patient
verbal explanation.
● Advise patient to take medication with
food if GI upset occurs.
● *Alert:* Tell patient to report unusual symptoms immediately and to stop drug and
notify prescriber about visual disturbances
or migraine.
● Teach woman how to perform routine
breast self-examination.
● Advise patient to immediately report
to prescriber any breast abnormalities,
vaginal bleeding, swelling, yellowed
skin or eyes, dark urine, clay-colored
stools, shortness of breath, chest pain, or
pregnancy.
● Advise patient that injection must be
given every 3 months to maintain adequate
contraceptive effects.

• Tell woman to immediately report to prescriber a suspected pregnancy.
• Advise patient that amenorrhea is possible with prolonged use.

methotrexate (amethopterin, MTX)
meth-oh-TREX-ate

methotrexate sodium
Methotrexate LPF, Rheumatrex, Trexall

Pharmacologic class: folic acid antagonist
Pregnancy risk category X

AVAILABLE FORMS
Injection: 25 mg/ml in 2-ml, 4-ml, 8-ml, 10-ml, 20-ml, and 40-ml preservative-free single-use vials; 25 mg/ml in 2-ml and 10-ml vials containing benzyl alcohol
Lyophilized powder: 20-mg, 1,000-mg vials, preservative-free; 2.5-mg/ml, 25-mg/ml vials
Tablets (scored): 2.5 mg, 5 mg, 7.5 mg, 10 mg, 15 mg

INDICATIONS & DOSAGES
➤ **Trophoblastic tumors (choriocarcinoma, hydatidiform mole)**
Adults: 15 to 30 mg P.O. or I.M. daily for 5 days. Repeat after 1 or more weeks, based on response or toxicity. Number of courses is three to maximum of five.
➤ **Acute lymphocytic leukemia**
Adults and children: 3.3 mg/m^2 daily P.O., I.V., or I.M. with 40 to 60 mg/m^2 prednisone daily for 4 to 6 weeks or until remission occurs; then 20 to 30 mg/m^2 P.O. or I.M. weekly in two divided doses or 2.5 mg/kg I.V. every 14 days.
➤ **Meningeal leukemia**
Adults and children: 12 mg/m^2 or less (maximum 15 mg) intrathecally every 2 to 5 days until CSF is normal; then one additional dose. Or, for children, use dosages based on age.
Children age 3 and older: 12 mg intrathecally every 2 to 5 days.

Children ages 2 to 3: 10 mg intrathecally every 2 to 5 days.
Children ages 1 to 2: 8 mg intrathecally every 2 to 5 days.
Children younger than age 1: 6 mg intrathecally every 2 to 5 days.
➤ **Burkitt lymphoma (stage I, II, or III)**
Adults: 10 to 25 mg P.O. daily for 4 to 8 days, with 1-week rest intervals.
➤ **Lymphosarcoma (stage III)**
Adults: 0.625 to 2.5 mg/kg daily P.O., I.M., or I.V.
➤ **Osteosarcoma**
Adults: Initially, 12 g/m^2 I.V. as 4-hour infusion. Give subsequent doses 15 g/m^2 I.V. as 4-hour I.V. infusion at postoperative weeks 4, 5, 6, 7, 11, 12, 15, 16, 29, 30, 44, and 45. Give with leucovorin, 15 mg P.O. every 6 hours for 10 doses, beginning 24 hours after start of methotrexate infusion.
➤ **Breast cancer**
Adults: 40 mg/m^2 I.V. on days 1 and 8 of each cycle, combined with cyclophosphamide and fluorouracil.
Adjust-a-dose: In patients older than age 60, give 30 mg/m^2.
➤ **Mycosis fungoides**
Adults: 2.5 to 10 mg P.O. daily; or 50 mg I.M. weekly; or 25 mg I.M. twice weekly.
➤ **Psoriasis**
Adults: 10 to 25 mg P.O., I.M., or I.V. as single weekly dose; or 2.5 to 5 mg P.O. every 12 hours for three doses weekly. Dosage shouldn't exceed 30 mg per week.
➤ **Rheumatoid arthritis**
Adults: Initially, 7.5 mg P.O. weekly, either in single dose or divided as 2.5 mg P.O. every 12 hours for three doses once weekly. Dosage may be gradually increased to maximum of 20 mg weekly.

ADMINISTRATION
P.O.
• Give drug when patient has an empty stomach.
• Tablets may contain lactose. If needed, give with OTC lactose enzyme supplement.
I.V.
• Preparing and giving parenteral drug may be mutagenic, teratogenic, or carcinogenic. Follow facility policy to reduce risks.

- Dilution of drug depends on product, and infusion guidelines vary, depending on dose.
- Reconstitute 20-mg vial to a concentration no greater than 25 mg/ml. Reconstitute 1-g vial to a concentration of 50 mg/ml.
- If giving infusion, dilute total dose in D_5W.
- Reconstitute solutions without preservatives with normal saline solution or D_5W immediately before use, and discard unused drug.
- **Incompatibilities:** Bleomycin, chlorpromazine, droperidol, gemcitabine, idarubicin, ifosfamide, midazolam, nalbuphine, promethazine, propofol.

I.M.
- Preparing and giving parenteral drug may be mutagenic, teratogenic, or carcinogenic. Follow facility policy to reduce risks.

ACTION

Reversibly binds to dihydrofolate reductase, blocking reduction of folic acid to tetrahydrofolate, a cofactor necessary for purine, protein, and DNA synthesis.

Route	Onset	Peak	Duration
P.O.	Unknown	1–2 hr	Unknown
I.V.	Immediate	Immediate	Unknown
I.M.	Unknown	30 min–1 hr	Unknown
Intrathecal	Unknown	Unknown	Unknown

Half-life: For doses below 30 mg/m^2, about 3 to 10 hours; for doses of 30 mg/m^2 and above, 8 to 15 hours.

ADVERSE REACTIONS

CNS: *arachnoiditis within hours of intrathecal use, leukoencephalopathy, seizures,* subacute neurotoxicity possibly beginning a few weeks later, demyelination, malaise, fatigue, dizziness, headache, aphasia, hemiparesis, fever, drowsiness.
EENT: pharyngitis, blurred vision.
GI: gingivitis, *stomatitis, diarrhea,* abdominal distress, anorexia, GI ulceration and *bleeding,* enteritis, *nausea, vomiting.*
GU: nephropathy, *tubular necrosis, renal failure,* hematuria, menstrual dysfunction, defective spermatogenesis, infertility, abortion, cystitis.

Hematologic: *anemia, leukopenia, thrombocytopenia.*
Hepatic: *acute toxicity, chronic toxicity,* including cirrhosis and, *hepatic fibrosis.*
Metabolic: *diabetes,* hyperuricemia.
Musculoskeletal: arthralgia, myalgia, osteoporosis in children on long-term therapy.
Respiratory: *pulmonary fibrosis; pulmonary interstitial infiltrates;* pneumonitis; dry, nonproductive cough.
Skin: *urticaria,* pruritus, hyperpigmentation, erythematous rashes, ecchymoses, rash, photosensitivity reactions, alopecia, acne, psoriatic lesions aggravated by exposure to sun.
Other: chills, reduced resistance to infection, *septicemia, sudden death.*

INTERACTIONS

Drug-drug. *Acitretin:* May increase the risk of hepatitis. Avoid using together.
Acyclovir: Use with intrathecal methotrexate may cause neurologic abnormalities. Monitor patient closely.
Digoxin: May decrease digoxin level. Monitor digoxin level closely.
Folic acid derivatives: Antagonizes methotrexate effect. Avoid using together, except for leucovorin rescue with high-dose methotrexate therapy.
Fosphenytoin, phenytoin: May decrease phenytoin and fosphenytoin levels. Monitor drug levels closely.
Hepatotoxic drugs: May increase risk of hepatotoxicity. Monitor patient closely.
NSAIDs, phenylbutazone, salicylates: May increase methotrexate toxicity. Avoid using together.
Oral antibiotics: May decrease absorption of methotrexate. Monitor patient closely.
Penicillins, sulfonamides, trimethoprim: May increase methotrexate level. Monitor patient for methotrexate toxicity.
Probenecid: May impair excretion of methotrexate, causing increased level, effect, and toxicity of methotrexate. Monitor methotrexate level closely and adjust dosage accordingly.
Procarbazine: May increase risk of nephrotoxicity. Monitor patient closely.
Theophylline: May increase theophylline level. Monitor theophylline level closely.
Thiopurines: May increase thiopurine level. Monitor patient closely.

Vaccines: May make immunizations ineffective; may cause risk of disseminated infection with live-virus vaccines. Postpone immunization, if possible.

Drug-food. *Any food:* May delay absorption and reduce peak level of methotrexate. Instruct patient to take drug on an empty stomach.

Drug-lifestyle. *Alcohol use:* May increase hepatotoxicity. Discourage use together.

Sun exposure: May cause photosensitivity reactions. Advise patient to avoid excessive sunlight exposure.

EFFECTS ON LAB TEST RESULTS

● May increase uric acid level. May decrease hemoglobin level.

● May decrease WBC, RBC, and platelet counts.

● May alter results of laboratory assay for folate, which interferes with detection of folic acid deficiency.

CONTRAINDICATIONS & CAUTIONS

● Contraindicated in patients hypersensitive to drug and in those with psoriasis or rheumatoid arthritis who also have alcoholism, alcoholic liver, chronic liver disease, immunodeficiency syndromes, or blood dyscrasias.

● Contraindicated in pregnant or breast-feeding women.

● Use cautiously and at modified dosage in patients with impaired hepatic or renal function, bone marrow suppression, aplasia, leukopenia, thrombocytopenia, or anemia.

● Use cautiously in very young, elderly, or debilitated patients and in those with infection, peptic ulceration, or ulcerative colitis.

NURSING CONSIDERATIONS

● *Alert:* Drug may be given daily or once weekly, depending on the disease. To avoid administration errors, know your patient's dosing schedule.

● Monitor pulmonary function tests periodically and fluid intake and output daily. Encourage fluid intake of 2 to 3 L daily.

● Monitor uric acid level.

● Drug distributes readily into pleural effusions and other third-space compartments, such as ascites, leading to prolonged systemic level and risk of toxicity. Use drug cautiously in these patients.

● *Alert:* Alkalinize urine by giving sodium bicarbonate tablets or fluids to prevent precipitation of drug, especially at high doses. Maintain urine pH above 7. If BUN level is 20 to 30 mg/dl or creatinine level is 1.2 to 2 mg/dl, reduce dosage. If BUN level exceeds 30 mg/dl or creatinine level is higher than 2 mg/dl, stop drug and notify prescriber.

● Watch for increases in AST, ALT, and alkaline phosphatase levels, which may signal hepatic dysfunction.

● Watch for signs and symptoms of bleeding (especially GI) and infection.

● To prevent bleeding, avoid all I.M. injections when platelet count is below $50,000/mm^3$.

● Give blood transfusions for cumulative anemia. Patient may receive injections of RBC colony-stimulating factors to promote RBC production and decrease need for blood transfusions.

● Leucovorin rescue is needed with doses of more than 100 mg and starts 24 hours after therapy starts. Leucovorin is continued until methotrexate level falls below 5×10^{-8} M. Consult specialized references for specific recommendations for leucovorin dosage. Monitor methotrexate level and adjust leucovorin dose.

● The WBC and platelet count nadirs usually occur on day 7.

● For intrathecal administration, use preservative-free form.

PATIENT TEACHING

● Advise patient to watch for signs and symptoms of infection (fever, sore throat, fatigue) and bleeding (easy bruising, nosebleeds, bleeding gums, tarry stools). Tell patient to take temperature daily.

● Teach and encourage diligent mouth care to reduce risk of superinfection in the mouth.

● Instruct patient how to take leucovorin. Stress the importance of taking as prescribed until instructed by prescriber to stop.

● Tell patient to use highly protective sunblock when exposed to sunlight.

● Warn both men and women to avoid conception during and for at least

---

12 weeks after therapy because of risk of abortion, birth defects, or fetal death.
- Advise woman to stop breast-feeding during therapy.

methylprednisolone
meth-ill-pred-NISS-oh-lone

Medrol, Medrol Dosepak, Meprolone Unipak

methylprednisolone acetate
Depo-Medrol

methylprednisolone sodium succinate
A-Methapred, Solu-Medrol

Pharmacologic class: glucocorticoid
Pregnancy risk category C

AVAILABLE FORMS
methylprednisolone
Tablets: 2 mg, 4 mg, 8 mg, 16 mg, 24 mg, 32 mg
methylprednisolone acetate
Injection (suspension): 20 mg/ml, 40 mg/ml, 80 mg/ml
methylprednisolone sodium succinate
Injection: 40-mg vial, 125-mg vial, 500-mg vial, 1,000-mg vial, 2,000-mg vial

INDICATIONS & DOSAGES
➤ **Severe inflammation or immunosuppression**
Adults: 2 to 60 mg base P.O. usually in four divided doses. Or, initially, 24 mg (six 4-mg tablets) on the first day; taper by 4 mg per day until 21 tablets have been given. Or, 10 to 80 mg acetate I.M. daily, or 10 to 250 mg succinate I.M. or I.V. up to six times daily. Or, 4 to 40 mg acetate into smaller joints or 20 to 80 mg acetate into larger joints. Intralesional use is usually 20 to 60 mg acetate. Repeat intralesional and intra-articular injections every 1 to 5 weeks.
Children: 0.117 to 1.66 mg/kg or 3.3 to 50 mg/m^2 P.O. daily in three or four divided doses. Or, 0.03 to 0.2 mg/kg or 1 to 6.25 mg/m^2 succinate I.M. once daily or b.i.d.

➤ **Congenital adrenogenital syndrome**
Children: 40 mg acetate I.M. every 2 weeks.
➤ **Shock**
Adults: 100 to 250 mg succinate I.V. every 2 to 6 hours. Or, 30 mg/kg I.V. initially; repeat every 4 to 6 hours as needed. Give over 3 to 15 minutes. Continue therapy for 2 to 3 days or until patient is stable.

ADMINISTRATION
P.O.
- Give drug with milk or food when possible. Critically ill patients may need to take drug with an antacid or H$_2$-receptor antagonist.
I.V.
- Use only methylprednisolone sodium succinate, never the acetate form.
- Reconstitute according to manufacturer's directions using supplied diluent, or use bacteriostatic water for injection with benzyl alcohol.
- Compatible solutions include D$_5$W, normal saline solution, and dextrose 5% in normal saline solution.
- For direct injection, inject diluted drug into vein or free-flowing compatible I.V. solution over at least 1 minute.
- For intermittent or continuous infusion, dilute solution according to manufacturer's instructions and give over prescribed duration. If used for continuous infusion, change solution every 24 hours.
- For shock, give massive doses over at least 10 minutes to prevent arrhythmias and circulatory collapse.
- Discard reconstituted solution after 48 hours.
- **Incompatibilities:** Allopurinol, aminophylline, calcium gluconate, ciprofloxacin, cytarabine, diltiazem, docetaxel, doxapram, etoposide, filgrastim, gemcitabine, glycopyrrolate, nafcillin, ondansetron, paclitaxel, penicillin G sodium, potassium chloride, propofol, sargramostim, vinorelbine, vitamin B complex with C.
I.M.
- Give injection deeply into gluteal muscle. Avoid subcutaneous injection because atrophy and sterile abscesses may occur.
- Dermal atrophy may occur with large doses of acetate form. Use several small

injections rather than a single large dose, and rotate injection sites.

ACTION
Not clearly defined. Decreases inflammation, mainly by stabilizing leukocyte lysosomal membranes; suppresses immune response; stimulates bone marrow; and influences protein, fat, and carbohydrate metabolism.

Route	Onset	Peak	Duration
P.O.	Rapid	2–3 hr	30–36 hr
I.V.	Rapid	Immediate	1 wk
I.M.	6–48 hr	4–8 days	4–8 days
Intra-articular	Rapid	7 days	1–5 wk

Half-life: 18 to 36 hours.

ADVERSE REACTIONS
CNS: *euphoria, insomnia,* psychotic behavior, ***pseudotumor cerebri,*** vertigo, headache, paresthesia, ***seizures.***
CV: ***arrhythmias, heart failure,*** hypertension, edema, thrombophlebitis, ***thromboembolism, cardiac arrest, circulatory collapse after rapid use of large I.V. dose.***
EENT: cataracts, glaucoma.
GI: *peptic ulceration,* GI irritation, increased appetite, ***pancreatitis,*** nausea, vomiting.
GU: menstrual irregularities.
Metabolic: hypokalemia, hyperglycemia, carbohydrate intolerance, hypercholesterolemia, hypocalcemia.
Musculoskeletal: growth suppression in children, muscle weakness, osteoporosis.
Skin: hirsutism, delayed wound healing, acne, various skin eruptions.
Other: cushingoid state, susceptibility to infections, ***acute adrenal insufficiency after increased stress or abrupt withdrawal after long-term therapy.***
After abrupt withdrawal (may be fatal after prolonged use): rebound inflammation, fatigue, weakness, arthralgia, fever, dizziness, lethargy, depression, fainting, orthostatic hypotension, dyspnea, anorexia, ***hypoglycemia.***

INTERACTIONS
Drug-drug. *Aspirin, indomethacin, other NSAIDs:* May increase risk of GI distress and bleeding. Use together cautiously.

Barbiturates, carbamazepine, phenytoin, rifampin: May decrease corticosteroid effect. Increase corticosteroid dosage.
Cyclosporine: May increase toxicity. Monitor patient closely.
Ketoconazole and macrolide antibiotics: May decrease methylprednisolone clearance. Decreased dose may be required.
Oral anticoagulants: May alter dosage requirements. Monitor PT and INR closely.
Potassium-depleting drugs such as thiazide diuretics: May enhance potassium-wasting effects of methylprednisolone. Monitor potassium level.
Salicylates: May decrease salicylate levels. Monitor patient for lack of salicylate effectiveness.
Skin-test antigens: May decrease response. Postpone skin testing until after therapy.
Toxoids, vaccines: May decrease antibody response and may increase risk of neurologic complications. Avoid using together.
Drug-herb. *Echinacea:* May increase immune-stimulating effects. Discourage use together.
Ginseng: May increase immune-regulating response. Discourage use together.

EFFECTS ON LAB TEST RESULTS
● May increase glucose and cholesterol levels and urine calcium levels. May decrease T_3, T_4, potassium, and calcium levels.
● May decrease ^{131}I uptake and protein-bound iodine levels in thyroid function tests. May cause false-negative results in nitroblue tetrazolium test for systemic bacterial infections. May alter reactions to skin tests.

CONTRAINDICATIONS & CAUTIONS
● Contraindicated in patients hypersensitive to drug or its ingredients, in those with systemic fungal infections, in premature infants (acetate and succinate), and in patients receiving immunosuppressive doses together with live virus vaccines.
● Use cautiously in patients with GI ulceration or renal disease, hypertension, osteoporosis, diabetes mellitus, hypothyroidism, cirrhosis, diverticulitis, nonspecific ulcerative colitis, recent intestinal anastomoses, thromboembolic disorders, seizures, active hepatitis, myasthenia gravis, heart failure,

tuberculosis, ocular herpes simplex, emotional instability, and psychotic tendencies or in breast-feeding women.

NURSING CONSIDERATIONS
• Medrol may contain tartrazine. Watch for allergic reaction to tartrazine in patients with sensitivity to aspirin.
• Drug may be used for alternate-day therapy.
• Determine whether patient is sensitive to other corticosteroids. Most adverse reactions to corticosteroids are dose- or duration-dependent. For better results and less toxicity, give a once-daily dose in the morning.
• *Alert:* Different salts aren't interchangeable.
• *Alert:* Don't give Solu-Medrol intrathecally because severe adverse reactions may occur.
• If immediate onset of action is needed, don't use acetate form.
• Always adjust to lowest effective dose.
• Monitor patient's weight, blood pressure, electrolyte level, and sleep patterns. Euphoria may initially interfere with sleep, but patients typically adjust to therapy in 1 to 3 weeks.
• Monitor patient for cushingoid effects, including moon face, buffalo hump, central obesity, thinning hair, hypertension, and increased susceptibility to infection.
• Measure growth and development periodically in children during high-dose or prolonged treatment.
• Drug may mask or worsen infections, including latent amebiasis.
• Watch for depression or psychotic episodes, especially in high-dose therapy.
• Diabetic patient may need increased insulin; monitor glucose level.
• Watch for an enhanced response to drug in patients with hypothyroidism or cirrhosis.
• Unless contraindicated, give low-sodium diet that's high in potassium and protein. Give potassium supplements as needed.
• Elderly patients may be more susceptible to osteoporosis with prolonged use.
• Taper off dosage after long-term therapy.
• *Look alike–sound alike:* Don't confuse Solu-Medrol with Solu-Cortef or methylprednisolone with medroxyprogesterone.

PATIENT TEACHING
• Tell patient not to stop drug abruptly or without prescriber's consent.
• Instruct patient to take oral form of drug with milk or food.
• Teach patient signs and symptoms of early adrenal insufficiency: fatigue, muscle weakness, joint pain, fever, anorexia, nausea, shortness of breath, dizziness, and fainting.
• Instruct patient to carry or wear medical identification indicating his need for supplemental systemic glucocorticoids during stress. This card should contain prescriber's name, name of drug, and dosage taken.
• Warn patient on long-term therapy about cushingoid effects (moon face, buffalo hump) and the need to notify prescriber about sudden weight gain or swelling.
• Advise patient receiving long-term therapy to consider exercise or physical therapy. Also, tell patient to ask prescriber about vitamin D or calcium supplement.
• Instruct patient to avoid exposure to infections (such as chickenpox or measles) and to contact prescriber if such exposure occurs.

SAFETY ALERT!

milrinone lactate
MILL-ri-none

Primacor

Pharmacologic class: bipyridine phosphodiesterase inhibitor
Pregnancy risk category C

AVAILABLE FORMS
Injection: 1 mg/ml
Injection (premixed): 200 mcg/ml in D_5W

INDICATIONS & DOSAGES
➤ **Short-term treatment of acutely decompensated heart failure**
Adults: Give first loading dose of 50 mcg/kg I.V. slowly over 10 minutes; then give continuous I.V. infusion of 0.375 to 0.75 mcg/kg/minute. Titrate infusion dose based on clinical and hemodynamic responses. Don't exceed 1.13 mg/kg/day.
Adjust-a-dose: If creatinine clearance is 50 ml/minute, infusion rate is

0.43 mcg/kg/minute; if 40 ml/minute, infusion rate is 0.38 mcg/kg/minute; if 30 ml/minute, infusion rate is 0.33 mcg/kg/minute; if 20 ml/minute, infusion rate is 0.28 mcg/kg/minute; if 10 ml/minute, infusion rate is 0.23 mcg/kg/minute; and if 5 ml/minute, infusion rate is 0.2 mcg/kg/minute. Don't exceed 1.13 mg/kg/day.

ADMINISTRATION
I.V.
• Give loading dose undiluted as a direct injection over 10 minutes.
• Prepare I.V. infusion solution using half-normal saline solution, normal saline solution, or D₅W. Prepare the 100-mcg/ml solution by adding 180 ml of diluent per 20-mg (20-ml) vial, the 150-mcg/ml solution by adding 113 ml of diluent per 20-mg (20-ml) vial, and the 200-mcg/ml solution by adding 80 ml of diluent per 20-mg (20-ml) vial.
• **Incompatibilities:** Bumetanide, furosemide, imipenem and cilastatin sodium, procainamide, torsemide.

ACTION
Produces inotropic action by increasing cellular levels of cAMP and vasodilation by relaxing vascular smooth muscle.

Route	Onset	Peak	Duration
I.V.	5–15 min	1–2 hr	3–6 hr

Half-life: 2½ to 3¾ hours.

ADVERSE REACTIONS
CNS: headache.
CV: VENTRICULAR ARRHYTHMIAS, *ventricular ectopic activity,* **sustained ventricular tachycardia, ventricular fibrillation,** hypotension, nonsustained ventricular tachycardia.

INTERACTIONS
None significant.

EFFECTS ON LAB TEST RESULTS
• May cause abnormal liver function test results.

CONTRAINDICATIONS & CAUTIONS
• Contraindicated in patients hypersensitive to drug.

• Contraindicated for use in patients with severe aortic or pulmonic valvular disease in place of surgery and during acute phase of MI.
• Use cautiously in patients with atrial flutter or fibrillation because drug slightly shortens AV node conduction time and may increase ventricular response rate.

NURSING CONSIDERATIONS
• In patients with atrial flutter or fibrillation, give digoxin before milrinone therapy. Drug is typically given with digoxin and diuretics.
• Improved cardiac output may increase urine output. Reduce diuretic dosage when heart failure improves. Potassium loss may cause digitalis toxicity.
• Monitor fluid and electrolyte status, blood pressure, heart rate, and renal function during therapy. Excessive decrease in blood pressure requires stopping or slowing rate of infusion.
• Correct hypoxemia.

PATIENT TEACHING
• Instruct patient to report adverse reactions to prescriber promptly, especially angina.
• Tell patient that drug may cause headache, which can be treated with analgesics.
• Tell patient to report discomfort at I.V. insertion site.

modafinil
moe-DAFF-in-ill

Provigil

Pharmacologic class: analeptic
Pregnancy risk category C
Controlled substance schedule IV

AVAILABLE FORMS
Tablets: 100 mg, 200 mg

INDICATIONS & DOSAGES
➤ **To improve wakefulness in patients with excessive daytime sleepiness caused by narcolepsy, obstructive sleep apnea-hypoapnea syndrome, and shift-work sleep disorder**

Adults: 200 mg P.O. daily, as single dose in the morning. Patients with shift-work sleep disorder should take dose about 1 hour before the start of their shift.
Adjust-a-dose: In patients with severe hepatic impairment, give 100 mg P.O. daily, as single dose in the morning.

ADMINISTRATION
P.O.
● Give drug without regard for food; however, food may delay effect of drug.

ACTION
Unknown. Similar to action of sympathomimetics, including amphetamines, but drug is structurally distinct from amphetamines and doesn't alter release of dopamine or norepinephrine to produce CNS stimulation.

Route	Onset	Peak	Duration
P.O.	Unknown	2–4 hr	Unknown

Half-life: 15 hours.

ADVERSE REACTIONS
CNS: *headache, nervousness, dizziness, insomnia,* fever, depression, anxiety, cataplexy, paresthesia, dyskinesia, hypertonia, confusion, syncope, amnesia, emotional lability, ataxia, tremor, mania, hallucination, *suicidal ideation.*
CV: *arrhythmias,* hypotension, hypertension, vasodilation, chest pain.
EENT: *rhinitis,* pharyngitis, epistaxis, amblyopia, abnormal vision.
GI: *nausea,* diarrhea, dry mouth, anorexia, vomiting, mouth ulcer, gingivitis, thirst.
GU: abnormal urine, urine retention, abnormal ejaculation, albuminuria.
Hematologic: eosinophilia.
Metabolic: hyperglycemia.
Musculoskeletal: joint disorder, neck pain, neck rigidity.
Respiratory: asthma, dyspnea, lung disorder.
Skin: sweating.
Other: herpes simplex, chills.

INTERACTIONS
Drug-drug. *Carbamazepine, phenobarbital, rifampin, and other inducers of CYP3A4:* May alter modafinil level. Monitor patient closely.

Cyclosporine, theophylline: May reduce levels of these drugs. Use together cautiously.
Diazepam, phenytoin, propranolol, other drugs metabolized by CYP2C19: May inhibit CYP2C19 and lead to higher levels of drugs metabolized by this enzyme. Use together cautiously; adjust dosage as needed.
Hormonal contraceptives: May reduce contraceptive effectiveness. Advise patient to use alternative or additional method of contraception during modafinil therapy and for 1 month after drug is stopped.
Itraconazole, ketoconazole, other inhibitors of CYP3A4: May alter modafinil level. Monitor patient closely.
Methylphenidate: May cause 1-hour delay in modafinil absorption. Separate dosage times.
Phenytoin, warfarin: May inhibit CYP2C9 and increase phenytoin and warfarin levels. Monitor patient closely for toxicity.
Tricyclic antidepressants (such as clomipramine, desipramine): May increase tricyclic antidepressant level. Reduce dosage of these drugs.

EFFECTS ON LAB TEST RESULTS
● May increase glucose, GGT, and AST levels.
● May increase eosinophil count.

CONTRAINDICATIONS & CAUTIONS
● Contraindicated in patients hypersensitive to drug and in those with a history of left ventricular hypertrophy or ischemic ECG changes, chest pain, arrhythmias, or other evidence of mitral valve prolapse linked to CNS stimulant use.
● Use cautiously in patients with recent MI or unstable angina and in those with history of psychosis.
● Use cautiously and give reduced dosage to patients with severe hepatic impairment, with or without cirrhosis.
● Use cautiously in patients taking MAO inhibitors.
● Safety and efficacy in patients with severe renal impairment haven't been determined.

NURSING CONSIDERATIONS
● Monitor hypertensive patients closely.

• Although single daily 400-mg doses have been well tolerated, the larger dose is no more beneficial than the 200-mg dose.

PATIENT TEACHING
• *Alert:* Advise patient to stop drug and notify prescriber if rash, peeling skin, trouble swallowing or breathing, or other symptoms of allergic reaction occur. Rare cases of serious rash including Stevens-Johnson syndrome, toxic epidermal necrolysis, and drug rash with eosinophilia and hypersensitivity have been reported.
• Advise woman to notify prescriber about planned, suspected, or known pregnancy, or if she's breast-feeding.
• Caution patient that use of hormonal contraceptives (including depot or implantable contraceptives) together with modafinil tablets may reduce contraceptive effectiveness. Recommend an alternative method of contraception during modafinil therapy and for 1 month after drug is stopped.
• Instruct patient to confer with prescriber before taking prescription or OTC drugs to avoid drug interactions.
• Tell patient to avoid alcohol while taking drug.
• Warn patient to avoid activities that require alertness or good coordination until CNS effects of drug are known.

---

mometasone furoate
moe-MEH-tah-zone

Asmanex Twisthaler

Pharmacologic class: glucocorticoid
Pregnancy risk category C

AVAILABLE FORMS
Inhalation powder: 220 mcg/inhalation

INDICATIONS & DOSAGES
➤ **Maintenance therapy for asthma; asthma in patients who take an oral corticosteroid**
Adults and children age 12 and older who previously used a bronchodilator or inhaled corticosteroid: Initially, 220 mcg by oral inhalation every day in the evening. Maximum, 440 mcg/day.

Adults and children age 12 and older who take an oral corticosteroid:
440 mcg b.i.d. by oral inhalation. Maximum, 880 mcg/day. Reduce oral corticosteroid dosage by no more than 2.5 mg/day at weekly intervals, beginning at least 1 week after starting mometasone. After stopping oral corticosteroid, reduce mometasone dose to lowest effective amount.

ADMINISTRATION
Inhalational
• Have patient breathe deeply and rapidly during administration.
• Have patient rinse his mouth after administration.

ACTION
Unknown, although corticosteroids inhibit many cells and mediators involved in inflammation and the asthmatic response.

Route	Onset	Peak	Duration
Inhalation	Unknown	1–2½ hr	Unknown

Half-life: 5 hours.

ADVERSE REACTIONS
CNS: *headache,* depression, fatigue, insomnia, pain.
EENT: *allergic rhinitis, pharyngitis,* dry throat, dysphonia, earache, epistaxis, nasal irritation, sinus congestion, sinusitis.
GI: abdominal pain, anorexia, dyspepsia, flatulence, gastroenteritis, nausea, oral candidiasis, vomiting.
GU: dysmenorrhea, menstrual disorder, UTI.
Musculoskeletal: arthralgia, back pain, myalgia.
Respiratory: *upper respiratory tract infection,* respiratory disorder.
Other: accidental injury, flulike symptoms, infection.

INTERACTIONS
Drug-drug. *Ketoconazole:* May increase mometasone level. Use together cautiously.

EFFECTS ON LAB TEST RESULTS
None reported.

CONTRAINDICATIONS & CAUTIONS

• Contraindicated in patients hypersensitive to drug or its ingredients and in those with status asthmaticus or other acute forms of asthma or bronchospasm (as primary treatment).

• Use cautiously in patients at high risk for decreased bone mineral content (those with a family history of osteoporosis, prolonged immobilization, long-term use of drugs that reduce bone mass), patients switching from a systemic to an inhaled corticosteroid, and patients with active or dormant tuberculosis, untreated systemic infections, ocular herpes simplex, or immunosuppression.

• Use cautiously in breast-feeding women.

NURSING CONSIDERATIONS

• *Alert:* Don't use for acute bronchospasm.

• Wean patient slowly from a systemic corticosteroid after he switches to mometasone. Monitor lung function tests, beta-agonist use, and asthma symptoms.

• *Alert:* If patient is switching from an oral corticosteroid to an inhaled form, watch closely for evidence of adrenal insufficiency, such as fatigue, lethargy, weakness, nausea, vomiting, and hypotension.

• After an oral corticosteroid is withdrawn, hypothalamic-pituitary-adrenal (HPA) function may not recover for months. If patient has trauma, stress, infection, or surgery during this HPA recovery period, he is particularly vulnerable to adrenal insufficiency or adrenal crisis.

• Because an inhaled corticosteroid can be systemically absorbed, watch for cushingoid effects.

• Assess patient for bone loss during long-term use.

• Watch for evidence of localized mouth infections, glaucoma, and immunosuppression.

• Use drug only if benefits to mother justify risks to fetus. If a woman takes a corticosteroid during pregnancy, monitor neonate for hypoadrenalism.

• Monitor elderly patients for increased sensitivity to drug effects.

PATIENT TEACHING

• Instruct patient on proper use and routine care of the inhaler.

• Tell patient to use drug regularly and at the same time each day. If he uses it only once daily, tell him to do so in the evening.

• Caution patient not to use drug for immediate relief of an asthma attack or bronchospasm.

• Inform patient that maximal benefits might not occur for 1 to 2 weeks or longer after therapy starts; instruct him to notify his prescriber if his condition fails to improve or worsens.

• Tell patient that if he has bronchospasm after taking drug, he should immediately use a fast-acting bronchodilator. Urge him to contact prescriber immediately if bronchospasm doesn't respond to the fast-acting bronchodilator.

• *Alert:* If patient has been weaned from an oral corticosteroid, urge him to contact prescriber immediately if an asthma attack occurs or if he is experiencing a period of stress. The oral corticosteroid may need to be resumed.

• Warn patient to avoid exposure to chickenpox or measles and to notify prescriber if such contact occurs.

• Long-term use of an inhaled corticosteroid may increase the risk of cataracts or glaucoma; tell patient to report vision changes.

• Advise patient to write the date on a new inhaler on the day he opens it and to discard the inhaler after 45 days or when the dose counter reads "00."

montelukast sodium
mon-tell-OO-kast

Singulair

Pharmacologic class: leukotriene-receptor antagonist
Pregnancy risk category B

AVAILABLE FORMS
Oral granules: 4-mg packet
Tablets (chewable): 4 mg, 5 mg
Tablets (film-coated): 10 mg

INDICATIONS & DOSAGES
➤ **Asthma, seasonal allergic rhinitis, perennial allergic rhinitis**
Adults and children age 15 and older: 10 mg P.O. once daily in evening.

Children ages 6 to 14: Give 5 mg chewable tablet P.O. once daily in evening.
Children ages 2 to 5: Give 4 mg chewable tablet or 1 packet of 4-mg oral granules P.O. once daily in the evening.
Children ages 12 to 23 months (asthma only): 1 packet of 4-mg oral granules P.O. once daily in the evening.
Children ages 6 to 23 months (perennial allergic rhinitis only): 1 packet of 4-mg oral granules P.O. once daily in the evening.

➤ **Prevention of exercise-induced bronchospasm**
Adults and children age 15 and older: 10 mg P.O. at least 2 hours before exercise. Patients already taking a daily dose shouldn't take an additional dose. Also, an additional dose shouldn't be taken within 24 hours of a previous dose.

ADMINISTRATION
P.O.
● Don't dissolve oral granules in liquid; let the patient take a drink after receiving the granules.
● Give oral granules without regard for food.

ACTION
Reduces early and late-phase bronchoconstriction from antigen challenge.

Route	Onset	Peak	Duration
P.O. (chewable, granules)	Unknown	2–2½ hr	24 hr
P.O. (film-coated)	Unknown	3–4 hr	24 hr

Half-life: 2¾ to 5½ hours.

ADVERSE REACTIONS
CNS: *headache,* asthenia, dizziness, fatigue, fever.
EENT: dental pain, nasal congestion.
GI: abdominal pain, dyspepsia, infectious gastroenteritis.
GU: pyuria.
Hematologic: systemic eosinophilia.
Respiratory: cough.
Skin: rash.
Other: influenza, trauma.

INTERACTIONS
Drug-drug. *Phenobarbital, rifampin:* May decrease bioavailability of montelukast because of hepatic metabolism induction. Monitor patient for effectiveness.

EFFECTS ON LAB TEST RESULTS
● May increase ALT and AST levels.

CONTRAINDICATIONS & CAUTIONS
● Contraindicated in patients hypersensitive to drug or its ingredients.
● Use cautiously and with appropriate monitoring in patients whose dosages of systemic corticosteroids are reduced.

NURSING CONSIDERATIONS
● Assess patient's underlying condition, and monitor him for effectiveness.
● *Alert:* Don't abruptly substitute drug for inhaled or oral corticosteroids. Dose of inhaled corticosteroids may be reduced gradually.
● Drug isn't indicated for use in patients with acute asthmatic attacks, status asthmaticus, or as monotherapy for management of exercise-induced bronchospasm. Continue appropriate rescue drug for acute worsening.

PATIENT TEACHING
● Inform caregiver that the oral granules may be given directly into the child's mouth, dissolved in 1 teaspoon of cold or room-temperature baby formula or breast milk, or mixed in a spoonful of applesauce, carrots, rice, or ice cream.
● Tell caregiver not to open packet until ready to use and, after opening, to give the full dose within 15 minutes. Tell her that if she's mixing the drug with food, not to store excess for future use and to discard the unused portion.
● Advise patient to take drug daily, even if asymptomatic, and to contact his prescriber if asthma isn't well controlled.
● Warn patient not to reduce or stop taking other prescribed antiasthmatics without prescriber's approval.
● Advise patient to seek medical attention if short-acting inhaled bronchodilators are needed more often than usual during drug therapy.
● Warn patient that drug isn't beneficial in acute asthma attacks or in exercise-induced

bronchospasm, and advise him to keep appropriate rescue drugs available.
• Advise patient with known aspirin sensitivity to continue to avoid using aspirin and NSAIDs during drug therapy.
• Advise patient with phenylketonuria that chewable tablet contains phenylalanine.

morphine hydrochloride
MOR-feen

Doloral†, M.O.S†, M.O.S.-S.R†

morphine sulfate
Astramorph PF, Avinza, DepoDur, Duramorph, Infumorph, Kadian, M-Eslon†, Morphine H.P†, MS Contin, MSIR, Oramorph SR, RMS Uniserts, Roxanol, Statex†

Pharmacologic class: opioid
Pregnancy risk category C
Controlled substance schedule II

AVAILABLE FORMS
morphine hydrochloride
Oral solution: 1 mg/ml†, 5 mg/ml†, 10 mg/ml†, 20 mg/ml†, 50 mg/ml†
Suppositories: 10 mg†, 20 mg†, 30 mg†
Syrup: 1 mg/ml*†, 5 mg/ml*†, 10 mg/ml*†, 20 mg/ml*†, 50 mg/ml*†
Tablets: 10 mg†, 20 mg†, 40 mg†, 60 mg†
Tablets (extended-release): 30 mg†, 60 mg†
morphine sulfate
Capsules: 15 mg, 30 mg
Capsules (extended-release beads): 30 mg, 60 mg, 90 mg, 120 mg
Capsules (extended-release pellets): 10 mg, 20 mg, 30 mg, 50 mg, 60 mg, 80 mg, 100 mg, 200 mg
Injection (with preservative): 0.5 mg/ml, 1 mg/ml, 2 mg/ml, 4 mg/ml, 5 mg/ml, 8 mg/ml, 10 mg/ml, 15 mg/ml, 25 mg/ml, 50 mg/ml
Injection (without preservative): 0.5 mg/ml, 1 mg/ml, 10 mg/ml, 15 mg/ml, 25 mg/ml
Oral solution: 10 mg/5 ml, 20 mg/5 ml, 20 mg/ml (concentrate), 100 mg/5 ml (concentrate)
Soluble tablets: 10 mg, 15 mg, 30 mg

Suppositories: 5 mg, 10 mg, 20 mg, 30 mg
Tablets: 15 mg, 30 mg
Tablets (extended-release): 15 mg, 30 mg, 60 mg, 100 mg, 200 mg

INDICATIONS & DOSAGES
➤ Severe pain
Adults: 5 to 20 mg subcutaneously or I.M. or 2.5 to 15 mg I.V. every 4 hours p.r.n. Or, 5 to 30 mg P.O. or 10 to 20 mg P.R. every 4 hours p.r.n.
  For continuous I.V. infusion, give loading dose of 15 mg I.V.; then continuous infusion of 0.8 to 10 mg/hour.
  For extended-release tablet, give 15 or 30 mg P.O., every 8 to 12 hours.
  For extended-release Kadian capsules used as a first opioid, give 20 mg P.O. every 12 hours or 40 mg P.O. once daily; increase conservatively in opioid-naive patients.
  For epidural injection, give 5 mg by epidural catheter; then, if pain isn't relieved adequately in 1 hour, give supplementary doses of 1 to 2 mg at intervals sufficient to assess effectiveness. Maximum total epidural dose shouldn't exceed 10 mg/24 hours.
  For intrathecal injection, a single dose of 0.2 to 1 mg may provide pain relief for 24 hours (only in the lumbar area). Don't repeat injections.
Children: 0.1 to 0.2 mg/kg subcutaneously or I.M. every 4 hours. Maximum single dose, 15 mg.
➤ Moderate to severe pain requiring continuous, around-the-clock opioid
Adults: Individualize dosage of Avinza. For patients with no tolerance to opioids, begin with 30 mg Avinza P.O. daily; adjust dosage by no more than 30 mg every 4 days. When converting from another oral morphine form, individualize the dosage schedule according to patient's schedule.
➤ Single-dose, epidural extended pain relief after major surgery
Adults: Inject 10 to 15 mg (maximum 20 mg) DepoDur via lumbar epidural administration before surgery or after clamping of umbilical cord during cesarean section. May be injected undiluted or may be diluted up to 5 ml total volume with preservative-free normal saline solution.

ADMINISTRATION
P.O.
• Oral solutions of various concentrations and an intensified oral solution (20 mg/ml) are available. Carefully note the strength given.
• Give morphine sulfate without regard to food.
• Oral capsules may be carefully opened and the entire contents poured into cool, soft foods, such as water, orange juice, applesauce, or pudding; patient should consume mixture immediately.
• Don't crush, break, or chew extended-release forms.
S.L.
• For S.L. use, measure oral solution with tuberculin syringe. Give dose a few drops at a time to allow maximal S.L. absorption and minimize swallowing.
I.V.
• For direct injection, dilute 2.5 to 15 mg in 4 or 5 ml of sterile water for injection and give slowly over 4 to 5 minutes.
• For continuous infusion, mix drug with D_5W to yield 0.1 to 1 mg/ml, and give by a continuous infusion device.
• In adults with severe, chronic pain, maintenance I.V. infusion is 0.8 to 80 mg/hour; sometimes higher doses are needed.
• Don't mix DepoDur with other drugs. Once DepoDur is given, don't give any other drugs into epidural space for at least 48 hours. Don't use in-line filter during administration.
• Store DepoDur in refrigerator. Unopened vials can be stored at room temperature for up to 7 days. After drug is withdrawn from vial, it can be stored at room temperature for up to 4 hours before use.
• **Incompatibilities:** Aminophylline, amobarbital, cefepime, chlorothiazide, fluorouracil, haloperidol, heparin sodium, meperidine, pentobarbital, phenobarbital sodium, phenytoin sodium, prochlorperazine, promethazine hydrochloride, sodium bicarbonate, thiopental.
I.M.
• Document injection site.
• Store injection solution at room temperature and protect from light.
• Solution may darken with age. Don't use if injection is darker than pale yellow, discolored, or contains precipitate.

Subcutaneous
• Document injection site.
• Store injection solution at room temperature and protect from light.
• Solution may darken with age. Don't use if injection is darker than pale yellow, discolored, or contains precipitate.
Rectal
• Refrigeration of rectal suppository isn't needed.

ACTION
Unknown. Binds with opioid receptors in the CNS, altering perception of and emotional response to pain.

Route	Onset	Peak	Duration
P.O.	30 min	1–2 hr	4–12 hr
P.O. (extended-release)	1–2 hr	3–4 hr	12–24 hr
I.V.	5 min	20 min	4–5 hr
I.M.	10–30 min	30–60 min	4–5 hr
Subcut	10–30 min	50–90 min	4–5 hr
P.R.	20–60 min	20–60 min	4–5 hr
Epidural	15–60 min	15–60 min	24 hr
Intrathecal	15–60 min	30–60 min	24 hr

Half-life: 2 to 3 hours.

ADVERSE REACTIONS
CNS: *dizziness, euphoria, lightheadedness, nightmares, sedation, somnolence,* **seizures,** depression, hallucinations, nervousness, physical dependence, syncope.
CV: *bradycardia, cardiac arrest, shock,* hypertension, hypotension, tachycardia.
GI: *constipation, nausea, vomiting,* anorexia, biliary tract spasms, dry mouth, ileus.
GU: urine retention.
Hematologic: *thrombocytopenia.*
Respiratory: *apnea, respiratory arrest, respiratory depression.*
Skin: diaphoresis, edema, pruritus and skin flushing.
Other: decreased libido.

INTERACTIONS
Drug-drug. *Cimetidine:* May increase respiratory and CNS depression when

given with morphine sulfate. Monitor patient closely.

CNS depressants, general anesthetics, hypnotics, MAO inhibitors, other opioid analgesics, sedatives, tranquilizers, tricyclic antidepressants: May cause respiratory depression, hypotension, profound sedation, or coma. Use together with caution, reduce morphine dose, and monitor patient response.

Drug-lifestyle. *Alcohol use:* May cause additive CNS effects. Warn patient to avoid alcohol.

EFFECTS ON LAB TEST RESULTS

● May increase amylase level. May decrease hemoglobin level (morphine sulfate).

● May decrease platelet count.

● May cause abnormal liver function test values (morphine sulfate).

CONTRAINDICATIONS & CAUTIONS

● Contraindicated in patients hypersensitive to drug and in those with conditions that would preclude I.V. administration of opioids (acute bronchial asthma or upper airway obstruction).

● Contraindicated in patients with GI obstruction.

● Use with caution in elderly or debilitated patients and in those with head injury, increased intracranial pressure, seizures, chronic pulmonary disease, prostatic hyperplasia, severe hepatic or renal disease, acute abdominal conditions, hypothyroidism, Addison's disease, and urethral stricture.

● Use with caution in patients with circulatory shock, biliary tract disease, CNS depression, toxic psychosis, acute alcoholism, delirium tremens, and seizure disorders.

NURSING CONSIDERATIONS

● Reassess patient's level of pain at least 15 and 30 minutes after giving parenterally and 30 minutes after giving orally.

● Keep opioid antagonist (naloxone) and resuscitation equipment available.

● Monitor circulatory, respiratory, bladder, and bowel functions carefully. Drug may cause respiratory depression, hypotension, urine retention, nausea, vomiting, ileus, or altered level of consciousness regardless

of the route. If respirations drop below 12 breaths/minute, withhold dose and notify prescriber.

● Preservative-free preparations are available for epidural and intrathecal use.

● When drug is given epidurally, monitor patient closely for respiratory depression up to 24 hours after the injection. Check respiratory rate and depth every 30 to 60 minutes for 24 hours. Watch for pruritus and skin flushing.

● Morphine is drug of choice in relieving MI pain; may cause transient decrease in blood pressure.

● An around-the-clock regimen best manages severe, chronic pain.

● Morphine may worsen or mask gallbladder pain.

● Constipation is commonly severe with maintenance dose. Ensure that stool softener and/or stimulant laxative is ordered.

● Taper morphine sulfate therapy gradually when stopping therapy.

● *Look alike–sound alike:* Don't confuse morphine with hydromorphone or Avinza with Invanz.

PATIENT TEACHING

● When drug is used after surgery, encourage patient to turn, cough, deep-breathe, and use incentive spirometer to prevent lung problems.

● Caution ambulatory patient about getting out of bed or walking. Warn outpatient to avoid driving and other potentially hazardous activities that require mental alertness until drug's adverse CNS effects are known.

● *Alert:* Drinking alcohol or taking drugs containing alcohol while taking extended-release capsules may cause additive CNS effects. Warn patient to read labels on OTC drugs carefully and not to use alcohol in any form.

● Tell patient to swallow morphine sulfate whole or to open capsule and sprinkle beads or pellets on a small amount of applesauce immediately before taking.

● *Alert:* Warn patient not to crush, break, or chew extended-release forms.

moxifloxacin hydrochloride
mocks-ah-FLOX-a-sin

Avelox, Avelox I.V.

Pharmacologic class: fluoroquinolone
Pregnancy risk category C

AVAILABLE FORMS
Injection: 400 mg/250 ml
Tablets (film-coated): 400 mg

INDICATIONS & DOSAGES
➤ **Acute bacterial sinusitis caused
by** *Streptococcus pneumoniae,
Haemophilus influenzae,* **or** *Moraxella
catarrhalis*
Adults: 400 mg P.O. or I.V. every 24 hours
for 10 days.
➤ **Complicated skin and skin
structure infections caused by
methicillin-susceptible** *Staphylococcus aureus, Escherichia coli, Klebsiella
pneumoniae,* **or** *Enterobacter cloacae*
Adults: 400 mg P.O. or I.V. every 24 hours
for 7 to 21 days.
➤ **Complicated intra-abdominal
infection caused by** *E. coli, Bacteroides
fragilis, Streptococcus anginosis, Streptococcus constellatus, Enterococcus
faecalis, Proteus mirabilis, Clostridium
perfringens, Bacteroides thetaiotaomi-
cron,* **or** *Peptostreptococcus species*
Adults: 400 mg P.O. or I.V. every 24 hours
for 5 to 14 days. Start with the I.V. form;
switch to P.O. when appropriate.
➤ **Community-acquired pneumonia
from multidrug-resistant** *S. pneumoniae* **(resistance to two or more of
the following antibiotics: penicillin,
second-generation cephalosporins,
macrolides, trimethoprim-
sulfamethoxazole, tetracyclines),**
*S. aureus, M. catarrhalis, H. influenzae,
H. parainfluenzae, K. pneumoniae,
Chlamydia pneumoniae, Legionella
pneumophila,* **or** *Mycoplasma pneumoniae*
Adults: 400 mg P.O. or I.V. every 24 hours
for 7 to 14 days.
➤ **Acute bacterial worsening of
chronic bronchitis caused by**
S. pneumoniae, H. influenzae,

*H. parainfluenzae, K. pneumoniae, S.
aureus,* **or** *M. catarrhalis*
Adults: 400 mg P.O. or I.V. every 24 hours
for 5 days.
➤ **Uncomplicated skin-structure or
skin infection caused by** *S. aureus* **or**
S. pyogenes
Adults: 400 mg P.O. or I.V. every 24 hours
for 7 days.

ADMINISTRATION
P.O.
● Give drug without regard for food. Give
at same time each day.
● Space doses of antacids, sucralfate,
multivitamins, and products containing
aluminum, magnesium, iron, and zinc to
avoid decreasing drug's therapeutic effects.
● Store drug at controlled room tempera-
ture.
I.V.
● Don't use if particulate matter is visible.
● Flush I.V. line with a compatible solution
such as D_5W, normal saline, or Ringer's
lactate solution before and after use.
● Give only by infusion over 1 hour. Avoid
rapid or bolus infusion.
● **Incompatibilities:** Other I.V. drugs.

ACTION
Interferes with action of enzymes needed
for bacterial replication. Inhibits topoiso-
merases I (DNA gyrase) and IV, impairing
bacterial DNA replication, transcription,
repair, and recombination.

Route	Onset	Peak	Duration
P.O., I.V.	Unknown	1–3 hr	Unknown

Half-life: About 12 hours.

ADVERSE REACTIONS
CNS: dizziness, headache, asthenia, pain,
malaise, insomnia, nervousness, anxiety,
confusion, somnolence, tremor, vertigo,
paresthesia.
CV: *prolonged QT interval,* chest pain,
hypertension, palpitations, peripheral
edema, tachycardia.
GI: *pseudomembranous colitis,* abdominal pain, anorexia, constipation, diarrhea,
dyspepsia, dry mouth, flatulence, GI disorder, glossitis, nausea, oral candidiasis,
stomatitis, taste perversion, vomiting.
GU: vaginal candidiasis, vaginitis.

Reactions may be *common,* uncommon, *life-threatening,* or COMMON AND LIFE-THREATENING.
Interaction may have a *rapid onset* or **delayed onset.**

Hematologic: *leukopenia, thrombocytopenia, thrombocytosis,* eosinophilia.
Hepatic: abnormal liver function, cholestatic jaundice.
Musculoskeletal: arthralgia, back pain, leg pain, myalgia, tendon rupture.
Respiratory: dyspnea.
Skin: injection site reaction, pruritus, rash (maculopapular, purpuric, pustular), sweating.
Other: allergic reaction, candidiasis.

INTERACTIONS
Drug-drug. *Aluminum hydroxide, aluminum-magnesium hydroxide, calcium carbonate, didanosine, magnesium hydroxide, multivitamins, products containing zinc:* May interfere with GI absorption of moxifloxacin. Give moxifloxacin 4 hours before or 8 hours after these products.
Class IA antiarrhythmics (such as procainamide, quinidine), class III antiarrhythmics (such as amiodarone, sotalol): May increase risk of cardiac arrhythmias. Avoid using together.
Drugs that prolong QT interval, such as antipsychotics, erythromycin, tricyclic antidepressants: May have additive effect. Avoid using together.
NSAIDs: May increase risk of CNS stimulation and seizures. Avoid using together.
Sucralfate: May decrease absorption of moxifloxacin, reducing anti-infective response. If use together can't be avoided, give at least 6 hours apart.
Warfarin: May increase anticoagulant effects. Monitor PT and INR closely.
Drug-lifestyle. *Sun exposure:* May cause photosensitivity reactions. Advise patient to avoid excessive sunlight exposure.

EFFECTS ON LAB TEST RESULTS
● May increase GGT, amylase, and LDH levels. May decrease hemoglobin level.
● May increase eosinophil count. May decrease PT and WBC count. May increase or decrease platelet count.

CONTRAINDICATIONS & CAUTIONS
● Contraindicated in patients hypersensitive to drug or other fluoroquinolones and in those with prolonged QT interval or uncorrected hypokalemia.
● Use cautiously in patients with ongoing proarrhythmic conditions, such as

clinically significant bradycardia or acute myocardial ischemia.
● Use cautiously in patients who may have CNS disorders and in those with other risk factors that may lower the seizure threshold or predispose them to seizures.
● Safety and efficacy in children, adolescents younger than age 18, and pregnant or breast-feeding women haven't been established.

NURSING CONSIDERATIONS
● **Alert:** Monitor patient for adverse CNS effects, including seizures, dizziness, confusion, tremors, hallucinations, depression, and suicidal thoughts. If these occur, stop drug and notify prescriber.
● Monitor patient for hypersensitivity reactions, including anaphylaxis.
● If diarrhea develops during therapy, send stool specimen for *Clostridium difficile* test.
● Rupture of the Achilles and other tendons is linked to fluoroquinolone use. If pain, inflammation, or tendon rupture occurs, stop drug and notify prescriber.

PATIENT TEACHING
● Instruct patient to take drug once daily, at the same time each day, without regard to meals.
● Tell patient to finish entire course of therapy, even if symptoms are relieved.
● Advise patient to drink plenty of fluids.
● Tell patient to space antacids, sucralfate, multivitamins, and products containing aluminum, magnesium, iron, and zinc to avoid decreasing drug's therapeutic effects.
● Instruct patient to contact prescriber and stop drug if he experiences allergic reaction, rash, heart palpitations, fainting, or persistent diarrhea.
● Direct patient to contact prescriber, stop drug, rest, and refrain from exercise if he experiences pain, inflammation, or tendon rupture.
● Warn patient that drug may cause dizziness and light-headedness. Tell patient to avoid hazardous activities, such as driving or operating machinery, until effects of drug are known.
● Instruct patient to avoid excessive sunlight exposure and ultraviolet light and to report photosensitivity reactions to prescriber.

neomycin sulfate
nee-o-MYE-sin

Neo-fradin

Pharmacologic class: aminoglycoside
Pregnancy risk category D

AVAILABLE FORMS
Oral solution: 125 mg/5 ml
Tablets: 500 mg

INDICATIONS & DOSAGES
➤ **Infectious diarrhea caused by
enteropathogenic** *Escherichia coli*
Adults: 50 mg/kg daily P.O. in four divided
doses for 2 to 3 days; maximum of 3 g/day.
Children: 50 to 100 mg/kg daily P.O. in
divided doses every 4 to 6 hours for 2 to
3 days.
➤ **To suppress intestinal bacteria
before surgery**
Adults: After saline cathartic, 1 g P.O.
every hour for four doses; then 1 g every
4 hours for the balance of the 24 hours.
Or, 88 mg/kg in six equally divided doses
every 4 hours. Or, 1 g neomycin with 1 g
erythromycin base at 1 p.m., 2 p.m., and
11 p.m. on day before 8 a.m. surgery.
Children: After saline cathartic, 40 to
100 mg/kg daily P.O. in divided doses
every 4 to 6 hours. Or, 88 mg/kg in equally
divided doses every 4 hours.
➤ **Adjunctive treatment for hepatic
coma**
Adults: 1 to 3 g P.O. q.i.d. for 5 to 6 days;
or 200 ml of 1% solution. For patients
with chronic hepatic insufficiency, 4 g/day
indefinitely may be needed.
Children: 50 to 100 mg/kg/day P.O. in
divided doses for 5 to 6 days.

ADMINISTRATION
P.O.
● For preoperative disinfection, provide a
low-residue diet and a cathartic immediately before therapy.

ACTION
Inhibits protein synthesis by binding
directly to the 30S ribosomal subunit;
bactericidal.

Route	Onset	Peak	Duration
P.O.	Unknown	1–4 hr	8 hr

Half-life: 2 to 3 hours.

ADVERSE REACTIONS
EENT: *ototoxicity.*
GI: nausea, vomiting, diarrhea, malabsorption syndrome, *Clostridium
difficile*–related colitis.
GU: *nephrotoxicity,* possible increase in
urinary excretion of casts.

INTERACTIONS
Drug-drug. *Acyclovir, amphotericin B,
cephalosporins, cidofovir, cisplatin,
methoxyflurane, vancomycin, other aminoglycosides:* May increase nephrotoxicity.
Monitor renal function test results.
*Atracurium, pancuronium, rocuronium,
vecuronium:* May increase effects of nondepolarizing muscle relaxants, including
prolonged respiratory depression. Use together only when necessary, and expect to
reduce dosage of nondepolarizing muscle
relaxants.
Digoxin: May decrease digoxin absorption.
Monitor digoxin level.
I.V. loop diuretics (such as furosemide):
May increase ototoxicity. Monitor patient's
hearing.
Oral anticoagulants: May inhibit vitamin
K–producing bacteria; may increase
anticoagulant effect. Monitor PT and INR.

EFFECTS ON LAB TEST RESULTS
● May increase BUN, creatinine, and
nonprotein nitrogen levels.

CONTRAINDICATIONS & CAUTIONS
● Contraindicated in patients hypersensitive to other aminoglycosides and in those
with intestinal obstruction.
● Use cautiously in elderly patients and
in those with impaired renal function,
neuromuscular disorders, or ulcerative
bowel lesions.

NURSING CONSIDERATIONS
● *Alert:* Monitor renal function: urine output, specific gravity, urinalysis, BUN and
creatinine levels, and creatinine clearance.
Report to prescriber evidence of declining
renal function.

• **Alert:** Evaluate patient's hearing before and during prolonged therapy. Notify prescriber if patient has tinnitus, vertigo, or hearing loss. Deafness may start several weeks after drug is stopped.

• Watch for signs and symptoms of super-infection, such as fever, chills, and increased pulse rate.

• **Alert:** Neuromuscular blockage and respiratory paralysis have been reported after administration of aminoglycosides. Monitor patient closely.

• For adjunctive treatment for hepatic coma, decrease patient's dietary protein and assess neurologic status frequently during therapy.

• The ototoxic and nephrotoxic properties of drug limit its usefulness.

PATIENT TEACHING
• Instruct patient to report adverse reactions promptly.
• Encourage patient to maintain adequate fluid intake.

---

nifedipine
nye-FED-i-peen

Adalat CC, Adalat XL†,
Apo-Nifed†, Nifedical XL,
Nu-Nifed†, Procardia XL

Pharmacologic class: calcium channel blocker
Pregnancy risk category C

AVAILABLE FORMS
Capsules: 10 mg, 20 mg
Tablets (extended-release): 20 mg†, 30 mg, 60 mg, 90 mg

INDICATIONS & DOSAGES
➤ **Vasospastic angina (Prinzmetal's or variant angina), classic chronic stable angina pectoris**
Adults: Initially, 10 mg short-acting capsule P.O. t.i.d. Usual effective dosage range is 10 to 20 mg t.i.d. Some patients may require up to 30 mg q.i.d. Maximum daily dose is 180 mg. Adjust dosage over 7 to 14 days to evaluate response. Or, 30 to 60 mg (extended-release tablets, except Adalat CC) P.O. once daily. Maximum

daily dose is 120 mg. Adjust dosage over 7 to 14 days to evaluate response.
➤ **Hypertension**
Adults: 30 or 60 mg P.O. extended-release tablet once daily. Adjusted over 7 to 14 days. Doses larger than 90 mg (Adalat CC) and 120 mg (Procardia XL) aren't recommended.

ADMINISTRATION
P.O.
• Don't give immediate-release capsules within 1 week of acute MI or in acute coronary syndrome.
• **Alert:** Don't use capsules S.L. to rapidly reduce severe high blood pressure because the result may be fatal.
• Give extended-release tablets whole; don't break or crush tablet.
• Don't give drug with grapefruit juice.
• Protect capsules from direct light and moisture and store at room temperature.

ACTION
Thought to inhibit calcium ion influx across cardiac and smooth muscle cells, decreasing contractility and oxygen demand. Drug may also dilate coronary arteries and arterioles.

Route	Onset	Peak	Duration
P.O.	20 min	30–60 min	4–8 hr
P.O. (extended)	20 min	6 hr	24 hr

Half-life: 2 to 5 hours.

ADVERSE REACTIONS
CNS: *dizziness, light-headedness, headache, weakness,* somnolence, syncope, nervousness.
CV: *flushing, peripheral edema, **heart failure, MI,*** hypotension, palpitations.
EENT: nasal congestion.
GI: *nausea,* diarrhea, constipation, abdominal discomfort.
Musculoskeletal: muscle cramps.
Respiratory: dyspnea, ***pulmonary edema,*** cough.
Skin: rash, pruritus.

INTERACTIONS
Drug-drug. *Antiretrovirals, cimetidine, verapamil:* May decrease nifedipine metabolism. Monitor blood pressure

closely and adjust nifedipine dosage as needed.

Azole antifungals, erythromycin, quinupristin, and dalfopristin: May increase the effects of nifedipine. Monitor blood pressure closely and decrease nifedipine dosage as needed.

Digoxin: May cause elevated digoxin level. Monitor digoxin level.

Diltiazem: May increase the effects of nifedipine. Monitor patient closely.

Fentanyl: May cause severe hypotension. Monitor blood pressure.

Phenytoin: May reduce phenytoin metabolism. Monitor phenytoin level.

Propranolol, other beta blockers: May cause hypotension and heart failure. Use together cautiously.

Quinidine: May decrease levels and effects of quinidine while increasing effects of nifedipine. Monitor heart rate and adjust nifedipine dose as needed.

Rifamycins: May decrease nifedipine levels. Monitor patient.

Tacrolimus: May increase tacrolimus levels and risk for toxicity. Decrease tacrolimus dose as needed.

Drug-herb. *Ginkgo:* May increase effects of drug. Discourage use together.

Ginseng: May increase drug levels with possible toxicity. Discourage use together.

Melatonin, St. John's wort: May interfere with antihypertensive effect. Discourage use together.

Drug-food. *Grapefruit juice:* May increase bioavailability of drug. Discourage use together.

EFFECTS ON LAB TEST RESULTS
● May increase ALT, AST, alkaline phosphatase, and LDH levels.

CONTRAINDICATIONS & CAUTIONS
● Contraindicated in patients hypersensitive to drug.
● Use cautiously in patients with heart failure or hypotension and in elderly patients. Use extended-release tablets cautiously in patients with severe GI narrowing.

NURSING CONSIDERATIONS
● Monitor blood pressure regularly, especially in patients who take beta blockers or antihypertensives.

● Watch for symptoms of heart failure.
● *Look alike–sound alike:* Don't confuse nifedipine with nimodipine or nicardipine.

PATIENT TEACHING
● If patient is kept on nitrate therapy while nifedipine dosage is being adjusted, urge continued compliance. Patient may take S.L. nitroglycerin, as needed, for acute chest pain.
● Tell patient that chest pain may worsen briefly as therapy starts or dosage increases.
● Instruct patient to swallow extended-release tablets without breaking, crushing, or chewing them.
● Advise patient to avoid taking drug with grapefruit juice.
● Reassure patient taking the extended-release tablet that the wax mold may be passed in the stools. Assure him that drug has already been completely absorbed.
● Tell patient to protect capsules from direct light and moisture and to store at room temperature.

SAFETY ALERT!

nitroglycerin (glyceryl trinitrate)
nye-troe-GLIH-ser-in

Deponit, Minitran, Nitrek, Nitro-Bid, Nitro-Dur, Nitrogard, Nitrolingual, NitroQuick, Nitrostat, NitroTab, Nitro-Time, NTS, Trinipatch†

Pharmacologic class: nitrate
Pregnancy risk category C

AVAILABLE FORMS
Aerosol (translingual): 0.4 mg/metered spray
Capsules (sustained-release): 2.5 mg, 6.5 mg, 9 mg
Injection: 5 mg/ml; 100 mcg/ml, 200 mcg/ml, 400 mcg/ml
Tablets (S.L.): 0.3 mg ($^1/_{200}$ grain), 0.4 mg ($^1/_{150}$ grain), 0.6 mg ($^1/_{100}$ grain)
Tablets (sustained-release): 2.6 mg, 6.5 mg, 9 mg, 13 mg
Topical: 2% ointment
Transdermal: 0.1 mg/hour, 0.2 mg/hour, 0.3 mg/hour, 0.4 mg/hour, 0.6 mg/hour, 0.8 mg/hour release rate

INDICATIONS & DOSAGES
➤ **To prevent chronic anginal attacks**
Adults: 2.5 or 2.6 mg sustained-release capsule or tablet every 8 to 12 hours. Increase to an effective dose in 2.5- or 2.6-mg increments b.i.d. to q.i.d. Or, use 2% ointment: Start dosage with $^1/_2$-inch ointment, increasing by $^1/_2$-inch increments until desired results are achieved. Range of dosage with ointment is $^1/_2$ to 5 inches. Usual dose is 1 to 2 inches every 6 to 8 hours. Or, transdermal patch 0.2 to 0.4 mg/hour once daily.

➤ **Acute angina pectoris; to prevent or minimize anginal attacks before stressful events**
Adults: 1 S.L. tablet ($^1/_{200}$ grain, $^1/_{150}$ grain, $^1/_{100}$ grain) dissolved under the tongue or in the buccal pouch as soon as angina begins. Repeat every 5 minutes, if needed, for 15 minutes. Or, one or two sprays Nitrolingual into mouth, preferably onto or under the tongue. Repeat every 3 to 5 minutes, if needed, to a maximum of three doses within a 15-minute period. Or, 1 to 3 mg transmucosally every 3 to 5 hours while awake.

➤ **Hypertension from surgery, heart failure after MI, angina pectoris in acute situations, to produce controlled hypotension during surgery (by I.V. infusion)**
Adults: Initially, infuse at 5 mcg/minute, increasing as needed by 5 mcg/minute every 3 to 5 minutes until response occurs. If a 20-mcg/minute rate doesn't produce a response, increase dosage by as much as 20 mcg/minute every 3 to 5 minutes. Up to 100 mcg/minute may be needed.

ADMINISTRATION
P.O.
● Give 30 minutes before or 1 to 2 hours after meals.
● Drug must be swallowed whole and not chewed.
I.V.
● Dilute with D_5W or normal saline solution for injection. Concentration shouldn't exceed 400 mcg/ml.

● Always give with an infusion control device and titrate to desired response.
● Regular polyvinyl chloride tubing can bind up to 80% of drug, making it necessary to infuse higher dosages. A special nonabsorbent polyvinyl chloride tubing is available from the manufacturer. Always mix in glass bottles and avoid using a filter.
● Use the same type of infusion set when changing lines.
● When changing the concentration of infusion, flush the administration set with 15 to 20 ml of the new concentration before use. This will clear the line of the old drug solution.
● **Incompatibilities:** Alteplase, bretylium, hydralazine, levofloxacin, phenytoin sodium.
Topical
● To apply ointment, measure the prescribed amount on the application paper; then place the paper on any nonhairy area. Don't rub in. Cover with plastic film to aid absorption and to protect clothing. Remove all excess ointment from previous site before applying the next dose. Avoid getting ointment on fingers.
Transdermal
● Patch can be applied to any nonhairy part of the skin except distal parts of the arms or legs. (Absorption won't be maximal at distal sites.) Patch may cause contact dermatitis.
● Remove patch before defibrillation. Because of the aluminum backing on the patch, the electric current may cause arcing that can damage the paddles and burn the patient.
● When stopping transdermal treatment of angina, gradually reduce the dosage and frequency of application over 4 to 6 weeks.
S.L.
● Give tablet at first sign of attack. Patient should wet the tablet with saliva, place it under tongue until absorbed. Dose may be repeated every 5 minutes for a maximum of three doses. If drug doesn't provide relief, contact prescriber.
Buccal
● The tablet should be placed between the lip and gum above the incisors or between the cheek and gum. Tablets shouldn't be swallowed or chewed.

Translingual
● Patient using translingual aerosol form shouldn't inhale the spray but should release it onto or under the tongue. He should wait about 10 seconds or so before swallowing.

ACTION
A nitrate that reduces cardiac oxygen demand by decreasing left ventricular end-diastolic pressure (preload) and, to a lesser extent, systemic vascular resistance (afterload). Also increases blood flow through the collateral coronary vessels.

Route	Onset	Peak	Duration
P.O.	20–45 min	Unknown	3–8 hr
I.V.	Immediate	Immediate	3–5 min
Topical	30 min	Unknown	2–12 hr
Trans-dermal	30 min	Unknown	24 hr
S.L.	1–3 min	Unknown	30–60 min
Buccal	3 min	Unknown	3–5 hr
Trans-lingual	2–4 min	Unknown	30–60 min

Half-life: About 1 to 4 minutes.

ADVERSE REACTIONS
CNS: *headache, dizziness,* syncope, weakness.
CV: *orthostatic hypotension, tachycardia, flushing, palpitations.*
EENT: S.L. burning.
GI: nausea, vomiting.
Skin: cutaneous vasodilation, contact dermatitis, rash.
Other: hypersensitivity reactions.

INTERACTIONS
Drug-drug. *Alteplase:* May decrease tissue plasminogen activator–antigen level. Avoid using together; if unavoidable, use lowest effective dose of nitroglycerin.
Antihypertensives: May increase hypotensive effect. Monitor blood pressure closely.
Heparin: I.V. nitroglycerin may interfere with anticoagulant effect of heparin. Monitor PTT.
Sildenafil, tadalafil, vardenafil: May cause severe hypotension. Use of nitrates in any form with these drugs is contraindicated.

Drug-lifestyle. *Alcohol use:* May increase hypotension. Discourage use together.

EFFECTS ON LAB TEST RESULTS
● May falsely decrease values in cholesterol determination tests using the Zlatkis-Zak color reaction.

CONTRAINDICATIONS & CAUTIONS
● Contraindicated in patients with early MI (oral and sublingual), severe anemia, increased intracranial pressure, angle-closure glaucoma, orthostatic hypotension, allergy to adhesives (transdermal), or hypersensitivity to nitrates.
● I.V. nitroglycerin is contraindicated in patients hypersensitive to I.V. form, with cardiac tamponade, restrictive cardiomyopathy, or constrictive pericarditis.
● Use cautiously in patients with hypotension or volume depletion.

NURSING CONSIDERATIONS
● Closely monitor vital signs during infusion, particularly blood pressure, especially in a patient with an MI. Excessive hypotension may worsen the MI.
● Monitor blood pressure and intensity and duration of drug response.
● Drug may cause headaches, especially at beginning of therapy. Dosage may be reduced temporarily, but tolerance usually develops. Treat headache with aspirin or acetaminophen.
● Tolerance to drug can be minimized with a 10- to 12-hour nitrate-free interval. To achieve this, remove the transdermal system in the early evening and apply a new system the next morning or omit the last daily dose of a buccal, sustained-release, or ointment form. Check with the prescriber for alterations in dosage regimen if tolerance is suspected.
● *Look alike–sound alike:* Don't confuse Nitro-Bid with Nicobid or nitroglycerin with nitroprusside.

PATIENT TEACHING
● Caution patient to take nitroglycerin regularly, as prescribed, and to have it accessible at all times.
● *Alert:* Advise patient that stopping drug abruptly causes spasm of the coronary arteries.

Reactions may be *common,* uncommon, *life-threatening,* or COMMON AND LIFE-THREATENING.
Interaction may have a *rapid onset* or *delayed onset*.

• Teach patient how to give the prescribed form of nitroglycerin.
• Tell patient to take S.L. tablet at first sign of attack. Patient should wet the tablet with saliva, place it under tongue until absorbed, and then sit down and rest. Dose may be repeated every 5 minutes for a maximum of three doses. If drug doesn't provide relief, he should obtain medical help promptly.
• Advise patient who complains of a tingling sensation with S.L. drug to try holding tablet in cheek.
• Tell patient to take oral tablets on an empty stomach either 30 minutes before or 1 to 2 hours after meals, to swallow oral tablets whole, and not to chew tablets.
• Remind patient using translingual aerosol form that he shouldn't inhale the spray but should release it onto or under the tongue. Tell him to wait about 10 seconds or so before swallowing.
• Tell patient to place the buccal tablet between the lip and gum above the incisors or between the cheek and gum. Tablets shouldn't be swallowed or chewed.
• Tell patient to take an additional dose before anticipated stress or at bedtime if chest pain occurs at night.
• Urge patient using skin patches to dispose of them carefully because enough medication remains after normal use to be hazardous to children and pets.
• Advise patient to avoid alcohol.
• To minimize dizziness when standing up, tell patient to rise slowly. Advise him to go up and down stairs carefully and to lie down at the first sign of dizziness.
• *Alert:* Advise patient that use of sildenafil, tadalafil, or vardenafil with any nitrate may cause life-threatening low blood pressure. Use together is contraindicated.
• Tell patient to store drug in cool, dark place in a tightly closed container. Tell him to remove cotton from container because it absorbs drug.
• Tell patient to store S.L. tablets in original container or other container specifically approved for this use and to carry the container in a jacket pocket or purse, not in a pocket close to the body.

SAFETY ALERT!

nitroprusside sodium
nye-troe-PRUSS-ide

Nipride†, Nitropress

Pharmacologic class: vasodilator
Pregnancy risk category C

AVAILABLE FORMS
Injection: 50 mg/vial in 2-ml and 5-ml vials

INDICATIONS & DOSAGES
➤ **To lower blood pressure quickly in hypertensive emergencies, to produce controlled hypotension during anesthesia, to reduce preload and afterload in cardiac pump failure or cardiogenic shock (may be used with or without dopamine)**
Adults and children: Begin infusion at 0.25 to 0.3 mcg/kg/minute I.V. and gradually titrate every few minutes to a maximum infusion rate of 10 mcg/kg/minute.
Adjust-a-dose: Patients also taking other antihypertensives are extremely sensitive to nitroprusside. Titrate dosage accordingly. Use with caution in patients with severe renal impairment or hepatic insufficiency; use minimum effective dose.

ADMINISTRATION
I.V.
• Prepare solution by dissolving 50 mg in 2 to 3 ml of D_5W injection or according to manufacturer's instructions. Further dilute concentration in 250, 500, or 1,000 ml of D_5W to provide solutions with 200, 100, or 50 mcg/ml, respectively. Reconstitute ADD-Vantage vials labeled as containing 50 mg of drug according to manufacturer's directions.
• Because drug is sensitive to light, wrap solution in foil or other opaque material; it's not necessary to wrap the tubing. Fresh solution has a faint brownish tint. Discard if highly discolored after 24 hours.
• Use an infusion pump. Drug is best given via piggyback through a peripheral line with no other drug. Don't titrate rate of main I.V. line while drug is being infused. Even a small bolus can cause severe hypotension.

• Check blood pressure every 5 minutes during titration at start of infusion and every 15 minutes thereafter.
• If severe hypotension occurs, stop infusion; effects of drug quickly reverse. Notify prescriber.
• If possible, start an arterial pressure line. Regulate drug flow to desired blood pressure response.
• **Incompatibilities:** Amiodarone, atracurium besylate, bacteriostatic water for injection, levofloxacin. Don't mix with other I.V. drugs or preservatives.

ACTION
Relaxes arteriolar and venous smooth muscle.

Route	Onset	Peak	Duration
I.V.	Immediate	1–2 min	10 min

Half-life: 2 minutes.

ADVERSE REACTIONS
CNS: *headache, dizziness, **increased intracranial pressure,** loss of consciousness,* apprehension, restlessness.
CV: ***bradycardia,*** hypotension, tachycardia, palpitations, ECG changes, flushing.
GI: *nausea, abdominal pain,* ileus.
Hematologic: ***methemoglobinemia.***
Metabolic: acidosis, hypothyroidism.
Musculoskeletal: *muscle twitching.*
Skin: *diaphoresis,* pink color, rash.
Other: ***thiocyanate toxicity, cyanide toxicity,*** venous streaking, irritation at infusion site.

INTERACTIONS
Drug-drug. *Antihypertensives:* May cause sensitivity to nitroprusside. Adjust dosage. *Ganglionic-blocking drugs, general anesthetics, negative inotropic drugs, other antihypertensives:* May cause additive effects. Monitor blood pressure closely. *Sildenafil, vardenafil:* May increase hypotensive effects. Avoid use together.

EFFECTS ON LAB TEST RESULTS
• May increase creatinine level.
• May decrease RBC and WBC counts.

CONTRAINDICATIONS & CAUTIONS
• Contraindicated in patients hypersensitive to drug.

• Contraindicated in those with compensatory hypertension (such as in arteriovenous shunt or coarctation of the aorta), inadequate cerebral circulation, acute heart failure with reduced peripheral vascular resistance, congenital optic atrophy, or tobacco-induced amblyopia.
• Use with extreme caution in patients with increased intracranial pressure.
• Use cautiously in patients with hypothyroidism, hepatic or renal disease, hyponatremia, or low vitamin B level.

NURSING CONSIDERATIONS
• Obtain baseline vital signs before giving drug; find out parameters prescriber wants to achieve.
• Keep patient in supine position when starting therapy or titrating drug.
• *Alert:* Giving excessive doses of 500 mcg/kg delivered faster than 2 mcg/kg/minute or using maximum infusion rate of 10 mcg/kg/minute for more than 10 minutes can cause cyanide toxicity. If patient is at risk, check thiocyanate level every 72 hours. Level higher than 100 mcg/ml may be toxic. If profound hypotension, metabolic acidosis, dyspnea, headache, loss of consciousness, ataxia, or vomiting occurs, stop drug immediately and notify prescriber.
• *Look alike–sound alike:* Don't confuse nitroprusside with nitroglycerin.

PATIENT TEACHING
• Instruct patient to report adverse reactions promptly.
• Tell patient to alert nurse if discomfort occurs at I.V. insertion site.

---

norfloxacin
nor-FLOX-a-sin

Noroxin

Pharmacologic class: fluoroquinolone
Pregnancy risk category C

AVAILABLE FORMS
Tablets (film-coated): 400 mg

INDICATIONS & DOSAGES
➤ **Complicated or uncomplicated UTI from susceptible strains of**

Enterococcus faecalis, Escherichia coli, E. cloacae, Klebsiella pneumoniae, Enterobacter aerogenes, Proteus mirabilis, P. vulgaris, Pseudomonas aeruginosa, Citrobacter freundii, Staphylococcus agalactiae, S. aureus, S. epidermidis, S. saprophyticus, **or** *Serratia marcescens*
Adults: 400 mg P.O. every 12 hours for 7 to 10 days (uncomplicated infection). Or, 400 mg P.O. every 12 hours for 10 to 21 days (complicated infection).

➤ **Prostatitis**
Adults: 400 mg P.O. every 12 hours for 28 days.

➤ **Cystitis caused by** *E. coli, K. pneumoniae,* **or** *P. mirabilis*
Adults: 400 mg P.O. every 12 hours for 3 days.

Adjust-a-dose: If creatinine clearance is 30 ml/minute or less, give 400 mg once daily for above indications.

➤ **Acute, uncomplicated urethral and cervical gonorrhea**
Adults: 800 mg P.O. as a single dose, then doxycycline therapy to treat any coexisting chlamydial infection.

ADMINISTRATION
P.O.
● Obtain specimen for culture and sensitivity testing before starting therapy.
● Give drug 1 hour before or 2 hours after meals because food may hinder absorption.
● Space doses of iron products and antacids when taking norfloxacin.
● Make sure that patient drinks several glasses of water throughout the day to maintain hydration and adequate urine output.

ACTION
Inhibits bacterial DNA synthesis, mainly by blocking DNA gyrase; bactericidal.

Route	Onset	Peak	Duration
P.O.	Unknown	15–120 min	Unknown

Half-life: 3 to 4 hours.

ADVERSE REACTIONS
CNS: *seizures,* depression, dizziness, fatigue, fever, headache, insomnia, somnolence.

GI: *pseudomembranous colitis,* abdominal pain, anorexia, constipation, dry mouth, diarrhea, flatulence, heartburn, nausea, vomiting.
GU: crystalluria.
Hematologic: *leukopenia, neutropenia, thrombocytopenia,* eosinophilia.
Musculoskeletal: back pain.
Skin: hyperhidrosis, photosensitivity, rash.
Other: *anaphylaxis,* hypersensitivity reactions.

INTERACTIONS
Drug-drug. *Aluminum hydroxide, aluminum–magnesium hydroxide, calcium carbonate, magnesium hydroxide:* May decrease norfloxacin level. Give antacid at least 6 hours before or 2 hours after norfloxacin.
Cyclosporine: May increase cyclosporine level. Monitor cyclosporine level.
Iron salts: May decrease absorption of norfloxacin, reducing anti-infective response. Give at least 2 hours apart.
Nitrofurantoin: May antagonize norfloxacin effect. Monitor patient closely.
Oral anticoagulants: May increase anticoagulant effect. Monitor PT and INR.
Probenecid: May increase norfloxacin level by decreasing its excretion. May give probenecid for this reason, but monitor high-risk patient for toxicity.
Sucralfate: May decrease absorption of norfloxacin, reducing anti-infective response. If use together can't be avoided, give at least 6 hours apart.
Theophylline: May impair theophylline metabolism, increasing drug level and risk of toxicity. Monitor patient closely.
Drug-herb. *Dong quai, St. John's wort:* May cause photosensitivity reactions. Advise patient to avoid excessive sunlight exposure.

EFFECTS ON LAB TEST RESULTS
● May increase BUN, creatinine, ALT, AST, and alkaline phosphatase levels. May decrease hematocrit.
● May increase eosinophil count. May decrease neutrophil count.

CONTRAINDICATIONS & CAUTIONS
• Contraindicated in patients hypersensitive to drug or other fluoroquinolones.
• Use cautiously in patients with conditions such as cerebral arteriosclerosis who may be predisposed to seizure disorders.
• Use cautiously and monitor renal function in those with renal impairment.
• Safety and efficacy in children younger than age 18 haven't been established.

NURSING CONSIDERATIONS
• Tendon rupture may occur in patients receiving quinolones. Stop drug if pain or inflammation occurs or tendon ruptures.
• Monitor patient for adverse CNS effects, including dizziness, headache, seizures, or depression. Stop drug and notify prescriber if these effects occur.
• Monitor patient for hypersensitivity reactions. Stop drug and initiate supportive therapy as indicated.
• *Look alike–sound alike:* Don't confuse Noroxin with Neurontin or Floxin.

PATIENT TEACHING
• Tell patient to take drug as prescribed, even after he feels better.
• Advise patient to take drug 1 hour before or 2 hours after meals because food may hinder absorption.
• Advise patient to appropriately space iron products and antacids when taking norfloxacin.
• Warn patient not to exceed the recommended dosages and to drink several glasses of water throughout the day to maintain hydration and adequate urine output.
• Warn patient to avoid hazardous tasks that require alertness until effects of drug are known.
• Instruct patient to avoid exposure to sunlight, wear protective clothing, and use sunscreen while outdoors.
• Tell patient to report pain, inflammation, or tendon rupture, and to refrain from exercise until diagnosis of rupture or tendinitis is excluded.

ofloxacin
oh-FLOX-a-sin

Floxin

Pharmacologic class: fluoro-quinolone
Pregnancy risk category C

AVAILABLE FORMS
Tablets: 200 mg, 300 mg, 400 mg

INDICATIONS & DOSAGES
➤ **Acute bacterial worsening of chronic bronchitis, uncomplicated skin and skin-structure infections, and community-acquired pneumonia**
Adults: 400 mg P.O. every 12 hours for 10 days.
➤ **Sexually transmitted infections, such as acute uncomplicated urethral and cervical gonorrhea, nongonococcal urethritis and cervicitis, and mixed infections of urethra and cervix**
Adults: For acute uncomplicated gonorrhea, 400 mg P.O. once as a single dose; for cervicitis and urethritis, 300 mg P.O. every 12 hours for 7 days.
➤ **Cystitis from *Escherichia coli, Klebsiella pneumoniae,* or other organisms**
Adults: 200 mg P.O. every 12 hours for 3 days (*E. coli* or *K. pneumoniae*), 200 mg P.O. every 12 hours for 7 days (other organisms).
➤ **Complicated UTI**
Adults: 200 mg P.O. every 12 hours for 10 days.
➤ **Prostatitis from *E. coli***
Adults: 300 mg P.O. every 12 hours for 6 weeks.
➤ **Pelvic inflammatory disease**
Adults: 400 mg P.O. every 12 hours with metronidazole for 10 to 14 days.
➤ **To prevent inhalation anthrax** ◆
Adults: 400 mg P.O. b.i.d. Continue therapy for 60 days if no vaccine is available. If vaccine is available, continue for 28 to 45 days and until three doses of the vaccine have been given.
➤ **Traveler's diarrhea**
Adults: 300 mg P.O. b.i.d. for 3 days.

Adjust-a-dose: For patients with creatinine clearance less than 20 ml/minute, give first dose as recommended; then give subsequent doses at 50% of recommended dose every 24 hours. For patients with hepatic impairment, don't exceed 400 mg/day.

ADMINISTRATION
P.O.
• Give drug without regard for meals but not at the same time as antacids and vitamins.
• Give drug with plenty of fluids.

ACTION
Interferes with DNA gyrase, which is needed for synthesis of bacterial DNA. Spectrum of action includes many gram-positive and gram-negative aerobic bacteria, including *Enterobacteriaceae* and *Pseudomonas aeruginosa.*

Route	Onset	Peak	Duration
P.O.	Unknown	15–120 min	Unknown

Half-life: 4 to 7½ hours.

ADVERSE REACTIONS
CNS: *seizures,* dizziness, drowsiness, fatigue, fever, headache, insomnia, lethargy, malaise, nervousness, sleep disorders, visual disturbances.
CV: chest pain, phlebitis.
GI: *nausea, pseudomembranous colitis,* abdominal pain or discomfort, anorexia, constipation, diarrhea, dry mouth, dysgeusia, flatulence, vomiting.
GU: genital pruritus, glucosuria, hematuria, proteinuria, vaginal discharge, vaginitis.
Hematologic: *leukopenia, neutropenia,* anemia, eosinophilia, leukocytosis.
Metabolic: *hypoglycemia,* hyperglycemia.
Musculoskeletal: body pain, tendon rupture.
Skin: photosensitivity, pruritus, rash.
Other: *anaphylactoid reaction,* hypersensitivity reactions.

INTERACTIONS
Drug-drug. *Aluminum hydroxide, aluminum–magnesium hydroxide, calcium carbonate, magnesium hydroxide:* May decrease effects of ofloxacin. Give antacid at least 6 hours before or 2 hours after ofloxacin.
Antidiabetics: May affect glucose level, causing hypoglycemia or hyperglycemia. Monitor patient closely.
Didanosine (chewable or buffered tablets or pediatric powder for oral solution): May interfere with GI absorption of ofloxacin. Separate doses by 2 hours.
Iron salts: May decrease absorption of ofloxacin, reducing anti-infective response. Separate doses by at least 2 hours.
Sucralfate: May decrease absorption of ofloxacin, reducing anti-infective response. If use together can't be avoided, separate doses by at least 6 hours.
Theophylline: May increase theophylline level. Monitor patient closely and adjust theophylline dosage as needed.
Warfarin: May prolong PT and INR. Monitor PT and INR.
Drug-lifestyle. *Sun exposure:* May cause photosensitivity reactions. Advise patient to avoid excessive sunlight exposure.

EFFECTS ON LAB TEST RESULTS
• May increase BUN, creatinine, and liver enzyme levels. May decrease hemoglobin level and hematocrit. May increase or decrease glucose level.
• May increase erythrocyte sedimentation rate and eosinophil count. May decrease neutrophil count. May increase or decrease WBC count.
• May produce false-positive opioid assay results.

CONTRAINDICATIONS & CAUTIONS
• Contraindicated in patients hypersensitive to drug or other fluoroquinolones.
• Use cautiously in pregnant patients and in those with seizure disorders, CNS diseases, such as cerebral arteriosclerosis, hepatic disorders, or renal impairment.
• Ofloxacin appears in breast milk in levels similar to those found in plasma. Safety hasn't been established in breast-feeding women.
• Safety and efficacy in children younger than age 18 haven't been established.

NURSING CONSIDERATIONS
• *Alert:* Patients treated for gonorrhea should be tested for syphilis. Drug isn't effective against syphilis, and treating

gonorrhea may mask or delay syphilis symptoms.

• Periodically assess organ system functions during prolonged therapy.

• Monitor patient for overgrowth of non-susceptible organisms.

• Monitor renal and hepatic studies and CBC in prolonged therapy.

• Monitor patient for adverse CNS effects, including dizziness, headache, seizures, or depression. Stop drug and notify prescriber if these effects occur.

• Monitor patient for hypersensitivity reactions. Stop drug and initiate supportive therapy, as indicated.

PATIENT TEACHING

• Tell patient to drink plenty of fluids during drug therapy and to finish the entire prescription, even if he starts feeling better.

• Tell patient drug may be taken without regard to meals, but he shouldn't take antacids and vitamins at the same time as ofloxacin.

• Warn patient that dizziness and light-headedness may occur. Advise caution when driving or operating hazardous machinery until effects of drug are known.

• Warn patient that hypersensitivity reactions may follow first dose; he should stop drug at first sign of rash or other allergic reaction and call prescriber immediately.

• Advise patient to avoid prolonged exposure to direct sunlight and to use a sunscreen when outdoors.

---

omalizumab
oh-mah-LIZ-uh-mab

Xolair

Pharmacologic class: DNA-derived humanized immunoglobulin monoclonal antibody
Pregnancy risk category B

AVAILABLE FORMS
Powder for injection: 150 mg in 5-ml vial

INDICATIONS & DOSAGES
➤ **Moderate to severe persistent asthma in patients with positive skin test or in vitro reactivity to a perennial aeroallergen and whose symptoms aren't adequately controlled by inhaled corticosteroids**
Adults and adolescents age 12 and older: 150 to 375 mg subcutaneously every 2 or 4 weeks. Dose and frequency vary with pretreatment immunoglobulin E (IgE) level (international units/ml) and patient weight. Divide doses larger than 150 mg among more than one injection site.

ADMINISTRATION
Subcutaneous
• Prepare with sterile water for injection only.

• The lyophilized product takes 15 to 20 minutes to dissolve.

• The fully reconstituted product will appear clear or slightly opalescent and may have a few small bubbles or foam around the edge of the vial.

• Because the solution is slightly viscous, it may take 5 to 10 seconds to give.

• Use reconstituted solution within 4 hours if at room temperature or within 8 hours if refrigerated.

ACTION
Inhibits binding of IgE to high-affinity receptor, on surface of mast cells and basophils, which limits release of allergic response mediators.

Route	Onset	Peak	Duration
Subcut	Unknown	7–8 days	Unknown

Half-life: About 26 days.

ADVERSE REACTIONS
CNS: *headache,* dizziness, fatigue, pain.
EENT: *pharyngitis, sinusitis,* earache.
Musculoskeletal: arm pain, arthralgia, fracture, leg pain.
Respiratory: *upper respiratory tract infection.*
Skin: *injection site reaction,* dermatitis, pruritus.
Other: *viral infections.*

INTERACTIONS
None reported.

EFFECTS ON LAB TEST RESULTS
• May increase IgE level.

CONTRAINDICATIONS & CAUTIONS
• Contraindicated in patients severely hypersensitive to drug.
• Safety and effectiveness haven't been established in children younger than age 12.
• Drug should be given only in a health care setting under direct medical supervision because of the risk of anaphylaxis.

NURSING CONSIDERATIONS
• *Alert:* Don't use this drug to treat acute bronchospasm or status asthmaticus.
• Don't abruptly stop systemic or inhaled corticosteroid when omalizumab therapy starts; taper the dose gradually and under supervision.
• Injection site reactions may occur, such as bruising, redness, warmth, burning, stinging, itching, hives, pain, induration, and inflammation. Most occur within 1 hour after the injection, last fewer than 8 days, and decrease in frequency with subsequent injections.
• *Alert:* Observe patient for at least 2 hours after the injection, and keep drugs available to respond to anaphylactic reactions. These reactions usually occur within 2 hours of subcutaneous injection; however, delayed reactions may occur up to 24 hours after administration. If the patient has a severe hypersensitivity reaction, stop treatment.
• Drug increases IgE level, so it can't be used to determine appropriate dosage during therapy or for 1 year after therapy ends.
• Patient medication guide must be given with each dose.

PATIENT TEACHING
• Tell patients not to stop or reduce the dosage of any other asthma drugs unless directed by the prescriber. Patient medication guide must be given with each dose.
• Explain that patient may not notice an immediate improvement in asthma after therapy starts.

oseltamivir phosphate
oz-el-TAM-ah-ver

Tamiflu

Pharmacologic class: selective neuraminidase inhibitor
Pregnancy risk category C

AVAILABLE FORMS
Capsules: 30 mg, 45 mg, 75 mg
Oral suspension: 12 mg/ml after reconstitution

INDICATIONS & DOSAGES
➤ **Uncomplicated, acute illness caused by influenza infection in patients who have had symptoms for 2 days or less**
Adults and adolescents age 13 and older: 75 mg P.O. b.i.d. for 5 days.
Children age 1 and older who weigh more than 40 kg (88 lb): 75 mg oral suspension P.O. b.i.d. for 5 days.
Children age 1 and older who weigh 23 to 40 kg (51 to 88 lb): 60 mg oral suspension P.O. b.i.d. for 5 days.
Children age 1 and older who weigh 15 to 23 kg (33 to 51 lb): 45 mg oral suspension P.O. b.i.d. for 5 days.
Children age 1 and older who weigh 15 kg (33 lb) or less: 30 mg oral suspension P.O. b.i.d. for 5 days.
Adjust-a-dose: For adults and adolescents with creatinine clearance of 10 to 30 ml/minute, reduce dosage to 75 mg P.O. once daily for 5 days.
➤ **To prevent influenza after close contact with infected person within 2 days of exposure**
Adults and adolescents age 13 and older: 75 mg P.O. once daily for at least 10 days.
Children age 1 and older who weigh more than 40 kg (88 lb): 75 mg P.O. once daily for 10 days.
Children age 1 and older who weigh 23 to 40 kg (51 to 88 lb): 60 mg P.O. once daily for 10 days.

Children age 1 and older who weigh 15 to 23 kg (33 to 51 lb): 45 mg P.O. once daily for 10 days.

Children age 1 and older who weigh 15 kg (33 lb) or less: 30 mg oral suspension P.O. once daily for 10 days.

Adjust-a-dose: For adults and adolescents with creatinine clearance of 10 to 30 ml/minute, reduce dosage to 75 mg P.O. every other day or 30 mg once daily.

➤ **To prevent influenza during a community outbreak**

Adults and adolescents age 13 and older: 75 mg P.O. once daily for up to 6 weeks.

ADMINISTRATION
P.O.
• Give drug with meals to decrease GI adverse effects.

• Store at controlled room temperature (59° F to 86° F [15° C to 30° C]).

• Capsules may be opened and mixed with sweetened liquids such as chocolate syrup.

ACTION
Inhibits influenza A and B virus enzyme neuraminidase, which is thought to play a role in viral particle aggregation and release from the host cell and appears to interfere with viral replication.

Route	Onset	Peak	Duration
P.O.	Unknown	Unknown	Unknown

Half-life: 1 to 10 hours.

ADVERSE REACTIONS
CNS: dizziness, fatigue, headache, insomnia, vertigo.
GI: abdominal pain, diarrhea, nausea, vomiting.
Respiratory: bronchitis, cough.

INTERACTIONS
None significant.

EFFECTS ON LAB TEST RESULTS
None reported.

CONTRAINDICATIONS & CAUTIONS
• Contraindicated in patients hypersensitive to drug or its components.

• Use cautiously in patients with chronic cardiac or respiratory diseases, or any medical condition that may require imminent hospitalization. Also use cautiously in patients with renal failure.

• It's unknown if drug or its metabolite appears in breast milk. Use only if benefits to patient outweigh risks to infant.

NURSING CONSIDERATIONS
• Drug must be given within 2 days of onset of symptoms.

• Safety and effectiveness of repeated treatment courses haven't been established.

PATIENT TEACHING
• Instruct patient to begin treatment as soon as possible after appearance of flu symptoms.

• Inform patient that drug may be taken with or without meals. If nausea or vomiting occurs, he can take drug with food or milk.

• Tell patient that, if a dose is missed, he should take it as soon as possible. However, if next dose is due within 2 hours, tell him to skip the missed dose and take the next dose on schedule.

• Advise patient to complete the full course of treatment, even if symptoms resolve.

• Alert patient that drug isn't a replacement for the annual influenza vaccination. Patients for whom vaccine is indicated should continue to receive the vaccine each fall.

---

paroxetine hydrochloride
pah-ROX-a-teen

Paxil, Paxil CR

Pharmacologic class: SSRI
Pregnancy risk category D

AVAILABLE FORMS
Suspension: 10 mg/5 ml
Tablets: 10 mg, 20 mg, 30 mg, 40 mg
Tablets (controlled-release): 12.5 mg, 25 mg, 37.5 mg

INDICATIONS & DOSAGES
➤ **Depression**
Adults: Initially, 20 mg P.O. daily, preferably in morning, as indicated. If patient doesn't improve, increase dose by 10 mg daily at intervals of at least 1 week to a

---

maximum of 50 mg daily. If using controlled-release form, initially, 25 mg P.O. daily. Increase dose by 12.5 mg daily at weekly intervals to a maximum of 62.5 mg daily.
Elderly patients: Initially, 10 mg P.O. daily, preferably in morning, as indicated. If patient doesn't improve, increase dose by 10 mg daily at weekly intervals, to a maximum of 40 mg daily. If using controlled-release form, start therapy at 12.5 mg P.O. daily. Don't exceed 50 mg daily.

➤ **Obsessive-compulsive disorder (OCD)**
Adults: Initially, 20 mg P.O. daily, preferably in morning. Increase dose by 10 mg daily at weekly intervals. Recommended daily dose is 40 mg. Maximum daily dose is 60 mg.

➤ **Panic disorder**
Adults: Initially, 10 mg P.O. daily. Increase dose by 10 mg at no less than weekly intervals to maximum of 60 mg daily. Or, 12.5 mg Paxil CR P.O. as a single daily dose, usually in the morning, with or without food; increase dose at intervals of at least 1 week by 12.5 mg daily, up to a maximum of 75 mg daily.
Adjust-a-dose: In elderly or debilitated patients and in those with severe renal or hepatic impairment, the first dose of Paxil CR is 12.5 mg daily; increase if indicated. Dosage shouldn't exceed 50 mg daily.

➤ **Social anxiety disorder**
Adults: Initially, 20 mg P.O. daily, preferably in morning. Dosage range is 20 to 60 mg daily. Adjust dosage to maintain patient on lowest effective dose. Or, 12.5 mg Paxil CR P.O. as a single daily dose, usually in the morning, with or without food. Increase dosage at weekly intervals in increments of 12.5 mg daily, up to a maximum of 37.5 mg daily.

➤ **Generalized anxiety disorder**
Adults: 20 mg P.O. daily initially, increasing by 10 mg per day weekly up to 50 mg daily.
Adjust-a-dose: For debilitated patients or those with renal or hepatic impairment taking immediate-release form, initially, 10 mg P.O. daily, preferably in morning. If patient doesn't respond after full antidepressant effect has occurred, increase dose by 10 mg per day at weekly intervals to a maximum of 40 mg daily. If using

controlled-release form, start therapy at 12.5 mg daily. Don't exceed 50 mg daily.

➤ **Posttraumatic stress disorder**
Adults: Initially, 20 mg P.O. daily. Increase dose by 10 mg daily at intervals of at least 1 week. Maximum daily dose is 50 mg P.O.

➤ **Premenstrual dysphoric disorder (PMDD)**
Adults: Initially, 12.5 mg Paxil CR P.O. as a single daily dose, usually in the morning, with or without food, daily or during the luteal phase of the menstrual cycle. Dose changes should occur at intervals of at least 1 week. Maximum dose is 25 mg P.O. daily.

➤ **Premature ejaculation ♦**
Adults: 10 to 40 mg P.O. daily. Or, 20 mg P.O. as needed 3 to 4 hours before planned intercourse.

➤ **Diabetic neuropathy ♦**
Adults: 40 mg P.O. daily.

ADMINISTRATION
P.O.
• Give drug without regard for food.
• Don't split or crush controlled-release tablets.

ACTION
Thought to be linked to drug's inhibition of CNS neuronal uptake of serotonin.

Route	Onset	Peak	Duration
P.O.	Unknown	2–8 hr	Unknown
P.O. (controlled-release)	Unknown	6–10 hr	Unknown

Half-life: About 24 hours.

ADVERSE REACTIONS
CNS: *asthenia, dizziness, headache, insomnia, somnolence, tremor, nervousness,* **suicidal behavior,** anxiety, paresthesia, confusion, agitation.
CV: palpitations, vasodilation, orthostatic hypotension.
EENT: lump or tightness in throat.
GI: *dry mouth, nausea, constipation, diarrhea,* flatulence, vomiting, dyspepsia, dysgeusia, increased or decreased appetite, abdominal pain.
GU: *ejaculatory disturbances, sexual dysfunction,* urinary frequency, other urinary disorders.

Musculoskeletal: myopathy, myalgia, myasthenia.
Skin: *diaphoresis,* rash, pruritus.
Other: *decreased libido,* yawning.

INTERACTIONS

Drug-drug. *Amphetamines, buspirone, dextromethorphan, dihydroergotamine, lithium salts, meperidine, other SSRIs or SSNRIs (duloxetine, venlafaxine),* **tramadol,** *trazodone, tricyclic antidepressants, tryptophan:* May increase the risk of serotonin syndrome. Avoid combining drugs that increase the availability of serotonin in the CNS; monitor patient closely if used together.
Cimetidine: May decrease hepatic metabolism of paroxetine, leading to risk of adverse reactions. Dosage adjustments may be needed.
Digoxin: May decrease digoxin level. Use together cautiously.
MAO inhibitors, such as phenelzine, selegiline, tranylcypromine: May cause serotonin syndrome. Avoid using within 14 days of MAO inhibitor therapy.
Phenobarbital, phenytoin: May alter pharmacokinetics of both drugs. Dosage adjustments may be needed.
Procyclidine: May increase procyclidine level. Watch for excessive anticholinergic effects.
Sumatriptan: May cause weakness, hyperreflexia, and incoordination. Monitor patient closely.
Theophylline: May decrease theophylline clearance. Monitor theophylline level.
Thioridazine: May prolong QTc interval and increase risk of serious ventricular arrhythmias, such as torsades de pointes, and sudden death. Avoid using together.
Tricyclic antidepressants: May inhibit tricyclic antidepressant metabolism. Dose of tricyclic antidepressant may need to be reduced. Monitor patient closely.
Triptans: May cause serotonin syndrome (restlessness, hallucinations, loss of coordination, fast heartbeat, rapid changes in blood pressure, increased body temperature, overactive reflexes, nausea, vomiting, and diarrhea). Use cautiously, especially at the start of therapy and at dosage increases.
Warfarin: May cause bleeding. Use together cautiously.

Drug-herb. *St. John's wort:* May increase sedative-hypnotic effects. Discourage use together.
Drug-lifestyle. *Alcohol use:* May alter psychomotor function. Discourage use together.

EFFECTS ON LAB TEST RESULTS
None reported.

CONTRAINDICATIONS & CAUTIONS
• Contraindicated in patients hypersensitive to drug, within 14 days of MAO inhibitor therapy, and in those taking thioridazine.
• Contraindicated in children and adolescents younger than age 18 for major depressive disorders.
• Use cautiously in patients with history of seizure disorders or mania and in those with other severe, systemic illness.
• Use cautiously in patients at risk for volume depletion and monitor them appropriately.
• Using drug in the first trimester may increase the risk of congenital fetal malformations; using drug in the third trimester may cause neonatal complications at birth. Consider the risk versus benefit of therapy.

NURSING CONSIDERATIONS
• Patients taking drug may be at increased risk for developing suicidal behavior, but this hasn't been definitively attributed to use of the drug.
• Patients taking Paxil CR for PMDD should be periodically reassessed to determine the need for continued treatment.
• If signs or symptoms of psychosis occur or increase, expect prescriber to reduce dosage. Record mood changes. Monitor patient for suicidal tendencies, and allow only a minimum supply of drug.
• *Alert:* Drug may increase the risk of suicidal thinking and behavior in children, adolescents, and young adults ages 18 to 24 during the first 2 months of treatment, especially in those with major depressive disorder or other psychiatric disorder.
• Monitor patient for complaints of sexual dysfunction. In men, they include anorgasmy, erectile difficulties, delayed ejaculation or orgasm, or impotence; in women, they include anorgasmia or difficulty with orgasm.

• *Alert:* Don't stop drug abruptly. Withdrawal or discontinuation syndrome may occur if drug is stopped abruptly. Symptoms include headache, myalgia, lethargy, and general flulike symptoms. Taper drug slowly over 1 to 2 weeks.

• *Alert:* Combining triptans with an SSRI or an SSNRI may cause serotonin syndrome. Signs and symptoms may include restlessness, hallucinations, loss of coordination, fast heartbeat, rapid changes in blood pressure, increased body temperature, overactive reflexes, nausea, vomiting, and diarrhea. Serotonin syndrome may be more likely to occur when starting or increasing the dose of triptan, SSRI, or SSNRI.

• *Look alike–sound alike:* Don't confuse paroxetine with paclitaxel, or Paxil with Doxil, paclitaxel, Plavix, or Taxol.

PATIENT TEACHING

• Tell patient that drug may be taken with or without food, usually in morning.

• Tell patient not to break, crush, or chew controlled-release tablets.

• Warn patient to avoid activities that require alertness and good coordination until effects of drug are known.

• Advise woman of childbearing age to contact prescriber if she becomes pregnant or plans to become pregnant during therapy or if she's currently breast-feeding.

• Tell patient to avoid alcohol and to consult prescriber before taking other prescription or OTC drugs or herbal medicines.

• Instruct patient not to stop taking drug abruptly.

SAFETY ALERT!

pemetrexed
peh-meh-TREX-ed

Alimta

Pharmacologic class: folate antagonist
Pregnancy risk category D

AVAILABLE FORMS
Injection: 500 mg in single-use vials

INDICATIONS & DOSAGES

➤ **Malignant pleural mesothelioma, with cisplatin, in patients whose disease is unresectable or who aren't candidates for surgery**
Adults: 500 mg/m^2 I.V. over 10 minutes on day 1 of each 21-day cycle. Starting 30 minutes after pemetrexed infusion ends, give cisplatin 75 mg/m^2 I.V. over 2 hours.

➤ **Locally advanced or metastatic non–small-cell lung cancer after chemotherapy**
Adults: 500 mg/m^2 I.V. over 10 minutes on day 1 of each 21-day cycle.

Adjust-a-dose: In patients who develop toxic reactions, adjust dosage according to the table.

Toxic reaction	Dosage change
– Grade 3 (severe or undesirable) or grade 4 (life-threatening or disabling) diarrhea	Give 75% of previous pemetrexed and cisplatin doses.
– Diarrhea that warrants hospitalization	
– Any grade 3 toxicity (except mucositis and increased transaminase levels)	
– Any grade 4 toxicity (except mucositis)	
– Platelet count $\geq$ 50,000/mm^3 and absolute neutrophil count < 500/mm^3	
Platelet count < 50,000/mm^3	Give 50% of previous pemetrexed and cisplatin doses.
Grade 3 or 4 mucositis	Give 50% of previous pemetrexed dose and 100% of previous cisplatin dose.
Grade 2 (moderate) neurotoxicity	Give 100% of previous pemetrexed dose and 50% of previous cisplatin dose.
– Grade 3 or 4 neurotoxicity	Stop therapy.
– Any grade 3 or 4 toxicity (except increased transaminase levels) present after two dose reductions	

ADMINISTRATION
I.V.
● Reconstitute 500-mg vial with 20 ml of preservative-free normal saline solution to yield 25 mg/ml.
● Swirl vial gently until powder is completely dissolved. Solution should be clear and colorless to yellow or yellow-green.
● Calculate appropriate dose, and further dilute with 100 ml normal saline solution.
● Give over 10 minutes.
● Reconstituted solution and dilution are stable for 24 hours refrigerated or at room temperature.
● **Incompatibilities:** Calcium-containing diluents including Ringer's or lactated Ringer's for injection; other drugs or diluents.

ACTION
Disturbs cell replication by inhibiting several folate-dependent enzymes involved in nucleotide synthesis. When given with other antineoplastics, drug inhibits growth of mesothelioma cell lines.

Route	Onset	Peak	Duration
I.V.	Unknown	Unknown	Unknown

Half-life: 3½ hours.

ADVERSE REACTIONS
CNS: *depression, fatigue, fever, neuropathy.*
CV: *cardiac ischemia,* *chest pain, edema,* ***emboli,*** *thrombosis.*
EENT: *pharyngitis.*
GI: *anorexia, constipation, diarrhea, nausea, stomatitis, vomiting,* esophagitis, painful, difficult swallowing.
GU: *renal failure.*
Hematologic: *anemia,* LEUKOPENIA, NEUTROPENIA, THROMBOCYTOPENIA.
Metabolic: dehydration.
Musculoskeletal: arthralgia, *myalgia.*
Respiratory: *dyspnea.*
Skin: *alopecia, rash.*
Other: allergic reaction, *infection.*

INTERACTIONS
Drug-drug. *Nephrotoxic drugs, probenecid:* May delay pemetrexed clearance. Monitor patient.
NSAIDs: May decrease pemetrexed clearance in patients with mild to moderate renal insufficiency. For NSAIDs with short half-lives, avoid use for 2 days before, during, and 2 days after pemetrexed therapy. For NSAIDs with long half-lives, avoid use for 5 days before, during, and 2 days after pemetrexed therapy.

EFFECTS ON LAB TEST RESULTS
● May increase ALT, AST, and creatinine levels. May decrease hemoglobin level and hematocrit.
● May decrease absolute neutrophil, platelet, and WBC counts.

CONTRAINDICATIONS & CAUTIONS
● Contraindicated in patients with a history of severe hypersensitivity reaction to drug or its ingredients. Don't use in patients with creatinine clearance less than 45 ml/minute.

NURSING CONSIDERATIONS
● Patient shouldn't start a new cycle of treatment unless absolute neutrophil count is 1,500 cells/mm^3 or more, platelet count is 100,000 cells/mm^3 or more, and creatinine clearance is 45 ml/minute or more.
● Patients with pleural effusion and ascites may need to have effusion drained before therapy.
● Monitor renal function, CBC, platelet count, hemoglobin level, hematocrit, and liver function test values.
● Assess patient for neurotoxicity, mucositis, and diarrhea. Severe symptoms may warrant dosage adjustment.
● *Alert:* To reduce the occurrence and severity of cutaneous reactions, give a corticosteroid, such as dexamethasone 4 mg P.O. b.i.d., the day before, the day of, and the day after giving this drug.
● *Alert:* To reduce toxicity, patient should take 350 to 1,000 mcg of folic acid daily, 5 days before therapy until 21 days after therapy.
● *Alert:* Give vitamin B$_{12}$ 1,000 mcg I.M. once during the week before the first dose and every three cycles thereafter. After the first cycle, vitamin injections may be given on the first day of the cycle.

PATIENT TEACHING
● Inform patient that he may receive corticosteroids and vitamins before pemetrexed to help minimize its adverse effects.

• Tell patient to avoid NSAIDs for several days before, during, and after treatment.
• Urge patient to report adverse effects, especially fever, sore throat, infection, diarrhea, fatigue, and limb pain.
• It's unknown if drug appears in breast milk. Advise patient to stop breast-feeding during treatment.

penicillin G benzathine (benzathine benzylpenicillin)

pen-i-SILL-in

Bicillin L-A, Permapen

Pharmacologic class: natural penicillin
Pregnancy risk category B

AVAILABLE FORMS

Injection: 600,000 units/ml; 1.2 million units/2 ml; 2.4 million units/4 ml

INDICATIONS & DOSAGES

➤ Congenital syphilis
Children younger than age 2: 50,000 units/kg (up to 2.4 million units) I.M. as a single dose.

➤ Group A streptococcal upper respiratory tract infections
Adults: 1.2 million units I.M. as a single injection.
Children who weigh 27 kg (59.5 lb) or more: 900,000 units I.M. as a single injection.
Children who weigh less than 27 kg: 300,000 to 600,000 units I.M. as a single injection.

➤ To prevent poststreptococcal rheumatic fever
Adults and children: 1.2 million units I.M. once monthly or 600,000 units I.M. every 2 weeks.

➤ Syphilis of less than 1 year duration
Adults: 2.4 million units I.M. as a single dose.
Children: 50,000 units/kg I.M. as a single dose. Don't exceed adult dosage.

➤ Syphilis of more than 1 year duration
Adults: 2.4 million units I.M. weekly for 3 weeks.
Children: 50,000 units/kg I.M. weekly for 3 weeks. Don't exceed adult dosage.

ADMINISTRATION

I.M.
• Before giving drug, ask patient about allergic reactions to penicillin.
• Obtain specimen for culture and sensitivity tests before giving first dose. Begin therapy while awaiting results.
• Shake well before injecting.
• Give drug at least 1 hour before a bacteriostatic antibiotic.
• Inject deep into upper outer quadrant of buttocks in adults and in midlateral thigh in infants and small children. Rotate injection sites. Avoid injection into or near major nerves or blood vessels to prevent permanent neurovascular damage.
• Injection may be painful, but ice applied to the site may ease discomfort.

ACTION

Inhibits cell-wall synthesis during bacterial multiplication.

Route	Onset	Peak	Duration
I.M.	Unknown	13–24 hr	1–4 wk

Half-life: 30 to 60 minutes.

ADVERSE REACTIONS

CNS: ***seizures,*** agitation, anxiety, confusion, depression, dizziness, fatigue, hallucinations, lethargy, neuropathy, pain.
GI: ***pseudomembranous colitis,*** enterocolitis, nausea, vomiting.
GU: interstitial nephritis, nephropathy.
Hematologic: ***agranulocytosis, leukopenia, thrombocytopenia,*** anemia, eosinophilia, hemolytic anemia.
Skin: exfoliative dermatitis, maculopapular rash.
Other: ***anaphylaxis,*** hypersensitivity reactions, sterile abscess at injection site.

INTERACTIONS

Drug-drug. *Aminoglycosides:* Physical and chemical incompatibility. Give separately.
Colestipol: May decrease penicillin G benzathine level. Give penicillin G benzathine 1 hour before or 4 hours after colestipol.
Hormonal contraceptives: May decrease hormonal contraceptive effectiveness.

Advise use of additional form of contraception during therapy.
Probenecid: May increase penicillin level. Probenecid may be used for this purpose.
Tetracycline: May antagonize penicillin G benzathine effects. Avoid using together.

EFFECTS ON LAB TEST RESULTS
• May decrease hemoglobin level.
• May increase eosinophil count. May decrease platelet, WBC, and granulocyte counts. May cause positive Coombs' test results.
• May falsely decrease aminoglycoside level. May cause false-positive CSF protein test results. May alter urine glucose testing using cupric sulfate (Benedict's reagent).

CONTRAINDICATIONS & CAUTIONS
• Contraindicated in patients hypersensitive to drug or other penicillins.
• Use cautiously in patients allergic to other drugs, especially to cephalosporins, because of possible cross-sensitivity.

NURSING CONSIDERATIONS
• *Alert:* Bicillin L-A is the only penicillin G benzathine product indicated for sexually transmitted infections. Don't substitute Bicillin C-R because it may not be effective.
• *Alert:* Inadvertent I.V. use may cause cardiac arrest and death. Never give I.V.
• Drug's extremely slow absorption time makes allergic reactions difficult to treat.
• If large doses are given or if therapy is prolonged, bacterial or fungal superinfection may occur, especially in elderly, debilitated, or immunosuppressed patients.
• *Look alike–sound alike:* Don't confuse drug with Polycillin, penicillamine, or the various types of penicillin.

PATIENT TEACHING
• Tell patient to report adverse reactions promptly.
• Inform patient that fever and increased WBC count are the most common reactions.
• Warn patient that I.M. injection may be painful but that ice applied to the site may ease discomfort.

---

pentoxifylline
pen-tox-IH-fi-leen

Trental

Pharmacologic class: xanthine derivative
Pregnancy risk category C

AVAILABLE FORMS
Tablets (extended-release): 400 mg

INDICATIONS & DOSAGES
➤ **Intermittent claudication from chronic occlusive vascular disease**
Adults: 400 mg P.O. t.i.d. with meals. May decrease to 400 mg b.i.d. if GI and CNS adverse effects occur.

ADMINISTRATION
P.O.
• Give drug whole; don't crush or split tablet.
• Give drug with meals to minimize GI upset.

ACTION
Unknown. Improves capillary blood flow, probably by increasing RBC flexibility and lowering blood viscosity.

Route	Onset	Peak	Duration
P.O.	Unknown	1 hr	Unknown

Half-life: About 30 to 45 minutes.

ADVERSE REACTIONS
CNS: dizziness, headache.
GI: dyspepsia, nausea, vomiting.

INTERACTIONS
Drug-drug. *Anticoagulants:* May increase anticoagulant effect. Monitor PT.
Antihypertensives: May increase hypotensive effect. May need to adjust dosage.
Theophylline: May increase theophylline level. Monitor patient closely.
Drug-lifestyle. *Smoking:* May cause vasoconstriction. Advise patient to avoid smoking.

EFFECTS ON LAB TEST RESULTS
None reported.

CONTRAINDICATIONS & CAUTIONS
• Contraindicated in patients intolerant to this drug or to methylxanthines, such as caffeine, theophylline, and theobromine, and in those with recent cerebral or retinal hemorrhage.

NURSING CONSIDERATIONS
• Drug is useful in patients who aren't good surgical candidates.
• Elderly patients may be more sensitive to drug's effects.
• *Look alike–sound alike:* Don't confuse Trental with Trandate.

PATIENT TEACHING
• Advise patient to take drug with meals to minimize GI upset.
• Instruct patient to swallow tablet whole, without breaking, crushing, or chewing.
• Tell patient to report GI or CNS adverse reactions; prescriber may reduce dosage.
• Urge patient not to stop drug during the first 8 weeks of therapy unless directed by prescriber.

SAFETY ALERT!

phenylephrine hydrochloride
fen-ill-EF-rin

Neo-Synephrine

Pharmacologic class: adrenergic
Pregnancy risk category C

AVAILABLE FORMS
Injection: 10 mg/ml (1%)

INDICATIONS & DOSAGES
➤ **Hypotensive emergencies during spinal anesthesia**
Adults: 0.2 mg I.V.; subsequent doses should be no more than 0.1 to 0.2 mg over the previous dose; don't exceed 0.5 mg in a single dose.
Children: 0.044 to 0.088 mg/kg I.M. or subcutaneously.
➤ **Prevention of hypotension during spinal anesthesia**
Adults: 2 to 3 mg I.M. or subcutaneously 3 to 4 minutes before injection of spinal anesthesia.

➤ **To prolong spinal anesthesia**
Adults: 2 to 5 mg added to anesthetic solution.
➤ **Vasoconstrictor for regional anesthesia**
Adults: 1 mg phenylephrine added to each 20 ml local anesthetic.
➤ **Mild to moderate hypotension**
Adults: 2 to 5 mg I.M. (dose ranges from 1 to 10 mg) or subcutaneously; repeat in 1 or 2 hours as needed and tolerated. First dose shouldn't exceed 5 mg. Or, 0.1 to 0.5 mg slow I.V., not to be repeated more often than 10 to 15 minutes.
Children: 0.1 mg/kg or 3 mg/m^2 I.M. or subcutaneously; repeat in 1 or 2 hours as needed and tolerated.
➤ **Severe hypotension and shock (including drug-induced)**
Adults: 10 mg in 250 to 500 ml of D_5W or normal saline solution for injection. I.V. infusion started at 100 to 180 mcg/minute; then decrease to maintenance infusion of 40 to 60 mcg/minute when blood pressure stabilizes.
➤ **Paroxysmal supraventricular tachycardia**
Adults: Initially, 0.5 mg rapid I.V.; increase in increments of 0.1 to 0.2 mg. Use cautiously. Maximum single dose is 1 mg.

ADMINISTRATION
I.V.
• For direct injection, dilute 10 mg (1 ml) with 9 ml sterile water for injection to provide 1 mg/ml. Infusions are usually prepared by adding 10 mg of drug to 500 ml of D_5W or normal saline solution for injection. The first I.V. infusion rate is usually 100 to 180 mcg/minute; maintenance rate is usually 40 to 60 mcg/minute.
• Use a central venous catheter or large vein, as in the antecubital fossa, to minimize risk of extravasation. Use a continuous infusion pump to regulate infusion flow rate.
• During infusion, frequently monitor ECG, blood pressure, cardiac output, central venous pressure, pulmonary artery wedge pressure, pulse rate, urine output, and color and temperature of limbs. Titrate infusion rate according to findings and prescriber guidelines. Maintain blood pressure slightly below patient's normal level. In previously normotensive patients,

maintain systolic blood pressure at 80 to
100 mm Hg; in previously hypertensive
patients, maintain systolic blood pressure
at 30 to 40 mm Hg below usual level.
• Avoid abrupt withdrawal after prolonged
I.V. infusions.
• To treat extravasation, infiltrate site
promptly with 10 to 15 ml of normal
saline solution for injection containing 5 to
10 mg phentolamine. Use a fine needle.
• **Incompatibilities:** Alkaline solutions,
iron salts, other metals, phenytoin sodium,
thiopental sodium.
I.M.
• Don't give drug if solution is discolored
or has particulate matter.
• Document injection site.
• Discard unused solution.
Subcutaneous
• Don't give drug if solution is discolored
or has particulate matter.
• Document injection site.
• Discard unused solution.

ACTION
Stimulates alpha receptors in the sympathetic nervous system, causing vasoconstriction.

Route	Onset	Peak	Duration
I.V.	Immediate	Unknown	15–20 min
I.M.	10–15 min	Unknown	30–120 min
Subcut	10–15 min	Unknown	50–60 min

Half-life: 2 to 3 hours.

ADVERSE REACTIONS
CNS: *headache,* excitability, restlessness,
anxiety, nervousness, dizziness, weakness.
CV: *bradycardia, arrhythmias,* hyperten-
sion.
Respiratory: *asthmatic episodes.*
Skin: tissue sloughing with extravasation.
Other: *anaphylaxis,* tachyphylaxis and
decreased organ perfusion with continued
use.

INTERACTIONS
Drug-drug. *Alpha blockers, phenothi-
azines:* May decrease pressor response.
Monitor patient closely.
Atropine, guanethidine, oxytocics: May
increase pressor response. Monitor patient.
Beta blockers: May block cardiostimula-
tion. Monitor patient closely.

*Halogenated hydrocarbon anesthetics,
sympathomimetics:* May cause serious
arrhythmias. Use together with caution.
*MAO inhibitors (phenelzine, tranyl-
cypromine):* May cause severe headache,
hypertension, fever, and hypertensive
crisis. Avoid using together.
Tricyclic antidepressants: May potentiate
pressor response and cause arrhythmias.
Use together cautiously.

EFFECTS ON LAB TEST RESULTS
• May cause false-normal tonometry
reading.

CONTRAINDICATIONS & CAUTIONS
• Contraindicated in patients hypersensitive to drug and in those with severe
hypertension or ventricular tachycardia.
• Use with caution in elderly patients and
in patients with heart disease, hyperthyroidism, severe atherosclerosis, bradycardia, partial heart block, myocardial
disease, or sulfite sensitivity.

NURSING CONSIDERATIONS
• Drug causes little or no CNS stimulation.
• Drug may lower intraocular pressure in
normal eyes or in open-angle glaucoma.
• Drug is used in OTC eyedrops and cold
preparations for decongestant effects.

PATIENT TEACHING
• Tell patient to report adverse reactions
promptly.
• Instruct patient to report discomfort at
I.V. insertion site.

pirbuterol acetate
peer-BYOO-ter-ole

Maxair Autohaler

Pharmacologic class: beta₂ agonist
Pregnancy risk category C

AVAILABLE FORMS
Inhaler: 0.2 mg/metered dose

INDICATIONS & DOSAGES
➤ **To prevent and reverse bronchospasm; asthma**
Adults and children age 12 and older: 1
or 2 inhalations (0.2 to 0.4 mg), repeated

every 4 to 6 hours. Don't exceed 12 inhalations daily.

ADMINISTRATION
Inhalational
● If more than one inhalation is ordered, wait 1 minute between inhalations.
● Have patient hold his breath for 10 seconds after inhalation, then exhale slowly.
● Give corticosteroid inhaler 5 minutes after bronchodilator.

ACTION
Relaxes bronchial smooth muscle by stimulating beta$_2$ receptors.

Route	Onset	Peak	Duration
Inhalation	5 min	30–60 min	5 hr

Half-life: About 2 hours.

ADVERSE REACTIONS
CNS: tremor, nervousness, dizziness, insomnia, headache, vertigo.
CV: tachycardia, palpitations, chest tightness.
EENT: dry or irritated throat.
GI: nausea, vomiting, diarrhea, dry mouth.
Respiratory: cough.

INTERACTIONS
Drug-drug. *Beta blockers, propranolol:* May decrease bronchodilating effects. Avoid using together.
MAO inhibitors, tricyclic antidepressants: May potentiate action of beta agonist on vascular system. Use together cautiously.

EFFECTS ON LAB TEST RESULTS
None reported.

CONTRAINDICATIONS & CAUTIONS
● Contraindicated in patients hypersensitive to drug.
● Use cautiously in patients unusually responsive to sympathomimetic amines and patients with CV disorders, hyperthyroidism, diabetes, and seizure disorders.

NURSING CONSIDERATIONS
● Monitor patient for increased pulse or blood pressure during therapy.

● Stop drug immediately and notify prescriber if paradoxical bronchospasm occurs.
● The likelihood of paradoxical bronchospasm is increased with the first use of a new canister.
● Notify prescriber of decreasing effectiveness of the drug.

PATIENT TEACHING
● Give the following instructions for using Autohaler:
−Remove mouthpiece cover by pulling down lip on back cover. Inspect mouthpiece for foreign objects. Locate "Up" arrows and air vents.
−Hold Autohaler upright so that arrows point up; raise lever until it snaps into place.
−Hold Autohaler around the middle, and shake gently several times.
−Continue to hold upright, and be careful not to block air vents at bottom. Exhale normally before use.
−Seal lips around mouthpiece. Inhale deeply through mouthpiece with steady, moderate force to trigger release of the drug. You'll hear a click and feel a soft puff when drug is released. Continue to take a full, deep breath.
−Take Autohaler away from mouth when done inhaling. Hold breath for 10 seconds; then exhale slowly.
−Continue to hold Autohaler upright while lowering lever. Lower lever after each puff. If additional puffs are ordered, wait 1 minute before repeating process to obtain the next puff.
● Have patient clean inhaler per manufacturer's instructions.
● If patient also uses a corticosteroid inhaler, tell him to use the bronchodilator first, and then wait about 5 minutes before using the corticosteroid. This allows the bronchodilator to open air passages for maximal effectiveness of the corticosteroid.
● Instruct patient to call prescriber if bronchospasm increases after using drug.
● Advise patient to seek medical attention if a previously effective dosage doesn't control symptoms; this may signal worsening of disease.

prednisone
PRED-ni-sone

Deltasone, Liquid Pred*,
Meticorten, Orasone, Panasol-S,
Prednicen-M, Prednisone
Intensol*, Sterapred, Sterapred
DS, Winpred†

Pharmacologic class: adrenocorticoid
Pregnancy risk category C

AVAILABLE FORMS
Oral solution: 5 mg/5 ml*, 5 mg/ml
(concentrate)*
Syrup: 5 mg/5 ml*
Tablet: 1 mg, 2.5 mg, 5 mg, 10 mg, 20 mg,
50 mg
Tablet (film-coated): 5 mg

INDICATIONS & DOSAGES
➤ **Severe inflammation, immuno-suppression**
Adults: 5 to 60 mg P.O. daily in single dose
or as two to four divided doses. Maintenance dose given once daily or every other
day. Dosage must be individualized.
Children: 0.14 to 2 mg/kg or 4 to
60 mg/m² daily P.O. in four divided doses.
➤ **Contact dermatitis; poison ivy**
Adults: Initially, 30 mg (six 5-mg tablets);
taper by 5 mg daily until 21 tablets have
been given.
➤ **Acute exacerbations of multiple sclerosis**
Adults: 200 mg P.O. daily for 7 days; then
80 mg P.O. every other day for 1 month.
➤ **Advanced pulmonary tuberculosis**
Adults: 40 to 60 mg P.O. daily; taper over 4
to 8 weeks.
➤ **Tuberculosis meningitis**
Adults: 1 mg/kg P.O. daily for 30 days;
taper over several weeks.
➤ **Adjunctive treatment in *Pneumocystis carinii* pneumonia in patients with AIDS** ◆
Adults and children age 13 and older:
40 mg P.O. b.i.d. for 5 days; then 40 mg
P.O. daily for 5 days; then 20 mg P.O.
daily for 11 days or until completion of
anti-infective therapy.

ADMINISTRATION
P.O.
● Unless contraindicated, give drug with
food to reduce GI irritation. Patient may
need another drug to prevent GI irritation.
● Solution may be diluted in juice or other
flavored diluent or semisolid food such as
applesauce before using.

ACTION
Not clearly defined. Decreases inflammation, mainly by stabilizing leukocyte
lysosomal membranes; suppresses immune
response; stimulates bone marrow; and
influences protein, fat, and carbohydrate
metabolism.

Route	Onset	Peak	Duration
P.O.	Variable	Variable	Variable

Half-life: 18 to 36 hours.

ADVERSE REACTIONS
CNS: *euphoria, insomnia,* psychotic
behavior, *pseudotumor cerebri,* vertigo,
headache, paresthesia, *seizures.*
CV: *heart failure,* hypertension, edema,
arrhythmias, thrombophlebitis, *thromboembolism.*
EENT: cataracts, glaucoma.
GI: *peptic ulceration, pancreatitis,* GI
irritation, increased appetite, nausea,
vomiting.
GU: menstrual irregularities, increased
urine calcium level.
Metabolic: hypokalemia, hyperglycemia,
carbohydrate intolerance, hypercholesterolemia, hypocalcemia.
Musculoskeletal: growth suppression in
children, muscle weakness, osteoporosis.
Skin: hirsutism, delayed wound healing,
acne, various skin eruptions.
Other: cushingoid state, susceptibility to
infections, *acute adrenal insufficiency,*
after increased stress or abrupt withdrawal
after long-term therapy.
After abrupt withdrawal: rebound inflammation, fatigue, weakness, arthralgia,
fever, dizziness, lethargy, depression,
fainting, orthostatic hypotension, dyspnea,
anorexia, *hypoglycemia. After prolonged
use, sudden withdrawal may be fatal.*

INTERACTIONS

Drug-drug. *Aspirin, indomethacin, other NSAIDs:* May increase risk of GI distress and bleeding. Use together cautiously.
Barbiturates, carbamazepine, fosphenytoin, phenytoin, rifampin: May decrease corticosteroid effect. Increase corticosteroid dosage.
Cyclosporine: May increase toxicity and cause seizures. Monitor patient closely.
Oral anticoagulants: May alter dosage requirements. Monitor PT and INR closely.
Potassium-depleting drugs, such as thiazide diuretics and amphotericin B: May enhance potassium-wasting effects of prednisone. Monitor potassium level.
Salicylates: May decrease salicylate level. Monitor patient for lack of salicylate effectiveness.
Skin-test antigens: May decrease response. Postpone skin testing until therapy is completed.
Toxoids, vaccines: May decrease antibody response and may increase risk of neurologic complications. Avoid using together.

EFFECTS ON LAB TEST RESULTS

● May increase glucose and cholesterol levels. May decrease T_3, T_4, potassium, and calcium levels.
● May decrease ^{131}I uptake and protein-bound iodine values in thyroid function tests. May cause false-negative results in nitroblue tetrazolium test for systemic bacterial infections. May alter reactions to skin tests.

CONTRAINDICATIONS & CAUTIONS

● Contraindicated in patients hypersensitive to drug or its ingredients, in those with systemic fungal infections, and in those receiving immunosuppressive doses together with live-virus vaccines.
● Use cautiously in patients with recent MI, GI ulcer, renal disease, hypertension, osteoporosis, diabetes mellitus, hypothyroidism, cirrhosis, active hepatitis, diverticulitis, nonspecific ulcerative colitis, recent intestinal anastomoses, thromboembolic disorders, seizures, myasthenia gravis, heart failure, tuberculosis, ocular herpes simplex, emotional instability, and psychotic tendencies or in breast-feeding women.

NURSING CONSIDERATIONS

● Determine whether patient is sensitive to other corticosteroids.
● Drug may be used for alternate-day therapy.
● Always adjust to lowest effective dose.
● Most adverse reactions to corticosteroids are dose- or duration-dependent.
● For better results and less toxicity, give a once-daily dose in the morning.
● Monitor patient's blood pressure, sleep patterns, and potassium level.
● Weigh patient daily; report sudden weight gain to prescriber.
● Monitor patient for cushingoid effects, including moon face, buffalo hump, central obesity, thinning hair, hypertension, and increased susceptibility to infection.
● Watch for depression or psychotic episodes, especially during high-dose therapy.
● Diabetic patient may need increased insulin; monitor glucose level.
● Elderly patients may be more susceptible to osteoporosis with long-term use.
● Drug may mask or worsen infections, including latent amebiasis.
● Unless contraindicated, give low-sodium diet that's high in potassium and protein. Give potassium supplements as needed.
● Gradually reduce dosage after long-term therapy.
● *Look alike–sound alike:* Don't confuse prednisone with prednisolone or primidone.

PATIENT TEACHING

● Tell patient not to stop drug abruptly or without prescriber's consent.
● Instruct patient to take drug with food or milk.
● Teach patient signs and symptoms of early adrenal insufficiency: fatigue, muscle weakness, joint pain, fever, anorexia, nausea, shortness of breath, dizziness, and fainting.
● Instruct patient to carry or wear medical identification indicating his need for supplemental systemic glucocorticoids during stress. It should include prescriber's name and name and dosage of drug.
● Warn patient on long-term therapy about cushingoid effects (moon face, buffalo hump) and the need to notify prescriber about sudden weight gain or swelling.

• Advise patient receiving long-term therapy to consider exercise or physical therapy. Also, tell patient to ask prescriber about vitamin D or calcium supplement.
• Tell patient to report slow healing.
• Advise patient receiving long-term therapy to have periodic eye examinations.
• Instruct patient to avoid exposure to infections and to contact prescriber if exposure occurs.

promethazine hydrochloride
proe-METH-a-zeen

Phenadoz, Phenergan*

Pharmacologic class: phenothiazine
Pregnancy risk category C

AVAILABLE FORMS
Injection: 25 mg/ml, 50 mg/ml
Suppositories: 12.5 mg, 25 mg, 50 mg
Syrup: 6.25 mg/5 ml*
Tablets: 12.5 mg, 25 mg, 50 mg

INDICATIONS & DOSAGES
➤ **Motion sickness**
Adults: 25 mg P.O. or P.R. taken 30 minutes to 1 hour before departure. May repeat dose 8 to 12 hours later p.r.n.
Children older than age 2: 12.5 to 25 mg or 0.5 mg/kg P.O. or P.R. 30 minutes to 1 hour before departure. May repeat dose 8 to 12 hours later p.r.n.
➤ **Nausea and vomiting**
Adults: 12.5 to 25 mg P.O., I.M., or P.R. every 4 to 6 hours p.r.n.
Children older than age 2: Give 12.5 to 25 mg P.O. or P.R. every 4 to 6 hours p.r.n. Or, 6.25 to 12.5 mg I.M. every 4 to 6 hours p.r.n.
➤ **Rhinitis, allergy symptoms**
Adults: 25 mg P.O. or P.R. at bedtime; or, 12.5 mg P.O. or P.R. t.i.d. and at bedtime.
Children older than age 2: Give 25 mg P.O. or P.R. at bedtime; or, 6.25 to 12.5 mg P.O. or P.R. t.i.d. Alternatively, 0.5 mg/kg at bedtime or 0.125 mg/kg p.r.n.
➤ **Nighttime sedation**
Adults: 25 to 50 mg P.O., I.V., I.M., or P.R. at bedtime.
Children older than age 2: Give 12.5 to 25 mg P.O., I.M., or P.R. at bedtime.

➤ **Adjunct to analgesics for routine preoperative or postoperative sedation**
Adults: 25 to 50 mg I.V., I.M., P.O. or P.R.
Children older than age 2: Give 0.5 to 1.1 mg/kg P.O., I.M., or P.R.

ADMINISTRATION
P.O.
• Reduce GI distress by giving drug with food or milk.
I.V.
• If solution is discolored or contains a precipitate, discard.
• Give injection through a free-flowing I.V. line.
• Don't give at a concentration above 25 mg/ml or a rate above 25 mg/minute.
• **Incompatibilities:** Aldesleukin, allopurinol, aminophylline, amphotericin B, cephalosporins, chloramphenicol sodium succinate, chloroquine phosphate, chlorothiazide, diatrizoate, dimenhydrinate, doxorubicin liposomal, foscarnet, furosemide, heparin sodium, hydrocortisone sodium succinate, iodipamide meglumine (52%), iothalamate, ketorolac, methohexital, morphine, nalbuphine, penicillin G potassium and sodium, pentobarbital sodium, phenobarbital sodium, phenytoin sodium, thiopental, vitamin B complex.
I.M.
• I.M. injection is the preferred parenteral route. Inject deep I.M. into large muscle mass. Rotate injection sites.
• Don't give subcutaneously.
Rectal
• If suppository is too soft, place wrapped in refrigerator for 15 minutes or run under cold water.

ACTION
Phenothiazine derivative that competes with histamine for H_1-receptor sites on effector cells. Prevents, but doesn't reverse, histamine-mediated responses. At high doses, drug also has local anesthetic effects.

Route	Onset	Peak	Duration
P.O.	15–60 min	Unknown	< 12 hr
I.V.	3–5 min	Unknown	< 12 hr
I.M., P.R.	20 min	Unknown	< 12 hr

Half-life: Unknown.

ADVERSE REACTIONS

CNS: *drowsiness, sedation,* confusion, sleepiness, dizziness, disorientation, extrapyramidal symptoms.
CV: hypotension, hypertension.
EENT: *dry mouth,* blurred vision.
GI: nausea, vomiting.
GU: urine retention.
Hematologic: *leukopenia, agranulocytosis, thrombocytopenia.*
Metabolic: hyperglycemia.
Respiratory: *respiratory depression, apnea.*
Skin: photosensitivity, rash.

INTERACTIONS

Drug-drug. *Anticholinergics, tricyclic antidepressants:* May increase anticholinergic effects. Avoid using together.
CNS depressants: May increase sedation. Use together cautiously. If used together, reduce opiate dose by at least 25% to 50%, and reduce barbiturate dose by at least 50%.
Epinephrine: May block or reverse effects of epinephrine. Use other pressor drugs instead.
Levodopa: May decrease antiparkinsonian action of levodopa. Avoid using together.
Lithium: May reduce GI absorption or enhance renal elimination of lithium. Avoid using together.
MAO inhibitors: May increase extrapyramidal effects. Avoid using together.
Quinolones: May cause life-threatening arrhythmias. Avoid using together.
Drug-herb. *Yohimbe:* May increase risk of herb toxicity. Ask patient about use of herbal remedies, and recommend caution.
Drug-lifestyle. *Alcohol use:* May increase sedation. Discourage use together.
Sun exposure: May cause photosensitivity reactions. Advise patient to avoid extensive sunlight exposure and to use sunblock.

EFFECTS ON LAB TEST RESULTS

• May increase hemoglobin level and hematocrit.
• May decrease WBC, platelet, and granulocyte counts.
• May prevent, reduce, or mask positive result in diagnostic skin test. May cause false-positive or false-negative pregnancy test result. May interfere with blood grouping in the ABO system.

CONTRAINDICATIONS & CAUTIONS

• Contraindicated in patients hypersensitive to drug, those who have experienced adverse reactions to phenothiazines, breast-feeding women, children younger than age 2, comatose patients, and acutely ill or dehydrated children.
• Use cautiously in patients with asthma or pulmonary, hepatic, or CV disease and in those with intestinal obstruction, prostatic hyperplasia, bladder-neck obstruction, angle-closure glaucoma, seizure disorders, CNS depression, and stenosing or peptic ulcerations.

NURSING CONSIDERATIONS

• Monitor patient for neuroleptic malignant syndrome: altered mental status, autonomic instability, muscle rigidity, and hyperpyrexia.
• Stop drug 4 days before diagnostic skin testing because antihistamines can prevent, reduce, or mask positive skin test response.
• Drug is used as an adjunct to analgesics, usually to increase sedation; it has no analgesic activity.
• Drug may be mixed with meperidine in same syringe.
• In patients scheduled for a myelogram, stop drug 48 hours before procedure. Don't resume drug until 24 hours after procedure because of the risk of seizures.

PATIENT TEACHING

• Tell patient to take oral form with food or milk.
• When treating motion sickness, tell patient to take first dose 30 to 60 minutes before travel; dose may be repeated in 8 to 12 hours, if necessary. On succeeding days of travel, patient should take dose upon arising and with evening meal.
• Warn patient to avoid alcohol and hazardous activities that require alertness until CNS effects of drug are known.
• Inform patient that sugarless gum, hard candy, or ice chips may relieve dry mouth.
• Warn patient about possible photosensitivity reactions. Advise use of a sunblock.

pseudoephedrine hydrochloride
soo-dow-e-FED-rin

Cenafed ◊, Decofed ◊, Dimetapp
Decongestant Pediatric ◊,
Dimetapp, Maximum Strength,
Non-Drowsy ◊, Genaphed ◊,
PediaCare Infants' Decongestant
Drops ◊, Sudafed ◊, Triaminic ◊

pseudoephedrine sulfate
Drixoral Non-Drowsy Formula ◊

Pharmacologic class: adrenergic
Pregnancy risk category C

AVAILABLE FORMS
pseudoephedrine hydrochloride
Capsules: 30 mg ◊, 60 mg ◊
Drops: 7.5 mg/0.8 ml ◊
Oral solution: 15 mg/5 ml ◊, 30 mg/5 ml ◊
Tablets: 30 mg ◊, 60 mg ◊
Tablets (chewable): 15 mg ◊
Tablets (extended-release): 120 mg ◊,
240 mg ◊
pseudoephedrine sulfate
Tablets (extended-release): 120 mg
(60 mg immediate-release, 60 mg delayed-
release) ◊

INDICATIONS & DOSAGES
➤ **To decongest nose and eustachian
tube**
Adults and children older than age 12:
Give 60 mg P.O. every 4 to 6 hours; or
120 mg P.O. extended-release tablet every
12 hours; or 240 mg P.O. extended-release
tablet once daily. Maximum dosage is
240 mg daily.
Children ages 6 to 12: Give 30 mg P.O.
every 4 to 6 hours. Maximum dosage is
120 mg daily.
Children ages 2 to 5: Give 15 mg P.O.
every 4 to 6 hours. Maximum dosage
is 60 mg daily, or 4 mg/kg/day or
125 mg/m^2/day P.O. in divided doses
q.i.d.
➤ **To prevent otitic barotraumas
during air travel or underwater
diving ◆**
Adults: 120 mg extended-release tablet
P.O. 30 minutes before air travel or 60 mg
P.O. 30 minutes before underwater diving.

ADMINISTRATION
P.O.
● Don't crush or break extended-release
forms.

ACTION
Stimulates alpha receptors in the respiratory tract, constricting blood vessels,
shrinking swollen nasal mucous membranes, increasing airway patency, and
reducing tissue hyperemia, edema, and
nasal congestion.

Route	Onset	Peak	Duration
P.O.	30 min	30–60 min	4–12 hr

Half-life: Unknown.

ADVERSE REACTIONS
CNS: *anxiety, nervousness,* dizziness,
headache, insomnia, transient stimulation,
tremor.
CV: *palpitations,* **arrhythmias, CV col-
lapse,** tachycardia.
GI: anorexia, dry mouth, nausea, vomit-
ing.
GU: difficulty urinating.
Respiratory: *respiratory difficulties.*
Skin: pallor.
Other: diaphoresis.

INTERACTIONS
Drug-drug. *Antihypertensives:* May
inhibit hypotensive effect. Monitor blood
pressure closely.
*MAO inhibitors (phenelzine, tranyl-
cypromine):* May cause severe headache,
hypertension, fever, and hypertensive
crisis. Avoid using together.
Methyldopa, reserpine: May increase
pressor response. Monitor patient closely.

EFFECTS ON LAB TEST RESULTS
None reported.

CONTRAINDICATIONS & CAUTIONS
● Contraindicated in patients with severe
hypertension or severe coronary artery
disease, in those receiving MAO inhibitors,
and in breast-feeding women. Extended-
release forms are contraindicated in children younger than age 12.

• Use cautiously in patients with hypertension, cardiac disease, diabetes, glaucoma, hyperthyroidism, and prostatic hyperplasia.

NURSING CONSIDERATIONS
• Elderly patients are more sensitive to drug's effects. Extended-release tablets shouldn't be given to elderly patients until safety with short-acting preparations has been established.

PATIENT TEACHING
• Tell patient not to crush or break extended-release forms.
• Warn against using OTC products containing other sympathomimetics.
• Instruct patient not to take drug within 2 hours of bedtime because it can cause insomnia.
• Tell patient to stop drug and notify prescriber if he becomes unusually restless.

SAFETY ALERT!

reteplase, recombinant
RET-ah-place

Retavase

Pharmacologic class: tissue plasminogen activator
Pregnancy risk category C

AVAILABLE FORMS
Injection: 10.4 units (18.1 mg)/vial. Supplied in a kit with components for reconstitution for two single-use vials

INDICATIONS & DOSAGES
➤ **To manage acute MI**
Adults: Double-bolus injection of 10 + 10 units. Give each bolus I.V. over 2 minutes. If complications, such as serious bleeding or anaphylactoid reaction, don't occur after first bolus, give second bolus 30 minutes after start of first.

ADMINISTRATION
I.V.
• Reconstitute drug according to manufacturer's instructions using items provided in kit and sterile water for injection, without preservatives. Make sure reconstituted solution is colorless; resulting concen-

tration is 1 unit/ml. If foaming occurs, let vial stand for several minutes. Inspect for precipitation. Use within 4 hours of reconstitution; discard unused portions.
• Give as a double-bolus injection. If bleeding or anaphylactoid reaction occurs after first bolus, notify prescriber; second bolus may be withheld.
• **Incompatibilities:** Other I.V. drugs.

ACTION
Enhances cleavage of plasminogen to generate plasmin, which leads to fibrinolysis.

Route	Onset	Peak	Duration
I.V.	Unknown	Unknown	Unknown

Half-life: 13 to 16 minutes.

ADVERSE REACTIONS
CNS: *intracranial hemorrhage.*
CV: *arrhythmias, cholesterol embolization, hemorrhage.*
GI: *hemorrhage.*
GU: hematuria.
Hematologic: *bleeding tendency,* anemia.
Other: bleeding at puncture sites, hypersensitivity reactions.

INTERACTIONS
Drug-drug. *Heparin, oral anticoagulants, platelet inhibitors (abciximab, aspirin, dipyridamole, eptifibatide, tirofiban):* May increase risk of bleeding. Use together cautiously.

EFFECTS ON LAB TEST RESULTS
• May increase PT, PTT, and INR.
• May alter coagulation study results.

CONTRAINDICATIONS & CAUTIONS
• Contraindicated in patients with active internal bleeding, known bleeding diathesis, history of stroke, recent intracranial or intraspinal surgery or trauma, severe uncontrolled hypertension, intracranial neoplasm, arteriovenous malformation, or aneurysm.
• Use cautiously in patients with previous puncture of noncompressible vessels; in those with recent (within 10 days) major surgery, obstetric delivery, organ biopsy, GI or GU bleeding, or trauma; in those with cerebrovascular disease, systolic blood pressure 180 mm Hg or

higher or diastolic pressure 110 mm Hg or higher, and conditions that may lead to left heart thrombus, including mitral stenosis, acute pericarditis, subacute bacterial endocarditis, and hemostatic defects.
• Use cautiously in those with diabetic hemorrhagic retinopathy, septic thrombophlebitis, and other conditions in which bleeding would be difficult to manage.
• Use cautiously in patients age 75 and older and in breast-feeding women.

NURSING CONSIDERATIONS
• Drug remains active in vitro and can lead to degradation of fibrinogen in sample, changing coagulation study results. Collect blood samples with chloromethylketone at 2-micromolar concentrations.
• Drug may be given to menstruating women.
• Carefully monitor ECG during treatment. Coronary thrombolysis may cause arrhythmias linked with reperfusion. Be prepared to treat bradycardia or ventricular irritability.
• Closely monitor patient for bleeding. Avoid I.M. injections, invasive procedures, and nonessential handling of patient. Bleeding is the most common adverse reaction and may occur internally or at external puncture sites. If local measures don't control serious bleeding, stop anticoagulant and notify prescriber. Withhold second bolus of reteplase.
• Potency is expressed in units specific to reteplase and isn't comparable with other thrombolytics.
• Avoid use of noncompressible puncture sites during therapy. If an arterial puncture is needed, use an arm vessel that can be compressed manually. Apply pressure for at least 30 minutes; then apply a pressure dressing. Check site frequently.

PATIENT TEACHING
• Explain use and administration of drug to patient and family.
• Tell patient to report adverse reactions immediately.

ribavirin
rye-ba-VYE-rin

Copegus, Rebetol, Ribaspheres, Virazole

Pharmacologic class: synthetic nucleoside
Pregnancy risk category X

AVAILABLE FORMS
Capsules: 200 mg, 400 mg, 600 mg
Oral solution: 40 mg/ml
Powder to be reconstituted for inhalation: 6 g in 100-ml glass vial
Tablets: 200 mg

INDICATIONS & DOSAGES
➤ **Hospitalized infants and young children infected by respiratory syncytial virus (RSV)**
Infants and young children: Solution in concentration of 20 mg/ml delivered via the Viratek Small Particle Aerosol Generator (SPAG-2) and mechanical ventilator or oxygen hood, face mask, or oxygen tent at a rate of about 12.5 L of mist/minute. Treatment is given for 12 to 18 hours/day for at least 3 days, and no longer than 7 days.
➤ **Chronic hepatitis C**
Adults who weigh more than 75 kg (165 lb): 1,200 mg Rebetol P.O. divided b.i.d. (600 in morning, 600 mg in evening) with interferon alfa-2b, 3 million units subcutaneously three times weekly. Or, 1,200 mg Copegus with 180 mcg of peginterferon alfa-2a.
Adults who weigh 75 kg or less: 1,000 mg Rebetol P.O. daily in divided dose (400 mg in morning, 600 mg in evening) with interferon alfa-2b 3 million units subcutaneously three times weekly. Or, 1,000 mg Copegus with 180 mcg of peginterferon alfa-2a.
Children age 3 and older who weigh 50 to 61 kg (110 to 134 lb): 400 mg P.O. (Rebetol) every morning and 400 mg P.O. every evening with interferon alfa-2b, 3 million units/m^2 subcutaneously three times weekly.
Children age 3 and older who weigh 37 to 49 kg (81 to 108 lb): 200 mg P.O. (Rebetol) every morning and 400 mg P.O.

every evening with interferon alfa-2b, 3 million units/m² subcutaneously three times weekly.

Children age 3 and older who weigh 25 to 36 kg (55 to 79 lb): 200 mg P.O. (Rebetol) every morning and 200 mg P.O. every evening with interferon alfa-2b, 3 million units/m² subcutaneously three times weekly.

➤ **Chronic hepatitis C (regardless of genotype) in HIV-infected patients who haven't previously been treated with interferon**

Adults: 800 mg Copegus P.O. daily given in two divided doses with peginterferon alfa-2a 180 mcg subcutaneously weekly for 48 weeks.

Adjust-a-dose: In patient with no cardiac history and hemoglobin level less than 10 g/dl, reduce dosage to 600 mg daily (200 mg in a.m., 400 mg in p.m.) for adults and 7.5 mg/kg daily for children. If hemoglobin level is less than 8.5 g/dl, stop drug. In patient with cardiac history and whose hemoglobin level falls 2 g/dl or more during any 4-week period, reduce dosage to 600 mg daily (200 mg in a.m., 400 mg in p.m.) for adults and 7.5 mg/kg daily for children. If hemoglobin level is less than 12 g/dl after 4 weeks of reduced dosage, stop drug.

ADMINISTRATION

Inhalational
- Give by the Viratek SPAG-2 only. Don't use any other aerosol-generating device.
- Use sterile USP water for injection, not bacteriostatic water. Water used to reconstitute this drug must not contain any antimicrobial product.
- Discard solutions placed in the SPAG-2 unit at least every 24 hours before adding newly reconstituted solution.
- Store reconstituted solutions at room temperature for 24 hours.

P.O.
- Give drug without regard for meals at the same time every day.

ACTION

Inhibits viral activity by an unknown mechanism, possibly by inhibiting RNA and DNA synthesis by depleting intracellular nucleotide pools.

Route	Onset	Peak	Duration
Inhalation	Unknown	Unknown	Unknown
P.O.	Unknown	2 hr	Unknown

Half-life: First phase, 9¼ hours; second phase, 40 hours.

ADVERSE REACTIONS

CV: *bradycardia, cardiac arrest,* hypotension.
EENT: conjunctivitis, rash or erythema of eyelids.
Hematologic: anemia, reticulocytosis.
Respiratory: *apnea, bronchospasm,* bacterial pneumonia, *pneumothorax, pulmonary edema,* worsening respiratory state.

INTERACTIONS

Drug-drug. *Acetaminophen, antacids that contain magnesium, aluminum, or simethicone, aspirin, cimetidine:* May affect drug level. Monitor patient.
Didanosine: May increase toxicity. Avoid using together.
Stavudine, zidovudine: May decrease antiretroviral activity. Use together cautiously.

EFFECTS ON LAB TEST RESULTS

- May increase ALT, AST, and bilirubin levels. May decrease hemoglobin level.
- May increase reticulocyte count.

CONTRAINDICATIONS & CAUTIONS

- Aerosol form contraindicated in patients hypersensitive to drug, and women who are or may become pregnant during exposure to aerosolized ribavirin.
- Oral form is contraindicated in patients hypersensitive to drug, pregnant women, men whose partners are pregnant or may become pregnant within 6 months, patients with thalassemia major or sickle cell anemia, patients with a history of significant or unstable cardiac disease, and patients whose creatinine clearance is less than 50 ml/minute.
- Use cautiously in elderly patients and patients with hepatic or renal insufficiency.

NURSING CONSIDERATIONS

Aerosol form
- *Alert:* The long-term and cumulative effects to health care personnel exposed

to this form aren't known. Eye irritation and headache may occur. Advise pregnant women to avoid unnecessary exposure.
● *Alert:* Monitor ventilator function frequently. Drug may precipitate in ventilator, causing equipment to malfunction with serious consequences.
● This form is indicated only for severe lower respiratory tract infection caused by RSV. Although you should begin treatment while awaiting test results, an RSV infection must be documented eventually.
● Most infants and children with RSV infection don't require treatment with antivirals because the disease is commonly mild and self-limiting. Premature infants or those with cardiopulmonary disease experience RSV in its severest form and benefit most from treatment with ribavirin aerosol.

Oral form
● Don't start therapy until a negative pregnancy test is confirmed in patient or partner of patient; they should take a pregnancy test every month during therapy and for 6 months afterward.
● Women or female partner of patient should use two reliable forms of contraception before and during treatment and for 6 months afterward.
● Report pregnancies that occur during treatment by calling 800-727-7064 for capsules and 800-593-2214 for tablets.
● Monitor hematologic status, liver function, and thyroid-stimulating hormone level at baseline and throughout therapy.
● Ribavirin alone is ineffective for treating chronic hepatitis C.
● *Alert:* Monitor patient for suicidal ideation, severe depression, hemolytic anemia, bone marrow suppression, autoimmune and infective disorders, pulmonary dysfunction, pancreatitis, and diabetes.
● Stop drug if pulmonary infiltrates or severe pulmonary impairment occur.

PATIENT TEACHING
● Inform parents of need for drug, and answer any questions.
● Encourage parents to immediately report any subtle change in child.
● Inform patient that oral form may be taken without regard to meals but should be taken in a consistent manner.

---

rifabutin
rif-ah-BYOO-tin

Mycobutin

Pharmacologic class: semisynthetic ansamycin
Pregnancy risk category B

AVAILABLE FORMS
Capsules: 150 mg

INDICATIONS & DOSAGES
➤ **To prevent disseminated** *Mycobacterium avium* **complex in patients with advanced HIV infection**
Adults: 300 mg P.O. daily as a single dose or divided b.i.d.

ADMINISTRATION
P.O.
● For patient who has difficulty swallowing, mix drug with soft foods such as applesauce.
● Patient experiencing GI adverse effects, such as nausea or vomiting, may divide total daily dose into two doses and take with food.

ACTION
Inhibits DNA-dependent RNA polymerase in susceptible bacteria, blocking bacterial protein synthesis.

Route	Onset	Peak	Duration
P.O.	Unknown	2–4 hr	Unknown

Half-life: About 2 days.

ADVERSE REACTIONS
CNS: headache, fever.
EENT: eye inflammation.
GI: dyspepsia, eructation, flatulence, diarrhea, nausea, vomiting, abdominal pain, anorexia, taste perversion.
GU: discolored urine.
Hematologic: *neutropenia, leukopenia, thrombocytopenia,* eosinophilia.
Musculoskeletal: myalgia.
Skin: *rash.*

INTERACTIONS
Drug-drug. *Benzodiazepines, beta blockers, buspirone,* **corticosteroids,**

---

cyclosporine, delavirdine, doxycycline, fluconazole, hydantoins, indinavir, itraconazole, ketoconazole, losartan, macrolides, methadone, morphine, nelfinavir, quinidine, quinine, **tacrolimus,** theophylline, tricyclic antidepressants, zolpidem: May decrease effectiveness of these drugs. Monitor patient for drug effects.
Hormonal contraceptives: May decrease contraceptive effectiveness. Tell patient to use another form of birth control.
Indinavir: May increase rifabutin level. Decrease rifabutin dosage by 50%.
Ritonavir: May increase the risk of rifabutin hematologic toxicity. Use together is contraindicated.
Voriconazole: May decrease therapeutic effects of voriconazole while increasing the risk of rifabutin adverse effects. Use together is contraindicated.
Warfarin: May decrease effectiveness of warfarin. May require higher dosages of anticoagulants. Monitor PT and INR.
Drug-food. *High-fat foods:* May reduce rate but not extent of absorption. Discourage use together.

EFFECTS ON LAB TEST RESULTS
• May increase aminotransferase level.
• May decrease neutrophil, WBC, and platelet counts.

CONTRAINDICATIONS & CAUTIONS
• Contraindicated in patients hypersensitive to drug or other rifamycin derivatives, such as rifampin, and in patients with active tuberculosis because single-drug therapy with rifabutin increases risk of inducing bacterial resistance to both rifabutin and rifampin.
• Use cautiously in patients with neutropenia and thrombocytopenia.

NURSING CONSIDERATIONS
• In patients with neutropenia or thrombocytopenia, obtain baseline hematologic studies and repeat periodically.
• **Look alike–sound alike:** Don't confuse rifabutin with rifampin or rifapentine.

PATIENT TEACHING
• Instruct patient to take drug for as long as prescribed, exactly as directed, even after feeling better.

• Tell patient experiencing GI adverse effects, such as nausea or vomiting, to divide total daily dose into 2 doses and to take with food.
• Tell patient that drug may cause brownish orange staining of urine, feces, sputum, saliva, tears, and skin. Tell him to avoid wearing soft contact lenses because they may be permanently stained.
• Instruct patient to report sensitivity to light, excessive tears, or eye pain immediately.
• Advise patient to report tingling and joint stiffness, swelling, or tenderness.

rifampin (rifampicin)
RIF-am-pin

Rifadin, Rimactane, Rofact†

Pharmacologic class: semisynthetic rifamycin
Pregnancy risk category C

AVAILABLE FORMS
Capsules: 150 mg, 300 mg
Powder for injection: 600 mg

INDICATIONS & DOSAGES
➤ **Pulmonary tuberculosis, with other antituberculotics**
Adults: 10 mg/kg P.O. or I.V. daily in single dose. Give oral doses 1 hour before or 2 hours after meals with a full glass of water. Maximum daily dose is 600 mg.
Children age 5 and older: 10 to 20 mg/kg P.O. or I.V. daily in single dose. Give oral doses 1 hour before or 2 hours after meals with a full glass of water. Maximum daily dose is 600 mg. Give with other antituberculotics.
➤ **Meningococcal carriers**
Adults: 600 mg P.O. or I.V. every 12 hours for 2 days; or 600 mg P.O. or I.V. once daily for 4 days.
Children ages 1 month to 12 years: 10 mg/kg P.O. or I.V. every 12 hours for 2 days, not to exceed 600 mg/day; or 20 mg/kg once daily for 4 days.
Neonates: 5 mg/kg P.O. or I.V. every 12 hours for 2 days.

➤ *Mycobacterium avium* **complex** ◆
Adults: 600 mg P.O. or I.V. daily as part of
a multiple-drug regimen.

ADMINISTRATION

P.O.
● Give drug with at least one other antituberculotic.
● For best absorption, give capsules 1 hour
before or 2 hours after meals.
● For the patient who can't tolerate capsules on an empty stomach, give drug with
meals and a full glass of water.
I.V.
● Reconstitute drug with 10 ml of sterile
water for injection to yield 60 mg/ml.
● Add to 100 ml of D₅W and infuse over
30 minutes, or add to 500 ml of D₅W and
infuse over 3 hours.
● When dextrose is contraindicated, dilute
with normal saline solution for injection.
● Once prepared, dilutions in D₅W are
stable for up to 4 hours and dilutions in
normal saline solution are stable for up to
24 hours at room temperature.
● **Incompatibilities:** Diltiazem, minocycline, other I.V. solutions.

ACTION

Inhibits DNA-dependent RNA polymerase,
which impairs RNA synthesis; bacteri-
dal.

Route	Onset	Peak	Duration
P.O.	Unknown	2–4 hr	Unknown
I.V.	Unknown	Unknown	Unknown

Half-life: 1¼ to 5 hours.

ADVERSE REACTIONS

CNS: headache, fatigue, drowsiness,
behavioral changes, dizziness, mental
confusion, generalized numbness, ataxia.
CV: *shock.*
EENT: visual disturbances, exudative
conjunctivitis.
GI: *pancreatitis, pseudomembranous
colitis,* epigastric distress, anorexia, nausea, vomiting, abdominal pain, diarrhea,
flatulence, sore mouth and tongue.
GU: *acute renal failure,* hemoglobinuria,
hematuria, menstrual disturbances.

Hematologic: *thrombocytopenia, tran-
sient leukopenia,* eosinophilia, hemolytic
anemia.
Hepatic: *hepatotoxicity.*
Metabolic: hyperuricemia.
Musculoskeletal: osteomalacia.
Respiratory: shortness of breath, wheez-
ing.
Skin: pruritus, urticaria, rash.
Other: flulike syndrome, discoloration of
body fluids, porphyria exacerbation.

INTERACTIONS

Drug-drug. *Acetaminophen, amiodarone,
analgesics, anticonvulsants, barbiturates, beta blockers, cardiac glycosides,
chloramphenicol, clofibrate,* **corticosteroids, cyclosporine,** *dapsone, delavirdine, diazepam, digoxin, disopyramide,
doxycycline, enalapril, fluoroquinolones,
hormonal contraceptives, hydantoins,
losartan, methadone, mexiletine, midazolam, nifedipine, ondansetron, opioids, progestins, propafenone, quinidine,* **ritonavir,**
sulfonylureas, **tacrolimus,** *theophylline,
tocainide, triazolam, tricyclic antidepressants, verapamil, zidovudine, zolpidem:*
May decrease effectiveness of these drugs.
Monitor effectiveness.
Anticoagulants: May increase requirements for anticoagulant. Monitor PT and
INR closely and adjust dosage of anticoagulants.
Halothane: May increase risk of hepatotoxicity. Monitor liver function test results.
Isoniazid: May increase risk of hepatotoxicity. Monitor liver function test results.
*Ketoconazole, para-aminosalicylate
sodium:* May interfere with absorption of
rifampin. Separate doses by 8 to 12 hours.
Macrolide antibiotics, protease inhibitors:
May inhibit rifampin metabolism but increase metabolism of other drug. Monitor
patient for clinical and adverse effects.
Probenecid: May increase rifampin levels.
Use together cautiously.
Voriconazole: May decrease voriconazole's
therapeutic effects while increasing the
risk of rifampin adverse effects. Use
together is contraindicated.
Drug-lifestyle. *Alcohol use:* May increase
risk of hepatotoxicity. Discourage use
together.

Reactions may be *common,* uncommon, *life-threatening*, or COMMON AND LIFE-THREATENING.
Interaction may have a *rapid onset* or **delayed onset**.

EFFECTS ON LAB TEST RESULTS
● May increase ALT, AST, alkaline phosphatase, bilirubin, and uric acid levels. May decrease hemoglobin level.
● May increase eosinophil counts. May decrease platelet and WBC counts.
● May alter standard folate and vitamin B_{12} assay results.

CONTRAINDICATIONS & CAUTIONS
● Contraindicated in patients hypersensitive to rifampin or related drugs.
● Use cautiously in patients with liver disease.

NURSING CONSIDERATIONS
● Monitor hepatic function, hematopoietic studies, and uric acid levels. Drug's systemic effects may asymptomatically raise liver function test results and uric acid level.
● Watch for and report to prescriber signs and symptoms of hepatic impairment.
● Drug may cause hemorrhage in neonates and mother when drug is given during last few weeks of pregnancy. Monitor clotting parameters closely, and treat with vitamin K as needed.
● *Look alike–sound alike:* Don't confuse rifampin with rifabutin or rifapentine.

PATIENT TEACHING
● Instruct patient who can't tolerate capsules on an empty stomach to take drug with meals and a full glass of water.
● Advise patient who is unable to swallow capsules whole that an oral suspension can be prepared by the pharmacist.
● Warn patient that he may feel drowsy and that drug can turn body fluids red-orange and permanently stain contact lenses.
● Advise a woman using hormonal contraceptive to consider another form of birth control.
● Advise patient to contact prescriber if he experiences fever, loss of appetite, malaise, nausea, vomiting, dark urine, or yellow discoloration of the eyes or skin.
● Advise patient to avoid alcohol during drug therapy.

rifapentine
rif-ah-PIN-ten

Priftin

Pharmacologic class: synthetic rifamycin
Pregnancy risk category C

AVAILABLE FORMS
Tablets (film-coated): 150 mg

INDICATIONS & DOSAGES
➤ **Pulmonary tuberculosis (TB), with at least one other antituberculotic to which the isolate is susceptible**
Adults: During intensive phase of short-course therapy, 600 mg P.O. twice weekly for 2 months, with an interval between doses of at least 3 days (72 hours). During continuation phase of short-course therapy, 600 mg P.O. once weekly for 4 months, combined with isoniazid or another drug to which the isolate is susceptible.

ADMINISTRATION
P.O.
● Give drug with pyridoxine (vitamin B_6) in malnourished patients; in those predisposed to neuropathy, such as alcoholics and diabetics; and in adolescents.
● *Alert:* Give drug with appropriate daily companion drugs. Compliance with all drug regimens, especially with daily companion drugs on the days when rifapentine isn't given, is crucial for early sputum conversion and protection from relapse of TB.

ACTION
Inhibits DNA-dependent RNA polymerase in susceptible strains of *Mycobacterium tuberculosis.* Demonstrates bactericidal activity against the organism both intracellularly and extracellularly.

Route	Onset	Peak	Duration
P.O.	Unknown	5–6 hr	Unknown

Half-life: 13 hours.

ADVERSE REACTIONS
CNS: headache, dizziness, pain.
CV: hypertension.

GI: anorexia, nausea, vomiting, dyspepsia, diarrhea.
GU: pyuria, proteinuria, hematuria, urinary casts.
Hematologic: *leukopenia, neutropenia,* anemia, *thrombocytosis.*
Metabolic: *hyperuricemia.*
Musculoskeletal: arthralgia.
Respiratory: hemoptysis.
Skin: rash, pruritus, acne, maculopapular rash.

INTERACTIONS

Drug-drug. *Antiarrhythmics (disopyramide, mexiletine, quinidine, tocainide), antibiotics (chloramphenicol, clarithromycin, dapsone, doxycycline, fluoroquinolones), anticonvulsants (phenytoin), antifungals (fluconazole, itraconazole, ketoconazole), barbiturates, benzodiazepines (diazepam), beta blockers, calcium channel blockers (diltiazem, nifedipine, verapamil), cardiac glycosides, clofibrate,* **corticosteroids,** *haloperidol, HIV protease inhibitors (indinavir, nelfinavir, ritonavir, saquinavir), hormonal contraceptives,* **immunosuppressants (cyclosporine, tacrolimus),** *levothyroxine, opioid analgesics (methadone), oral anticoagulants (warfarin), oral hypoglycemics (sulfonylureas), progestins, quinine, reverse transcriptase inhibitors (delavirdine, zidovudine), sildenafil, theophylline, tricyclic antidepressants (amitriptyline, nortriptyline):* May decrease activity of these drugs because of cytochrome P-450 enzyme metabolism. May need to adjust dosage.
Ritonavir: May decrease ritonavir levels. Carefully monitor patient's response.

EFFECTS ON LAB TEST RESULTS

• May increase uric acid, ALT, and AST levels. May decrease hemoglobin level.
• May increase platelet count. May decrease neutrophil and WBC counts.
• May alter folate and vitamin B_{12} assay results.

CONTRAINDICATIONS & CAUTIONS

• Contraindicated in patients hypersensitive to rifamycins (rifapentine, rifampin, or rifabutin).
• Use drug cautiously and with frequent monitoring in patients with liver disease.

NURSING CONSIDERATIONS

• Rifamycin antibiotics may cause hepatotoxicity. Obtain baseline liver function test results before therapy.
• If used during the last 2 weeks of pregnancy, drug may lead to postnatal hemorrhage in mother or infant. Monitor clotting parameters closely if drug is used at that time.
• *Look alike–sound alike:* Don't confuse rifapentine with rifabutin or rifampin.

PATIENT TEACHING

• Stress importance of strict compliance with this drug regimen and that of daily companion drugs, as well as needed follow-up visits and laboratory tests.
• Advise woman to use nonhormonal birth control methods.
• Tell patient to take drug with food if nausea, vomiting, or GI upset occurs.
• Instruct patient to report to prescriber fever, appetite loss, malaise, nausea, vomiting, darkened urine, yellowish skin and eyes, joint pain or swelling, or excessive loose stools or diarrhea.
• Instruct patient to protect pills from excessive heat.
• Tell patient that drug may turn body fluids red-orange and permanently stain contact lenses.

---

salmeterol xinafoate
sal-MEE-ter-ol

Serevent Diskus

Pharmacologic class: long-acting selective beta₂ agonist
Pregnancy risk category C

AVAILABLE FORMS
Inhalation powder: 50 mcg/blister

INDICATIONS & DOSAGES
➤ **Long-term maintenance of asthma; to prevent bronchospasm in patients with nocturnal asthma or reversible obstructive airway disease who need regular treatment with short-acting beta agonists**
Adults and children age 4 and older:
1 inhalation (50 mcg) every 12 hours, morning and evening.

➤ **To prevent exercise-induced bronchospasm**
Adults and children age 4 and older:
1 inhalation (50 mcg) at least 30 minutes before exercise. Additional doses shouldn't be taken for at least 12 hours.

➤ **COPD or emphysema**
Adults: 1 inhalation (50 mcg) b.i.d. in the morning and evening, about 12 hours apart.

ADMINISTRATION
Inhalational
● Give drug 30 to 60 minutes before exercise to prevent exercise-induced bronchospasm.
● Don't use a spacer device with this drug.

ACTION
Unclear. Selectively activates beta$_2$ receptors, which results in bronchodilation; also, blocks the release of allergic mediators from mast cells lining the respiratory tract.

Route	Onset	Peak	Duration
Inhalation	10–20 min	3 hr	12 hr

Half-life: 5½ hours; xinafoate salt, 11 days.

ADVERSE REACTIONS
CNS: headache, sinus headache, tremor, nervousness, giddiness, dizziness.
CV: *ventricular arrhythmias,* tachycardia, palpitations.
EENT: *nasopharyngitis,* pharyngitis, nasal cavity or sinus disorder.
GI: nausea, vomiting, diarrhea, heartburn.
Musculoskeletal: joint and back pain, myalgia.
Respiratory: *upper respiratory tract infection,* **bronchospasm,** cough, lower respiratory tract infection.
Other: hypersensitivity reactions.

INTERACTIONS
Drug-drug. *Beta agonists, other methylxanthines, theophylline:* May cause adverse cardiac effects with excessive use. Monitor patient.
MAO inhibitors: May cause risk of severe adverse CV effects. Avoid use within 14 days of MAO inhibitor therapy.
Tricyclic antidepressants: May cause risk of moderate to severe adverse CV effects. Use together with caution.

EFFECTS ON LAB TEST RESULTS
None reported.

CONTRAINDICATIONS & CAUTIONS
● Contraindicated in patients hypersensitive to drug or its ingredients.
● Use cautiously in patients unusually responsive to sympathomimetics and those with coronary insufficiency, arrhythmias, hypertension, other CV disorders, thyrotoxicosis, or seizure disorders.

NURSING CONSIDERATIONS
● Drug isn't indicated for acute bronchospasm.
● *Alert:* Monitor patient for rash and urticaria, which may signal a hypersensitivity reaction.
● *Look alike–sound alike:* Don't confuse Serevent with Serentil.

PATIENT TEACHING
● Remind patient to take drug at about 12-hour intervals for optimal effect and to take drug even when feeling better.
● If patient is taking drug to prevent exercise-induced bronchospasm, tell him to take it 30 to 60 minutes before exercise.
● *Alert:* Tell patient drug shouldn't be used to treat acute bronchospasm. He must use a short-acting beta agonist, such as albuterol, to treat worsening symptoms.
● *Alert:* Rare serious asthma episodes or asthma-related deaths may occur in patients using salmeterol. Black patients may be at greater risk.
● Tell patient to contact prescriber if the short-acting agonist no longer provides sufficient relief or if he needs more than 4 inhalations daily. This may be a sign that the asthma symptoms are worsening. Tell him not to increase the dosage of salmeterol.
● If patient takes an inhaled corticosteroid, he should continue to use it regularly. Warn patient not to take other drugs without prescriber's consent.
● If patient takes the inhalation powder (in a multidose inhaler), instruct him not to exhale into the device. He should activate and use it only in a level, horizontal position.
● Tell patient not to use the dry-powder multidose inhaler with a spacer.

• Instruct patient never to wash the mouth-piece or any part of the dry-powder multi-dose inhaler; it must be kept dry.

SAFETY ALERT!

streptokinase
strep-to-KIN-ase

Streptase

Pharmacologic class: plasminogen activator
Pregnancy risk category C

AVAILABLE FORMS
Injection: 250,000 international units; 750,000 international units; 1.5 million international units in vials for reconstitution

INDICATIONS & DOSAGES
➤ **Arteriovenous-cannula occlusion**
Adults: 250,000 international units in 2 ml I.V. solution by I.V. pump infusion into each occluded limb of the cannula over 25 to 35 minutes. Clamp off cannula for 2 hours. Then aspirate contents of cannula, flush with normal saline solution, and reconnect.
➤ **Venous thrombosis, pulmonary embolism, arterial thrombosis, and embolism**
Adults: Loading dose is 250,000 international units by I.V. infusion over 30 minutes. Sustaining dose is 100,000 international units/hour I.V. infusion for 72 hours for deep vein thrombosis and 100,000 international units/hour over 24 to 72 hours by I.V. infusion pump for pulmonary embolism and arterial thrombosis or embolism.
➤ **Lysis of coronary artery thrombi following acute MI**
Adults: Infuse 1.5 million international units I.V. over 30 to 60 minutes.

ADMINISTRATION
I.V.
• Reconstitute drug in each vial with 5 ml of normal saline solution for injection or D_5W solution. Further dilute to 45 ml (if needed, total volume may be increased to 500 ml in a glass or 50 ml in a plastic container). Don't shake; roll gently to mix.

Solution may precipitate after reconstituting; discard if large amounts are present.
• Filter solution with 0.8-micron or larger filter.
• Use immediately after reconstitution. If refrigerated, solution can be used for direct I.V. administration within 8 hours.
• Use an infusion pump to start a continuous infusion of heparin 1 to 4 hours after stopping streptokinase. Starting heparin 12 hours after intracoronary streptokinase may minimize bleeding risk.
• Store powder at room temperature.
• **Incompatibilities:** Dextrans. Don't mix with other drugs or give other drugs through the same I.V. line.

ACTION
Converts plasminogen to plasmin by directly cleaving peptide bonds at two sites, causing fibrinolysis.

Route	Onset	Peak	Duration
I.V.	Immediate	20 min–2 hr	4–24 hr

Half-life: First phase, 18 minutes; second phase, 83 minutes.

ADVERSE REACTIONS
CNS: polyradiculoneuropathy, headache, *fever.*
CV: *reperfusion arrhythmias,* hypotension, vasculitis, flushing.
EENT: periorbital edema.
GI: nausea.
Hematologic: *bleeding,* moderately decreased hematocrit.
Respiratory: minor breathing difficulty, *bronchospasm, pulmonary edema.*
Skin: urticaria, pruritus.
Other: phlebitis at injection site, hypersensitivity reactions, *anaphylaxis,* delayed hypersensitivity reactions, *angioedema,* shivering.

INTERACTIONS
Drug-drug. *Anticoagulants:* May increase risk of bleeding. Monitor patient closely. *Antifibrinolytic drugs (such as aminocaproic acid):* May inhibit and reverse streptokinase activity. Avoid using together. *Aspirin, dipyridamole, drugs affecting platelet activity (abciximab, eptifibatide, tirofiban), indomethacin, NSAIDs,*

phenylbutazone: May increase risk of bleeding. Monitor patient closely.

EFFECTS ON LAB TEST RESULTS

- May decrease hematocrit, plasminogen, and fibrinogen levels.
- May increase PT, PTT, and INR.

CONTRAINDICATIONS & CAUTIONS

- Contraindicated in patients with active internal bleeding; recent (within 2 months) cerebrovascular accident, or intracranial or intraspinal surgery; intracranial neoplasm; severe uncontrolled hypertension, or any patient with a history of an allergic reaction to the drug.
- Contraindicated with I.M. injections and other invasive procedures.
- Use cautiously in patients with recent (within 10 days) major surgery, obstetric delivery, organ biopsy, previous puncture of noncompressible vessels, serious GI bleeding, or trauma including cardiopulmonary resuscitation.
- Use cautiously in patients with a systolic blood pressure of 180 mm Hg or greater or a diastolic blood pressure of 110 mm Hg or greater, a high likelihood of left heart thrombus (mitral stenosis with atrial fibrillation), subacute bacterial endocarditis, hemostatic defects including those secondary to severe hepatic or renal disease, age older than 75 years, pregnancy, cerebrovascular disease, diabetic hemorrhagic retinopathy, septic thrombophlebitis or occluded AV cannula at seriously infected site, or any other condition in which bleeding constitutes a significant hazard or would be particularly difficult to manage because of its location.

NURSING CONSIDERATIONS

- For acute MI, give as soon as possible after symptom onset. The greatest benefit in mortality reduction was observed when streptokinase was given within 4 hours, but significant benefit has been reported up to 24 hours.
- For pulmonary embolism, deep vein thrombosis, arterial thrombosis, or embolism, institute treatment as soon as possible after thrombotic event onset, preferably within 7 days.
- Drug may be given to menstruating women.

- Only prescribers with experience managing thrombotic disease should give drug and only where clinical and laboratory monitoring can be performed.
- Before using drug to clear an occluded AV cannula, try flushing with heparinized saline solution.
- Keep aminocaproic acid available to treat bleeding and corticosteroids to treat allergic reactions.
- Before starting therapy, draw blood for coagulation studies, hematocrit, platelet count, and type and crossmatching. Rate of infusion depends on thrombin time and drug resistance.
- To check for hypersensitivity in acutely ill patients or patients with known allergies, give 100 international units I.D.; a wheal-and-flare response within 20 minutes means patient is probably allergic. Monitor vital signs frequently.
- For patient who has had a streptococcal infection or has been treated with streptokinase or anistreplase in the last 2 years, use a different thrombolytic.
- Combined therapy with low-dose aspirin (162.5 mg) or dipyridamole has improved short- and long-term results.
- Monitor patient for excessive bleeding every 15 minutes for first hour, every 30 minutes for second through eighth hours, and then every 4 hours. If bleeding is evident, stop therapy and notify prescriber. Pretreatment with heparin or drugs that affect platelets causes high risk of bleeding but may improve long-term results.
- Monitor pulse, color, and sensation of arms and legs every hour.
- Keep involved limb in straight alignment to prevent bleeding from infusion site.
- Monitor blood pressure closely.
- Avoid unnecessary handling of patient; pad side rails. Bruising is more likely during therapy.
- Keep a laboratory flow sheet on patient's chart to monitor PTT, PT, thrombin time, hemoglobin level, and hematocrit. Monitor vital signs and neurologic status.
- Avoid I.M. injection. Keep venipuncture sites to a minimum; use pressure dressing on puncture sites for at least 15 minutes.
- *Alert:* Watch for signs of hypersensitivity and notify prescriber immediately if any occur. Antihistamines or corticosteroids

---

may be used for mild allergic reactions. If a severe reaction occurs, stop infusion immediately and notify prescriber.

PATIENT TEACHING
• Explain use and administration of drug to patient and family.
• Tell patient to promptly report adverse reactions, such as bleeding and bruising.

---

streptomycin sulfate
strep-toe-MYE-sin

Pharmacologic class: aminoglycoside
Pregnancy risk category D

AVAILABLE FORMS
Injection: 1-g/2.5-ml ampules

INDICATIONS & DOSAGES
➤ **Streptococcal endocarditis**
Adults: 1 g every 12 hours I.M. for 1 week; then 500 mg I.M. every 12 hours for 1 week, given with penicillin.
Adjust-a-dose: In patients older than age 60, give 500 mg I.M. every 12 hours for entire 2 weeks, with penicillin.
➤ **Second-line treatment of tuberculosis (TB), given with other antituberculotics**
Adults: 15 mg/kg (maximum of 1 g) I.M. daily, continued long enough to prevent relapse. For intermittent use, 25 to 30 mg/kg (maximum of 1.5 g) two to three times weekly.
Children: 20 to 40 mg/kg (maximum of 1 g) I.M. daily. Give with other antituberculotics, except capreomycin; continue until sputum test result becomes negative. For intermittent use, 25 to 30 mg/kg (maximum of 1.5 g) two to three times weekly.
Adults older than 59: Give 10 mg/kg I.M. daily.
➤ **Enterococcal endocarditis**
Adults: 1 g I.M. every 12 hours for 2 weeks; then 500 mg I.M. every 12 hours for 4 weeks, given with penicillin.
➤ **Tularemia**
Adults: 1 to 2 g I.M. daily in divided doses injected deep into upper outer quadrant of buttocks; continued for 7 to 14 days or until patient is afebrile for 5 to 7 days.

ADMINISTRATION
I.M.
• Obtain specimen for culture and sensitivity tests before giving, except when treating TB. Begin therapy while awaiting results.
• Obtain blood for peak level 1 to 2 hours after I.M. injection; obtain blood for trough level just before next dose. Don't use a heparinized tube; heparin is incompatible with aminoglycosides.
• To avoid irritation, protect hands when preparing drug.
• Inject deep into upper outer quadrant of buttocks or midlateral thigh. Rotate injection sites.
• In children, give injection in midlateral thigh, if possible, to minimize possibility of damaging sciatic nerve.

ACTION
Inhibits protein synthesis by binding directly to the 30S ribosomal subunit; bactericidal.

Route	Onset	Peak	Duration
I.M.	Unknown	1–2 hr	Unknown

Half-life: 2 to 3 hours.

ADVERSE REACTIONS
CNS: *neuromuscular blockade,* vertigo, facial paresthesia.
EENT: *ototoxicity.*
GI: vomiting, nausea.
GU: *nephrotoxicity,* increase in urinary excretion of casts.
Hematologic: *leukopenia, thrombocytopenia, hemolytic anemia,* eosinophilia.
Respiratory: *apnea.*
Skin: exfoliative dermatitis.
Other: *anaphylaxis,* hypersensitivity reactions.

INTERACTIONS
Drug-drug. *Acyclovir, amphotericin B, cephalosporins, cidofovir, cisplatin, methoxyflurane, vancomycin, other aminoglycosides:* May increase nephrotoxicity. Monitor renal function test results.
Atracurium, pancuronium, rocuronium, vecuronium: May increase effects of nondepolarizing muscle relaxants, including prolonged respiratory depression. Use together only when necessary, and expect to

---

reduce dosage of nondepolarizing muscle relaxant.

General anesthetics: May increase neuromuscular blockade. Monitor patient closely.

I.V. loop diuretics such as furosemide: May increase ototoxicity. Monitor patient's hearing.

Penicillins: May inactivate streptomycin, decreasing the therapeutic effects. Don't mix together.

EFFECTS ON LAB TEST RESULTS
● May increase BUN, creatinine, and nonprotein nitrogen levels. May decrease hemoglobin level.
● May increase eosinophil count. May decrease WBC and platelet counts.
● May cause false-positive reaction in copper sulfate tests for urine glucose, such as Benedict's reagent and Diastix.

CONTRAINDICATIONS & CAUTIONS
● Contraindicated in patients hypersensitive to drug or other aminoglycosides.
● Use cautiously in elderly patients and in patients with impaired renal function or neuromuscular disorders.

NURSING CONSIDERATIONS
● **Alert:** Evaluate patient's hearing before therapy and for 6 months afterward. Notify prescriber if patient has hearing loss, feels fullness in ears, or hears roaring noises.
● Drug has been given off-label as I.V. infusion over 30 to 60 minutes without unusual adverse effects in patients who can't tolerate I.M. injections.
● Watch for signs and symptoms of superinfection, such as continued fever, chills, and increased pulse rate.
● **Alert:** Monitor renal function: urine output, specific gravity, urinalysis, BUN and creatinine levels, and creatinine clearance. Report to prescriber evidence of declining renal function. Nephrotoxicity occurs less frequently with streptomycin than with other aminoglycosides.
● When drug is used as primary treatment of TB, stop therapy when sputum test result becomes negative.
● Total dose for TB shouldn't exceed 120 g over the course of therapy unless there are no other treatment options.

PATIENT TEACHING
● Instruct patient to report adverse reactions promptly.
● Encourage patient to maintain adequate fluid intake.
● Emphasize need for blood tests to monitor levels and determine effectiveness of therapy.

---

tacrolimus
tack-ROW-lim-us

Prograf

Pharmacologic class: macrolide
Pregnancy risk category C

AVAILABLE FORMS
Capsules: 0.5 mg, 1 mg, 5 mg
Injection: 5 mg/ml

INDICATIONS & DOSAGES
➤ **To prevent organ rejection in allogenic liver, kidney, or heart transplant**
Adults: For patients who can't take drug orally, give 0.03 to 0.05 mg/kg/day (liver or kidney) or 0.01 mg/kg/day (heart) I.V. as continuous infusion at least 6 hours after transplant. Switch to oral therapy as soon as possible, with first dose 8 to 12 hours after stopping I.V. infusion. For renal transplant, give oral dose within 24 hours of transplantation after renal function has recovered. Initial P.O. dosages: For liver transplant, give 0.1 to 0.15 mg/kg daily in two divided doses every 12 hours; for kidney transplant, give 0.2 mg/kg daily in two divided doses every 12 hours; for heart transplant, give 0.075 mg/kg daily in two divided doses every 12 hours. Adjust dosages based on patient response.
Children (liver transplant only): Initially, 0.03 to 0.05 mg/kg daily I.V.; then 0.15 to 0.2 mg/kg daily P.O. on schedule similar to that of adults, adjusted as needed.
Adjust-a-dose: Give lowest recommended P.O. and I.V. dosages to patients with renal or hepatic impairment.

ADMINISTRATION

P.O.
- Give drug 1 hour before or 2 hours after a meal.
- Don't give with grapefruit juice.

I.V.
- Dilute drug with normal saline solution for injection or D_5W injection to 0.004 to 0.02 mg/ml before use.
- Monitor patient continuously during first 30 minutes and frequently thereafter for signs and symptoms of anaphylaxis.
- Store diluted infusion solution for up to 24 hours in glass or polyethylene containers. Don't store drug in a polyvinyl chloride container because of decreased stability and potential for extraction of phthalates.
- **Incompatibilities:** Solutions or I.V. drugs with a pH above 9, such as acyclovir and ganciclovir.

ACTION

Exact mechanism unknown. Inhibits T-cell activation, which results in immunosuppression.

Route	Onset	Peak	Duration
P.O., I.V.	Unknown	1½–3 hr	Unknown

Half-life: 33 to 56 hours.

ADVERSE REACTIONS

CNS: *asthenia, delirium, fever, headache, insomnia, pain, paresthesia, tremor,* **coma.**
CV: *peripheral edema,* hypertension.
GI: *abdominal pain, anorexia, ascites, constipation, diarrhea, nausea, vomiting.*
GU: *abnormal renal function, oliguria, UTI.*
Hematologic: THROMBOCYTOPENIA, anemia, leukocytosis.
Metabolic: *hyperglycemia,* HYPER-KALEMIA, *hypokalemia,* HYPOMAGNE-SEMIA.
Musculoskeletal: *back pain.*
Respiratory: *atelectasis, dyspnea, pleural effusion.*
Skin: *burning, photosensitivity, pruritus, rash,* alopecia.

INTERACTIONS

Drug-drug. *Azole antifungals, bromocriptine, cimetidine, clarithromycin, cyclosporine, danazol, diltiazem, erythromycin, methylprednisolone, metoclopramide, nicardipine, verapamil:* May increase tacrolimus level. Watch for adverse effects.
Carbamazepine, phenobarbital, phenytoin, **rifamycins:** May decrease tacrolimus level. Monitor effectiveness of tacrolimus.
Cyclosporine: May increase risk of excess nephrotoxicity. Avoid using together.
Immunosuppressants (except adrenal corticosteroids): May oversuppress immune system. Monitor patient closely, especially during times of stress.
Inducers of cytochrome P-450 enzyme system: May increase tacrolimus metabolism and decrease blood levels. Dosage adjustment may be needed.
Inhibitors of cytochrome P-450 enzyme system (phenobarbital, phenytoin, rifampin): May decrease tacrolimus metabolism and increase blood level. Dosage adjustment may be needed.
Live-virus vaccines: May interfere with immune response to live-virus vaccines. Postpone routine immunizations.
Nephrotoxic drugs, such as aminoglycosides, amphotericin B, cisplatin, cyclosporine: May cause additive or synergistic effects. Monitor patient closely. Don't use tacrolimus simultaneously with cyclosporine. Stop cyclosporine at least 24 hours before starting tacrolimus.
Potassium-sparing diuretics: May cause severe hyperkalemia. Don't use together.
Sirolimus: May increase risk of wound healing complications, renal impairment, and insulin-dependent post-transplant diabetes mellitus in heart transplant patients. Avoid using together.
Drug-herb. *St. John's wort:* May decrease drug level. Discourage use together.
Drug-food. *Any food:* May inhibit drug absorption. Urge patient to take drug on empty stomach.
Grapefruit juice: May increase drug level. Discourage patient from taking together.

EFFECTS ON LAB TEST RESULTS

- May increase BUN, creatinine, and glucose levels. May decrease magnesium and hemoglobin levels. May increase or decrease potassium level and cause abnormal liver function test values.
- May decrease WBC and platelet counts.

CONTRAINDICATIONS & CAUTIONS
● Contraindicated in patients hypersensitive to drug.
● I.V. form is contraindicated in patients hypersensitive to castor oil derivatives.

NURSING CONSIDERATIONS
● *Alert:* Patient has increased risk for infections, lymphomas, and other malignant diseases. Use only after other treatments have failed.
● *Alert:* Because of risk of anaphylaxis, use injection only in patients who can't take oral form. Keep epinephrine 1:1,000 and oxygen available.
● Children with normal renal and hepatic function may need higher dosages than adults.
● Patients with hepatic or renal dysfunction should receive lowest dosage possible.
● Use with adrenal corticosteroids for all indications. For heart transplant patients, also use with azathioprine or mycophenolate mofetil.
● Don't use tacrolimus simultaneously with cyclosporine. Stop either drug at least 24 hours before initiating the other.
● Monitor patient for signs and symptoms of neurotoxicity and nephrotoxicity, especially if patient is receiving a high dose or has renal or hepatic dysfunction.
● Monitor patient for signs and symptoms of hyperkalemia, such as palpitations and muscle weakness or cramping. Obtain potassium levels regularly. Avoid potassium-sparing diuretics during drug therapy.
● Monitor patient's glucose level regularly. Also monitor patient for signs and symptoms of hyperglycemia, such as dizziness, confusion, and frequent urination. Treatment of hyperglycemia may be needed. Insulin-dependent posttransplant diabetes may occur; in some cases, it's reversible.

PATIENT TEACHING
● Advise patient to check with prescriber before taking other drugs during therapy.
● Urge patient to report adverse reactions promptly.
● Tell diabetic patient that glucose levels may increase.

terbutaline sulfate
ter-BYOO-ta-leen

Brethine

Pharmacologic class: beta$_2$ agonist
Pregnancy risk category B

AVAILABLE FORMS
Injection: 1 mg/ml
Tablets: 2.5 mg, 5 mg

INDICATIONS & DOSAGES
➤ **Bronchospasm in patients with reversible obstructive airway disease**
Adults and children age 12 and older: 0.25 mg subcutaneously. Repeat in 15 to 30 minutes, p.r.n. Maximum, 0.5 mg in 4 hours. If patient fails to respond to second dose, consider other measures.
Adults and adolescents older than age 15: Give 2.5 to 5 mg P.O. t.i.d. every 6 hours while awake. Maximum, 15 mg daily.
Children ages 12 to 15: Give 2.5 mg P.O. t.i.d. every 6 hours while awake. Maximum, 7.5 mg daily.

ADMINISTRATION
P.O.
● Give drug without regard for food.
Subcutaneous
● Give subcutaneous injections into the side of the deltoid.
● Protect drug from light. Don't use if discolored.

ACTION
Relaxes bronchial smooth muscle by stimulating beta$_2$ receptors.

Route	Onset	Peak	Duration
P.O.	30 min	2–3 hr	4–8 hr
Subcut	15 min	30 min	1½ –4 hr

Half-life: Unknown.

ADVERSE REACTIONS
CNS: *nervousness, tremor, drowsiness, dizziness, headache,* weakness.
CV: *palpitations,* **arrhythmias,** tachycardia, flushing.

GI: *vomiting, nausea,* heartburn.
Metabolic: hypokalemia.
Respiratory: *paradoxical bronchospasm with prolonged use,* dyspnea.
Skin: diaphoresis.

INTERACTIONS
Drug-drug. *Cardiac glycosides, cyclopropane, halogenated inhaled anesthetics, levodopa:* May increase risk of arrhythmias. Monitor patient closely, and avoid using together with levodopa.
CNS stimulants: May increase CNS stimulation. Avoid using together.
MAO inhibitors: When given with sympathomimetics, may cause severe hypertension (hypertensive crisis). Avoid using together.
Propranolol, other beta blockers: May block bronchodilating effects of terbutaline. Avoid using together.

EFFECTS ON LAB TEST RESULTS
• May decrease potassium level.

CONTRAINDICATIONS & CAUTIONS
• Contraindicated in patients hypersensitive to drug or sympathomimetic amines.
• Use cautiously in patient with CV disorders, hyperthyroidism, diabetes, or seizure disorders.

NURSING CONSIDERATIONS
• Drug may reduce the sensitivity of spirometry for the diagnosis of bronchospasm.
• *Look alike–sound alike:* Don't confuse terbutaline with tolbutamide or terbinafine.

PATIENT TEACHING
• Make sure patient and caregivers understand why patient needs drug.
• Remind patient to separate oral doses by 6 hours.

theophylline
thee-OFF-i-lin

Immediate-release liquids
Elixophyllin*

Immediate-release tablets
Theolair

Timed-release tablets
Theochron, Uniphyl

Timed-release capsules
TheoCap, Theo-24

Pharmacologic class: xanthine derivative
Pregnancy risk category C

AVAILABLE FORMS
Capsules (extended-release): 100 mg, 125 mg, 200 mg, 300 mg, 400 mg
D_5W injection: 200 mg in 50 ml or 100 ml; 400 mg in 100 ml, 250 ml, 500 ml, or 1,000 ml; 800 mg in 500 ml or 1,000 ml
Elixir: 27 mg/5 ml*
Syrup: 80 mg/15 ml*
Tablets: 125 mg, 250 mg
Tablets (extended-release): 100 mg, 200 mg, 300 mg, 400 mg, 450 mg, 600 mg

INDICATIONS & DOSAGES
Extended-release preparations shouldn't be used to treat acute bronchospasm.
➤ **Oral theophylline for acute bronchospasm in patients not currently receiving theophylline**
Adult nonsmokers and children older than age 16: Give 5 mg/kg P.O.; then 3 mg/kg every 6 hours for two doses. Maintenance dosage is 3 mg/kg every 8 hours.
Children ages 9 to 16: Give 5 mg/kg P.O.; then 3 mg/kg every 4 hours for three dosages. Maintenance dosage is 3 mg/kg every 6 hours.
Children ages 6 months to 9 years: 5 mg/kg P.O.; then 4 mg/kg every 4 hours for three doses. Maintenance dosage is 4 mg/kg every 6 hours.

Adjust-a-dose: For otherwise healthy adult smokers, 5 mg/kg P.O.; then 3 mg/kg every 4 hours for three doses. Maintenance dosage is 3 mg/kg every 6 hours. For older adults and patients with cor pulmonale, 5 mg/kg P.O.; then 2 mg/kg every 6 hours for two doses. Maintenance dosage is 2 mg/kg every 8 hours. For adults with heart failure or liver disease, 5 mg/kg P.O.; then 2 mg/kg every 8 hours for two doses. Maintenance dosage is 1 to 2 mg/kg every 12 hours.

➤ **Parenteral theophylline for patients not currently receiving theophylline**
Loading dose: 4.7 mg/kg I.V. slowly; then maintenance infusion.
Adult nonsmokers and children older than age 16: Give 0.55 mg/kg/hour I.V. for 12 hours; then 0.39 mg/kg/hour.
Children ages 9 to 16: Give 0.79 mg/kg/hour I.V. for 12 hours; then 0.63 mg/kg/hour.
Children ages 6 months to 9 years: 0.95 mg/kg/hour I.V. for 12 hours; then 0.79 mg/kg/hour.
Adjust-a-dose: For otherwise healthy adult smokers, 0.79 mg/kg/hour I.V. for 12 hours; then 0.63 mg/kg/hour. For older adults and patients with cor pulmonale, 0.47 mg/kg/hour I.V. for 12 hours; then 0.24 mg/kg/hour. For adults with heart failure or liver disease, 0.39 mg/kg/hour I.V. for 12 hours; then 0.08 to 0.16 mg/kg/hour.
➤ **Oral and parenteral theophylline for acute bronchospasm in patients currently receiving theophylline**
Adults and children: Ideally, dose is based on current theophylline level. Each 0.5 mg/kg I.V. or P.O. loading dose will increase drug level by 1 mcg/ml. In emergencies, when theophylline level can't be readily obtained, some prescribers recommend a 2.5-mg/kg P.O. dose of rapidly absorbed form if patient develops no obvious signs or symptoms of theophylline toxicity.
➤ **Chronic bronchospasm**
Adults and children: Initially, 16 mg/kg or 400 mg P.O. daily, whichever is less, given in three or four divided doses at 6- to 8-hour intervals. Or, 12 mg/kg or 400 mg P.O. daily, whichever is less, in an extended-release preparation given in two or three divided doses at 8- or 12-hour

intervals. Dosage may be increased, as tolerated, at 2- to 3-day intervals to the following maximums: adults and children older than age 16, 13 mg/kg or 900 mg P.O. daily, whichever is less; children ages 12 to 16, 18 mg/kg P.O. daily; children ages 9 to 12, 20 mg/kg P.O. daily; children younger than age 9, 24 mg/kg P.O. daily.

ADMINISTRATION
P.O.
● Give drug with full glass of water after meals, if needed, to relieve GI symptoms, although taking with food delays absorption.
● Give drug around-the-clock, using extended-release product at bedtime.
● Don't dissolve or crush extended-release products. Small children unable to swallow these can ingest (without chewing) the contents of capsules sprinkled over soft food.
I.V.
● Use commercially available infusion solution, or mix in D₅W solution.
● Use infusion pump for continuous infusion.
● **Incompatibilities:** Ascorbic acid, ceftriaxone, cimetidine, hetastarch, phenytoin.

ACTION
Inhibits phosphodiesterase, the enzyme that degrades cAMP, resulting in relaxation of smooth muscle of the bronchial airways and pulmonary blood vessels.

Route	Onset	Peak	Duration
P.O.	15–60 min	1–2 hr	Unknown
P.O. (extended)	15–60 min	4–7 hr	Unknown
I.V.	15 min	15–30 min	Unknown

Half-life: Adults, 7 to 9 hours; smokers, 4 to 5 hours; children, 3 to 5 hours; premature infants, 20 to 30 hours.

ADVERSE REACTIONS
CNS: *restlessness, dizziness, insomnia, seizures,* headache, irritability, muscle twitching.
CV: *palpitations, sinus tachycardia, arrhythmias,* extrasystoles, flushing, marked hypotension.
GI: *nausea, vomiting,* diarrhea, epigastric pain.

Metabolic: urinary catecholamines.
Respiratory: *respiratory arrest,* tachypnea.

INTERACTIONS
Drug-drug. *Adenosine:* May decrease antiarrhythmic effect. Higher doses of adenosine may be needed.
Allopurinol, calcium channel blockers, **cimetidine,** *disulfiram, influenza virus vaccine, interferon,* **macrolides (such as erythromycin),** *methotrexate,* **mexiletine,** *oral contraceptives,* **quinolones (such as ciprofloxacin):** May decrease hepatic clearance of theophylline; may increase theophylline level. Monitor levels closely and adjust theophylline dose.
Barbiturates, ketoconazole, nicotine, **phenytoin, rifamycins:** May enhance metabolism and decrease theophylline level; may increase phenytoin metabolism. Monitor patient for decreased therapeutic effect; monitor levels and adjust dosage.
Carbamazepine, isoniazid, loop diuretics: May increase or decrease theophylline level. Monitor theophylline level.
Carteolol, pindolol, propranolol, timolol: May act antagonistically, reducing the effects of one or both drugs; may reduce elimination of theophylline. Monitor theophylline level and patient closely.
Ephedrine, other sympathomimetics: May exhibit synergistic toxicity with these drugs, predisposing patient to arrhythmias. Monitor patient closely.
Lithium: May increase lithium excretion. Monitor patient closely.
Tetracyclines: May enhance the adverse effects of theophylline. Monitor patient closely.
Drug-herb. *Cacao tree:* May inhibit drug metabolism. Discourage use together.
Cayenne: May increase risk of drug toxicity. Advise patient to use together cautiously.
Ephedra: May increase risk of adverse reactions. Discourage use together.
Guarana: May cause additive CNS and CV effects. Discourage use together.
Ipriflavone: May increase risk of drug toxicity. Advise patient to use together cautiously.
St. John's wort: May decrease drug level. Discourage use together.

Drug-food. *Any food:* May cause accelerated drug release from extended-release products. Tell patient to take extended-release products on an empty stomach.
Caffeine: May decrease hepatic clearance of drug and increase drug level. Monitor patient for toxicity.
Drug-lifestyle. *Smoking:* May increase elimination of drug, increasing dosage requirements. Monitor drug response and level.

EFFECTS ON LAB TEST RESULTS
● May increase free fatty acid level and blood glucose.
● May falsely elevate theophylline level in the presence of acetaminophen, furosemide, phenylbutazone, probenecid, theobromine, caffeine, tea, chocolate, and cola, depending on assay used.

CONTRAINDICATIONS & CAUTIONS
● Contraindicated in patients hypersensitive to xanthine compounds (caffeine, theobromine) and in those with active peptic ulcer or poorly controlled seizure disorders.
● Use cautiously in young children, infants, neonates, elderly patients, and those with COPD, cardiac failure, cor pulmonale, renal or hepatic disease, peptic ulceration, hyperthyroidism, diabetes mellitus, glaucoma, severe hypoxemia, hypertension, compromised cardiac or circulatory function, angina, acute MI, or sulfite sensitivity.

NURSING CONSIDERATIONS
● Dosage may need to be increased in cigarette smokers and in habitual marijuana smokers because smoking causes drug to be metabolized faster.
● Monitor vital signs; measure and record fluid intake and output. Expect improved quality of pulse and respirations.
● Patients metabolize xanthines at different rates; dosage is determined by monitoring response, tolerance, pulmonary function, and drug level. Drug levels range from 10 to 20 mcg/ml; toxicity may occur at levels above 20 mcg/ml.
● *Alert:* Evidence of toxicity includes tachycardia, anorexia, nausea, vomiting, diarrhea, restlessness, irritability, and

headache. If these signs occur, check drug level and adjust dosage, as indicated.

● *Look alike–sound alike:* Don't confuse extended-release form with regular-release form.

● *Look alike–sound alike:* Don't confuse Theolair with Thyrolar.

PATIENT TEACHING

● Supply instructions for home care and dosage schedule.

● Warn patient not to dissolve, crush, or chew extended-release products. Small children unable to swallow these can ingest (without chewing) the contents of capsules sprinkled over soft food.

● Tell patient to relieve GI symptoms by taking oral drug with full glass of water after meals, although food in stomach delays absorption.

● Warn patient to take drug regularly, only as directed. Patients tend to want to take extra "breathing pills."

● Inform elderly patient that dizziness is common at start of therapy.

● Urge patient to tell prescriber about any other drugs taken. OTC drugs or herbal remedies may contain ephedrine or theophylline salts; excessive CNS stimulation may result.

● If a smoker quits, tell him to inform prescriber. Dosage reduction may be needed to prevent toxicity.

---

ticarcillin disodium and clavulanate potassium

tie-kar-SIL-in and KLAV-yoo-lan-nayt

Timentin

Pharmacologic class: extended-spectrum penicillin, beta-lactamase inhibitor
Pregnancy risk category B

AVAILABLE FORMS

Injection: 3 g ticarcillin and 100 mg clavulanic acid in 3.1-g vials
Premixed: 3.1 g/100 ml

INDICATIONS & DOSAGES

➤ **Gynecologic infection**
Women who weigh 60 kg (132 lb) or more: For moderate infections, 200 mg/kg (ticar-

cillin component) I.V. daily in divided doses every 6 hours. For severe infections, 300 mg/kg (ticarcillin component) I.V. daily in divided doses every 4 hours.
Women who weigh less than 60 kg: 200 to 300 mg/kg (ticarcillin component) I.V. daily in divided doses every 4 to 6 hours.

➤ **Lower respiratory tract, urinary tract, bone and joint, intra-abdominal, or skin and skin-structure infection and septicemia caused by beta-lactamase–producing strains of bacteria or by ticarcillin-susceptible organisms**
Adults and children who weigh more than 60 kg (132 lb): 3.1 g (Timentin) by I.V. infusion every 4 to 6 hours.
Adults and children ages 3 months to 16 years who weigh less than 60 kg: 200 mg/kg (ticarcillin component) I.V. daily in divided doses every 6 hours. For severe infections, 300 mg/kg (ticarcillin component) I.V. daily in divided doses every 4 hours.
Adjust-a-dose: If creatinine clearance is 30 to 60 ml/minute, dosage is 2 g I.V. every 4 hours; if clearance is 10 to 29 ml/minute, 2 g I.V. every 8 hours; if clearance is less than 10 ml/minute, 2 g I.V. every 12 hours; if clearance is less than 10 ml/minute and patient has hepatic dysfunction, 2 g I.V. every 24 hours. For patients receiving peritoneal dialysis or hemodialysis, give a loading dose of 3.1 g I.V. and then maintenance doses of 3.1 g I.V. every 12 hours for patients receiving peritoneal dialysis or 2 g I.V. every 12 hours for patients receiving hemodialysis. Supplement with 3.1 g after each hemodialysis session.

ADMINISTRATION
I.V.

● Before giving, ask patient about allergic reactions to penicillin.

● Obtain specimen for culture and sensitivity tests. Begin therapy while awaiting results.

● Give drug at least 1 hour before a bacteriostatic antibiotic.

● Reconstitute drug with 13 ml of sterile water for injection or normal saline solution for injection. Further dilute to a maximum of 10 to 100 mg/ml (based on drug component).

● Infuse over 30 minutes.
● **Incompatibilities:** Aminoglycosides, amphotericin B, azithromycin, cisatracurium, other anti-infectives, sodium bicarbonate, topotecan, vancomycin.

ACTION
Inhibits cell-wall synthesis during bacterial multiplication.

Route	Onset	Peak	Duration
I.V.	Immediate	Immediate	Unknown

Half-life: 1 hour.

ADVERSE REACTIONS
CNS: *seizures,* headache, giddiness, neuromuscular excitability.
CV: phlebitis, vein irritation.
EENT: taste and smell disturbances.
GI: *pseudomembranous colitis,* diarrhea, flatulence, epigastric pain, nausea, stomatitis, vomiting.
Hematologic: *leukopenia, neutropenia, thrombocytopenia,* anemia, eosinophilia, hemolytic anemia.
Metabolic: hypernatremia, hypokalemia.
Skin: *Stevens-Johnson syndrome,* pain at injection site, pruritus, rash.
Other: *anaphylaxis,* hypersensitivity reactions, overgrowth of nonsusceptible organisms.

INTERACTIONS
Drug-drug. *Hormonal contraceptives:* May decrease contraceptive effectiveness. Advise use of another form of contraception during therapy.
Oral anticoagulants: May increase risk of bleeding. Monitor PT and INR.
Probenecid: May increase ticarcillin level. Probenecid may be used for this purpose.

EFFECTS ON LAB TEST RESULTS
● May increase ALT, AST, alkaline phosphatase, LDH, and sodium levels. May decrease potassium and hemoglobin levels.
● May increase eosinophil count. May decrease platelet, WBC, and granulocyte counts.
● May alter results of turbidimetric tests that use sulfosalicylic acid, trichloroacetic acid, acetic acid, or nitric acid.

CONTRAINDICATIONS & CAUTIONS
● Contraindicated in patients hypersensitive to drug or other penicillins.
● Use cautiously in patients with other drug allergies, especially to cephalosporins because of possible cross-sensitivity, and in those with impaired renal function, hemorrhagic conditions, hypokalemia, or sodium restriction. Drug contains 4.5 mEq sodium/g.

NURSING CONSIDERATIONS
● Check CBC and platelet counts frequently. Drug may cause thrombocytopenia.
● Monitor PT and INR in patients taking oral anticoagulants.
● Monitor potassium and sodium levels.
● If large doses are given or if therapy is prolonged, bacterial or fungal superinfection may occur, especially in elderly, debilitated, or immunosuppressed patients.

PATIENT TEACHING
● Tell patient to report adverse reactions promptly.
● Instruct patient to report discomfort at I.V. site.
● Advise patient to limit salt intake during drug therapy because of high sodium content.

---

tiotropium bromide
tye-oh-TROH-pee-um

Spiriva

Pharmacologic class: anticholinergic
Pregnancy risk category C

AVAILABLE FORMS
Capsules for inhalation: 18 mcg

INDICATIONS & DOSAGES
➤ **Maintenance treatment of bronchospasm in COPD, including chronic bronchitis and emphysema**
Adults: 1 capsule (18 mcg) inhaled orally once daily using the HandiHaler inhalation device.

ADMINISTRATION
Inhalational
• Give capsules only by oral inhalation with the HandiHaler device.
• Open capsule blister immediately before use.
• Capsules aren't for oral ingestion.

ACTION
Competitive, reversible inhibition of muscarinic receptors leads to bronchodilation.

Route	Onset	Peak	Duration
Inhalation	30 min	3 hr	> 24 hr

Half-life: 5 to 6 days.

ADVERSE REACTIONS
CNS: depression, paresthesia.
CV: *angina pectoris,* chest pain, edema.
EENT: *sinusitis,* cataract, dysphonia, epistaxis, glaucoma, laryngitis, pharyngitis, rhinitis.
GI: *dry mouth,* abdominal pain, constipation, dyspepsia, gastroesophageal reflux, stomatitis, vomiting.
GU: UTI.
Metabolic: hypercholesterolemia, hyperglycemia.
Musculoskeletal: arthritis, leg pain, myalgia, skeletal pain.
Respiratory: *upper respiratory tract infection,* cough.
Skin: rash.
Other: *accidental injury,* allergic reaction, candidiasis, flulike syndrome, herpes zoster, infections.

INTERACTIONS
Drug-drug. *Anticholinergics:* May increase the risk of adverse reactions. Avoid using together.

EFFECTS ON LAB TEST RESULTS
• May increase cholesterol and glucose levels.

CONTRAINDICATIONS & CAUTIONS
• Contraindicated in patients hypersensitive to atropine, its derivatives, ipratropium, or any component of the product.
• Use cautiously in women who are pregnant or breast-feeding, patients with creatinine clearance of 50 ml/minute or less, or patients with angle-closure glaucoma, prostatic hyperplasia, or bladder neck obstruction.

NURSING CONSIDERATIONS
• *Alert:* Use drug for maintenance treatment of COPD, not for acute bronchospasm.
• Watch for evidence of hypersensitivity (especially angioedema) and paradoxical bronchospasm.
• *Look alike–sound alike:* Don't confuse Spiriva with Inspra.

PATIENT TEACHING
• Inform patient that drug is for maintenance treatment of COPD and not for immediate relief of breathing problems.
• *Alert:* Explain that capsules are for inhalation and shouldn't be swallowed.
• Provide full instructions for the HandiHaler device.
• Tell patient not to get powder in his eyes.
• Review signs and symptoms of hypersensitivity (especially angioedema) and paradoxical bronchospasm. Tell patient to stop the drug and contact the prescriber if they occur.
• Advise patient to report eye pain, blurred vision, visual halos, colored images, or red eyes immediately.
• Tell patient to keep capsules in sealed blisters and to remove each capsule just before use. Caution against storing capsules in the HandiHaler device.
• Instruct patient to store capsules at 77° F (25° C) and not to expose them to extreme temperatures or moisture.

tobramycin sulfate
toe-bra-MYE-sin

TOBI

Pharmacologic class: aminoglycoside
Pregnancy risk category D

AVAILABLE FORMS
Multidose vials (pediatric): 10 mg/ml, 40 mg/ml
Nebulizer solution (for inhalation): 300 mg/5 ml
Prefilled syringe (pediatric): 40 mg/ml

Premixed parenteral injection for infusion: 60 mg or 80 mg in normal saline solution

INDICATIONS & DOSAGES
➤ **Serious infection by sensitive strains of** *Escherichia coli, Proteus, Klebsiella, Enterobacter, Serratia, Morganella morganii, Staphylococcus aureus, Citrobacter, Pseudomonas,* **or** *Providencia*
Adults: 3 mg/kg/day I.M. or I.V. in divided doses. For life-threatening infections, give up to 5 mg/kg/day in divided doses every 6 to 8 hours; reduce to 3 mg/kg daily as soon as clinically indicated.
Children: 6 to 7.5 mg/kg/day I.M. or I.V., divided t.i.d. or q.i.d.
Neonates younger than age 1 week or premature infants: Up to 4 mg/kg/day I.V. or I.M. in two equal doses every 12 hours.
Adjust-a-dose: For patients with renal impairment, give loading dose of 1 mg/kg; then give decreased doses at 8-hour intervals or same dose at prolonged intervals. For patients with severe cystic fibrosis, initial dose is 10 mg/kg/day I.V. or I.M., divided q.i.d.
➤ **To manage cystic fibrosis patients with** *Pseudomonas aeruginosa*
Adults and children age 6 and older: 300 mg via nebulizer every 12 hours for 28 days. Continue cycle of 28 days on drug and 28 days off.

ADMINISTRATION
I.V.
● Obtain specimen for culture and sensitivity tests before giving. Begin therapy while awaiting results.
● For adults, dilute in 50 to 100 ml of normal saline solution or D_5W; use a smaller volume for children.
● Infuse over 20 to 60 minutes.
● After infusion, flush line with normal saline solution or D_5W.
● Obtain blood for peak level 30 minutes after infusion stops; draw blood for trough level just before next dose. Don't collect blood in a heparinized tube because of incompatibility.
● **Incompatibilities:** Allopurinol; amphotericin B; azithromycin; beta lactam antibiotics; cefepime; clindamycin; dextrose 5% in Isolyte E, M, or P; heparin sodium; hetastarch; indomethacin; propofol; sargramostim; solutions containing alcohol.
I.M.
● Obtain specimen for culture and sensitivity tests before giving. Begin therapy while awaiting results.
● Obtain blood for peak level 1 hour after I.M. injection; draw blood for trough level just before next dose. Don't collect blood in a heparinized tube because of incompatibility.
Inhalational
● Obtain specimen for culture and sensitivity tests before giving. Begin therapy while awaiting results.
● Give nebulizer solution over 10 to 15 minutes using handheld Pari LC Plus reusable nebulizer with DeVilbiss Pulmo-Aide compressor.

ACTION
Generally bactericidal. Inhibits protein synthesis by binding directly to the 30S ribosomal subunit.

Route	Onset	Peak	Duration
I.V.	Immediate	30 min	8 hr
I.M.	Unknown	30–60 min	8 hr
Inhalation	Unknown	Unknown	Unknown

Half-life: 2 to 3 hours.

ADVERSE REACTIONS
CNS: *seizures,* headache, lethargy, confusion, disorientation, fever.
EENT: *ototoxicity, hoarseness, pharyngitis.*
GI: vomiting, nausea, diarrhea.
GU: *nephrotoxicity,* possible increase in urinary excretion of casts.
Hematologic: anemia, eosinophilia, *leukopenia, thrombocytopenia, agranulocytosis.*
Metabolic: electrolyte imbalances.
Musculoskeletal: muscle twitching.
Respiratory: *bronchospasm.*
Skin: rash, urticaria, pruritus.

INTERACTIONS
Drug-drug. *Acyclovir, amphotericin B, cephalosporins, cidofovir, cisplatin, methoxyflurane, vancomycin, other*

aminoglycosides: May increase nephrotoxicity. Monitor renal function test results.

Atracurium, pancuronium, rocuronium, vecuronium: May increase effects of nondepolarizing muscle relaxants, including prolonged respiratory depression. Use together only when necessary, and expect to reduce dosage of nondepolarizing muscle relaxant.

Dimenhydrinate: May mask symptoms of ototoxicity. Monitor patient's hearing.

General anesthetics: May increase neuromuscular blockade. Monitor patient for increased clinical effects.

I.V. loop diuretics such as furosemide: May increase ototoxicity. Monitor patient's hearing.

Parenteral penicillins: May inactivate tobramycin in vitro. Don't mix together.

EFFECTS ON LAB TEST RESULTS
• May increase BUN, creatinine, nonprotein nitrogen, and urine urea levels. May decrease calcium, magnesium, and potassium levels.
• May increase eosinophil count. May decrease WBC, platelet, and granulocyte counts.

CONTRAINDICATIONS & CAUTIONS
• Contraindicated in patients hypersensitive to drug or other aminoglycosides.
• Use cautiously in patients with impaired renal function or neuromuscular disorders and in elderly patients.

NURSING CONSIDERATIONS
• Weigh patient and review renal function studies before therapy.
• **Alert:** Evaluate patient's hearing before and during therapy. If patient complains of tinnitus, vertigo, or hearing loss, notify prescriber.
• Don't dilute or mix with dornase alpha in a nebulizer.
• Unrefrigerated drug, which is normally slightly yellow, may darken with age. This change doesn't indicate a change in product quality.
• Avoid exposing ampules to intense light.
• **Alert:** Peak levels over 12 mcg/ml and trough levels over 2 mcg/ml may increase the risk of toxicity. Reserve higher peak levels for cystic fibrosis patients, who need a greater lung penetration.

• **Alert:** Monitor renal function: urine output, specific gravity, urinalysis, creatinine clearance, and BUN and creatinine levels. Notify prescriber about signs and symptoms of decreasing renal function.
• Watch for signs and symptoms of superinfection, such as continued fever, chills, and increased pulse rate.
• If no response occurs in 3 to 5 days, therapy may be stopped and new specimens obtained for culture and sensitivity testing.
• **Look alike–sound alike:** Don't confuse tobramycin with Trobicin.

PATIENT TEACHING
• Instruct patient to report adverse reactions promptly.
• Caution patient not to perform hazardous activities if adverse CNS reactions occur.
• Encourage patient to maintain adequate fluid intake.
• Teach patient how to use and maintain nebulizer.
• Tell patient using several inhaled therapies to use this drug last.
• Instruct patient not to use if the solution is cloudy or contains particles or if it has been stored at room temperature for longer than 28 days.

---

treprostinil sodium
tra-PROS-tin-ill

Remodulin

Pharmacologic class: vasodilator
Pregnancy risk category B

AVAILABLE FORMS
Injection: 1 mg/ml, 2.5 mg/ml, 5 mg/ml, 10 mg/ml in 20-ml vials

INDICATIONS & DOSAGES
➤ **To reduce symptoms caused by exercise in patients with New York Heart Association class II to IV pulmonary arterial hypertension (PAH)**
Adults: Initially, 1.25 nanogram/kg/minute by continuous subcutaneous infusion. If patient doesn't tolerate initial dose, reduce infusion rate to 0.625 nanogram/kg/minute. Increase by 1.25 nanogram/kg/minute each week for the first 4 weeks

and then by no more than 2.5 nanogram/ kg/minute each week for the remaining duration of infusion. Maximum infusion rate is 40 nanogram/kg/minute. May be given I.V. through a central catheter if subcutaneous route isn't tolerated.

Adjust-a-dose: In patients with mild or moderate hepatic insufficiency, initially, 0.625 nanogram/kg ideal body weight per minute, and increase cautiously.

➤ **To decrease the rate of clinical deterioration in patients requiring transition from epoprostenol sodium (Flolan)**

Adults: Start treprostinil at 10% of the current epoprostenol dose; increase dose as the epoprostenol dose is reduced. Decrease epoprostenol dose in 20% increments and increase treprostinil in 20% increments, always maintaining a total dose of 110% of epoprostenol starting dose. Once epoprostenol is at 20% of starting dose and treprostinil is at 90%, decrease epoprostenol to 5% and increase treprostinil to 110%. Finally, stop epoprostenol and maintain treprostinil dose at 110% of epoprostenol starting dose plus an additional 5% to 10% as needed. Change rate based on individual patient response. Treat worsening of PAH symptoms with increases in treprostinil dose. Treat adverse effects associated with prostacyclin and prostacyclin analogs with decreases in epoprostenol dose.

ADMINISTRATION
I.V.
- Give I.V. through a central venous catheter only if subcutaneous route isn't tolerated.
- Dilute with either sterile water for injection or normal saline solution.
- Inspect for particulate matter and discoloration before giving.
- Give by continuous infusion through a surgically placed indwelling central venous catheter, using an infusion pump designed for I.V. drug delivery.
- To avoid potential interruptions in drug delivery, make sure patient has immediate access to a backup infusion pump and infusion sets.
- Diluted drug is stable at room temperature for up to 48 hours.

- **Incompatibilities:** Other I.V. drugs.
Subcutaneous
- Preferred route is continuous subcutaneous infusion via a self-inserted subcutaneous catheter, using an infusion pump designed for subcutaneous drug delivery.
- The infusion pump should be small and lightweight; adjustable to about 0.002 ml/hour; have occlusion/no-delivery, low-battery, programming-error, and motor-malfunction alarms; have delivery accuracy of ± 6% or better; and be positive-pressure driven.
- The reservoir should be made of polyvinyl chloride, polypropylene, or glass.

ACTION
Directly vasodilates pulmonary and systemic arterial vascular beds and inhibits platelet aggregation.

Route	Onset	Peak	Duration
I.V.	Unknown	Unknown	Unknown
Subcut	Rapid	Unknown	Unknown

Half-life: 2 to 4 hours.

ADVERSE REACTIONS
CNS: dizziness, fatigue, *headache.*
CV: *vasodilation, right ventricular heart failure,* chest pain, edema, hypotension.
GI: *diarrhea, nausea.*
Musculoskeletal: *jaw pain.*
Respiratory: dyspnea.
Skin: *infusion site pain, infusion site reaction, rash,* pallor, pruritus.

INTERACTIONS
Drug-drug. *Anticoagulants:* May increase risk of bleeding. Monitor patient closely for bleeding.
Antihypertensives, diuretics, vasodilators: May worsen reduction in blood pressure. Monitor blood pressure.

EFFECTS ON LAB TEST RESULTS
None reported.

CONTRAINDICATIONS & CAUTIONS
- Contraindicated in patients hypersensitive to drug or structurally related compounds.
- Use cautiously in patients with hepatic or renal impairment and in elderly patients.

NURSING CONSIDERATIONS
• Assess the patient's ability to accept, place, and care for a subcutaneous catheter and to use an infusion pump.
• During use, a single reservoir syringe can be given for up to 72 hours at 98.6° F (37° C).
• Don't use a single vial longer than 14 days after the initial introduction to the vial.
• Start treatment in setting where adequate monitoring and emergency care are available.
• Increase dose if patient doesn't improve or symptoms worsen, and decrease if drug effects become excessive or unacceptable infusion site symptoms develop.
• Avoid abrupt withdrawal or sudden large dose reductions because PAH symptoms may worsen.

PATIENT TEACHING
• Inform patient that he'll need to continue therapy for a prolonged period, possibly years.
• Tell patient that subsequent disease management may require I.V. therapy.
• Inform patient that many side effects, such as labored breathing, fatigue, and chest pain, may be related to the underlying disease.
• Tell patient that the most common local reactions are pain, redness, tissue hardening, and rash at the infusion site.
• Tell patient that a backup infusion pump must be available to avoid interruption in therapy.

---

triamcinolone acetonide
trye-am-SIN-oh-lone

Azmacort, Nasacort AQ, Nasacort HFA

Pharmacologic class: glucocorticoid
Pregnancy risk category C

AVAILABLE FORMS
Inhalation aerosol: 100 mcg/metered spray
Nasal spray: 55 mcg/metered spray, 50 mcg/metered spray

INDICATIONS & DOSAGES
➤ **Persistent asthma**
Adults and children older than age 12:
Give 2 inhalations t.i.d. to q.i.d. Maximum, 16 inhalations daily. In some patients, maintenance can be achieved when total daily dose is given b.i.d.
Children ages 6 to 12: Give 1 to 2 inhalations t.i.d. to q.i.d. Maximum, 12 inhalations daily.
➤ **Nasal treatment of symptoms of seasonal and perennial allergic rhinitis**
Adults and children older than age 12:
Give 2 sprays Nasacort AQ in each nostril daily; may decrease to 1 spray per nostril daily. Or, 2 sprays Nasacort HFA in each nostril once daily. May increase to 4 sprays into each nostril once daily. Adjust to minimum effective dosage.
Children ages 6 to 12: Initially, give 1 spray Nasacort AQ in each nostril daily. If no response occurs, increase to 2 sprays in each nostril daily. Or, 2 sprays Nasacort HFA into each nostril once daily. Adjust to minimum effective dosage.

ADMINISTRATION
Inhalational
• Shake well before using.
• Have patient rinse mouth after use.
Intranasal
• Have patient clear nasal passages before use.

ACTION
May decrease inflammation through inhibitory activities against cell types such as mast cells and macrophages and against mediators such as leukotrienes.

Route	Onset	Peak	Duration
Inhalation (nasal)	12–24 hr	Several days	1–2 wk
Inhalation (oral)	1–4 wk	Unknown	Unknown

Half-life: 18 to 36 hours; 5.4 hours (HFA).

ADVERSE REACTIONS
CNS: *headache.*
EENT: *pharyngitis, sneezing,* dry or irritated nose or throat, hoarseness, rhinitis.
GI: dry or irritated tongue or mouth, oral candidiasis.

Respiratory: cough, wheezing.
Other: facial edema, *adrenal insufficiency,* hypothalamic-pituitary-adrenal function suppression.

INTERACTIONS
None significant.

EFFECTS ON LAB TEST RESULTS
None reported.

CONTRAINDICATIONS & CAUTIONS
• Contraindicated in patients hypersensitive to drug or its ingredients and in those with status asthmaticus.
• Use with extreme caution, if at all, in patients with tuberculosis of the respiratory tract, ocular herpes simplex, or untreated fungal, bacterial, or systemic viral infections.
• Because of risk of severe adverse effects, don't use in breast-feeding women. It's unknown if drug appears in breast milk.

NURSING CONSIDERATIONS
• Unlike other corticosteroids, drug has a spacer built into the drug-delivery device.
• Use cautiously in patients receiving systemic corticosteroids.
• Most adverse reactions to corticosteroids are dose- or duration-dependent.
• Patients who have recently been switched from systemic corticosteroids to oral inhaled corticosteroids may need to resume systemic corticosteroid therapy during periods of stress or severe asthma attacks.
• Taper oral therapy slowly.
• Store drug between 59° and 86° F (15° and 30° C).
• For nasal spray, if symptoms don't improve after 2 to 3 weeks, reevaluate the patient.
• *Look alike–sound alike:* Don't confuse triamcinolone with Triaminicin.

PATIENT TEACHING
Inhalation aerosol
• Inform patient that inhaled corticosteroids don't relieve emergency asthma attacks.
• Advise patient to warm canister to room temperature before using. Some patients carry canister in a pocket to keep it warm.
• If patient needs a bronchodilator, tell him to use it several minutes before

triamcinolone. Tell patient to allow 1 minute to elapse before repeat inhalations and to hold his breath for a few seconds to enhance drug action.
• Teach patient to check mucous membranes frequently for evidence of fungal infection. Advise patient to avoid exposure to chickenpox or measles and to contact provider if exposure occurs.
• Tell patient to prevent oral fungal infections by gargling or rinsing mouth with water after each use of the inhaler. Remind him not to swallow the water.
• Tell patient to keep inhaler clean and unobstructed and to wash it with warm water and dry it thoroughly after use.
• Instruct patient to contact prescriber if response to therapy decreases; dosage may need adjustment. Tell him not to exceed recommended dosage on his own.
• Instruct patient to wear or carry medical identification indicating his need for supplemental systemic glucocorticoids during periods of stress.
Nasal spray
• Advise patient to use at regular intervals for full therapeutic effect.
• Advise patient to clear nasal passages before use.
• Have patient follow manufacturer's recommendations for use and cleaning.

SAFETY ALERT!

urokinase
yoor-oh-KIN-ase

Abbokinase, Kinlytic

Pharmacologic class: enzyme
Pregnancy risk category B

AVAILABLE FORMS
Injection: 250,000 international units/vial

INDICATIONS & DOSAGES
➤ **Lysis of acute massive pulmonary embolism and of pulmonary embolism with unstable hemodynamics**
Adults: For I.V. infusion only by constant infusion pump. For priming dose, give 4,400 international units/kg with normal saline solution or D_5W solution, over 10 minutes, followed by 4,400

international units/kg/hour for 12 hours. Then give continuous I.V. infusion of heparin and oral anticoagulants.

➤ **Lysis of coronary artery thrombi following an acute MI ♦**
Adults: After bolus dose of heparin ranging from 2,500 to 10,000 units, infuse 6,000 international units/minute urokinase into occluded artery for up to 2 hours. Average total dose is 500,000 international units. Start drug within 6 hours after symptoms start.

➤ **Venous catheter occlusion ♦**
Adults: Instill 5,000 international units into occluded line.

ADMINISTRATION
I.V.
● Reconstitute according to manufacturer's directions using sterile water for injection. Gently roll vial; don't shake. Don't use bacteriostatic water for injection to reconstitute; it contains preservatives. Dilute further with normal saline solution or D_5W solution before infusion. Filter urokinase solutions through a 0.45-micron or smaller cellulose-membrane filter before administration. Discard unused solution. Total volume of fluid given by I.V. infusion shouldn't exceed 200 ml.
● Heparin by continuous infusion may be started concurrently or within 3 to 4 hours after urokinase has been stopped to prevent recurrent thrombosis.
● **Incompatibilities:** Other I.V. drugs.

ACTION
Converts plasminogen to plasmin by directly cleaving peptide bonds at two different sites, causing fibrinolysis.

Route	Onset	Peak	Duration
I.V.	Immediate	20 min–4 hr	12–24 hr

Half-life: 10 to 20 minutes.

ADVERSE REACTIONS
CNS: fever.
CV: *reperfusion arrhythmias,* tachycardia, transient hypotension or hypertension.
GI: nausea, vomiting.
Hematologic: *bleeding.*
Respiratory: *bronchospasm,* minor breathing difficulties.

Skin: phlebitis at injection site, rash.
Other: *anaphylaxis,* chills.

INTERACTIONS
Drug-drug. *Anticoagulants, aspirin, dipyridamole, indomethacin, NSAIDs, phenylbutazone, other drugs affecting platelet activity:* May increase risk of bleeding. Monitor patient.

EFFECTS ON LAB TEST RESULTS
● May decrease hematocrit.
● May increase PT, PTT, and INR.

CONTRAINDICATIONS & CAUTIONS
● Contraindicated in patients with a history of hypersensitivity to the drug; active internal bleeding; recent (within 2 months) cerebrovascular accident, or intracranial or intraspinal surgery; recent trauma including cardiopulmonary resuscitation; intracranial neoplasm, arteriovenous malformation, or aneurysm; severe uncontrolled hypertension, or known bleeding diatheses.
● Contraindicated with I.M. injections and other invasive procedures.
● Use cautiously in patients with recent (within 10 days) major surgery, obstetric delivery, organ biopsy, previous puncture of noncompressible vessels, or serious GI bleeding. Also use cautiously in patients with a high likelihood of left heart thrombus (mitral stenosis with atrial fibrillation), subacute bacterial endocarditis, hemostatic defects including those secondary to severe hepatic or renal disease, pregnancy, cerebrovascular disease, diabetic hemorrhagic retinopathy, or any other condition in which bleeding constitutes a significant hazard or would be particularly difficult to manage because of its location.

NURSING CONSIDERATIONS
● Give other drugs through separate I.V. line.
● Have aminocaproic acid and cross-matched and crosstyped RBCs, whole blood, plasma expanders (other than dextran) available for bleeding. Keep corticosteroids, epinephrine, and antihistamines available for allergic reactions.
● Drug may be given to menstruating women.

• Only prescribers with extensive experience in thrombotic disease management should use drug and only in facilities where clinical and laboratory monitoring can be performed.
• Monitor patient for excessive bleeding every 15 minutes for first hour; every 30 minutes for second through eighth hours; then once every 4 hours. Pretreatment with drugs affecting platelets places patient at high risk of bleeding.
• Monitor pulse, color, and sensation of arms and legs every hour.
• Although risk of hypersensitivity reactions is low, monitor patient.
• Keep a laboratory flow sheet on patient's chart to monitor PTT, PT, thrombin time, hemoglobin level, and hematocrit.
• Monitor vital signs and neurologic status. Don't take blood pressure in legs because doing so could dislodge a clot.
• Keep venipuncture sites to a minimum; use pressure dressing on puncture sites for at least 15 minutes.
• Avoid I.M. injections.
• Keep involved limb in straight alignment to prevent bleeding from infusion site.
• Because bruising is more likely during therapy, avoid unnecessary handling of patient, and pad side rails.
• Rarely, orolingual edema, urticaria, cholesterol embolization, and infusion reactions causing hypoxia, cyanosis, acidosis, and back pain may occur.

PATIENT TEACHING
• Explain use and administration of drug to patient and family.
• Instruct patient to report adverse reactions promptly.

SAFETY ALERT!

---

vinorelbine tartrate
vin-oh-REL-been

Navelbine

Pharmacologic class: semisynthetic vinca alkaloid
Pregnancy risk category D

AVAILABLE FORMS
Injection: 10 mg/ml, 50 mg/5 ml

INDICATIONS & DOSAGES
➤ **Alone or as adjunct therapy with cisplatin for first-line treatment of ambulatory patients with nonresectable advanced non–small-cell lung cancer (NSCLC); alone or with cisplatin in stage IV of NSCLC; with cisplatin in stage III of NSCLC**
Adults: 30 mg/m^2 I.V. weekly. In combination treatment, same dosage with 120 mg/m^2 of cisplatin given on days 1 and 29, and then every 6 weeks.
Adjust-a-dose: If granulocyte count is 1,000/mm^3 to 1,499/mm^3, give 50% of dose. If less than 1,000/mm^3, dose is withheld. If total bilirubin is 2.1 to 3 mg/dl, reduce dose by 50%; if more than 3 mg/dl, give 25% of dose.
➤ **Breast cancer** ◆
Adults: 20 to 30 mg/m^2 I.V. once weekly.

ADMINISTRATION
I.V.
• Drug may be a contact irritant; handle and give with care. Wear gloves. Avoid inhaling vapors and allowing contact with skin or mucous membranes, especially those of the eyes. In case of contact, wash with generous amounts of water for at least 15 minutes.
• Dilute drug before use to 1.5 to 3 mg/ml with D$_5$W or normal saline solution in a syringe. Or, dilute to 0.5 to 2 mg/ml in an I.V. bag.
• Give drug I.V. over 6 to 10 minutes into side port of a free-flowing I.V. line that is closest to I.V. bag; then flush with 75 to 125 ml or more of D$_5$W or normal saline solution.
• Monitor site for irritation and infiltration because drug can cause localized tissue damage, necrosis, and thrombophlebitis. If extravasation occurs, stop drug immediately and inject remaining dose into a different vein; notify prescriber.
• Drug may be stored for up to 24 hours at room temperature.
• **Incompatibilities:** Acyclovir, allopurinol, aminophylline, amphotericin B, ampicillin sodium, cefazolin, cefoperazone, ceftriaxone, cefuroxime, fluorouracil, furosemide, ganciclovir, methylprednisolone, mitomycin, piperacillin, sodium bicarbonate, thiotepa, trimethoprim-sulfamethoxazole.

Reactions may be *common*, uncommon, *life-threatening*, or COMMON AND LIFE-THREATENING.
Interaction may have a *rapid onset* or *delayed onset*.

ACTION
Exerts its primary antineoplastic effect by disrupting microtubule assembly, which in turn disrupts spindle formation and prevents mitosis.

Route	Onset	Peak	Duration
I.V.	Unknown	Unknown	Unknown

Half-life: About 27 to 43½ hours.

ADVERSE REACTIONS
CNS: *asthenia, fatigue, peripheral neuropathy.*
CV: chest pain.
GI: *anorexia, constipation, diarrhea, nausea, stomatitis, vomiting.*
Hematologic: anemia, **agranulocytosis, bone marrow suppression, granulocytopenia, thrombocytopenia,** LEUKOPENIA.
Hepatic: hyperbilirubinemia.
Musculoskeletal: arthralgia, jaw pain, loss of deep tendon reflexes, myalgia.
Respiratory: dyspnea, shortness of breath.
Skin: *alopecia, injection pain or reaction,* rash.

INTERACTIONS
Drug-drug. *Cisplatin:* May increase risk of bone marrow suppression when used with cisplatin. Monitor hematologic status closely.
Cytochrome P-450 inhibitors: May decrease metabolism of vinorelbine. Watch for increased adverse effects.
Mitomycin: May cause pulmonary reactions. Monitor respiratory status closely.
Paclitaxel: May increase risk of neuropathy. Monitor patient closely.

EFFECTS ON LAB TEST RESULTS
• May increase bilirubin level. May decrease hemoglobin level.
• May increase liver function test values. May decrease granulocyte, WBC, and platelet counts.

CONTRAINDICATIONS & CAUTIONS
• Contraindicated in patients with pretreatment granulocyte count below 1,000/mm³ and in patients hypersensitive to the drug.
• Use with caution in patients whose bone marrow may have been compromised by previous exposure to radiation therapy or chemotherapy or whose bone marrow is still recovering from chemotherapy.
• Use with caution in patients with hepatic impairment.
• Safety and effectiveness in children haven't been established.

NURSING CONSIDERATIONS
• Check patient's granulocyte count before giving; make sure count is 1,000/mm³ or higher before giving drug. If count is lower, withhold drug and notify prescriber. Granulocyte count nadir occurs between days 7 and 10.
• *Alert:* Drug is fatal if given intrathecally; it's for I.V. use only.
• Adjust dosage by hematologic toxicity or hepatic insufficiency, whichever results in the lower dosage. If granulocyte count falls below 1,500/mm³ but is greater than 1,000/mm³, reduce dosage by 50%. If three consecutive doses are skipped because of agranulocytosis, don't resume therapy.
• In patients with hepatic impairment, monitor liver enzyme levels.
• Patient may receive injections of WBC colony-stimulating factors to promote cell growth and decrease risk of infection.
• *Alert:* Monitor deep tendon reflexes; loss may represent cumulative toxicity.
• Monitor patient closely for hypersensitivity.
• As a guide to the effects of therapy, monitor patient's peripheral blood count and bone marrow.
• *Look alike–sound alike:* Don't confuse vinorelbine with vinblastine or vincristine.

PATIENT TEACHING
• Advise patient to report any pain or burning at site of injection.
• Instruct patient not to take other drugs, including OTC preparations, until approved by prescriber.
• Tell patient to report evidence of infection (fever, sore throat, fatigue) and bleeding (easy bruising, nosebleeds, bleeding gums, tarry stools). Tell him to take temperature daily.
• Advise patient to report increased shortness of breath, cough, abdominal pain, or constipation.
• Caution woman to avoid becoming pregnant during therapy.

warfarin sodium
WAR-far-in

Coumadin, Jantoven

Pharmacologic class: coumarin derivative
Pregnancy risk category X

AVAILABLE FORMS
Powder for injection: 2 mg/ml
Tablets: 1 mg, 2 mg, 2.5 mg, 3 mg, 4 mg, 5 mg, 6 mg, 7.5 mg, 10 mg

INDICATIONS & DOSAGES
➤ **Pulmonary embolism, deep vein thrombosis, MI, rheumatic heart disease with heart valve damage, prosthetic heart valves, chronic atrial fibrillation**
Adults: 2 to 5 mg P.O. or I.V. daily for 2 to 4 days; then dosage based on daily PT and INR. Usual maintenance dosage is 2 to 10 mg P.O. or I.V. daily.

ADMINISTRATION
P.O.
• Draw blood to establish baseline co-agulation parameters before therapy. PT and INR determinations are essential for proper control. INR range for chronic atrial fibrillation is usually 2 to 3.
• Give drug at same time daily.
I.V.
• Draw blood to establish baseline co-agulation parameters before therapy. PT and INR determinations are essential for proper control. INR range for chronic atrial fibrillation is usually 2 to 3.
• I.V. form may be ordered in rare in-stances when oral therapy can't be given.
• Reconstitute powder with 2.7 ml sterile water, or as instructed in manufacturer guidelines.
• Give as a slow bolus injection over 1 to 2 minutes into a peripheral vein.
• Because onset of action is delayed, heparin sodium is often given during the first few days of treatment of embolic disease. Blood for PT and INR may be drawn at any time during continuous heparin infusion.
• **Incompatibilities:** Aminophylline, ammonium chloride, bretylium tosylate, ceftazidime, cimetidine, ciprofloxacin, dobutamine, esmolol, gentamicin, heparin sodium, labetalol, lactated Ringer injection, metronidazole, promazine, Ringer injection, vancomycin.

ACTION
Inhibits vitamin K–dependent activation of clotting factors II, VII, IX, and X, formed in the liver.

Route	Onset	Peak	Duration
P.O.	Within 24 hr	4 hr	2–5 days
I.V.	Within 24 hr	< 4 hr	2–5 days

Half-life: 20 to 60 hours.

ADVERSE REACTIONS
CNS: *fever,* headache.
GI: *diarrhea,* anorexia, nausea, vomiting, cramps, mouth ulcerations, sore mouth, melena.
GU: enhanced uric acid excretion, hema-turia, excessive menstrual bleeding.
Hematologic: *hemorrhage.*
Hepatic: *hepatitis,* jaundice.
Skin: dermatitis, urticaria, necrosis, gangrene, alopecia, *rash.*

INTERACTIONS
Drug-drug. *Acetaminophen:* May increase bleeding with long-term therapy (more than 2 weeks) at high doses (more than 2 g/day) of acetaminophen. Monitor patient very carefully.
Allopurinol, **amiodarone, anabolic steroids,** *antidepressants,* **azole antifungals,** *aspirin, celecoxib, cephalosporins, chloramphenicol, cimetidine,* **danazol,** *diazoxide, diflunisal, disulfiram, erythromycin, ethacrynic acid,* **fibric acids, fluoxymesterone, fluoroquinolones,** *furosemide, glucagon, heparin, influenza virus vaccine, isoniazid,* **lansoprazole,** *meclofenamate, methimazole, methyldopa, methylphenidate,* **methyltestosterone, metronidazole, nalidixic acid,** *neomycin (oral),* **NSAIDs,** *omeprazole,* **oxandrolone,** *pentoxifylline, propafenone, propoxyphene, propylthiouracil, quinidine,* **salicylates,** *SSRIs,* **sulfinpyrazone,** *sulfamethoxazole and trimethoprim,* **sulfonamides,** *tamoxifen, tetracyclines, thiazides, thrombolytics,* **thyroid drugs,** *ticlopidine, tramadol, vitamin E, valproic*

acid, zafirlukast: May increase anticoagulant effect. Monitor patient carefully for bleeding. Reduce anticoagulant dosage as directed.

Anticonvulsants: May increase levels of phenytoin and phenobarbital. Monitor drug levels closely.

Ascorbic acid, **barbiturates,** *carbamazepine, clozapine, corticosteroids, corticotropin, cyclosporine, dicloxacillin, ethchlorvynol, griseofulvin, haloperidol, meprobamate, mercaptopurine, nafcillin, oral contraceptives containing estrogen, rifampin, spironolactone, sucralfate, thiazide diuretics, trazodone, vitamin K:* May decrease PT and INR with reduced anticoagulant effect. Monitor PT and INR carefully. Increase warfarin dosage, as needed.

Chloral hydrate, cyclophosphamide, HMG-CoA reductase inhibitors, phenytoin, propylthiouracil, ranitidine: May increase or decrease PT and INR. Monitor PT and INR carefully.

Cholestyramine: May decrease response when given too closely together. Give 6 hours after oral anticoagulants.

Sulfonylureas (oral antidiabetics): May increase hypoglycemic response. Monitor glucose levels.

Drug-herb. *Angelica (dong quai):* May significantly prolong PT and INR. Discourage use together.

Anise, arnica flower, asafoetida, bogbean, bromelain, capsicum, celery, chamomile, clove, dandelion, danshen, devil's claw, dong quai, fenugreek, feverfew, garlic, ginger, **ginkgo, ginseng,** *horse chestnut, horseradish, licorice, meadowsweet, motherwort, onion, papain, parsley, passion flower, quassia, red clover, Reishi mushroom, rue, sweet clover, turmeric, white willow:* May increase risk of bleeding. Discourage use together.

Coenzyme Q10, ginseng, St. John's wort: May reduce action of drug. Ask patient about use of herbal remedies, and advise caution.

Green tea: May decrease anticoagulant effect caused by vitamin K content of green tea. Advise patient to minimize variable consumption of green tea and other foods or nutritional supplements containing vitamin K.

Drug-food. *Foods, multivitamins, and other enteral products containing vitamin K:* May impair anticoagulation. Tell patient to maintain consistent daily intake of foods containing vitamin K.

Cranberry juice: May increase risk of severe bleeding. Discourage use together.

Drug-lifestyle. *Alcohol use:* May enhance anticoagulant effects. Tell patient to avoid large amounts of alcohol.

EFFECTS ON LAB TEST RESULTS
● May increase ALT and AST levels.
● May increase INR, PT, and PTT.
● May falsely decrease theophylline level.

CONTRAINDICATIONS & CAUTIONS
● Contraindicated in patients hypersensitive to drug and in those with bleeding from the GI, GU, or respiratory tract; aneurysm; cerebrovascular hemorrhage; severe or malignant hypertension; severe renal or hepatic disease; subacute bacterial endocarditis, pericarditis, or pericardial effusion; or blood dyscrasias or hemorrhagic tendencies.
● Contraindicated during pregnancy, threatened abortion, eclampsia, or preeclampsia, and after recent surgery involving large open areas, eye, brain, or spinal cord; recent prostatectomy; major regional lumbar block anesthesia, spinal puncture, or diagnostic or therapeutic invasive procedures.
● Avoid using in patients with a history of warfarin-induced necrosis; in unsupervised patients with senility, alcoholism, or psychosis; or in situations in which there are inadequate laboratory facilities for coagulation testing.
● Use cautiously in patients with diverticulitis, colitis, mild or moderate hypertension, or mild or moderate hepatic or renal disease; with drainage tubes in any orifice; with regional or lumbar block anesthesia; with heparin-induced thrombocytopenia and deep venous thrombosis; or in conditions that increase risk of hemorrhage.
● Use cautiously in breast-feeding women.

NURSING CONSIDERATIONS
● Avoid all I.M. injections.
● Regularly inspect patient for bleeding gums, bruises on arms or legs, petechiae,

nosebleeds, melena, tarry stools, hematuria, and hematemesis.
• Check for unexpected bleeding in breast-fed babies of women who take this drug.
• Monitor patient for purple-toes syndrome, characterized by a dark purple or mottled color of the toes; may occur 3 to 10 weeks, or even later after start of therapy.
• *Alert:* Withhold drug and call prescriber at once in the event of fever or rash (signs of severe adverse reactions).
• Effect can be neutralized by oral or parenteral vitamin K.
• Elderly patients and patients with renal or hepatic failure are especially sensitive to drug's effect.

PATIENT TEACHING
• Stress importance of complying with prescribed dosage and follow-up appointments. Tell patient to carry a card that identifies his increased risk of bleeding.
• Tell patient and family to watch for signs of bleeding or abnormal bruising and to call prescriber at once if they occur.
• Warn patient to avoid OTC products containing aspirin, other salicylates, or drugs that may interact with warfarin unless ordered by prescriber.
• Advise patient to consult with prescriber before initiating any herbal therapy; many herbs have anticoagulant, antiplatelet, or fibrinolytic properties.
• Tell patient to consult a prescriber before using miconazole vaginal cream or suppositories. Abnormal bleeding and bruising have occurred.
• Instruct woman to notify prescriber if menstruation is heavier than usual; she may need dosage adjustment.
• Tell patient to use electric razor when shaving and to use a soft toothbrush.
• Tell patient to read food labels. Food, nutritional supplements, and multivitamins that contain vitamin K may impair anticoagulation.
• Tell patient to eat a daily, consistent diet of food and drinks containing vitamin K, because eating varied amounts may alter anticoagulant effects.

zafirlukast
zah-FUR-luh-kast

Accolate

Pharmacologic class: leukotriene-receptor antagonist
Pregnancy risk category B

AVAILABLE FORMS
Tablets: 10 mg, 20 mg

INDICATIONS & DOSAGES
➤ **Prevention and long-term treatment of asthma**
Adults and children age 12 and older: Give 20 mg P.O. b.i.d.
Children ages 5 to 11: Give 10 mg P.O. b.i.d.

ADMINISTRATION
P.O.
• Give drug 1 hour before or 2 hours after meals.

ACTION
Selectively competes for leukotriene-receptor sites, blocking inflammatory action.

Route	Onset	Peak	Duration
P.O.	Rapid	3 hr	Unknown

Half-life: 10 hours.

ADVERSE REACTIONS
CNS: *headache,* asthenia, dizziness, pain, fever.
GI: abdominal pain, diarrhea, dyspepsia, gastritis, nausea, vomiting.
Musculoskeletal: back pain, myalgia.
Other: accidental injury, infection.

INTERACTIONS
Drug-drug. *Aspirin:* May increase zafirlukast level. Monitor patient for adverse effects.
Erythromycin, theophylline: May decrease zafirlukast level. Monitor patient for decreased effectiveness.
Warfarin: May increase PT. Monitor PT and INR, and adjust anticoagulant dosage.
Drug-food. *Food:* May reduce rate and extent of drug absorption. Advise patient

to take drug 1 hour before or 2 hours after a meal.

EFFECTS ON LAB TEST RESULTS
• May increase liver enzyme levels.

CONTRAINDICATIONS & CAUTIONS
• Contraindicated in patients hypersensitive to drug.
• Use cautiously in elderly patients and those with hepatic impairment.
• Use in pregnant women only if clearly needed. Don't use in breast-feeding women.

NURSING CONSIDERATIONS
• *Alert:* Reducing oral corticosteroid dose has been followed in rare cases by eosinophilia, vasculitic rash, worsening pulmonary symptoms, cardiac complications, or neuropathy, sometimes as Churg-Strauss syndrome.
• Drug isn't indicated to reverse bronchospasm in acute asthma attacks.

PATIENT TEACHING
• Tell patient that drug is used for long-term treatment of asthma and to keep taking it even if symptoms resolve.
• Advise patient to continue taking other antiasthmatics, as prescribed.
• Instruct patient to take drug 1 hour before or 2 hours after meals.

---

zanamivir
zan-AM-ah-ver

Relenza

Pharmacologic class: selective neuraminidase inhibitor
Pregnancy risk category C

AVAILABLE FORMS
Powder for inhalation: 5 mg/blister

INDICATIONS & DOSAGES
➤ **Uncomplicated acute illness caused by influenza virus A and B in patients who have had symptoms for no longer than 2 days**
Adults and children age 7 and older: 2 oral inhalations (one 5-mg blister per inhalation for total dose of 10 mg) b.i.d. using the

dry-powder inhalation device for 5 days. Give two doses on first day of treatment, allowing at least 2 hours to elapse between doses. Give subsequent doses about 12 hours apart (in the morning and evening) at about the same time each day.
➤ **Prevention of influenza in a household setting**
Adults and children age 5 and older: 2 oral inhalations (one 5-mg blister per inhalation for total dose of 10 mg) once daily for 10 days.
➤ **Prevention of influenza in a community setting**
Adults and adolescents: 2 oral inhalations (one 5-mg blister per inhalation for total dose of 10 mg) once daily for 28 days.

ADMINISTRATION
Inhalational
• Dry-powder inhaler should be kept level when patient loads and inhales drug. Patient should check inside the mouthpiece of the inhaler before each use to make sure it's free of foreign objects.
• Patient should exhale fully before putting the mouthpiece in his mouth; then, keeping the dry-powder inhaler level, he should close his lips around the mouthpiece and inhale steadily and deeply. Patient should hold his breath for a few seconds after inhaling to keep drug in lungs.

ACTION
Inhibits neuraminidase on the surface of the influenza virus, altering virus particle aggregation and release.

Route	Onset	Peak	Duration
Inhalation	Unknown	1–2 hr	Unknown

Half-life: $2\frac{1}{2}$ to $5\frac{1}{4}$ hours.

ADVERSE REACTIONS
CNS: dizziness, headache.
EENT: ear, nose, and throat infections, nasal signs and symptoms, sinusitis.
GI: diarrhea, nausea, vomiting.
Respiratory: *bronchospasm,* bronchitis, cough.
Skin: serious rash.
Other: *anaphylaxis.*

INTERACTIONS
None significant.

EFFECTS ON LAB TEST RESULTS
● May increase CK and liver enzyme levels.
● May decrease lymphocyte and neutrophil counts.

CONTRAINDICATIONS & CAUTIONS
● Contraindicated in patients hypersensitive to drug or its components.
● Not recommended for patients with severe or decompensated COPD, asthma, or other underlying respiratory disease.

NURSING CONSIDERATIONS
● For a patient with underlying respiratory disease, have a fast-acting bronchodilator readily available and carefully monitor respiratory status. Patients using an inhaled bronchodilator for asthma simultaneously with this drug should use the bronchodilator first.
● Start drug within 48 hours of symptoms or as prevention after household contact, within 36 hours, or community outbreak, within 5 days.
● Drug doesn't replace annual influenza vaccine.
● Monitor patient for bronchospasm and decline in lung function. Stop drug in such situations.

PATIENT TEACHING
● Tell patient to carefully read the instructions for the dry-powder inhalation device.
● Teach parents how to give the drug to a child and to properly supervise use.
● Advise patient to keep the dry-powder inhaler level when loading and inhaling drug. Tell him to always check inside the mouthpiece of the dry-powder inhaler before each use to make sure it's free of foreign objects.
● Tell patient to exhale fully before putting the mouthpiece in his mouth; then, keeping the dry-powder inhaler level, to close his lips around the mouthpiece and inhale steadily and deeply. Advise patient to hold his breath for a few seconds after inhaling to help drug stay in the lungs.
● Instruct patient simultaneously using a bronchodilator with this drug, to use the bronchodilator first. Tell patient to have a fast-acting bronchodilator readily available in case of wheezing.
● *Alert:* Advise all patients to immediately report worsening of respiratory symptoms, wheezing, shortness of breath, and bronchospasm.
● Advise patient that it's important to finish the entire treatment course.
● Tell patient that drug doesn't reduce the risk of transmitting the influenza virus to others.

Appendices & Index

Nurses carry a great deal of responsibility for administering drugs safely and correctly, for making sure the right patient gets the right drug, in the right dose, at the right time, and by the right route. By staying aware of potential trouble areas, you can minimize your risk of making medication errors and maximize the therapeutic effects of your patient's drug regimen.

Name game

Drugs with similar-sounding names can be easily confused. Even different-sounding names can look similar when written rapidly by hand on a prescription form. An example is Soriatane and Loxitane, which are both capsules. If the patient's drug order doesn't seem right for his diagnosis, call the prescriber to clarify the order.

Allergy alert

Once you've verified your patient's full name, check to see if he's wearing an allergy bracelet. If he is, the allergy bracelet should conspicuously display the name of the allergen. The allergy information should also be labeled on the front of the patient's chart and on his medication record. Whether the patient is wearing an allergy bracelet or not, take the time to double-check and ask the patient whether he has any allergies—even if he is in distress.

A patient who is severely allergic to peanuts could have an anaphylactic reaction to ipratropium bromide (Atrovent) aerosol given by metered-dose inhaler. Ask your patient (or his parents, if he's a child) whether he's allergic to peanuts before you give this drug. If you find that

he's allergic, you need to use the nasal spray and inhalation solution form of the drug. Because it doesn't contain soy lecithin, it's safe for patient's allergic to peanuts.

Compound errors

Many medication errors occur because of a compound problem—a mistake or group of mistakes that could have been caught at any of several steps along the way. For a drug to be given correctly, each member of the health care team must fill an appropriate role:
- The prescriber must write the order correctly and legibly.
- The pharmacist must evaluate whether the order is appropriate and fill it correctly.
- The nurse must evaluate whether the order is appropriate and give it correctly.

A breakdown anywhere along this chain of events can lead to a medication error. That's why it's important for these health care professionals to act as a real team. They should be encouraged to double-check each other in order to catch any problems that might arise before the problems affect the patient's health.

Route trouble

Many drug errors happen, at least in part, from problems related to the route of administration. The risk of error increases when a patient has several I.V. lines running for different purposes.

Risky abbreviations

Abbreviating drug names is risky. Abbreviations may not be commonly known and, in some cases, the same abbreviation may be used for different drugs or compounds. For example, epoetin alfa is commonly abbreviated EPO; however, some use the abbreviation EPO to stand for "evening primrose oil." Ask all prescribers to spell out drug names.

Unclear orders

Take the time to clarify orders. In one instance, a patient was supposed to receive one dose of the antineoplastic lomustine to treat brain cancer. (Lomustine is typically given in a single dose once every 6 weeks.) The doctor's order read, "Administer h.s." Because a nurse misinterpreted the order to mean every night, the patient received nine daily doses, developed severe thrombocytopenia and leukopenia, and died.

If you're unfamiliar with a drug, check a drug book before giving it to the patient. If a prescriber uses "h.s." and doesn't specify the frequency of administration, ask him to clarify the order. When documenting orders about bedtime doses, specify such instructions as "at bedtime nightly" or "at bedtime one dose today."

Color changes

If a familiar drug seems to have an unfamiliar appearance, investigate the cause. If the pharmacist cites a manufacturer change, ask him to double-check whether he has received verification from the manufacturer. Always document the appearance discrepancy, your actions, and the pharmacist's response in the patient record.

Stress levels

Committing a serious error can cause enormous stress and cloud your judg-

ment. If you're involved in a drug error, ask another professional to give the antidote.

Reconciling medications

Medication reconciliation is the process of comparing a patient's medication orders to all of the medications that the patient has been taking. This reconciliation is done to avoid medication errors, such as omissions, duplications, dosing errors, or drug interactions. Medication errors related to medication reconciliation are more likely to occur at the time of admission, upon transfer to another unit, or when the patient is discharged from the facility. Studies have shown that a medication reconciliation procedure can successfully reduce medication errors.

At discharge, it's important to provide both the patient and the next care provider with a complete list of current medications, including all prescription and over-the-counter medications as well as any vitamins, herbal medications, and nutraceuticals.

Be sure to provide a clearly written list that includes:

• the name of each medication and the reason for taking it

• all new medications and prehospital medications that the patient is to discontinue

• the correct dose and frequency, highlighting changes from the prehospital instructions

• a list of over-the-counter drugs that shouldn't be taken.

In addition to the reconciled list, it's important to ensure the availability of medications upon the patient's discharge and to determine whether the patient can read the medication labels correctly, afford the necessary medications, and get to the pharmacy to pick them up.

Common combination drugs: Indications and dosages

ANALGESICS

Alor 5/500
Azdone
Damason-P
Lortab ASA
Panasal 5/500
Controlled Substance Schedule (CSS) III

Generic components
500 mg aspirin and 5 mg hydrocodone bitartrate

Dosages
Moderate to moderately severe pain
Adults: 1 or 2 tablets every 4 hours. Maximum dosage, 8 tablets in 24 hours.

Anexsia 5/325
Norco 5/325
CSS III

Generic components
325 mg acetaminophen and 5 mg hydrocodone bitartrate

Dosages
Moderate to moderately severe pain
Adults: 1 to 2 tablets every 4 to 6 hours. Maximum dosage, 12 tablets in 24 hours.

Anexsia 5/500
Co-Gesic
Lorcet HD
Lortab 5/500
Panacet 5/500
Vicodin
CSS III

Generic components
500 mg acetaminophen and 5 mg hydrocodone bitartrate

Dosages
Moderate to moderately severe pain
Adults: 1 to 2 tablets every 4 to 6 hours. Maximum dosage, 8 tablets in 24 hours.

Anexsia 7.5/325
Norco 7.5/325
CSS III

Generic components
325 mg acetaminophen and 7.5 mg hydrocodone bitartrate

Dosages
Moderate to moderately severe pain
Adults: 1 to 2 tablets every 4 to 6 hours. Maximum dosage, 12 tablets in 24 hours.

Anexsia 7.5/650
Lorcet Plus
CSS III

Generic components
650 mg acetaminophen and 7.5 mg hydrocodone bitartrate

Dosages
Arthralgia, bone pain, dental pain, headache, migraine, moderate pain
Adults: 1 to 2 tablets every 4 hours. Maximum dosage, 6 tablets in 24 hours.

Anexsia 10/660
Vicodin HP
CSS III

Generic components
660 mg acetaminophen and 10 mg hydrocodone bitartrate

Dosages
Arthralgia, bone pain, dental pain, headache, migraine, moderate pain
Adults: 1 tablet every 4 to 6 hours. Maximum dosage, 6 tablets in 24 hours.

Capital with Codeine
Tylenol with Codeine Elixir
CSS V

Generic components
120 mg acetaminophen and 12 mg codeine phosphate/5 ml

Dosages
Mild to moderate pain
Adults: 15 ml every 4 hours.

Darvocet-A500
CSS IV

Generic components
500 mg acetaminophen and 100 mg propoxyphene napsylate

Dosages
Mild to moderate pain
Adults: 1 tablet every 4 hours. Maximum dosage, 8 tablets in 24 hours.

Darvocet-N50
CSS IV

Generic components
325 mg acetaminophen and 50 mg propoxyphene napsylate

Dosages
Mild to moderate pain
Adults: 2 tablets every 4 hours. Maximum dosage, 12 tablets in 24 hours.

Darvocet-N100
CSS IV

Generic components
650 mg acetaminophen and 100 mg propoxyphene napsylate

Dosages
Mild to moderate pain
Adults: 1 tablet every 4 hours. Maximum dosage, 6 tablets in 24 hours.

Empirin with Codeine
No. 3
CSS III

Generic components
325 mg aspirin and 30 mg codeine phosphate

Dosages
Fever and mild to moderate pain
Adults: 1 to 2 tablets every 4 hours. Maximum dosage, 12 tablets in 24 hours.

Empirin with Codeine
No. 4
CSS III

Generic components
325 mg aspirin and 60 mg codeine phosphate

Dosages
Fever and mild to moderate pain
Adults: 1 tablet every 4 hours. Maximum dosage, 6 tablets in 24 hours.

Endocet 5/325
Percocet 5/325
Roxicet
CSS II

Generic components
325 mg acetaminophen and 5 mg oxycodone hydrochloride

Dosages
Moderate to moderately severe pain
Adults: 1 tablet every 6 hours. Maximum dosage, 12 tablets in 24 hours.

Endocet 7.5/325
Percocet 7.5/325
CSS II

Generic components
325 mg acetaminophen and 7.5 mg oxycodone hydrochloride

Dosages
Moderate to moderately severe pain
Adults: 1 tablet every 6 hours. Maximum dosage, 8 tablets in 24 hours.

Endocet 7.5/500
Percocet 7.5/500
CSS II

Generic components
500 mg acetaminophen and 7.5 mg oxycodone hydrochloride

Dosages
Moderate to moderately severe pain
Adults: 1 tablet every 6 hours. Maximum dosage, 8 tablets in 24 hours.

Endocet 10/325
Percocet 10/325
CSS II

Generic components
325 mg acetaminophen and 10 mg oxycodone hydrochloride

Dosages
Moderate to moderately severe pain
Adults: 1 tablet every 6 hours. Maximum dosage, 6 tablets in 24 hours.

Fioricet with Codeine
CSS III

Generic components
325 mg acetaminophen, 50 mg butalbital, 40 mg caffeine, and 30 mg codeine phosphate

Dosages
Headache, mild to moderate pain
Adults: 1 to 2 capsules every 4 hours. Maximum dosage, 6 capsules in 24 hours.

Fiorinal with Codeine
CSS III

Generic components
325 mg aspirin, 50 mg butalbital, 40 mg caffeine, and 30 mg codeine phosphate

Dosages
Headache, mild to moderate pain
Adults: 1 to 2 tablets or capsules every 4 hours. Maximum dosage, 6 tablets or capsules in 24 hours.

Lorcet 10/650
CSS III

Generic components
650 mg acetaminophen and 10 mg hydrocodone bitartrate

Dosages
Moderate to moderately severe pain
Adults: 1 tablet every 4 to 6 hours. Maximum dosage, 6 tablets in 24 hours.

Lortab 2.5/500
CSS III

Generic components
500 mg acetaminophen and 2.5 mg hydrocodone bitartrate

Dosages
Moderate to moderately severe pain
Adults: 1 to 2 tablets every 4 to 6 hours. Maximum dosage, 8 tablets in 24 hours.

Lortab 7.5/500
CSS III

Generic components
500 mg acetaminophen and 7.5 mg hydrocodone bitartrate

Dosages
Moderate to moderately severe pain
Adults: 1 tablet every 4 to 6 hours. Maximum dosage, 8 tablets in 24 hours.

Lortab 10/500
CSS III

Generic components
500 mg acetaminophen and 10 mg hydrocodone bitartrate

Dosages
Moderate to moderately severe pain
Adults: 1 tablet every 4 to 6 hours. Maximum dosage, 6 tablets in 24 hours.

Lortab Elixir
CSS III

Generic components
167 mg acetaminophen and 2.5 mg/5 ml hydrocodone bitartrate

Dosages
Moderately severe pain
Adults: 15 ml every 4 to 6 hours. Maximum dosage, 90 ml/day.

Norco 325/10
CSS III

Generic components
325 mg acetaminophen and 10 mg hydrocodone bitartrate

Dosages
Moderate to moderately severe pain
Adults: 1 tablet every 4 to 6 hours. Maximum dosage, 6 tablets in 24 hours.

Percocet 2.5/325
CSS II

Generic components
325 mg acetaminophen and 2.5 mg oxycodone hydrochloride

Dosages
Moderate to moderately severe pain
Adults: 1 to 2 tablets every 4 to 6 hours. Maximum dosage, 12 tablets in 24 hours.

Percocet 10/650
CSS II

Generic components
650 mg acetaminophen and 10 mg oxycodone hydrochloride

Dosages
Moderate to moderately severe pain
Adults: 1 tablet every 4 hours. Maximum dosage, 6 tablets in 24 hours.

Percodan
CSS II

Generic components
325 mg aspirin, 4.5 mg oxycodone hydrochloride, and 0.38 mg oxycodone terephthalate

Dosages
Moderate to moderately severe pain
Adults: 1 tablet every 6 hours. Maximum dosage, 12 tablets in 24 hours.

Roxicet 5/500
Roxilox
Tylox
CSS II

Generic components
500 mg acetaminophen and 5 mg oxycodone hydrochloride

Dosages
Moderate to moderately severe pain
Adults: 1 tablet every 6 hours.

Roxicet Oral Solution
CSS II

Generic components
325 mg acetaminophen and 5 mg/5 ml oxycodone hydrochloride

Dosages
Moderate to moderately severe pain
Adults: 5 ml every 6 hours. Maximum dosage, 60 ml in 24 hours.

Talacen
CSS IV

Generic components
650 mg acetaminophen and 25 mg pentazocine hydrochloride

Dosages
Mild to moderate pain
Adults: 1 tablet every 4 hours. Maximum dosage, 6 tablets in 24 hours.

Talwin Compound
CSS IV

Generic components
325 mg aspirin and 12.5 mg pentazocine hydrochloride

Dosages
Moderate pain
Adults: 2 tablets every 6 to 8 hours. Maximum dosage, 8 tablets in 24 hours.

Talwin NX
CSS IV

Generic components
0.5 mg naloxone and 50 mg pentazocine hydrochloride

Dosages
Moderate to severe pain
Adults: 1 to 2 tablets every 3 to 4 hours. Maximum dosage, 12 tablets daily.

Tylenol with Codeine No. 2
CSS III

Generic components
300 mg acetaminophen and 15 mg codeine phosphate

Dosages
Fever, mild to moderate pain
Adults: 1 to 2 tablets every 4 hours. Maximum dosage, 12 tablets in 24 hours.

Tylenol with Codeine No. 3
CSS III

Generic components
300 mg acetaminophen and 30 mg codeine phosphate

Dosages
Fever, mild to moderate pain
Adults: 1 to 2 tablets every 4 hours. Maximum dosage, 12 tablets in 24 hours.

Tylenol with Codeine No. 4
CSS III

Generic components
300 mg acetaminophen and 60 mg codeine phosphate

Dosages
Fever, mild to moderate pain
Adults: 1 tablet every 4 hours. Maximum dosage, 6 tablets in 24 hours.

Tylox 5/500
CSS II

Generic components
500 mg acetaminophen and 5 mg oxycodone hydrochloride

Dosages
Moderate to moderately severe pain
Adults: 1 capsule every 6 hours. Maximum dosage, 8 capsules in 24 hours.

Vicodin ES
CSS III

Generic components
750 mg acetaminophen and 7.5 mg hydrocodone bitartrate

Dosages
Moderate to moderately severe pain
Adults: 1 tablet every 4 to 6 hours. Maximum dosage, 5 tablets in 24 hours.

Zydone 5/400
CSS III

Generic components
400 mg acetaminophen and 5 mg hydrocodone bitartrate

Dosages
Moderate to moderately severe pain
Adults: 1 to 2 tablets every 4 to 6 hours. Maximum dosage, 8 tablets in 24 hours.

Zydone 7.5/400
CSS III

Generic components
400 mg acetaminophen and 7.5 mg hydrocodone bitartrate

Dosages
Moderate to moderately severe pain
Adults: 1 tablet every 4 to 6 hours. Maximum dosage, 6 tablets in 24 hours.

Zydone 10/400
CSS III

Generic components
400 mg acetaminophen and 10 mg hydrocodone bitartrate

Dosages
Moderate to moderately severe pain
Adults: 1 tablet every 4 to 6 hours. Maximum dosage, 6 tablets in 24 hours.

ANTIBACTERIALS

Eryzole
Pediazole

Generic components
Granules for oral suspension

Erythromycin ethylsuccinate (equivalent of 200 mg erythromycin activity) and 600 mg sulfisoxazole per 5 ml when reconstituted according to manufacturer's directions.

Dosages
Acute otitis media
Children: 50 mg/kg/day erythromycin and 150 mg/kg/day sulfisoxazole in divided doses q.i.d. for 10 days. Give without regard to meals. Refrigerate after reconstitution; use within 14 days.

ANTIRETROVIRALS

Combivir

Generic components
Tablets
150 mg lamivudine and 300 mg zidovudine

Dosages
Adults and children age 12 and older who weigh more than 50 kg (110 lb): 1 tablet P.O. b.i.d.

Epzicom

Generic components
Tablets
600 mg abacavir with 300 mg lamivudine

Dosages
Adults: 1 tablet daily, taken without regard to food and in combination with other antiretrovirals.

Trizivir

Generic components
Tablets
300 mg abacavir sulfate, 150 mg lamivudine, and 300 mg zidovudine

Dosages
Adults and adolescents who weigh 40 kg (88 lb) or more: 1 tablet P.O. b.i.d., alone or with other antiretrovirals.

Truvada

Generic components
Tablets
200 mg emtricitabine with 300 mg tenofovir

Dosages
Adults and adolescents weighing more than 40 kg (88 lb): 1 tablet daily, taken without regard to food and in combination with other antiretrovirals.

RESPIRATORY TRACT DRUGS

Claritin-D

Generic components
Extended-release tablets
5 mg loratadine and 120 mg pseudoephedrine

Dosages
Adults: 1 tablet every 12 hours.

Claritin-D 24 Hour

Generic components
Extended-release tablets
10 mg loratadine and 240 mg pseudoephedrine

Dosages
Adults: 1 tablet every day.

Combivent

Generic components
Metered-dose inhaler
18 mcg ipratropium bromide and 90 mcg albuterol

Dosages
Bronchospasm with COPD in patients who require more than a single bronchodilator
Adults: Two inhalations q.i.d. Not for use during acute attack. Use cautiously with known sensitivity to atropine, soy, or peanuts.

Drugs by therapeutic class

Alkylating drugs
- chlorambucil (Leukeran)
- cisplatin (Platinol)
- cyclophosphamide (Cytoxan)
- ifosfamide (Ifex)

Aminoglycosides
- amikacin sulfate (Amikin)
- gentamicin sulfate
- neomycin sulfate (Neo-fradin)
- tobramycin sulfate (TOBI)

Antianginals
- amlodipine (Norvasc)
- diltiazem (Cardizem, Dilacor)
- nifedipine (Adalat, Procardia)
- nitroglycerin (Deponit, Nitro-Bid, Nitrol)

Antibiotic antineoplastics
- bleomycin (Blenoxane)
- doxorubicin (Adriamycin)

Anticoagulants
- dalteparin (Fragmin)
- enoxaparin (Lovenox)
- fondaparinux sodium (Arixtra)
- heparin
- warfarin (Coumadin)

Antidepressants
- clomipramine
- doxepin (Sinequan)
- paroxetine (Paxil)

Antihistamines
- cetirizine hydrochloride (Zyrtec)
- chlorpheniramine maleate (Chlor-Trimeton)
- clemastine fumarate (Dayhist)
- desloratadine (Clarinex)
- diphenhydramine hydrochloride (Benadryl)
- fexofenadine hydrochloride (Allegra)
- levocetirizine dihydrochloride (Xyzal)
- loratadine (Alavert)
- promethazine hydrochloride (Phenergan)

Antihypertensives
- captopril (Capoten)
- enalapril (Vasotec)
- nitroprusside (Nitropress)

Antimalarials
- hydroxychloroquine (Plaquenil)

Antimetabolites
- methotrexate (Rheumatrex)
- pemetrexed (Alimta)

Antimitotic drugs
- Vinorelbine (Navelbine)

Antituberculotics
- cycloserine (Seromycin)
- ethambutol hydrochloride (Myambutol)
- isoniazid (Nydrazid)
- rifabutin (Mycobutin)
- rifampin (Rifadin)
- rifapentine (Priftin)
- streptomycin sulfate

Antivirals
- acyclovir sodium (Zovirax)
- adefovir dipivoxil (Hepsera)
- amantadine hydrochloride (Symmetrel)
- cidofovir (Vistide)
- oseltamivir phosphate (Tamiflu)
- ribavirin (Virazole)
- zanamivir (Relenza)

Anxiolytics
- alprazolam (Xanax)
- lorazepam (Ativan)

Bronchodilators
- albuterol sulfate (Proventil, Ventolin)
- arformoterol tartrate (Brovana)
- epinephrine
- epinephrine bitartrate (AsthmaHaler Mist, Primatene Mist)
- epinephrine hydrochloride (AsthmaNefrin, Epi-pen)

- formoterol fumarate inhalation powder (Foradil Aerolizer)
- ipratropium bromide (Atrovent)
- isoproterenol hydrochloride (Isuprel)
- levalbuterol hydrochloride (Xopenex)
- pirbuterol acetate (Maxair Autohaler)
- salmeterol xinafoate (Serevent Diskus)
- terbutaline sulfate (Brethine)
- theophylline
- theophylline (Accurbron, Bronkodyl, Theo-bid)
- tiotropium bromide (Spiriva)

Central nervous system stimulants
- modafinil (Provigil)

Cephalosporins
- cefaclor (Ceclor)
- cefadroxil (Duricef)
- cefazolin sodium (Ancef)
- cefdinir (Omnicef)
- cefditoren pivoxil (Spectracef)
- cefepime hydrochloride (Maxipime)
- cefoperazone sodium (Cefobid)
- cefotaxime sodium (Claforan)
- cefoxitin sodium (Mefoxin)
- cefpodoxime pivoxil (Vantin)
- cefprozil (Cefzil)
- ceftazidime (Ceptaz)
- ceftizoxime sodium (Cefizox)
- ceftriaxone (Rocephin)
- cefuroxime axetil (Ceftin)
- cefuroxime sodium (Zinacef)
- cephalexin monohydrate (Keflex)
- loracarbef (Lorabid)

Diuretics
- acetazolamide (Diamox)
- bumetanide (Bumex)
- furosemide (Lasix)

Estrogens and progestins
- medroxyprogesterone

Fluoroquinolones
- ciprofloxacin (Cipro)
- gemifloxacin (Factive)
- levofloxacin (Levaquin)
- moxifloxacin hydrochloride (Avelox)
- norfloxacin (Noroxin)
- ofloxacin (Floxin)

Immunosuppressants
- azathioprine (Azasan, Imuran)
- cyclosporine (Gengraf, Neoral)
- infliximab (Remicade)
- tacrolimus (Prograf)

Inotropics
- digoxin (Lanoxin)
- milrinone (Primacor)

Miscellaneous anti-infectives
- azetreonam (Azactam)

Miscellaneous antineoplastics
- bevacizumab (Avastin)
- erlotinib (Tarceva)
- etoposide (Toposar)

Miscellaneous cardiovascular drugs
- pentoxifylline (Trental)
- phenylephrine hydrochloride (Neo-Synephrine)

Miscellaneous respiratory drugs
- acetylcysteine (Acetadote, Mucomyst)
- beclomethasone dipropionate (Beconase AQ, QVAR)
- benzonatate
- beractant (Survanta)
- budesonide (Pulmicort Turbuhaler, Pulmicort Respules, Rhinocort Aqua)
- calfactant (Infasurf)
- dextromethorphan hydrobromide
- flunisolide (AeroBid, Nasalide, Nasarel)
- flunisolide hemihydrate (AeroSpan HFA)
- fluticasone propionate (Flonase)
- fluticasone propionate and salmeterol inhalation powder (Advair Diskus)
- guaifenesin
- mometasone furoate (Asmanex Twisthaler)
- montelukast sodium (Singulair)
- omalizumab (Xolair)
- triamcinolone acetonide (Azmacort, Nasacort AQ)
- zafirlukast (Accolate)

Nasal drugs
- ciclesonide (Omnaris)
- pseudoephedrine hydrochloride (Sudafed)
- pseudoephedrine sulfate (Drixoral)

Opioid analgesics
- codeine sulfate
- codeine phosphate
- hydromorphone hydrochloride (Dilaudid)
- morphine (Duramorph)

Penicillins
- amoxicillin and clavulanate (Augmentin)
- amoxicillin trihydrate (Amoxil)
- ampicillin
- penicillin G benzathine (Bicillin)
- ticarcillin (Timentin)

Steroidal anti-inflammatories
- methylprednisolone (Medrol, Solu-Medrol)
- prednisone (Deltasone)

Thrombolytics
- alteplase (Activase)
- reteplase (Retavase)
- streptokinase (Streptase)
- urokinase (Abbokinase)

Vasodilators
- ambrisentan (Letairis)
- bosentan (Tracleer)
- iloprost (Ventavis)
- treprostinol (Remodulin)

Vasopressors
- dobutamine (Dobutrex)
- dopamine
- ephedrine sulfate

Selected references

Alho, O., et al. "Tonsillectomy Versus Watchful Waiting in Recurrent Streptococcal Pharyngitis in Adults: Randomised Controlled Trial," *British Medical Journal* 334(7600):939, May 2007.

Alsaghir, A.H., and Martin, C.M. "Effect of Prone Positioning in Patients with Acute Respiratory Distress Syndrome: A Meta-Analysis," *Critical Care Medicine* 36(2):603–09, February 2008.

Amati, M., et al. "Profiling Tumor-Associated Markers for Early Detection of Malignant Mesothelioma: An Epidemiologic Study," *Cancer Epidemiology, Biomarkers and Prevention* 17(1):163-70, January 2008.

Baren, J.M., et al. "Randomized Controlled Trial of Emergency Department Interventions to Improve Primary Care Follow-up for Patients with Acute Asthma," *Chest* 129(2):257–65, February 2006.

Bjelakovic, G., et al. "Mortality in Randomized Trials of Antioxidant Supplements for Primary and Secondary Prevention: Systematic Review and Meta-Analysis," *JAMA* 297(8):842–57, February 2007.

Blasi, F., et al. "Prulifloxacin: A Brief Review of its Potential in the Treatment of Acute Exacerbation of Chronic Bronchitis," *International Journal of Chronic Obstructive Pulmonary Disease* 2(1):27–31, December 2007.

Bonay, M., et al. "Cytokines in Pulmonary Emphysema: Can Results in Mice Be Translated to Humans?" *American Journal of Respiratory and Critical Care Medicine* 177(2):238, January 2008.

Chawla, R., et al. "Guidelines for Noninvasive Ventilation in Acute Respiratory Failure," *Indian Journal of Critical Care Medicine* 10(2):117–47, April-June 2006.

Currie, A.J., et al. "Targeting the Effector Site with IFN-(Alpha)(Beta)-Inducing TLR Ligands Reactivates Tumor-Resident CD8 T Cell Responses to Eradicate Established Solid Tumors," *Journal of Immunology* 180(3):1535–44, February 2008.

Diseases, 4th ed. Philadelphia: Lippincott Williams & Wilkins, 2006.

Doz, E., et al. "Cigarette Smoke-Induced Pulmonary Inflammation Is TLR4/MyD88 and IL-1R1/MyD88 Signaling Dependent," *Journal of Immunology* 180(2):1169–78, January 2008.

Drake, R., et al. *Gray's Atlas of Anatomy*, St. Louis: W.B. Saunders, 2008.

Lee, K.S., et al. "Modulation of Airway Remodeling and Airway Inflammation by Peroxisome Proliferator-Activated Receptor Gamma in a Murine Model of Toluene Diisocyanate-Induced Asthma," *Journal of Immunology* 177(8):5248–57, October 2006.

Nursing2009 Drug Handbook, Philadelphia: Lippincott Williams & Wilkins, 2009.

Porth, C.M. *Essentials of Pathophysiology: Concepts of Altered Health States,* 2nd ed. Philadelphia: Lippincott Williams & Wilkins, 2007.

Seeley, R.R., Stephens, T.D. and Tate, P. *Anatomy and Physiology*, 8th ed. New York: McGraw-Hill, 2007.

Smeltzer, S.C, et al. *Brunner and Suddarth's Textbook of Medical-Surgical Nursing*, 11th ed. Philadelphia: Lippincott Williams & Wilkins, 2006.

Index

i refers to an illustration; t refers to a table